Acupuncture Point Combinations

*For my mother, who gave me a love of the world of nature
that has sustained and inspired me through my life*

For Churchill Livingstone

Commissioning editor: Inta Ozols
Project editor: Valeria Bain
Project manager: Valeria Burgess
Project controllers: Nicola Haig/Pat Miller
Copy editor: Sara Firman
Design direction: Judith Wright
Sales promotion executive: Maria O'Connor

Acupuncture Point Combinations
The Key to Clinical Success

Jeremy Ross

Doctor of Acupuncture CAc(Nanjing) BSc CEd MNIMH TCM
Director, Swedish Institute for Alternative Medicine,
Stockholm, Sweden
Acupuncturist in Private Practice, Seattle, USA

Foreword by
Dan Bensky

Doctor of Osteopathy Dipl Oriental Med(Macau)
Director, Seattle Institute of Oriental Medicine, Seattle, USA

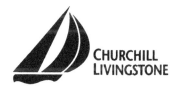

CHURCHILL
LIVINGSTONE

EDINBURGH LONDON NEW YORK OXFORD PHILADELPHIA ST LOUIS SYDNEY TORONTO 1998

CHURCHILL LIVINGSTONE
An imprint of Elsevier Limited

First published 1995
    Reprinted 1996 (twice), 1998, 1999, 2002, 2003, 2004, 2006, 2007 (twice), 2008, 2009

ISBN 978 0 443 05006 0

British Library Cataloguing in Publication Data
A catalogue record for this book is available from the British Library

Library of Congress Cataloguing in Publication Data
A catalogue record for this book is available from the Library of Congress

Note
Medical knowledge is constantly changing. As new information becomes available, changes
in treatment, procedures, equipment and the use of drugs become necessary. The
contributors and the publishers have taken care to ensure that the information given in this
text is accurate and up to date. However, readers are strongly advised to confirm that the
information, especially with regard to drug usage, complies with the latest legislation and
standards of practice.

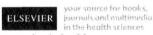

ELSEVIER   your source for books,
           journals and multimedia
           in the health sciences
www.elsevierhealth.com

Working together to grow
libraries in developing countries
www.elsevier.com | www.bookaid.org | www.sabre.org
ELSEVIER   BOOK AID   Sabre Foundation
           International

Printed and bound in the United Kingdom

Transferred to Digital Print 2010

The
publisher's
policy is to use
paper manufactured
from sustainable forests

Contents

Foreword

Practising acupuncture is simultaneously fascinating, fun, and frustrating. One reason is that it is quite rare to treat people using only one point per treatment. The decision on how and why to mix and match different points and techniques to the amazingly varied patient population that we see demands much of us. At least from the time of the *Inner Classic*, this has been a topic of interest and concern to acupuncturists. Jeremy Ross states in this book, that the practice of acupuncture is a constantly changing mix of empiricism, analysis, and intuition. From this perspective it is fascinating and useful to see how different people approach this aspect of the practice of acupuncture. Everyone who pays attention to their practice has their own ideas on how to combine points and their own pearls and tips for success. To have access to a seasoned practitioner's trove of knowledge and experience in this regard is a treat.

This book is an extensive, but personal integration of many strands of medicine. It draws on the extensive study, practice, and teaching experience of the author. Numerous and sundry constellations of points are discussed from many different angles so that practitioners of varying degrees of experience and understanding can utilize them effectively.

Approaches from the diverse systems used are all put in a very practical perspective. The relation of the information to the types of patients seen in modern clinics in the West is very clear. There are sections discussing the diagnosis and point combinations for a wide range of complaints which show his interest in applying traditional concepts to the needs of today. Some examples include malnutrition from dieting, long-term unemployment, excessive ambition, and excess food or alcohol in the evening. In every section Jeremy demonstrates an understanding of what type of information people need. One of the most helpful sections in this regard is his discussion of what to do when things do not progress as desired, either in a treatment session or over an entire course of treatment. Many of the ways in which acupuncture points are combined are described along with other clinically relevant information.

While not completely comprehensive, the range of ideas and approaches discussed in this book is quite broad. It is an eclectic combination of not only points but points of view. Besides the perspective of Chinese medicine, those of biomedicine and energy healing are well-represented. Jeremy also integrates the perspective of the self-help movement by, among other things, discussing a system often basic personality types and how to work with them.

Every section is marked by Jeremy's own particular stamp. Many of the concepts that he has found useful in this practice and in teaching are introduced. An example is irregularity as a rubric for such things as rebellion and hyperactive Liver yang. The system of the Four Imbalances is presented. This was designed by him as a system of differentiation that integrates acupuncture, energy work, and meditation using the same principles of treatment across systems. The generous use of illustrative case histories enables the reader to clearly and fully grasp these concepts.

Over all, this is an interesting and useful attempt to apply the concepts and traditions of Chinese medicine to the modern Western clinic.

Dan Bensky   1995

Preface

Success in any form of healing is founded not only on a mastery of theoretical principles and practical techniques, but also on compassion, a healing gift and an understanding of people. In acupuncture, the point combination is the medium or interface through which the practitioner can initiate healing in the patient. Clinical success in acupuncture depends on the choice of an effective point combination. This choice is based not only on accurate differentiation of the syndromes, but also on an understanding of the personality and life needs of the patient.

The point combinations given in this book, whether for personality types, lifestyle factors, or for the specific syndromes, are not meant as fixed formulas. They are given as guidelines which can be modified according to the patient's individual needs, the practioner's style of treatment, and also as the course of treatment progresses.

Acupuncture can often be used effectively as the sole method of therapy, or as a complement to Western medicine, with the patient in a passive role. However, many of the point combinations given in this book were evolved as part of an integrated system of acupuncture, Qi Gong, meditation and counselling. In this context, the point combination is seen as the stimulus which can initiate not only healing, but also an ongoing process of personal development.

Seattle 1995   J.R.

How this Book is Organized

This book is divided into three parts:

Part I   Theoretical principles of point combination
Part II Point combinations for the main acupuncture points
Part III Point combinations for diseases.

Part I Theoretical Principles of Point Combination

Part I is designed to enable practitioners to make their own successful point combinations. Familiarity with the basic acupuncture theories and techniques is assumed. Part I can be divided into two sections: Chapters 1–6 constitute the theoretical foundation, while Chapters 7–10 contain specific guidelines for point combinations.

Part II Point Combinations for the Main Acupuncture Points

Part II is the central core of this book. For each of the main points of acupuncture there is discussion of the different syndromes for which that point can be used, with an example point combination for each syndrome.

For each channel there is a table of point comparisons, to summarize the differences between the points on that channel, and to indicate when to use one point rather than another. There is also a table of point combinations for each channel, to illustrate which points on the channel combine well with each other and with points on other channels to treat different syndromes and ailments.

Part III Point Combinations for Diseases

The point combination tables given for each disorder in Part III are designed as a quick clinical reference guide. They can facilitate differentiation between the different syndromes of a disorder and indicate appropriate point combinations for each syndrome.

While some diseases, especially the psychological disorders, are considered in detail, Part III is essentially a series of summaries for easy clinical use. For fuller discussion of the treatment of diseases with herbal medicine and acupuncture, *The Practice of Chinese Medicine* by Giovanni Maciocia is highly recommended.
(Churchill Livingstone, Edinburgh, 1989)

Point combinations for organ syndromes

A point combination table for the syndromes of each organ system is given in the chapter on that organ system in Part II. The table and page references are as follows:

Organ system	Table no.	Page no.
Kidneys	13.3	174
Bladder	13.3	174
Spleen	15.4	209
Stomach	16.2	225
Liver	17.2	244
Gallbladder	17.2	244
Heart	19.2	274
Small Intestine	22.2	305
Lung	21.1	294
Large Intestine	22.2	305
Pericardium	19.2	274
Triple Energizer*	–	

*Not generally associated with syndromes of its own.

Point combinations have not been given for Substance syndromes, e.g. Deficient Blood or Stagnant Qi since these are too general and can be subdivided into more specific syndromes. For example, Deficient Blood can be subdivided into Deficient Spleen Blood, Deficient Liver Blood and Deficient Heart Blood, for which the point combinations are given in the tables for the specific organ syndromes.

Additional Syndromes

Some of the organ system syndromes given in this book are not generally recognized in classical Chinese texts, but arise from the clinical observations of the author. For example:

Stagnant Lung Qi
Stagnant Kidney Qi
Stagnant Heart Qi
Stagnant Spleen Qi
Kidney fear invades the Heart.

These additional syndromes are particularly useful in describing the psychological disorders.

Point combinations for disease factors

Chapter 3 on The Origins of Diseases contains three important point combination tables:

Table 3.2 Point combinations for Exterior factors, page
Table 3.3 Point combinations for the emotion groups, page
Table 3.4 Point combinations for lifestyle factors, page.

Nomenclature

Abbreviations for treatment methods

Rf Reinforcing method
gentle manipulation, producing a gentle needle sensation, used to tonify Deficiency

Rd Reducing method
strong manipulation, producing a strong needle sensation, used to disperse Excess

E Even method
intermediate manipulation, producing an intermediate-strength needle sensation, used for mixed syndromes

M moxa

B bleeding

El electroacupuncture

C cupping

The use of the different treatment methods to treat Deficiency, Excess, Stagnation and Irregularity is briefly discussed in Chapter 6 and summarized in Table 6.4.

Channel nomenclature

For the 12 Main channels and the 8 Extra channels, this book uses the nomenclature from the 1991 WHO publication *A Proposed Standard International Acupuncture Nomenclature*, WHO, Geneva.

Twelve Main channels

English name	Code
Lung	LU
Large Intestine	LI
Stomach	ST
Spleen	SP
Heart	HT
Small Intestine	SI
Bladder	BL
Kidney	KI
Pericardium	PC
Triple Energizer	TE
Gallbladder	GB
Liver	LR

'Triple Energizer' is used to translate the Pinyin 'San Jiao'. Previous translations were 'Triple Heater', 'Triple Warmer' and 'Triple Burner'.

Eight Extra channels

English name	Pinyin name	Code
Governor	Du	GV
Conception	Ren	CV
Thoroughfare	Chong	TV
Belt	Dai	BV
Yin Heel	Yin Qiao	Yin HV
Yang Heel	Yang Qiao	Yang HV
Yin Link	Yin Wei	Yin LV
Yang Link	Yang Wei	Yang LV

Note that the codes for the Extra channels reflect the altenative word for these meridians, vessel (V).

Point names

Point names have been put in lower case, broken up into their component elements, with appropriate Chinese accent on each element. For example, zú sān lǐ for ST.36.

Chinese concepts

English names have been used for the following Chinese concepts:

Tai Yang	Greater Yang	
Shao Yang	Lesser Yang	
Yang Ming	Bright Yang	Six Divisions
Tai Yin	Greater Yin	(Six Stages)
Shao Yin	Lesser Yin	
Jueh Yin	Terminal Yin	

Xue	Blood
Jin Ye	Body Fluids
Yuan Qi	Source Qi (Original Qi)
Wei Qi	Defensive Qi
Ying Qi	Nourishing Qi
Gu Qi	Food Qi
Zhen Qi	True Qi
Zhong Qi	Qi of the chest (Central Qi)
Xian Tian Zhi Qi	Prenatal Qi (Pre-Heaven Qi)
Hou Tian Zhi Qi	Postnatal Qi (Pre-Heaven Qi)

Zang Fu	Organ systems (of Chinese medicine)
Zang	Yin Organ systems
Fu	Yang Organ systems
Wu Xing	Five Elements
Xiang Sheng	Promotion cycle (Generating sequence)
Xiang Ke	Control cycle (Controlling sequence)
Jing	channel (meridian, vessel)

Shen	Heart Spirit
Yi	Intellect
Po	Corporeal Soul
Zhi	Will
Hun	Spiritual Soul

Ah Shi	Painful points
Yuan Xue	Source points
Luo Xue	Connecting points
Xi Xue	Accumulation points
Mu Xue	Alarm points (Front Collecting points)
Bei Shu Xue	Back Transporting points (Associated Effect points)
Hui Xue	Gathering points (Influential points)
Xia He Xue	Lower Sea points
Jiao Hui Xue	Crossing points (Meeting points, Intersecting points)
Wu Shu Xue	Transporting points
Wu Xing Shu Xue	Five Element points
Ba Mai Jiao Hui Xue	Extra channel Opening points (Extraordinary channel Confluent points)

Miscellaneous

Capitalization

English words beginning with a capital letter generally indicate translation of a Chinese concept. For example, 'Stomach' translates 'Wei', the Stomach organ system of Chinese medicine. The word 'stomach', starting with lower case, indicates the physical organ of Western medicine.

Spirit

The word 'Spirit', with a capital letter, represents the Chinese concept of 'Shen', the Heart Spirit, which is specifically associated with the Heart organ system of Chinese medicine. The word 'spirit', without a capital letter, indicates the energy or principle that vivifies all existence, not just the human body.

Measurement

The basis of point location measurement is given as the 'unit', otherwise known as the 'cun', or 'anatomical inch'.

Tones

The four tones of Mandarin Chinese are as follows:
 ̄ or first tone — begins *high* and is *held steady*.
 ́ or second tone — begins in the midrange and *rises*.
 ̌ or third tone — begins in the lower middle range and drops down before rising.
 ̀ or fourth tone — begins *high* and drops down *sharply*.

We have included the tone markings in the main text to enable the reader to pronounce the names of the points as accurately as possible. The tone markings reflect the way that the names are spoken, and the permutations of tone by context have been taken into consideration.

Acknowledgements

In writing this book, I am deeply grateful to all the many teachers and colleagues who have inspired me throughout my career, and to my students with whom I have developed so many ideas. However, the greatest appreciation of all goes to my patients, with whom over the years these point combinations were developed.

I would like to thank Angela Morris and Lindsey Dando for their work with the word processing.

Sources

The great majority of the point combinations given in this book derive from the author's twenty years of clinical experience. They have evolved from an interplay of study, intuition and empiricism, the final test always being whether a combination is successful in clinical practice. While many of the combinations discussed are based on classical formulas, this book makes no pretence to be a scholarly comparison of ancient texts. The combinations here have been developed for modern clinical practice and have been included because they are effective.

Most of the theoretical principles given for the combining of points are based on standard Chinese theory. However, whole sections of this book derive from the author's personal interpretation of Chinese medicine. This includes, for example, the sections on the life lessons of the 10 personality types in Part I and the chapters on psychological disorders in Part III.

Part I

Theoretical principles of point combination

Introduction 1

LEVELS OF ACUPUNCTURE

Acupuncture can operate at three main levels:

symptoms
syndromes
individuals.

SYMPTOMS

This book is not concerned with acupuncture at the first level, the treatment of symptoms, unless the underlying causes are also considered. It is assumed that the reader is familiar with the treatment of meridian problems, by the usual combination of Ah Shi points, local points and distal points on the meridians affected. Therefore there are no lists of points given separately for purely local problems such as ankle problems, knee problems, elbow problems and so on. Also there are no lists of points given to treat symptoms, since the lowest level of treatment in this book is the second level, the treatment of organ system syndromes.

SYNDROMES

In Part II, point combinations are given for the organ system syndromes associated with each of the main acupuncture points. For example, for SP.6, point combinations are given for nine main syndromes, associated with physical or psychological problems.

Part III contains point combinations for the organ syndromes associated with some of the diseases commonly treated by acupuncture. For example, for asthma, 10 syndromes are discussed.

INDIVIDUALS

The most effective acupuncture treatment is done when the point combination is tailored to meet the specific needs of an individual. Point combinations are given for some of the lifestyle factors in Chapter 3 and for the 10 psychological types in Chapter

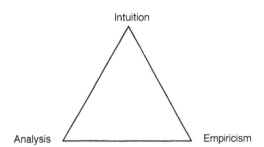

Fig. 1.1

4, and for various psychological disorders in Chapter 34. However, these combinations are only guidelines and may be modified or changed, according to individual requirement. Acupuncture at the level of the individual is based on a detailed understanding of the personality type and life problems, and involves a balance of empiricism, analysis and intuition.

ANALYSIS, INTUITION AND EMPIRICISM

The most effective combinations are created when each of the three faculties — empiricism, analysis and intuition — are well developed and in balance with each other.

EMPIRICISM

This is the practical, down-to-earth faculty of trial and error. The practitioner hears that certain combinations are successful and tries them out to find which ones are effective in different situations. The practitioner may not have any analytical or intuitive understanding of why the combinations are successful, but has simply determined this through experience and observation.

If empiricism is not balanced with intuition and analysis, it can easily lead to a mechanical approach to acupuncture, which ignores the needs of the patient and concentrates on temporary success by relieving symptoms. However, empiricism is vitally important to bring intuition and analysis down to earth and root them in reality. It can be easy to confuse true intuition with fantasy and euphoria, and it can be easy to be so preoccupied with the intellectual elegance of a treatment strategy that its effectiveness becomes of secondary importance. On the other hand, in the early years of practice, it can be easy to become so confused by theoretical complexity as to lose all self-confidence as a practitioner.

ANALYSIS

Perhaps the greatest emphasis in professional acupunc-

ture training in the West is on the development of the analytical faculty. Students spend a long time in memorizing information and in learning the theoretical principles of Chinese medicine. It is absolutely necessary that students learn and understand the theory as thoroughly as possible, otherwise they cannot differentiate the syndromes, or understand how to design effective point combinations for themselves. However, overemphasis of the analytical faculty can lead to the practitioner either becoming lost in a fascinating world of theory, or becoming limited by mental stress and confusion. This can reduce the ability to empathize with the patient and to be sensitive to their feelings and needs. It can also lead, in some cases, to a mental rigidity bordering on fanaticism, in which the facts are bent to fit the theory, rather than the theory made to fit the facts.

Most illness in the West is related to emotional imbalances. Human emotions are fluid, and to the knowledge of the author, no intellectual scheme has ever been made that is comprehensive enough and flexible enough to describe them satisfactorily. The faculty of intuition and the ability to feel and perceive the emotions of others with sympathy and sensitivity, is therefore invaluable to the practitioner.

INTUITION

During a consultation the practitioner may get a clear feeling or perception of the patient's emotional state, or of the overall pattern of their life. Similarly, during the treatment, the practitioner may get a strong feeling to use a certain point combination, which then proves to be effective. This is intuition.

Intuition is not a substitute for analysis, it is complementary to it. Intuition and analysis can be checked against each other, and both must be proved by empiricism. Otherwise it is very easy for the practitioners to confuse true intuition with fantasy, and with their own emotional peculiarities. Intuition is an ability which needs long and careful training, and it is hoped that in the future, this can be increasingly incorporated into acupuncture courses. It is especially important to integrate the development of intuition with the faculties of analysis and empiricism.

WESTERN, CHINESE AND ENERGY THEORIES

Professional acupuncture trainings in the West generally teach point combination in terms of the theoretical principles of Chinese medicine. However, there are two other theoretical systems that are increasingly being used

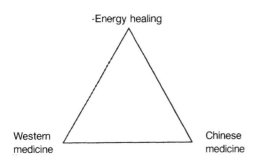

Fig. 1.2

as a basis for point selection: these are the systems of Western medicine and energy healing.

WESTERN MEDICINE

There is an increasing awareness of the relationship of acupuncture points to the segmental organization of the body. Acupuncture points can treat not only problems of the dermatome and myotome in which they are located, but also problems of the organ systems regulated by that pair of spinal nerves and their associated autonomic ganglia. Point combinations can be chosen on this basis. For example, GV.5, BL.22 and BL.51 can be combined for urinary frequency and back pain at the level of the first lumbar vertebra, or CV.13 and ST.20 for sour regurgitation and epigastric pain.

ENERGY HEALING

This system, whether labelled 'energy work', 'healing', Qi Gong, or whatever, is based on the ability of the practitioner to perceive the energy flows within the body of the patient, and to modify or direct them in order to rebalance the energies and effect healing.

The basic concept is that the solid material of the human body is permeated and surrounded by a field of energy, within which there are major and minor energy flows, corresponding in part to the acupuncture channel system. The central axis of these flows is constituted by the circulation of energy through the Governor–Conception channel system. The theory proposes that upon this central vertical axis are located the energy centres, or chakras, which are major focal points of energy flow. Each energy centre has its specific functions and pathologies, so that point combinations can be based on the GV or CV points located over the affected energy centres.

For example, the Throat centre governs communication, and the Heart centre governs the flow of feelings in close relationships. CV.23 and CV.17 can therefore be combined for feelings of constriction and discomfort in the throat and chest, associated to stress within relationships.

SUMMARY

There are obvious overlaps between the three systems of Chinese medicine, Western medicine and energy healing. The traditional functions of the GV, CV and Back Transporting points, bear close relationship to both Western segmental theory and to the concept of energy centres. The author feels that the future development of acupuncture may lie in an interplay and integration between the three systems.

ACUPUNCTURE, ENERGY WORK, MEDITATION AND COUNSELLING

The point combinations in this book are mainly based on the principles of Chinese medicine. However, the personal emphasis of the author is on selecting point combinations based on the energy centres, so that acupuncture can be readily combined with energy work and meditation.

For example, for depression associated with Deficiency of Kidneys and Heart, CV.4, CV.17 Rf might be used as the basis of the treatment, to strengthen the Dan Tian and Heart energy centres. The Extra channel pair of SP.4 + PC.6 could be added to emphasize the effect. The practitioner can then use the techniques of 'energy work' or Qi Gong, to enhance the acupuncture treatment, by focusing energy at the two Deficient centres, and by directing energy between the pairs of needles, e.g. between SP.4 and CV.4, or between CV.4 and CV.17. In addition, the patient can then be given Qi Gong or meditation exercises to strengthen and balance the affected energy centres, to begin a process of personal change and self-healing.

In this system, a common principle of treatment coordinates acupuncture point combinations, energy work and meditation.

Qi Gong exercises or meditations and visualizations given to the patient can be made specific for individual personality types or even organ system syndromes. For example, for the syndrome of Stagnant Lung Qi associated with suppressed grief, heavy smoking and bronchitis, the meditation can focus on the centre of the chest, use the theme of opening, moving and cleansing. The energy of the breath can be visualized as sparkling bright white light, the colour associated with the Metal element.

Counselling and psychotherapy can be integrated into this system, when the practitioner is trained and experienced in these modalities, and when appropriate to the patient's needs. Indeed, the author believes that one of the strongest developments of acupuncture in the future may be in the flexible combination with energy work, meditation and counselling. This relates the concept of the energy body and energy centres dealt with in the next chapter.

The energy body and the 2
energy centres

THE ENERGY BODY

THE GENERAL PERSPECTIVE

All objects have two aspects, that of apparently solid matter and that of energy. This applies to all objects, whether a table, a human being or a galaxy. For all objects, the solid matter is permeated and surrounded by a field of energy. The two aspects are inseparable, and are two facets of the same phenomenon.

The entire universe is a single continuous field of energy, with areas of varying density, the densest areas being perceived as solid matter. All material objects are therefore in connection with each other via the underlying field of energy. A human body can be seen as an isolated material object, separate from and unconnected to the objects that surround it. Alternatively, a human body can be seen as an energy field, which is connected with and inseparable from the energy fields of other bodies, and the larger energy field of the universe.

When individuals identify with the concept of the body as a separate material object, they can feel isolation, alienation and fear. These are the perceptions of ego, the lower self. When individuals experience the underlying unity between themselves and all life, they can experience a deep feeling of peace, love and understanding. The conscious awareness of the universal life force manifesting through an individual can be called the higher self.

THE HUMAN ENERGY BODY

The human energy body, sometimes called the etheric body, or etheric web, permeates and surrounds the solid physical body. It is the sum of the energy fields of the individual cells, tissues and organs, acting in coordination. It reflects the activity of the physical body, the thoughts and the emotions.

The acupuncture points and the acupuncture channels can be seen as an interface between the physical and energy bodies, having aspects of each. The so-called energy centres, or chakras, represent central areas for the coordination of energy flows within the energy body. The main energy centres are along the central vertical axis of the body, and are each usually associated with an endocrine gland, a group of spinal nerves and an autonomic nerve plexus. In other words, most of the energy centres correspond to the segmental organization of the body and the nervous system.

THE ENERGY CENTRES

FUNCTIONS

The exact number, location and function of the energy centres is a matter of opinion, or perhaps it is more accurate to say that different authors emphasize different aspects of the same phenomenon. The perspective adopted in this book relates to the location and individual functions of the acupuncture points on the Conception and Governor channels.

Table 2.1 Functions of the nine energy centres

Centre	Point	Function
Crown	GV.20	spiritual life, balance of the spirit in the physical body, emotions and mind
Brow	yìn táng	wisdom, clear perception, balance of intuition and analysis
Throat	CV.22–23	communication of ideas and feelings, creativity
Heart	CV.17	love, compassion
Solar Plexus	CV.14–15	sensitivity to emotional influences, survival of the ego
Spleen	CV.12	nourishment, whether physical, emotional or mental
Dan Tian	CV.4–6	storage and distribution of energy for the physical and energy bodies, focal point for movement, strength and will
Reproductive	CV.2–3	creativity and expression of self through sex and reproduction
Perineal	CV.1	survival, grounding of the spirit in the physical body, connection of the body with the energies of the earth

Nine energy centres are listed in Table 2.1, although there are others. Also, the aspect of the centres on the ventral surface has been emphasized, although the centres all have aspects on the dorsal surface, as shown in Figure 2.2 and Table 2.2 later.

THE ENERGY AXIS OF THE BODY

The Governor and Conception channels meet at CV.1 and are connected between GV.26 and CV.24, completing a circuit of energy flow through the midlines of the front and back of the head and body as shown in Figure 2.1.

DORSAL AND VENTRAL ASPECTS OF THE CENTRES

The energy centres lie within the body and have both dorsal and ventral aspects as shown in Figure 2.2.

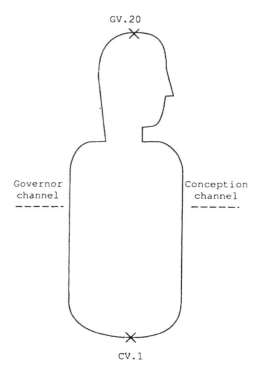

Fig. 2.1 The Governor–Conception channel energy cycle.

Usually, the dorsal and ventral aspects are located at approximately the same level, but the Dan Tian centre is a notable exception. The ventral aspect is at the level of CV.4–6, whilst the dorsal aspect is higher, at the level of GV.4. The functions of the dorsal and ventral aspects are similar, but the dorsal aspects generally have a more Yang function and are more related to spinal problems, whilst the ventral aspects generally have a more Yin function and are more related to abdominal problems.

Table 2.2 shows the correspondence in location of the dorsal centres to the Governor, inner Bladder and outer Bladder line points. There is a strong functional correspondence between the centres and these three lines of points. For example, the dorsal Dan Tian centre, GV.4, BL.23 and BL.52, are all concerned with the availability of stored energy, drive and ambition, and the balance between fear and the will.

While there is a strong correspondence between the ventral centres and the Conception points, there is not such a strong relationship between the Kidney and Stomach points and these ventral centres, as there is between the dorsal centres and the Bladder points.

POINTS AND CENTRES

The energy centres, the channels and the acupuncture points are all part of the energy circulation system of the body. The acupuncture points are located near the surface, and can affect both the local superficial levels of

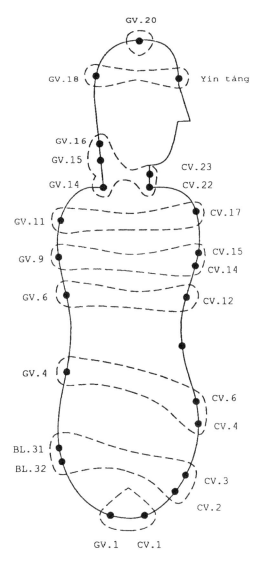

GV.20

GV.18   Yin táng

GV.16
GV.15
                CV.23
GV.14   CV.22

GV.11   CV.17

GV.9   CV.15
                         CV.14

GV.6   CV.12

GV.4

                         CV.6

                         CV.4

BL.31
BL.32

                         CV.3

                         CV.2

GV.1   CV.1

Fig. 2.2 Dorsal and ventral aspects of the energy cycle.

Table 2.2 Centres, points and vertebrae

Centre	CV point	GV point	Below vertebra	Inner BL point	Outer BL point
Crown	–	GV.20	–	–	–
Brow	–	yìn táng	–	–	–
Throat	CV.23	GV.15	C.1	–	–
	CV.22	GV.14	C.7	–	–
Heart	CV.17	GV.11	T.5	BL.15	BL.44
Solar Plexus	CV.14–15	GV.9	T.7	BL.17	BL.46
Spleen	CV.12	GV.6	T.11	BL.20	BL.49
Dan Tian	CV.4–6	GV.4	L.2	BL.23	BL.52
Reproductive	CV.2–3	–	mid-sacrum	BL.31-32	–
Perineal	CV.1	GV.1	tip of coccyx	–	–

nerves may influence not only the skin and muscles of their segment, but also the organ nearest to it. In addition to this physical function, the centres and the acupoints are seen to have effects on the mind and the emotions, dependent on the segment in which they are located. For example, BL.23 and the Dan Tian centre can influence the emotional aspect of fear and the mental aspect of focused concentration on goals.

CENTRES AND AUTONOMIC PLEXUSES

The centres may be linked to specific plexuses of the autonomic nervous system. For example, the Solar Plexus centre may be associated with the coeliac plexus. The various effects of Solar Plexus centre over-stimulation upon the different organ systems may be mediated partly by the secondary plexuses connected with the coeliac plexus. For example, the phrenic plexus to the diaphragm, the hepatic plexus to the liver, the gastric plexus to the stomach, the splenic plexus to the spleen, the suprarenal plexus to the adrenal glands, the renal plexus to the Kidneys, and so on.

CENTRES AND ENDOCRINE GLANDS

The exact relationship between the energy centres and the endocrine glands is not yet clear. Some relationships are more obvious, such as the Reproductive centre with the gonads, or the Spleen centre with the pancreas. Others are not clear because of uncertainty about the functions of the endocrine glands, for example the pineal and the thymus. The standard associations are shown in Table 2.3.

THE ENERGY CENTRES AND TREATMENT

Diagnosis can include perception of imbalances within

the skin and muscle and the inner organs. The energy centres are located deeper in the body and are not so much concerned with the superficial layers, as with the internal balance of energy.

CENTRES AND SEGMENTAL ORGANIZATION

In Western medicine, the body is seen to be organized on a segmental basis. Each segment consists of a vertebra, a pair of spinal nerves and the associated dermatome and myotome. There is considerable overlap between the dermatomes of consecutive spinal nerves, just as there is overlap in the functions of consecutive Governor and Bladder points on the back.

The energy centres and the acupuncture points appear to have a close correspondence in function to the spinal nerves in whose segment they occur. A pair of spinal

Table 2.3 Centres and endocrine glands

Centre	Gland
Crown	pineal
Brow	pituitary
Throat	thyroid
Heart	thymus
Solar Plexus	adrenals
Spleen	pancreas
Dan Tian	adrenals
Reproductive	gonads
Perineal	adrenals

and between the energy centres. Treatment can then focus on the correction of these imbalances, whether the treatment is acupuncture, Qi Gong, meditation, or counselling and psychotherapy.

ENERGY CENTRES AND ACUPUNCTURE

The Governor and Conception channels form the vertical axis for the energy circulation of the body. They are closely linked with the other Extra channels and with the Kidneys. The GV and CV points can be used together with the Extra channel Opening points, as the basis of a system of acupuncture focusing on the energy centres.

Example

A man of 40 had a condition of cold hands and feet that was aggravated by anxiety and improved by exercise. His pulse was hindered, irregular and moving. The diagnosis was that his attempts to control his anxiety had over-controlled his heart function and thus impaired peripheral circulation. When both the anxiety and control were relaxed, as in enjoyable work or exercise, the circulation improved.

The point combination was based on strengthening the Dan Tian centre to overcome fear, and calming the Solar Plexus centre to reduce anxiety and his control of heart function. The Opening points on the Thoroughfare and Yin Link channels were also used to regulate Heart–Kidney balance:

CV.4 Rf M; CV.14, PC.6, SP.4 E M

ENERGY CENTRES AND QI GONG

During an acupuncture treatment, the practitioner can consciously direct energy to a particular centre, or between pairs of needles. In the example just given, the practitioner could visualize energy flowing through the practitioner to strengthen the patient's Dan Tian centre, or could direct energy between pairs of needles, such as SP.4 and CV.4, or CV.14 and PC.6. The energy-directing techniques of Qi Gong can enhance the effectiveness of acupuncture treatment.

ENERGY CENTRES AND MEDITATION

Meditation techniques can treat Deficiency, Excess, Stagnation or Irregularity of energy in individual centres, and can also improve the balance between the centres. In the example just given, the patient could focus on the Dan Tian centre and the energy centres around KI.1 on the soles of the feet. These meditation exercises, done whether lying, sitting, standing or walking, can help to calm anxiety, and bring the awareness away from the head and chest, and into the physical body as a whole.

ENERGY CENTRES AND COUNSELLING

Counselling and psychotherapy can be focused on the known energy centre imbalances. Overactivity of the Solar Plexus centre can indicate oversensitivity to emotional influences, and deep insecurity, fear and anxiety. There may be fear of losing control of situations, emotions or mind. Counselling and psychotherapy can be combined with energy work, massage or acupuncture, directly on the imbalanced centre, or indirectly via another centre. In the example earlier, if CV.14 is too sensitive, or if the patient is too fearful to approach energy blocks, CV.4 can be strengthened first, to give the patient the calmness and strength to overcome fear.

BALANCING THE THREE MAIN CENTRES

Training in Qi Gong or meditation which is based on the energy centres, can be divided into three stages or levels:

basic	1 centre
intermediate	3 centres
advanced	9 centres.

The initial basic stage focuses on one centre, usually the Dan Tian centre, in order to take attention away from the head and upper body, so that the person becomes more grounded in the physical body. Once the person has embodied this basic training they can progress to exercises that strengthen each of the three centres and balance them with each other.

THE THREE CENTRES

The three centres chosen are usually the Brow centre, in the middle of the head, the Heart centre in the middle of the chest, and the Dan Tian centre in the middle of the lower abdomen. Each of these three centres can represent different faculties or energies as shown in Table 2.4.

Table 2.4 The three centres

Head	yìn táng	wisdom	thought	analysis
Heart	CV.17	compassion	feeling	intuition
Body	CV.4	strength	sensation	empiricism

The initial stage of all Qi Gong or meditation programmers is to relax deeply and experience a profound inner peace. In the Three Centre exercise, the next stage is to focus attention on the body centre to experience a feeling of inner strength and energy. The third stage is to bring the attention to the Heart centre and develop a feeling of compassion and peace. The fourth stage is to bring the attention to the Head centre and experience a feeling of openness and light. In the final stage, the attention returns to the Body centre, to bring awareness back to practical reality.

When the three centres are strong and in harmony, there is a balance between analysis, intuition and practicality. In other words, compassion is balanced with wisdom and strength.

COORDINATION WITH ACUPUNCTURE TREATMENT

• If there is weakness in the Dan Tian centre, CV.4 can be combined with points such as ST.36 and KI.3, which strengthen the energy of the physical body and also stabilize the emotions.

• If the will is weak, then KI.7 can be added with needle and moxa. If there is much fear, then SP.4 and PC.6 can be added with Even method.

• If there is weakness in the Heart centre, then the Source points LU.9 and HT.7 can be reinforced, and GV.11 and BL.15 may be added. If there is Stagnation of Qi in the Heart centre, then LU.7 and HT.6 can be used instead with Reducing method.

• If there is a weakness in the Heart centre with mental exhaustion and poor concentration, BL.1, BL.10 and BL.62 can be reinforced.

• If there is mental cloudiness, restlessness and confusion, then ST.8, ST.40 and ST.45 can be used with Even method.

These are just a few examples to illustrate how acupuncture combinations can be integrated with Qi Gong and meditation exercises. However, a word of caution: Qi Gong and meditation exercises should not be taught to patients unless practitioners are themselves trained and experienced in their use.

The origins of diseases 3

INTRODUCTION

In Chinese medicine the originating factors of disease are said to be constitution, the Exterior or climatic factors, the Interior or emotional factors, and the factors that are neither Exterior nor Interior, often called factors of lifestyle. However, in the discussion here, the origin of disease has been put in a broader philosophical context, which is based on the concept of the higher self.

THE HIGHER SELF

The universal life force, the spirit, manifests through each individual human being as the higher self, alternatively called the inner self. By getting in contact with the energies of the higher self, a person can become at one with their own life force and with that of others and all things. When there is a communion with the higher self, the individual can feel a deep inner source of peace, strength, love and wisdom. When a person lives in tune with the impulses of the higher self, the life force can unfold through the uniqueness of their individual personality in harmony with the unfolding of others and the world around them.

THE LOWER SELF

As each individual is born into this life, the ego, the lower self, is created as the conglomerate of selfish fears and desires, and negative patterns of thought, emotion and behaviour. The ego sees other people and the world as a threat to its existence, or as a means to the gratification of its selfish desires.

THE OPPOSING PULLS

Through the constant interplay of the higher and lower selves, the personality develops. The two selves represent opposite but complementary pulls upon the conscious mind. The higher self is an experience of unity, and an openness to other people, to the world and to life. This can feel very threatening to the lower self, to which openness represents vulnerability. The lower self is an experience of separation, of apartness, from other people and the world. The lower self represents duality — 'me and them' or, at best, 'us and them'.

THE PAIN OF SEPARATION

When there is a loss of contact with the energies of the higher self, there is pain and a deep inner dissatisfaction and longing. Instead of the peace, strength, love and wisdom of the inner self, there is an inner restlessness and unease, a feeling of powerlessness, fear and weakness, or of hatred and confusion.

THE COMPENSATIONS

People try in many ways to compensate for the pain of separation from the higher self. Some of the many forms of compensation are:

food	fame	drugs
possessions	overwork	illness
money	knowledge	insanity
sex	asceticism	crime
power	religion	cruelty
	fantasy	

These compensations may become addictions, it is only a matter of degree. However, compensations and addictions cannot be satisfied by more of the item, only by re-establishing contact with the higher self.

THE ORIGIN OF DISEASE

Most illness in modern society results from the lack of contact with the energies of the spirit. Instead of love, there is fear and hatred; of self, of others, and of the world. The sickness of society results from the deep unhappiness of individuals, from the sense of isolation and alienation of the lower self.

BEYOND DISEASE

Many times, disease can give a warning that there is an underlying life problem that needs solution. Often, the illness will subside if the person perceives the problem and makes the necessary changes in their patterns of thought and behaviour, realigning their personality with the positive energies of the higher self, and allowing the negative patterns of the ego to fade away.

Very often in modern society, patient and practitioner attempt to suppress the symptoms with medication, so that the patient learns nothing and does not progress. There is a time to treat symptoms, but there is also a time to deal with the deep origins of disease. If this is not done, then not only the individual, but also society, will remain sick.

LIFESTYLE

The Chinese category of lifestyle, sometimes called miscellaneous factors, mainly relates to the compensations for the pain of separation from the higher self. If these compensations are taken to excess, they can cause illness. For example, mental overwork can damage the Spleen, excess sex can damage the Kidneys, and lack of exercise can result in Deficient and Stagnant Qi.

Asceticism, the denial of the physical body, is an attractive compensation for some people (one example is anorexia), but it can damage the entire system and even cause death. The pursuit of power, from inner fear and insecurity, can result in great stress upon the Heart, and can also cause death, from myocardial infarction.

The type of compensation, or lifestyle factor, that is used to excess and that causes illness for a particular person will depend upon their psychological type.

PSYCHOLOGICAL TYPE

The Chinese category of Interior causes of disease, describes the emotions. The word personality will be used in this discussion to put the emotions into a wider context of the overall pattern of feelings, thoughts and behaviour. For example, anger can then be seen not merely as an isolated emotion, but as part of a pattern of frustration and blockage associated with poor planning and an underdeveloped intuitive faculty.

People can be classified into personality or psychological types in a multitude of ways, but in this book the main classification is into the 10 personality types of the Five Elements, each of the Five Elements having a Yin and Yang type as shown in Table 3.1. Each of the 10 types has a different potential for personal development, each has a different group of life lessons to be learned, and each feels the pain of separation from the higher self in a different way.

Table 3.1 The ten personality types

Yin types	Yang types
Yin Fire	Yang Fire
Yin Earth	Yang Earth
Yin Metal	Yang Metal
Yin Water	Yang Water
Yin Wood	Yang Wood

The 10 Five Element personality types, and their associated emotions, are discussed in detail in Chapter 4, and summarized in Tables 4.3 and 4.4. Another classification of psychological types is given in Chapter 10 on the Eight Extra channels, and summarized in Table 10.5.

EXTERIOR FACTORS

The climatic factors, or Exterior factors, are generally given as Wind, Cold, Heat, Damp, Dryness and Summer Heat. However, there is often confusion, since the term Exterior factor can be used in two different ways. Firstly, the term can be used to mean an actual environmental factor such as air movement — Wind, low external temperature — Cold, raised external temperature — Heat, and so on. Secondly, the term can be used to mean a pathological reaction of the body, for example, Wind Heat is a pathological pattern with fever and chills, and Heat is a pattern with fever only, regardless of whether the person was exposed to external air movement or raised temperature. Sometimes there is a close correspondence between the two meanings, for example, the pathological patterns of Wind Cold, Wind Dryness, Cold, Damp and Summer Heat, may follow exposure to the associated environmental factors.

The concepts of Wind Heat and Heat particularly, refer less to an environmental factor, and more to a pathological reaction of the body. In Western terms, Wind Heat and Heat refer mainly to infection by microorganisms, or in the case of Wind Heat, to allergic reactions. While Wind Heat is a reaction involving more the superficial levels of the body, Heat may involve progressively deeper levels of the body, as classified according to the Four Levels, for example. The term Exterior Heat is therefore rather dubious; it refers neither to raised external temperature, nor to a reaction limited to the surface of the body. Its only claim to the word Exterior is if the Western concept of external microorganisms is adopted. The most comparable Chinese concept is that of pestilences or epidemics. The term Exterior Heat is therefore used here to refer to acute fevers that do not appear to relate to Interior factors, but to microbial infections.

External invasion may relate to predisposing Interior factors. For example, Interior Cold may predispose to invasion by Exterior Cold; Interior Damp may predispose to Exterior Damp. However, the Interior equivalents of the Exterior factors are not discussed here since they relate to specific organ syndromes. For example, Interior Cold may relate to Deficient Yang of Kidneys, Heart or Spleen, and Interior Wind to Liver.

Table 3.2 Point combinations for Exterior factors

Syndrome	Signs and symptoms	Pulse	Tongue	Point combination
Wind Cold	common cold with acute cough, with white sputum, and chills predominant	superficial, tight	thin white coat	CV.22 Rd; LU.7, LI.4, BL.13 Rd M + KI.7, ST.36 Rf M for Deficient Defensive Qi
Wind Heat	common cold, with sore throat, and fever predominant	superficial, rapid	red tongue, thin yellow coat	GV.14, CV.22, LU.7, LI.4, TE.5 Rd + KI.6, Rf; KI.2 Rd for Deficiency Fire
Wind Dryness	acute, dry cough, with dry nose and throat, but not necessarily any signs of Heat	superficial	thin, dry, white or yellow coat	LU.7, LI.4 Rd; LU.5, KI.6 Rf
Cold	aversion to cold, feelings of cold following exposure to cold or consumption of cold food or drink, better with warmth	tight, maybe deep and slow	maybe pale, white coat	LI.4, KI.7, ST.36 Rf M + GV.14, BL.11 Rd M for Wind Cold + CV.4 or GV.4, BL.23 Rf M for Deficient Kidney Yang + CV.12 or GV.6, BL.20 Rf M for Deficient Spleen Yang
Damp	aversion to damp and cold, feelings of dullness and heaviness or ache in limbs, following exposure to damp conditions	maybe slippery	maybe pale, maybe greasy	CV.4, CV.12 Rf M; TE.6, SP.6, SP.9 Rd M alternate GV.4, GV.6, BL.20, BL.22, BL.23 E M + PC.6, ST.40 Rd for Phlegm + ST.25, ST.28 E M for Cold Damp in Intestines
Summer Heat	feelings of faintness, dizziness, fever and nausea following overexposure to sun or Summer Heat, maybe red itching skin	maybe superficial and flooding or empty or minute	maybe red, maybe yellow sl. greasy coat	GV.14, LI.4, LI.11 Rd; BL.40 B + PC.9 for syncope
Heat	fever of varying severity, with thirst and maybe delirium and red skin rash	rapid, full	dark red, dry, maybe yellow coat	GV.14, LI.4, LI.11 Rd + HT.9, PC.9 or shí xuān B for severe fever + ST.44, ST.45 Rd for Heat in Stomach and Intestines

Rd, Reducing method; Rf, Reinforcing method; E; Even method; M, moxa; B, bleeding.

Point combination for the Exterior factors are given in Table 3.2 for the commonest Exterior syndromes:

Cold	Wind Cold
Damp	Wind Heat
Summer Heat	Wind Dryness.

Heat has been included in Table 3.2, although it is perhaps not strictly an Exterior factor.

INTERIOR FACTORS

The Interior factors of disease, usually given as the emotions, in fact comprise the broader pattern of the personality, including feelings, thoughts and behaviour. Table 3.3 summarizes the 10 personality types of the Five Elements, including their emotional groups.

It is better to refer to the five emotion groups rather than the five emotions. For example, the emotion group of the Wood element includes not only anger, but also impatience, irritability, intolerance, hypersensitivity, uncertainty, self-doubt, frustration, depression and resentment.

Table 3.3 gives some examples of point combinations for the different emotion groups, but it must be emphasized that these combinations are only guidelines, to be modified according to individual need.

LIFESTYLE FACTORS

Those factors that are neither Exterior nor Interior, the lifestyle factors, are related to the particular excess compensations used by individuals, as discussed in the introduction to this chapter. Which compensations are used will depend on the personality type, as discussed in Chapter 4.

For example, a Yang Earth type is likely to use food as a compensation, and the resulting overeating, especially of sweet foods, is likely in this constitutional type to lead to obesity or catarrh. A Yang Wood type may use the compensation of aggressive fast driving, and the effect on this personality type of attempting this in modern traffic, is likely to be frustration, raised blood pressure, headache or trauma from accident.

Table 3.4 summarizes some common syndromes and ailments arising from some of the main lifestyle factors, with point combination examples for them. Again, these are guidelines only. In addition, in each case, acupuncture is best combined with self-help measures. For example, the point combination for Stomach Fire will be useless if the patient continues to consume excess cayenne pepper, vodka and strong coffee.

Only a selection of lifestyle factors is given in Table 3.4, for example, drugs, such as nicotine, alcohol, coffee, amphetamines, cocaine, heroin and LSD, have not been included.

Table 3.3 Point combinations for the emotion groups

Element	Type	Emotions	Point combinations
Fire Heart	Yin	sad, lonely, lacking interest in life, relationships and social activity	CV.4, CV.17, HT.8, PC.8, KI.3, ST.36 Rf
	Yang	overexcitable, overenthusiastic, irresponsible, socially or sexually overactive	CV.14, CV.17, HT.8, KI.1 Rd; HT.6, KI.6 Rf
Earth Spleen	Yin	worrying, with too much thinking and not enough action, feeling too tired and empty inside to care for self or others	GV.20, yin táng Rd; CV.4, CV.12, ST.36 Rf M; SP.6 Rf
	Yang	clinging, possessive, intrusive, limiting the independence of others by their overconcern	CV.4, CV.12, CV.17, ST.36, LR.1, LR.13 Rf M
Metal Lungs	Yin	withdrawn from active participation in life, fearful of loss, with insufficient energy to form lasting bonds	CV.4, CV.12, CV.17, LU.10, HT.8, ST.36 Rf M
	Yang	suppressing grief, dumping their negativity on to others, using new relationships merely to assuage unprocessed grief	CV.6, CV.17 E M; LU.7, SP.1, SP.21, LR.1, LR.14 E
Water Kidneys	Yin	fearful of life, lacking drive or ambition, easily discouraged by difficulty or danger, giving up on life	GV.20, CV.4, HT.8, KI.1, KI.7, BL.64 Rf M
	Yang	fearful of losing control, overambitious, ruthless, needing to obtain power over others to feel secure	GV.20, CV.14, PC.6, KI.1 Rd; CV.17, KI.6 Rf
Wood Liver	Yin	hypersensitive, uncertain, lacking self-confidence, unsure of their own identity and path in life, easily dominated by others, timid	CV.4, TE.4, GB.40, SP.6, ST.36 Rf; CV.14, GB.13 E
	Yang	aggressive, impatient, angry, intolerant and selfish, trying to expand their own ego without regard for others	GV.20, PC.8, KI.1, LR.2 Rd; LR.8, KI.6 Rf

Rf, Reinforcing method; Rd, Reducing method; E, Even method; M, moxa.

Table 3.4 Point combinations for lifestyle factors

Factor	Type	Example ailment	Syndrome	Point combination
Nutrition	malnutrition, e.g. from dieting	tiredness, muscular weakness	Deficient Qi and Blood	CV.12, LI.4, ST.36, SP 3 Rf M
	going too long without eating	faintness, headache, irritability	Deficient Spleen Qi Hyperactive Liver Yang	GV.20, GB.20, LR.3 E; CV.12, ST.36, SP.6 Rf
	eating whilst emotionally upset	gastritis, irritable bowel syndrome	Stagnant Liver Qi Hyperactive Liver Yang	CV.12, CV.14, PC.6, LR.3, LR.13, ST.36 E
	excessive eating	constipation, nausea, distension	Retention of food in stomach	CV.10, CV.13, PC.6, SP.4, ST.40 Rd
	excess cold food and drink	gastric distension and pain	Cold invades Stomach	CV.12, SP.4, ST.21, ST.36 Rf M
	excess greasy food and alcohol	nausea, headache	Liver–Gallbladder Damp Heat	PC.6, LI.4, GB.20, GB.34, LR.3, ST.40 Rd
	excess peppery food, coffee or spirits	gastritis	Stomach Fire	CV.12, PC.8, LI.11, ST.21, ST.44 Rd SP.6, KI.6 Rf
Exercise	excess strenuous exercise	exhaustion	Deficient Heart and Kidney Qi	GV.20, HT.7, ST.36, KI.7 Rf M
	insufficient regular exercise	frustration and depression	Stagnant Liver Qi	CV.6, CV.17, LU.7, LR.1, LR.3, LR.14 E
	excess exercise during menstruation	menorrhagia	Spleen not holding the Blood	CV.4, SP.1., SP.10, ST.36 Rf M
	strenuous exercise without adequate warm-up	muscle sprain	Stagnant Qi and Blood	Ah Shi points, local and distal points on the affected channel
Work	physical overwork	exhaustion, weak muscles	Deficient Spleen and Kidney Qi	CV.4, CV.12, LI.4, SP.6, ST.36, KI.3 Rf M
	stressful overwork	headaches, insomnia	Deficient Heart and Liver Yin	GV.20, HT.8, LR.2 Rd; HT.3, SP.6, KI.6 Rf
	excessive study, mental overwork	poor memory and concentration	Deficient Blood and Stagnant Stomach Qi	yìn táng, LI.1, SP.1, ST.45 E; CV.4, CV.12 SP.6, ST.36 Rf
	excessive ambition, unrealistic goals	total exhaustion, burnout	Excess Kidney Will and Deficient Kidney Qi	GV.20, KI.1 Rd; SP.6, ST.36, KI.7 Rf
	long-term unemployment	frustration, depression, lack of confidence	Stagnant Liver Qi	CV.6, PC.6, LR.3, LR.14 Rd; TE.4, GB.40 Rf M
	recent job loss or retirement	grief, depression, lack of social outlet	Stagnant Heart and Liver Qi	CV.6, CV.17 E M; LU.7, KI.6 E; KI.1 M
Lack of sleep	excess food or alcohol in evening	insomnia with feelings of heat or gastric discomfort	Stomach Fire and Liver Fire	GV.20, ān mián, PC.8, LR.2, ST.44 Rd; SP.6 F
	excess mental work into evening	insomnia with endless thoughts and worries	Stagnant Stomach Qi	GV.20, yìn táng, LI.4, SP.1, SP.6, ST.8, ST.45 E
	insufficient sleep — to sleep late and get up early	exhaustion, loss of work interest and efficiency	Deficient Kidney Qi and Yin	GV.20, CV.4, LI.4, ST.36, KI.6 Rf
Relationships	bereavement	shock, grief, depression	Stagnant Heart and Lung Qi	CV.6, CV.17 E M; LU.7, HT.6, KI.6 E
	difficulties in communication	throat or chest pain	Stagnant Heart Qi	CV.17, CV.23, PC.6, SP.4 Rd M; CV.4 Rf M

Table 3.4 (cont'd)

Factor	Type	Example ailment	Syndrome	Point combination
	difficulty in forming lasting bonds	fearfulness and withdrawal	Deficient Lung and Kidney Qi	CV.4, CV.17 Rf M; LU.7, KI.6, ST.36 Rf
	need for power in relationships	insecurity and paranoia	Deficient Kidney Qi	CV.4, CV.14, ST.36, KI.3, BL.64 Rf M; HT.7, SI.3 E
	clinging possessiveness	overeating and obesity	Stagnant Spleen Qi	CV.12, PC.6, SP.1, ST.40, LR.3, LR.13 E
Sex	excess sex	low back pain, tinnitus	Deficient Kidney Qi	CV.4, ST.29, ST.36, KI.3 Rf
	insufficient sex	depression, frustration, back pain	Stagnant Kidney, Liver and Heart Qi	CV.3, CV.6, CV.17, PC.6, KI.8, KI.13, LR. 3 E M
	sex whilst stressed	restlessness, nervous tension, inability to relax and fully enjoy sex	Deficient Heart and Liver Yin	CV.3, CV.14, CV.17, HT.7 E; SP.6, LR.8 Rf
	unsatisfactory sex	lack of orgasm, sadness, anger, resentment, bitterness	Stagnant Qi and Fire of Liver and Heart	CV.3, CV.6, CV.17, LU.7, HT.8, LR.2 Rd
Trauma	trauma sequelae	local pain or stiffness, area easily affected by Wind, Cold and Damp	Stagnant Qi and Blood	Ah Shi points, local and distal on the affected channels E M; LI.4, SP.8 Rd
	shock	shakiness, lack of confidence, withdrawal	Deficient Heart and Kidney Qi	GV.20, CV.4, CV.14, KI.3, ST.36 Rf M; HT.7 E
	accident prone (through inattention)	daydreaming, mental preoccupation	Deficient and Stagnant Spleen Qi	GV.20 yìn táng, LI.1, LI.4, SP.1, SP.6 E; ST.36 Rf M
	accident prone (through impatience)	inattention or recklessness through impatience	Hyperactive Liver Yang and Fire	GV.20, PC.8, TE.5, LR.2, GB.38 Rd; KI.6, SP.6 Rf

Rd, Reducing method; Rf, Reinforcing method; E, Even method; M, moxa.

ILLNESS ARISING FROM TREATMENT

This does not refer to the concept of 'healing crisis', but to either the side-effects of correct treatment, or the results of incorrect treatment.

SIDE-EFFECTS OF CORRECT TREATMENT

These are far more common in Western than in Chinese medicine. In Western medicine, correct treatment, whether pharmaceutical, surgical or radiological, can be accompanied by side-effects, which can range from mild to fatal. Side-effects have two main aspects. Firstly, a general reduction of the immunological and psychological resistance of the system, and second, specific effects.

Postsurgical shock and the after-effects of anaesthesia on the circulatory system may be treated by such point combinations as HT.7 and KI.3, or CV.4, CV.17, PC.6 and SP.4. Lowered resistance to infection following cortisone treatment can be treated with combinations such as LU.9, KI.7 and ST.36, or BL.13, BL.20 and BL.23. However, acupuncture combinations for the side-effects of specific drugs are outside the scope of this book.

INCORRECT TREATMENT

Whilst the use of moxa in some cases of Excess or Deficiency Heat can have unpleasant effects, acupuncture is a self-balancing treatment. Incorrect point combinations generally have no effect, whether adverse or beneficial. There are exceptions to this, for example, use of points like SP.4 and LI.4 in pregnancy can be unwise.

Incorrect treatment with Chinese herbs, and especially with Western medicine, can have more serious effects. It is not only incorrect treatment, but also overprescription that is so damaging to both health and national economies. For example, the psychotropic drugs, such as hypnotics, tranquillizers and antidepressants are grossly overprescribed, with problems of not only side-effects but also dependence and addiction.

Acupuncture can be used in many cases not only as an alternative to these drugs, but also to treat the side-effects and dependence. However, long-term acupuncture treatment must be based on the personality type of the patient, as discussed in Chapter 4. It is not enough simply to get the patient off the drug; the internal problem that caused them to go on the drug must be addressed, or they will return to drug use.

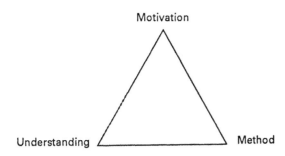

Fig. 3.1

ACUPUNCTURE AND SELF-HELP

From this chapter it is obvious that in many cases the benefits of acupuncture will be limited, unless patients make a determined effort to change themselves and their lives, or at least apply a modicum of self-help.

There are three main aspects of self-help: understanding, method and motivation.

UNDERSTANDING

The practitioner needs to build up an understanding of the personality and life pattern of the patient, in order to help the patient to a knowledge of self and an ability to see life in perspective. It may be necessary to do this slowly, a little at a time, since sudden self-awareness can often lead to self-disgust and loss of motivation. The gap between knowledge of self and acceptance of self can be one which is difficult to cross, and many patients need especial support at this stage.

METHOD

The practitioner needs to select methods of self-help that are appropriate to the patient's personality and lifestyle, and that are, as far as possible, enjoyable and rewarding. This applies not only to systems of nutrition, exercise and meditation, but also to techniques for reorganizing the patient's working and daily life.

Change can only occur at a speed that is acceptable to the patient, and it may be wise to give the patient only one project at a time and to wait until they have completed it before giving another. It is also often wise to start by giving the patient a task they can easily achieve, thus giving them confidence and not overtaxing them at the beginning.

MOTIVATION

The main problem is often lack of consistent motivation and many patients are discouraged by the inevitable set-backs, and give up. To some degree, this may be assisted by acupuncture treatment. For example, a Yin Water type may be easily discouraged by set-backs, and benefit from CV.4, KI.2, KI.7 Rf M. Alternatively, a Yang Wood type may become quickly impatient if the rate of progress seems too slow, and may benefit from GV.20, KI.1, LR.2 Rd.

However, in the end, motivation can only come from within the patient. The practitioner can give support and encouragement, but if the patient is not ready to make the consistent effort necessary for change, the practitioner must accept that. The problem is discussed in more detail in the introduction to the 10 personality types in the next chapter.

The ten personality types 4

Introduction

LIFE LESSONS

In the fabric of each individual life there are certain main threads or themes. These are the main issues or lessons to be dealt with in that life. When a person deals positively with these main themes, learning the lessons of their life and allowing their natural abilities to unfold, there may be many difficulties to be overcome, but there is satisfaction. In addition to the development of natural abilities, life lessons can involve rising above repeating negative patterns, such as anger and intolerance, fear of failure, or difficulty in expressing feelings in close personal relationships.

The 10 different personality types of the Five Elements each have their specific life lessons, although every individual is unique, and is often a complex mixture of the different Five Element types. These personality types and their life lessons, are summarized in Tables 4.2 and 4.3. The discussion of the 10 personality types that follows in this chapter, while based on traditional Chinese medicine, is the personal interpretation of the author.

UNUSED ABILITIES

If major abilities are unused, there may be an increasing internal pressure of dissatisfaction which can manifest in illness. For example, a man thinks he should be involved in healing, but his real abilities are in business and sales. Or a woman has drifted into administration, but her real abilities are in communication through writing.

Firstly the person has to perceive the problem, second find their true abilities within themselves, and third develop the strength of self and the perseverance to make the change. The disciplined development of intuition can be an enormous help in perceiving life problems in perspective, and in seeing the sequence of steps by which they can be solved.

REPEATING NEGATIVE PATTERNS

One person might repeatedly set themselves unrealistic goals and then overwork and become ill in trying to achieve them. Another person might, through insecurity, be overly clinging and possessive in relationships, thus driving partners away and reinforcing their own fears.

The first stage in learning such lessons is an increased self-awareness, so that the repeating pattern is clearly perceived. Second, the individual has to become so sated with repeating this same mistake, that they effect the necessary change in their personality to go beyond it. It may take many years to reach this point of satiation, in fact it may never happen, and the person may take their repeating pattern to their grave.

Sometimes the old negative patterns seem to fall away easily, often it requires constant daily discipline to go beyond them.

TRANSFORMING THE NEGATIVE

The way to rise above negative patterns is not to fight them, since this simply gives them more strength, but to put an increasing amount of energy into the positive patterns that are to replace them. Affirmations and creative visualization are two excellent ways to do this.

For example, for a Yang Liver type to berate themselves for their intolerance, or to try and force themselves to be tolerant by an effort of will, would be equally useless, only leading to more internal pressure. It is more effective quietly to visualize a scene where they are being kind and considerate to another person, and to put positive energy through that visualization each day.

THE ROLE OF THE PRACTITIONER

The practitioner can help the patient to a clearer understanding of their life lessons, and can act as a catalyst to self-awareness. The practitioner can teach the patient techniques of meditation, affirmation and creative visualization, and can help them to develop their intuition. But until the patient feels ready to change, until they reach the point of satiation with repeating their mistakes, the practitioner can do no more than offer support.

People can only change at their own speed. Some people do not want to change at all, in others change is very slow, and in others there are brief bursts of change followed by long periods of what seems to be stagnation. It is the role of the practitioner to act as a catalyst for change, when the catalyst is required.

POINT COMBINATIONS

The practitioner can use suitable point combinations for each of the 10 personality types to assist them in their personal growth. The basic combinations summarized in Table 4.3 are merely guidelines which must be varied according to the changing needs of the patient.

Table 4.1 The nature of the Five Elements

Fire	Fire represents the spirit, consciousness, the experience of unity in all life, love, affection and joy. It includes communication and expression of ideas and feelings. It is spontaneous, lively and social.
Earth	Earth represents solid matter, groundedness, stability and practicality. It represents nourishment, caring and concern for others. It represents the analytical mind and contemplation.
Metal	Metal is linked to the breath, to the energy body, and to the continuous rhythm of taking in and letting go. It is related to the formation, maintenance and dissolution of energy bonds, and the growth of wisdom. It is the ability to face the truth and become at one with it.
Water	Water represents energy storage and conservation, and at the same time the focused energy of the will directed at the achievement of goals. Water represents the major developmental changes of life, and yet it is also the limitations set by fear. Water represents inner strength and faith in self.
Wood	Wood represents intuition and the harmonious unfolding of an individual's potential. It can represent plans and decisions as an outer manifestation of that unfolding. It can represent the free-flow of self-expression, creativity and independence in harmony with the needs of others.

Table 4.2 The ten personality types of the five elements

Element	Yin type	Yang type	Balance
Fire Heart	serious, sad and melancholy; lacking interest in life, relationships and social activity, feeling lonely, unloved and unloveable	restless, overexcitable, overenthusiastic and manic, excessively talkative, socially or sexually overactive, foolish, irresponsible; tending to burnout, with exhaustion, depression, even suicide	experiencing love with themselves and allowing it to radiate out around them, but in calmness and peace; lively and happy, balancing spontaneity with contemplation, wisdom and sobriety
Earth Spleen	preoccupied with endless worries and mental arguments, with too much thinking and not enough action; having a feeling of emptiness within so that it is hard to nourish self or others	owing to fears and insecurities may use their caring to hold on to others, dominate their lives and limit their independence; may be clinging, possessive and intrusive into the lives of others	having a quiet, calm, logical mind that can freely translate thought into practical action, and a stable, pleasant personality which is sympathetic, supportive and caring, but not intrusive
Metal Lungs	having difficulty forming lasting bonds, or fearful of forming new relationships from fear of loss; withdrawn from active participation in life and living in the past	suppressing or holding on to their grief, liking to talk about it and offload their negativity on to others; using new relationships merely to assuage the unprocessed grief of a past one	allowing the process of grief, letting go of the past, gaining wisdom, and learning and growing from each attachment; participating in life and forming new bonds without inhibition by fear of loss
Water Kidneys	lacking energy, fearful, giving up on life and surrendering control of their own destiny; do not do enough, easily discouraged by difficulty or danger; lacking the determination to achieve goals	doing too much, ambitious and ruthless and lacking consideration for others, maybe reckless and foolhardy; suppressing fears but living in great stress from fear of loss of control; seeking safety by obtaining power and domination over others	having a firm will, but with concern for self and others, not discouraged by difficulty or danger but not foolhardy; acting from inner strength and faith in self, not as a compensation for insecurity and fear
Wood Liver	having a weak sense of self and insufficient personal force; unsure of their own identity and path in life; with difficulty expressing their own ego, so have weak boundaries, timid, lacking in confidence and plagued by self-doubt	feeling a pressure of inner uncertainty, so are impatient and irritable; intolerant and selfish, expanding their own egos without regard for others' needs; domineering, angry, aggressive and maybe violent, easily frustrated or depressed	confident and intuitive, having a clear vision of their own path in life, and the patience to allow it to unfold; strong and independent, but able to express their own personality in a smooth relaxed way, in harmony with the lives of others

Table 4.3 The life lessons of the Five Element types

Element	Yin type	Yang type	Point combination
Fire Heart	to conserve energy and build up strength, to use moderation and avoid extremes, to work in areas giving enjoyment and a quickening of the affections, to learn how to express feelings and needs	to learn when to stop, to turn attention inward and find stillness and peace, to balance love with contemplation and wisdom, to allow the inner fire of the spirit to radiate through them in sobriety	**Yin type** Deficiency CV.4, CV.17, KI.3, ST.36 Rf M; HT.7, PC.7 E; HT.8, PC.8 M alternate GV.4, GV.11, GV.20, BL.23, BL.44 Rf Stagnation CV.6, CV.17, SP.4 E M; CV.23, PC.6 E or Rd **Yang type** CV.14, CV.17, HT.8, KI.1 Rd; HT.6, KI.6 Rf
Earth Spleen	to come out of their inner world of thoughts, to fully inhabit their physical bodies and to use them in the real world, to gradually replace their negative thought patterns with a detailed structure of positive affirmations, to learn to nourish and care for self and others	to develop an inner strength, to control the fear and insecurity that makes them want to hold on to others, to find a source of love within themselves so that they do not feel the inner emptiness that makes them dependent on the presence of others	**Yin type** Lack of action GV.20, yìn táng Rd; SP.1, ST.45 M; CV.4, CV.12, ST.36 Rf M Lack of concern CV.12, CV.17, HT.8, SP.2, SP.3, ST.36 Rf M alternate BL.15, BL.20, BL.44, BL.49 Rf M **Yang type** CV.4, CV.12, CV.17, ST.36, LR.1, LR.13 Rf M
Metal Lungs	to strengthen the physical body and the Dan Tian, Spleen and Heart centres to strengthen the ability to form bonds and to reduce fear, to gain the strength and courage to let go, to learn to come out of themselves and be stirred again by the warmth of life	to learn to let go and allow grieving, to face the truth and to be honest with themselves and others, rather than using other people in a selfish way to palliate their grief; to learn to help with the sorrows of others and to put their griefs in perspective	**Yin type** Deficiency CV.4, CV.12, CV.17, LU.10, HT.8, ST.36 Rf M alternate GV.4, GV.12, BL.20, BL.23, BL.42, BL.44 Rf M Stagnation CV.6, CV.17 E M; LU.1, LU.6, LU.7, LI.4, KI.6, ST.40 E alternate BL.13, BL.15, BL.17, BL.42, BL.44 E **Yang type** CV.6, CV.17 E M; LU.7, LI.4, SP.1, SP.21, LR.1, LR.14 E

Table 4.3 (cont'd)

Element	Yin type	Yang type	Point combination
Water Kidneys	to conserve and strengthen their energy, not to attempt tasks beyond their capacity, but not to postpone or to leave tasks unfinished, to learn the lesson of action, to find inner strength to overcome the fear of failure	to learn to act from inner stillness and strength and not from inner restlessness and fear, to slow down and learn the balance of activity and rest, to learn to be as well as to do, to open up to love and learn consideration for self and others	**Yin type** GV.20, CV.4, HT.8, KI.1, KI.7, BL.64, ST.36 Rf M alternate GV.2, GV.4, GV.20, BL.23, BL.52 Rf M **Yang type** Excess GV.20, CV.14, PC.6, KI.1 Rd; CV.17, KI.6 Rf Deficiency GV.20, CV.4, KI.3, SP.6, ST.36 Rf; PC.6 Rd
Wood Liver	to find their inner strength and gain surety of self, to strengthen the projection of their energy to create stronger boundaries to reduce the intrusion and domination of others, to develop their intuition to give a greater sense of certainty and of their path in life	to slow down and to cultivate a discipline of inner peace, to act out of stillness and inner certainty, not out of impatience and inner stress, to learn to relax and surrender to and to develop their intuition so that they can flow harmoniously through life in tune with the needs of others	**Yin type** CV.4, TE.4, GB.40, SP.6, ST.36 Rf; CV.14, GB.13 E alternate GV.4, BL.19, BL.23, BL.48 Rf **Yang type** GV.20, yìn táng, PC.8, LR.2, KI.1 Rd; LR.8, KI.6

Rd, Reducing method; Rf, Reinforcing method; E, Even method; M, moxa.

Fire

THE NATURE OF FIRE

The Fire element can represent the spirit, the universal life force that vivifies matter and form. In human beings, the Heart Spirit vitalizes the physical body, the energy body, the emotions and the mind.

The spirit confers conscious awareness, consciousness of the life force as it manifests through self, through others and through all living things. This leads to an experience of unity, of communion, and of oneness of being with all life. The stronger the experience of oneness, the stronger the feeling of joy, of bliss, and of love for self, for others and for all things.

This experience of unity and love is the basis of all religious experience and of all the great religions. The manifestation of the spirit through an individual human being is the higher self. For each individual, contact with their higher self gives a deep inner experience of peace and love that can radiate out through all their lives. Identification with the ego, the lower self, can bring loss of contact with that experience of the spirit, and lead to a feeling of loss and alienation, that is the source of the troubles of the world and the ill health of individuals.

LOVE AND FEAR

Fear is the main block to the flow of love. The ego, the little self, is full of fear and sees the world and other people as threatening to its existence. To become open and loving seems the same as becoming vulnerable, and

is avoided. The person is then living without love, and living and loving seem separate. When living and loving become identical, the quest is over, the holy grail is found.

INNER EMPTINESS

When there is lack of contact with the fire of the spirit, with the experience of the higher self, the person feels an inner emptiness, which cannot be filled. People try in many ways to fill the void, to ease the pain of loss. There are many forms of compensation: drugs, sex, power, study, overwork, religion, money, material possessions, crime, illness, and more. All the patterns of lifestyle that cause illness arise from lack of love of self. Hatred of self, means hatred of others and of the world, causing the psychological and physical disorders of individuals and the ills of modern society.

CONFUSION ABOUT LOVE

With the experience of oneness with all things, comes the feeling of love and compassion for them. When this experience is lacking individuals tend to seek love outside themselves, in a relationship with another person. Some people, Fire types especially, tend to confuse love with passion. Love is selfless, a feeling of beauty and bliss, which invigorates the body and mind. Passion is simply an intense emotion, focused on another person, which can just as easily manifest in hatred as in love. If Fire type people do not experience love within themselves, they may seek pleasure, stimulation and sensation in sex and relationships with other people. They often create problems for themselves and others by their thoughtless, spontaneous, overenthusiastic and irresponsible behaviour.

FIRE AND WATER

The Fire element, the spirit, has an expansive energy, knowing no limits or boundaries. The Water element has a concentrative energy, limiting the spirit within the capabilities of an individual. Water controls Fire, and between them there is balance. The steady focused energy of the will is needed to balance the tendency of the Fire element to scatter its energy in all directions, and to move quickly from one object to another.

Just as fear controls excessive joy, so fear in its positive sense, as an awareness of limitations, moderates the flow of love within the boundaries of an individual's potential.

COMMUNICATION

The fire of the spirit welling up within an individual seeks expression in communication and sharing of ideas and feeling, of love and affection. Fire types often need to moderate their spontaneity, to contemplate the consequences of their speech and actions, to balance love with wisdom, and to have consideration for other people.

THE HEART CENTRE

The Heart energy centre is seen in most religions as the central focus for the flow of love through an individual. The harmony of the Dan Tian, Heart and Head centres represents the balance between will, love and wisdom that is the aim of self-development.

In terms of the organ systems, the expression of love, the quality of the heart organ system, is balanced by the qualities of the other four organ systems (Table 4.4).

Table 4.4 The qualities of the four organ systems

Wood	Liver	intuition
Water	Kidneys	will
Metal	Lungs	wisdom
Earth	Spleen	contemplation

YIN AND YANG FIRE TYPES

THE YIN FIRE TYPE

In the Yin type there is reduced manifestation of Fire in the individual due either to Deficiency or Stagnation. In the Deficiency type, there is simply a lack of Fire and love and joy. In the Stagnation type, the feeling is there, but is blocked.

In both types, there is a seriousness, a sadness, a melancholy, and a lack of interest in life, in relationships and in social activity. The person feels lonely, unloved and unloveable. However, the Stagnation type may recover for a time if the emotional blocks are loosed, for example, by laughter and social entertainment. But the relief may be only temporary since these people tend to difficulties in the flow and the expression of their emotions.

THE YANG FIRE TYPE

The Fire in the Yang type seems to burn too brightly, without proper control. The Yang Fire type tends to restless overexcitement, overenthusiasm and even to manic behaviour. There can be excessive talking, social or sexual overactivity, and a lack of consideration of the consequences of speech and action, resulting in foolish or irresponsible behaviour.

This type tends to burn out their energies, becoming exhausted and depressed, or even suicidal.

THE BALANCE

The extremes of foolishness, overexcitement and mania, or seriousness, apathy and depression, are both imbalanced. The balance for the Fire element lies in finding love within themselves and allowing it to radiate out around them, but in calmness and peace. Then they are lively and happy, balancing their spontaneity with contemplation, wisdom and strength.

LIFE LESSONS OF THE FIRE TYPES

THE YIN FIRE TYPE

Yin Fire types can be divided into two groups, those where there is reduced manifestation of Fire due to Deficiency, and those where this is due to Stagnation.

DEFICIENCY

This can be due to general constitutional Deficiency, to specific constitutional Deficiency of the Fire element, to burnout of the Fire element, or to lack of a suitable situation to encourage development of the Fire element.

For general constitutional Deficiency, the person needs to learn how slowly to build up strength and conserve energy. For constitutional Deficiency of the Fire element, the person needs to strengthen the heart and circulation with suitable nutrition and moderate exercise. To compensate for their internal lack of Fire, they may be drawn to heart stimulants, such as coffee or high doses of ginseng, but they should avoid these. Those whose Heart Fire is Deficient due to burnout need to learn the great lesson for Yang Fire types of moderation and sobriety. They need to learn to avoid the extremes in all things, and to find pleasure in balance and harmony. Those whose Fire is Deficient because it is underdeveloped need to allow themselves to be drawn to work and personal situations which give them enjoyment and a quickening of the affections, to open up the Heart centre.

STAGNATION

These people need to learn how to express their emotions, and how to communicate their needs to other people. They can be greatly helped by working in groups in counselling and psychotherapy, to gain fluency in communicating their feelings.

It may take continual daily discipline to try to express their needs and feelings to other people and not to let them stagnate inside themselves. It is like learning language, it is only by daily practice that fluency can develop. Sometimes writing down the feelings, or speaking them aloud when alone, can help to loosen the blocks.

THE YANG FIRE TYPE

These people may have great ability to inspire and encourage others, to communicate and to entertain, but they have to learn when to stop. Yang Fire types can exhaust themselves and others by ceaseless, overexcited, overenthusiastic rushed activity. They can create havoc in their own lives and in those of others, by hasty, thoughtless, irresponsible speech and behaviour. They need to turn their attention inward and learn to balance love with contemplation and wisdom. Then they can allow this inner fire of spirit to radiate out through them in sobriety.

POINT COMBINATIONS

Yin Fire type
Deficiency	CV.4, CV.17, KI.3, ST.36 Rf M; HT.7, PC.7 E; HT.8, PC.8 M alternate GV.4, GV.11, GV.20, BL.23, BL.44 Rf
Stagnation	CV.6, CV.17, SP.4 E M; CV.23, PC.6 E or Rd
Yang Fire type	CV.14, CV.17, HT.8, KI.1 Rd; HT.6, KI.6 Rf

Example

A man of 30 was diagnosed as having myalgic encephalitis. He was exhausted and easily overexcited. His pulse was empty, choppy, slightly irregular and changing in speed and volume.

The diagnosis was Deficiency Heart Fire with underlying Deficient Qi and Yin of Heart and Kidney. The point combination was:

GV.24, CV.14, CV.17 E; HT.6, KI.6 Rf; KI.1 massage

The Governor and Back Transporting points were avoided, since they had an adverse reaction in this patient.

He found Qi Gong exercises focusing on the Dan Tian centre and on the KI.1 areas, to be both strengthening and calming, but Qi Gong exercises using the Brow or Heart centres were avoided, since focusing attention in those two areas aggravated his feeling of unease.

Earth

THE NATURE OF EARTH

If the Fire element represents the spirit, then the Earth element represents the solid matter that the spirit vivifies, and through which it can manifest. If the spirit is not properly rooted in the solid physical body, the person can feel ungrounded and unreal, with unstable mind and emotions. Alternatively, if people try to deny their physical body, as in anorexia, they impair both their physiology and the flow of love through them into their lives.

EARTH AND THE MOTHER

The Earth element represents the mother, not only in the nourishment of the physical body, but also in the caring, enfolding and protection of the small child, so that it feels secure both physically and emotionally. If there are difficulties in the first year of life, and the mother is unable physically or emotionally to provide nourishment, or if the mother feels great fear and insecurity at this time, then, in a susceptible child, it may lead to patterns of insecurity that continue through its life.

The capacity of caring, of providing a warm, pleasant, solid and stable support for others, may be very strong in the Spleen type, or it may be lacking or underdeveloped. If the person feels empty in themselves, they may be unable to nurture others.

OVERCONCERN

Concern and caring for others is a natural part of life and a major role of the Earth element. However, if a person is

THE TEN PERSONALITY TYPES 27

insecure they may use concern for others as a means of holding them in their lives. They may be insecure, clinging and possessive in relationships, or they may try to dominate and intrude into the lives of others, using their concern. If they are rejected in this, they may feel very sorry for themselves and try to bind others to them by making them feel guilty.

EARTH AND THE CONTROL CYCLE

On the Control cycle of the Five Elements, Earth is controlled by Wood, and itself controls Water. Alternatively, anger controls sympathy, and sympathy controls fear. However, there may be back-control of Wood by Earth where excessive concern limits the independence and freedom of others, creating resentment. Or there may be back-control of Earth by Water, where fear limits the development of the ability to care for others.

Five Element treatments using the Control cycle can be used to relieve these imbalances.

CONTEMPLATION

Contemplation, thinking and analysis are attributes of the Earth element and of the rational mind. This is the part of the mind that deals with both day-to-day practical matters, and with the logic of abstract thought. It has been described as the left brain, as opposed to the right brain which deals with intuition, more the domain of the Liver and Heart.

If there is too much thinking and not enough action, the person may become lost in a world of obsessive thoughts, worries and mental arguments. In schizophrenia, the person's thoughts become divorced from the reality of their physical body and environment.

WORRY

A person can show sympathy and concern without trying to hold on to or limit the freedom of the individual for whom they are caring. But if sympathy and concern are mixed with fear and insecurity, then the person becomes attached to the one they are helping, needs their closeness and tries to cling on to them.

Worry is a compound of the emotions of insecurity and concern with the mental overactivity of the Earth element.

THE SPLEEN CENTRE

The Spleen energy centre, located within the body at the level of CV.12, has functions overlapping with that of the Spleen organ, in that it is responsible for the assimilation of energy into the body and its distribution throughout the system. Nourishment on the physical level links the Spleen centre to the Dan Tian centre and the Kidneys, which store the energy. Nourishment on the emotional level links the Spleen centre and the Heart Centre, and nourishment on the mental level links the Spleen and Brow centres.

Therefore, Deficiency of Qi can be treated by CV.4 + CV.12 Rf. Difficulty in finding sympathy and love for others can be treated with CV.12 + CV.17 Rf M, and mental congestion and overactivity can be treated with CV.12 + yìn táng Rd.

YIN AND YANG EARTH TYPES

THE YIN EARTH TYPE

There are two main types of Yin Earth personality, those with lack of action and those who lack concern.

LACK OF ACTION

This person lives in an internal world of thoughts and worries, where thought is not translated into action, indeed thought may be dissociated from reality. This group includes the overly intellectual, the worriers, the obsessives and the schizophrenics. They are not fully inhabiting the physical world or their physical body, although they may endlessly worry about them.

LACK OF CONCERN

These are people who feel an emptiness within themselves and find it hard to care for and nourish themselves or others. Sometimes, in the early childhood, sympathy is overcontrolled by fear, or else the Heart, the mother, cannot supply the love that the Spleen, the child, transmutes into sympathy.

THE YANG EARTH TYPE

The Yang Earth types often have a strong ability to care for others, but because of their own fears, insecurities and inner emptiness, they often use their caring to hold on to others or to dominate their lives.

They may use their sympathy and concern so strongly as to smother the development of those around them, limiting the development of their independence, self-confidence and their own creativity. Yang Earth types can use selflessness in a very selfish way.

Such is the relationship between Earth and Wood, that those cared for may become resentful of the limitations of their freedom, the carer may be resentful that they are rejected, and yet each remains locked in dependence on the other.

THE BALANCE

The balance for the Earth type is found in a quiet, calm, logical mind that can freely translate thought into practical action, and in a solid, stable and pleasant person, who is sympathetic, supportive and caring, but does not intrude into the lives of others.

LIFE LESSONS OF THE EARTH TYPES

THE YIN EARTH TYPE

The two main Yin Earth personalities have different life lessons.

LACK OF ACTION

These people need to learn to come out of their heads, to fully inhabit their physical bodies, and to fully use their physical bodies in the real outside world. For some, strenuous walks in the fields, woods and mountains can, by use of the physical body, and by an increasing rapport with the physical world of nature, start to bring consciousness of the real world.

For others, the use of a very detailed structure of positive affirmations can help to divert the energies of the mind from its worries and negative preoccupations into more positive channels. Focusing on the Dan Tian centre, and visualizing energy spreading from this centre to each part of the body can be a very helpful exercise. Exercises focusing on the head centres are best avoided.

LACK OF CONCERN

The first lesson is to learn to nourish and care for self. This can start with a pleasant balanced nutrition, with enjoyable meals. Not a diet, which implies punishment of self for being unworthy. Caring for self can include doing enjoyable things which are pleasant for mind and body, a visit to the theatre, an aromatherapy treatment, a holiday in the sun, and so on.

Unless a person feels that they themselves are worth

caring for, it may be difficult to care for others. Qi Gong exercises focusing on the Spleen centre with themes of nourishment and caring, can support acupuncture treatment. Later exercises can focus on the Heart centre.

THE YANG EARTH TYPE

This type needs to develop the inner strength to control the fear and insecurity that makes them want to hold on to others. They also need to find a source of love within themselves, so that they do not feel the inner emptiness that makes them dependent on the presence of other people.

Qi Gong exercises for the inner strength to control fear can focus on the Dan Tian centre, and to develop love of self, upon the Heart centre.

POINT COMBINATIONS

Yin Earth type

Lack of action	GV.20, yìn táng Rd; SP.1, ST.45 M; CV.4, CV.12, ST.36 Rf M
Lack of concern	CV.12, CV.17, HT.8, SP.2, SP.3, ST.36 Rf M
Yang Earth type	CV.4, CV.12, CV.17, ST.36, LR.1, LR.13 Rf M

Example

A man of 63, an intellectual, taking no physical exercise, complained of mental congestion and exhaustion and physical weakness. His pulse was thin, almost minute, choppy and slightly wiry.

The diagnosis was of Yin Earth type with Deficient Spleen Qi due to overactivity of the mind and underactivity of the body. The treatment was:

LI.4, BL.2 E; LI.1, BL.67, ST.36, ST.45 Rf M

LI.4 and ST.36 were to tonify Qi and Blood, LI.1 and ST.45 were used as points on the Bright Yang channels to clear and invigorate the mind, BL.2 and BL.67 were used as points to strengthen the brain and clear the mind.

Metal

THE NATURE OF METAL

CORPOREAL SOUL

In Chinese philosophy, the Po, the Corporeal Soul, is linked with the Lung organ system and the Metal element. The Corporeal Soul is said to be the densest, the most physical and the most material aspect of the soul of a human being. It is equivalent to the energy body of Western metaphysics, sometimes called the etheric body or etheric web. The Corporeal Soul or energy body, interpenetrates the physical body, and is said to be the foundation on which the physical body coalesces. It is inseparable from the physical body, and at death, both undergo dissolution.

SIGNIFICANCE OF THE BREATH

The Corporeal Soul, the energy body, is constantly vibrating with the rhythm of the breathing, as the energy of the breath enters and leaves the body, catalysing the energy flows within it.

Air and the breath have two aspects. The physical, molecular aspect, and the energy aspect of Qi or prana. The energy of the breath connects the individual with the fields of energy outside themselves. Each breath connects the inside with the outside, so that no human being can completely shut themselves off and withdraw from life. The breath is a ceaseless rhythm of taking in and letting go, taking in the necessary energy and molecules from outside, and letting go of the unnecessary, the wastes.

GRIEF

The Lungs, the Metal element, are involved with the rhythm of taking in and letting go, not only in breathing, but in the formation and dissolution of emotional attachments or bonds. These bonds are like threads of energy connecting the person to the object of attachment, which can be a material object, like a child's toy, or another human being. The severing or dissolution of these bonds causes the pain of loss and the emotion of grief.

FUNCTION OF GRIEF

Completed grief involves the clearing away of old bonds and attachments to make room for the new. It also throws the person back on themselves for a reappraisal of identity. Grief and the Metal element are like the sword of truth, cutting back the unessential, cutting away illusions, to confront the individual with reality.

WISDOM

Grief fulfils itself in wisdom. From each attachment, and from the clarifying pain of letting go of it, comes a new level of self-knowledge and awareness. This is wisdom.

When a person is as willing to let go of attachments as they are to form them, as freely as the rhythm of taking in and letting go of the breath, when they are as willing to accept the pain of grief as the understanding that it brings, then they are truly wise.

TYPES OF GRIEF

Attachment and grief can relate to many things, to bereavement and separation, to loss of a business or an outlet of creativity, to loss of a part of the body in an operation, to loss of femininity with age, to loss of an identity. Grief can relate to any situation where energy bonds have been formed between the person and the object of their attachment.

Grief can come from identification with the suffering of other people, with the many tragedies of the world, starvation, disease and the cruelty of man to man.

Grief, the difficulty of letting go, can also relate to the small, continual day-to-day releases of past preconceptions. For example, in a relationship, each partner needs to let go of their past images of the other person, as they change and reveal new aspects of their personality.

NEGATIVE ASPECTS OF GRIEF

Grief is a painful and disturbing emotion, which people may try to avoid. In some societies it is not wholly socially acceptable and tranquillizers may be prescribed to suppress it. However, unreleased grief produces the chronic pain of the tension between holding in and letting go. It can stagnate the Qi of the Lungs, causing respiratory problems such as dyspnoea and bronchitis. In the opinion of the author it can stagnate the Qi of the body, contributing to carcinoma.

Holding on to the lump of stagnant energy may substitute for holding on to the lost object of affections, but this encystment of energy within the body may result in the formation of physical lumps, such as uterine fibroids and carcinomas of the breasts. Other people may try to hold on to their memories, withdraw inside themselves, living in a world of the past and shutting themselves off from participation in the present. They may seem cold, dreamy or detached. They may be afraid of forming further attachments due to fear of the pain of loss; this effectively means they are afraid of life.

FEAR AND GRIEF

In the Five Element Promotion cycle, the child of grief is fear. Letting go means being alone, suffering a loss of identity and a little death. Grief can be closely bound to fear, fear of being alone, fear of the unknown, fear of letting go of attachments and the fear of death, fear of forming attachments and the fear of life.

If there is Deficient Kidney, the person may be too fearful of failure or loss to form bonds. It there is Deficient Lung Qi, the person may simply lack the energy to form bonds, or only be able to form weak bonds, so that they have difficulty in continuing relationships.

METAL AND THE ENERGY CENTRES

The Metal element and grief have different manifestations according to the energy centre.

BROW CENTRE

Completed grief can bring wisdom and a deeper perception and perspective. Unexpressed grief can cause mental dullness and confusion. The point of yìn táng can treat this.

THROAT CENTRE

This centre deals with communication and the expression of feelings, so that CV.22 can be used to help to release grief.

HEART CENTRE

The difference between Heart and Lungs in relationships, is that the Heart represents the exchange of feeling and affection, whilst the Lungs represent the forming, maintenance and dissolution of bonds of emotional attachment. Problems with both Heart and Lungs can block the Heart centre, prevent the free flow of love and affection between people, and contribute to diseases of the heart and circulatory systems, or to carcinoma of the breasts.

SOLAR PLEXUS CENTRE

Fear, anxiety and insecurity at separations can focus on the Solar Plexus centre, and these emotions can suppress grief, as well as causing physical problems such as restricted breathing or irritable bowel syndrome. CV.14 can help to relieve this situation.

SPLEEN CENTRE

Sympathy is the mother of grief, and the ability to care for and nourish another person is necessary for the formation of long-term attachments. CV.12 can assist this.

DAN TIAN CENTRE

Strengthening the Dan Tian centre can reduce the fear that prevents people from letting go of or starting relationships. It can also provide more energy for the formation of bonds. CV.4 can be used with Reinforcing method for this purpose, whilst CV.6 is better in combination with CV.17, with Even method, to move the Stagnant Qi of suppressed grief and depression.

REPRODUCTIVE CENTRE

Grief can stagnate the Reproductive centre and the process of sex and reproduction, causing irregular menstruation, cysts, fibroids, discharge or impotence.

The grief can be at the loss of a partner, children, a business, or it can be the grief of never having had children. CV.3 can be used in combination with CV.17 to treat these problems.

YIN AND YANG METAL TYPES

THE YIN METAL TYPE

Yin Metal personalities can be divided into two types, Deficiency and Stagnation.

DEFICIENCY

This type may have difficulties forming lasting bonds due to Deficient Qi of Lungs, and often also of Kidneys. They may be fearful of forming new relationships and withdraw from active participation in life, living in lonely dreams and memories of the past.

STAGNATION

These people may have more energy, and also more unexpressed grief. They may be reluctant to talk about their grief, to face or to express it, and they may try to suppress it with tranquillizers, alcohol or other drugs. Their internalization of grief can block satisfactory new relationships and sometimes lead to physical illness.

THE YANG METAL TYPE

The Yang Metal type is the least Yang and extrovert of all the Yang Five Element types. Violent public manifestation of grief, with sobbing, wailing, beating of the body, and the tearing of hair and clothes, is rare in Western society. It also tends to be sporadic and relatively brief, unlike the continuous hypomania of the Fire type or the continued intrusive possessiveness of the Earth personality.

It is natural to want to help someone who is grieving, but some Yang Metal personalities don't want to let go of their grief, they just want to talk about it and offload some of their misery on to others. They may also hold on to bitterness, resentment and regret about the past, and exhaust others with the endless repetition of their woes.

They may also use other people, by forming new relationships simply to assuage the pain of their grief, and not because they have any real regard for their new partner.

THE BALANCE

The balance lies in allowing the process of grief, in letting go of the past, in gaining wisdom and in learning and growing from each relationship or attachment, in participating fully in life and in forming new bonds, without being inhibited by fear of loss.

LIFE LESSONS OF THE METAL TYPES

THE YIN METAL TYPE

DEFICIENCY

If Qi is too weak to form bonds, then the first step is to strengthen the physical body by nutrition and moderate exercise. Qi Gong and acupuncture can focus on the Dan Tian, Spleen and Heart centres. Strengthening the Dan Tian centre can help to conserve energy and reduce fear, tonifying the Spleen centre can increase the ability to help and care for self and others, and strengthening the Heart centre can increase the flow of love and the desire to form bonds with others.

For those who have withdrawn into themselves, they need to learn to come slowly out of their sad and lonely world of ghosts, and become stirred again by the vibrancy of life. Joy controls grief, Fire controls Metal, and Five Element treatments on the Control cycle, with needles and much moxa, can be used to help these people.

STAGNATION

The lesson is letting go, in learning to externalize their emotions. Meditation can be helpful in going deeper and deeper into the self to find the strength and peace to face the truth, slowly and at their own speed. They need to learn that overactivity in the outer world may allow them partly to ignore their grief, but will not resolve it.

THE YANG METAL TYPE

These people need first to be aware of what they are doing, that is, refusing to look at their grief and let go of it, and using other people in a selfish and negative way. They have the energy and ability to form bonds, but may be self-indulgent in cherishing their grief, enjoying their self-pity, and not being honest with themselves and others. It may be useful for them to help to deal with the griefs and sorrows of others, to overcome their selfishness, become aware of the needs of others, and put their own griefs in perspective.

POINT COMBINATIONS

Yin Metal type

Deficiency	CV.4, CV.12, CV.17, LU.10, HT.8, ST.36 Rf M
	alternate GV.4, GV.12, BL.20, BL.23, BL.42, BL.44 Rf M
Stagnation	CV.6, CV.17 E M; LU.1, LU.6, LU.7, LI.4, KI.6. ST.40 E
	alternate BL.13, BL.15, BL.17, BL.42, BL.44 E
Yang Metal type	CV.6, CV.17 E M; LU.7, LI.4, SP.1, SP.21, LR.1, LR.14 E

Example

A woman of 35 tended to withdraw into herself, was unable to let go of much grief from unhappy past relationships, and tended to act in her new relationship as if it were one of her unsatisfactory old ones. Much of the repeated difficulties in her relationships with men came from a disturbed relationship with her father. Her pulse was thin, choppy, hindered and changing. The Lung position was sometimes empty and sometimes flooding.

The diagnosis was Deficiency and Stagnation of Lung Qi and Deficiency of Heart Fire. The point combination was:

CV.17, BL.13 E M; LU.1, LU.7 E; HT.8, LU.10, ST.36 Rf M

Water

THE NATURE OF WATER

STORAGE OF ENERGY

The Water element, the Kidney organ system and the Dan Tian energy centre, all relate to the storage and conservation of energy, so that it can be available when required. If this stored energy becomes depleted, then the person may be exhausted with no reserves of strength. Their emotional responses may be reduced, or they may become emotionally labile, since there is not enough Qi to hold the emotions stable. Since Qi gives the quality of adaptability, they may avoid or postpone necessary changes, since they do not have sufficient Qi for flexible behaviour.

WILL

The will is the ability to focus attention and energy upon a goal, with the concentration, determination and perseverance to achieve it. The stored energy of the Kidneys combines with the will to give drive and ambition.

If there is not enough Kidney energy, and if the will is weak, then the person has difficulty starting or completing tasks, is easily discouraged by set-backs, and is generally spineless in character. If there is not enough Kidney energy, and if the will is strong, the person may burn themselves out by attempting to achieve goals beyond their capacity. They may loathe themselves for their weakness and apparent failure.

If both energy and will are strong, the person may be dynamic and tireless with clear goals which they work hard and consistently to achieve. They may be charismatic leaders. However, they may be ruthless and inconsiderate of their own health and of the lives of others. If the strong energy and will is mixed with deep insecurity and fear, they may see the world as threatening, and become paranoid, suspicious, megalomaniac, aggressive, and obsessed with obtaining, maintaining and expanding power and control.

FEAR

Fear is a useful emotion in that it sets limitations and balances the expansive effect of the will and the Heart Spirit. But an excess of fear can paralyse action or create a constant stress upon the body that damages the Heart and the other organs. Fear is at the root of so many life problems, fear of failure, fear of loss of control, fear of responsibility, fear of being dependent, fear of being alone, fear of illness, fear of death, fear of sex, fear of life, and so on.

Fear is the mother of anger and the controller of joy. It also can inhibit sympathy and caring, and suppress the process of grieving and letting go.

STRENGTH

The experience of inner strength, of faith in life and faith in self, overcomes fear. Focusing on the Dan Tian centre in Qi Gong or mediation can give relief from fear. The use of CV.4 can assist this same effect.

WATER AND THE ENERGY CENTRES

Table 13.1 summarizes the Kidneys and the Lower Energy centres, and the effect of fear on the Heart centre is discussed on page 167.

YIN AND YANG WATER TYPES

THE YIN WATER TYPE

Through lack of energy or through fearfulness, the Yin Water type gives up on life and surrenders control of their own destiny. They simply do not do enough. Things seem too much effort, too difficult, too dangerous, and they lack the determination to achieve goals.

THE YANG WATER TYPE

The Yang Water type can be divided into two groups: Excess and Deficiency.

EXCESS

These people do too much. They are energetic, ambitious and ruthless, and sometimes reckless and foolhardy, even seeking dangerous situations. They may have great stress from the fear of losing control, and although they may try to suppress their fears, seeing them as a form of weakness, the constant emotional pressure may damage the heart and the physical body.

They may be cold and lonely people, seeking security in obtaining power over others, and dominating others with their will.

DEFICIENCY

These are people who either have constitutionally weak energy and strong will, or who once had strong energy and strong will, but who burned themselves out by overactivity. They can suffer great depression and loss of self-respect. They see themselves as failures and weaklings, but their problem is that they have set themselves inappropriate or unrealistic goals.

THE BALANCE

The balance is a firm will, but with concern for self and others, not discouraged by danger or difficulty, courageous but not foolhardy. The balance lies in action proceeding from inner strength and faith in self, and not as compensation for inner insecurities and fears.

LIFE LESSONS OF THE WATER TYPES

THE YIN WATER TYPE

The Yin water types have to learn the lesson of action. They need carefully to conserve their energy, and not to attempt tasks beyond their capacities. However, they need to discipline themselves not to delay, but to act. They tend to postpone tasks repeatedly so that these never get done, and they need daily self-discipline to go beyond this habit. Once they start a task they must learn to finish it without delay.

They need slowly and gradually to build up their self-confidence by completing tasks of increasing difficulty and challenge, but they must be careful not to go beyond their abilities or they become discouraged or depressed, and once again give up.

THE YANG WATER TYPE

Both Excess and Deficiency types need to find their source of inner strength and peace. They need to learn to act from inner stillness and strength, not from inner restlessness and fear. They need to learn how to be, as well as how to do, and they need to slow down and learn the need of a balance between activity and rest. There is a time to be busy, and a time to rest and store energy.

Those who are ruthless, without regard for others, need to learn consideration, compassion and love. They need to find strength within themselves so that they can open themselves up to love, and not see it as a dangerous vulnerability.

Meditation focusing on the Dan Tian centre can help to

control fear, so that they feel more secure, and less driven to gain power over others. CV.4 with Reinforcing method can be combined with CV.14 with Reducing method, to assist this.

DEFICIENCY

They have to learn that they are not weak failures, but that they need to readjust their goals. They need to learn that life can be enjoyed, it is for living, not merely for achieving an endless succession of goals.

POINT COMBINATIONS

Yin Water type   GV.20, CV.4, HT.8, KI.1, KI.7, BL.64, ST.36 Rf M
alternate GV.2, GV.4, GV.20, BL.23, BL.52 Rf M

Yang Water type
Excess   GV.20, CV.14, PC.6, KI.1 Rd; CV.17, KI.6 Rf
Deficiency   GV.20, CV.4, KI.3, SP.6, ST.36 Rf; PC.6 Rd

Example

A man of 38, was frustrated and depressed because of his tiredness and difficulty in maintaining a vigorous exercise routine. His pulse was slow, deep, empty, wiry and flooding. His tongue was pale and flabby.

The diagnosis was of Deficient Kidney Qi with Excess Kidney Will, and Stagnant Liver Qi. The flooding pulse in this case indicated the strain of excessive effort and pressure of will, and not Heat. The point combination was:

GV.20, PC.6, LR.3 E; SP.3, ST.36, KI.3 Rf M

CV.4, was not used initially, as in case this man exercised away his last reserves of energy. He was advised temporarily to reduce his exercise routine to give the acupuncture a chance to work, and to substitute two sessions of swimming per week for some of the jogging, since long-term that would increase his endurance and the strength of his muscles. The idea behind this was simply to get him to reduce his excessive exercise routine.

Wood

THE NATURE OF WOOD

INTUITION

The Hun, or Spiritual Soul, is related to the Wood element and to the Liver. It is associated with intuition, imagination, and the right side of the brain. Intuition is the ability to feel and perceive overall patterns in perspective. It is a complementary faculty to the analytical mind associated with the Spleen, and the left side of the brain.

Intuition can give a clear picture of the main threads of a person's life, or it can give a feeling of rightness about a particular course of action. It can give an insight into the potential unfolding of a personality, and it can give a strong sense of direction in life.

PLANS AND DECISIONS

The Wood element is linked to the ability to make plans and to make decisions. This ability is an extension into the analytical mind of the function of intuition to see an overall pattern and to know how it could unfold. The analytical ability of planning and decision-making, and the intuitive ability to perceive patterns of the past and present unfolding into the future, are complementary. But, when planning and decision-making have lost connection with the person's inner unfolding, then their life can become filled with difficulties and frustrations.

The problem of the modern world is partly that people are rarely trained in the intuitive faculty, and partly that it is difficult for mind, emotions and body to relax sufficiently for intuition to function.

INNER PRESSURE

Many Wood people feel an inner restless pressure of energy that seems to need release in action. This inner pressure tends to make them live and work at speed, and to become impatient, irritable and angry when progress becomes too slow to meet their mood. This pressure can give stress to themselves and to those who live and work around them.

If they surrender to this inner pressure, and the need for speedy action they can make many unwise decisions, that are not based on their own inner needs, but simply on their desire for a rapid decision, so that they can 'get on with it'. They are the kind of people likely to 'jump out of the frying pan into the fire'.

FRUSTRATION AND DEPRESSION

When Wood people cannot see their path in life, so that they have no satisfactory outlet for creativity, self-expression and self-growth, they can become frustrated and depressed. This can also happen if they lose contact with their intuition and make unsuitable plans and decisions. They are very sensitive to the feeling of being blocked and obstructed in their lives, but so often create these situations for themselves.

SUPPRESSION OF EMOTIONS

Many people, whether by nature Yin or Yang Wood types, suppress their anger and irritation, either because they fear the consequences of expression, or because they feel it is wrong. This is especially true of Wood–Earth types who wish to appear pleasant, caring and nice. However, the physical consequences of suppression of anger can range from headache and irritable bowel syndrome to myocardial infarction and cerebrovascular accident. Also, some degree of expression of anger can be necessary to establish boundaries, especially in those Yin Wood types who allow themselves to be dominated by other people.

SELF-EXPRESSION

The Wood element has an expansive energy, it is the element of birth, growth and self-expression. Indeed, some Yang Wood types try to use the people around them merely as a means to expand the self-expression of their own egos.

Many Wood people like movement, travel and change, because they hate the feeling of stasis, stagnation and depression, to which they are prone. They can be impatient for self-growth, personal change and development, often because their lack of patience and inability to use their intuition has put them in a situation of interwoven difficulties.

The Wood element can have a rather youthful aspect of impatience with constraint and limitation, desire for freedom and independence, and a feeling of rebellion and aggression towards restraining authority. The mature expression of the Wood element is the balance between freedom and responsibility.

YIN AND YANG WOOD TYPES

THE YIN WOOD TYPE

The Yin Wood type often has Deficient Kidney Qi, so that they have weak sense of self and insufficient personal force. They are unsure of their own identity and path in life, uncertain of their opinions and decisions, and find difficulty in expressing their own ego, so that they have weak boundaries and are easily influenced and dominated by others. They are timid, lack confidence, and are plagued by self-doubt.

THE YANG WOOD TYPE

Although energetic and forceful, they often lack connection with their own inner strength, and feel a pressure of insecurity and uncertainty, so that they are impatient and irritable with others. They may, on the other hand, be certain of self and know their own direction in life, or at least think they do. They may be intolerant of others less sure and quick than themselves, and may selfishly express and expand their own ego, regardless of the needs of others.

They tend to be domineering like the Yang Kidney type, but angry and aggressive or even violent, where the Kidney type would be coldly manipulating. They are prone to great impatience, frustration and depression when they feel blocked.

THE BALANCE

The balance manifests in the confident intuitive person, with a clear vision of their own path in life, and the patience to allow it to unfold. They are strong and independent, but able to express their own personality and creativity in a smooth and relaxed way, in harmony with the lives of others.

LIFE LESSONS OF THE WOOD TYPES

THE YIN WOOD TYPE

First of all, the Yin Wood type needs to contact and develop their own inner strength and surety of self. Meditation techniques focusing on the Dan Tian centre are helpful, especially if their weakness in Wood is linked to Deficient Kidneys. They need first to strengthen the Dan Tian centre, then to circulate its energy through their bodies, then to project it around themselves to strengthen their sense of boundaries, so that they are able to resist the intrusions of others.

The second main lesson is to develop and use their intuition, to make an increasingly strong connection to the ongoing pattern unfolding within them. This gives them a greater sense of certainty and direction, to overcome their tendency to hesitation, dithering and procrastination.

THE YANG WOOD TYPE

The first step is to slow down, and to cultivate a discipline of inner peace. To act out of stillness and certainty and not out of impatience and inner stress. They have to learn

to relax, to surrender, and let go of the pressure of their plans and decisions. Only by doing this can they develop their intuition which can allow them to flow smoothly through life, in harmony with it. They need to learn that things happen in their own time, and that life cannot be forced or hurried.

They need to accept that there are times of no apparent action and change, either in the outside world or in themselves. They need to accept times of rest, to be patient and to attune with their higher self, their intuition, to see the way they should go. They also have to overcome their natural selfishness, and learn love, compassion and consideration for others. They have to replace anger with calm, impatience with patience, and judgement with observation.

ANGER

Both Yin and Yang Wood types have to learn to deal with their anger, not to fear it or be disgusted by it, not to indulge in it, but when to express it and when to say nothing. By increasing strength of self, they are less vulnerable to impatience and touchiness. By decreasing the stress in their lives and living more harmoniously, they reduce the internal pressure that produces explosive anger. By slowing down and acting more from inner stillness and strength they can slowly reduce anger and impatience, but it takes a continual daily discipline and remembering.

POINT COMBINATIONS

Yin Wood type	CV.4, TE.4, GB.40, SP.6, ST.36 Rf; CV.14, GB.13 E alternate GV.4, BL.19, BL.23, BL.48 Rf
Yang Wood type	GV.20, yìn táng, PC.8, LR.2, KI.1 Rd; LR.8, KI.6 Rf

Example

A man of 30 was in some ways independent and in others emotionally dependent on his family. He was in some ways assertive, but in others lacking in confidence, needing much reassurance, and oversensitive to criticism or advice. He suffered from both migraines and depression. His pulse was empty, especially at the Kidney and Spleen positions, and thin and wiry in the Liver and Gallbladder positions.

The diagnosis was lack of confidence and hypersensitivity due to Deficient Qi of Kidney and Gallbladder, and of a tension between independence and dependence, due to Deficiency of Liver and Spleen. Liver is seen as ruling freedom and independence, and Spleen as ruling dependence due to the need to be cared for by others.

The point combination was:

CV.4, CV.12, GB.40, ST.36, KI.3 Rf; GV.20, GB.20 E
alternate BL.18, BL.19, BL.20, BL.23, Rf; BL.48, BL.49 E

This chapter has discussed the five Yin and the five Yang personality types. General discussion of the Yin–Yang is given in the next chapter.

Maintaining the balance 5 *of Yin and Yang*

Yang gives energy, movement and warmth; Yin gives solidity, nourishment, moisture, coolness and rest. The harmonious balance of Yin and Yang gives health and contentment.

Yin-Yang imbalance is at the root of much illness, whether physical or psychological. Excessive Yang, or Deficient Yin, means excessive activity, movement, heat and dryness, with lack of rest due to insufficient nourishment and grounding of the Heart Spirit. Excessive Yin, or Deficient Yang, means lack of physical, emotional and mental movement, with excessive Cold and Damp.

DEFICIENT YIN AND DEFICIENT YANG

People may inherit or develop a constitution which is basically Deficient Yin or Deficient Yang. This affects pathology. For example, Wind invasion of a Deficient Yin type person will tend to have a Wind Heat reaction in the body whilst Wind invasion of a Deficient Yang type will tend to have a Wind Cold reaction in the body. Between invasions, the Deficient Yin type may benefit from KI.6 + LU.5 Rf, while the Deficient Yang type may benefit from KI.7 + ST.36 Rf M.

Cultural differences will affect the number manifesting Deficient Yin or Deficient Yang signs in a population. For example, a rural society with physical overwork, exposure to Wind, Cold and Damp, and malnutrition, may tend to Deficient Yang. An industrial society with mental overwork and high levels of stress, greater intake of rich foods, and exposure to central heating, may tend more to Deficient Yin.

DEFICIENCY OF YIN IN MODERN SOCIETY

Modern life centres round ceaseless stressful activity. To a great extent, four things have been lost:

rest
sleep
intuition
inner strength.

The loss of these four things relates to the loss of the deep feelings of peace, calmness and tranquillity, that comes from contact with the inner self. The experience of the inner self is the experience of the balance between Yin and Yang. There is sense of inner peace, Yin, at the same time as an experience of energy and strength, Yang.

REST

True rest is rare in the modern world. Much of what people call rest is associated with mental overstimulation, whether drugs, television, video-games or whatever. The result of this is that Yin is not properly replenished, so that people become increasingly tired and restless. They may alternate between the use of stimulants such as coffee or amphetamines, to give them energy or excitement, and the use of tranquillizers and narcotics to give a temporary artificial calm.

SLEEP

In modern life, the world of daytime mental activity and stress has encroached into the world of sleep, so that sleep is often of poor quality, and the person does not awake refreshed in the morning. Indeed, the prevalence of insomnia and the widespread use of hypnotic drugs indicate the extent of this problem. Sleep is not merely a cessation of physical activity, it is a state of being which is necessary for the daily regeneration of mind and body. Lack of sleep means Deficient Yin, which in turn can cause insomnia in the night and restlessness in the day.

INTUITION

The world of sleep is allied with the right side of the brain, with dreaming, imagination and intuition. Analysis and intuition are complementary faculties, but the balance between them has been lost. In the modern world there is great overemphasis on analysis and great under-development of intuition. Loss of the intuitive ability greatly increases the level of uncertainty and stress, leading to further depletion of Yin.

Without intuition, it is difficult for people to see their path in life, and easy for them to become entangled in the long-term stressful consequences of unwise decisions.

INNER STRENGTH

Inner strength can be developed by the daily discipline or routine of deeply relaxing the mind to experience directly the balance of Yin–Yang. This simultaneous experience of peace and strength can then be allowed to flow out into the life. Thus, outer strength is based on inner strength and stillness.

Most people expend their energy in constant stressful activity in the external world, constantly seeking outside of themselves for the peace and strength that can only be found within. By doing this, they deplete their Yin, and shut themselves off from the source of their real strength.

TREATMENT OF DEFICIENT YIN

Deficient Yin can be treated symptomatically with points like SP.6 and KI.6, but this is not enough to both replenish Yin and prevent future Deficiency. A more thorough treatment of Deficient Yin has several aspects:

tonify Qi
tonify Yin
disperse Fire
calm the Spirit
develop inner peace and strength
readjust goals.

TONIFY QI

Deficient Yin is often based on Deficient Qi. If there is not enough Qi to hold things stable, the patient may alternate between Deficient Yin and Deficient Yang. Examples of this are manic depression and menopausal alternations between feelings of heat and feelings of cold.

Points such as ST.36 or SP.3 that tonify Qi and Blood can be used, in addition to neutral points, such as BL.23, CV.4 and KI.3 that stabilize the balance between Yin and Yang by strengthening Qi.

TONIFY YIN

Points like SP.6 and KI.6 can be used to strengthen Yin in general, and points like LU.5 and HT.6 can be used to tonify the Yin of specific organs.

DISPERSE FIRE

The system of reducing the Fire point and reinforcing the Water point is effective, e.g. KI.2 Rd + KI.10 Rf. If the Fire is more extreme, the system of reducing both Well point and Spring point can be adapted, e.g. KI.1 + KI.2 Rd.

CALM THE SPIRIT

In addition to the points just given, to tonify Yin and to disperse Fire, other points can be used to calm the Spirit, depending on the situation and on the energy centre affected. For example:

CV.14   for Deficient Yin with fear

CV.17	for Deficient Yin with overexcitement or anxiety
yìn táng	for Deficient Yin with mental restlessness
ān mián	for Deficient Yin + Deficient Blood with insomnia
GV.20	for Deficient Yin + Hyperactive Liver Yang
SP.1 + SP.2	for Deficient Yin with insomnia and dream-disturbed sleep.

DEVELOP INNER PEACE AND STRENGTH

This can only happen when patients realize that their greatest resources lie within themselves, and when they make a daily routine of relaxation and meditation exercises that allow them to contact these resources, and bring them out into their lives.

Acupuncture can open a window of opportunity, and the practitioner can give instruction and support, but it is only the patient's daily application that will lead them to a direct experience of the balance between Yin and Yang, the experience of unity.

READJUST GOALS

Many people in the modern world, set themselves goals that are inappropriate to their personality, beyond their capacity, or impossible within a given time limit. As a result they burn out their reserves of energy and suffer both exhaustion and depression — see Chapter 34.

Patient counselling is necessary if they are ever to rebuild the Qi and Yin, so that they understand themselves, both their abilities and limitations, select goals within their capacity, and allow themselves time to rest and recover.

Combinations such as GV.20 + KI.1 Rd can only be used to relax the will if the patient is likely to accept the sensation of exhaustion that may follow the use of these points — see Chapter 4 on the life lessons of the personality types.

YIN AND YANG PERSONALITY TYPES

Each of the Five Elements has a Yin and a Yang personality type. Each of these 10 types tends to characteristic illnesses and life problems. For each of the Five Elements there is a state of balance between Yin and Yang, and each of the 10 personality types can progress towards this balance by learning the particular lessons of their type. This is discussed in detail in Chapter 4, and

point combinations for the 10 personality types are summarized in Table 4.3.

FEMALE AND MALE

Each human being can focus their attention on their inner self, the Yin or female aspect, or on the outer world, the Yang or male aspect. The inner and outer aspects are complementary, and when an individual overemphasizes either of these aspects there is imbalance.

Yang must have its foundation in Yin. Activity in the outer world, Yang, needs to be founded on a strong contact with the inner self, Yin. Exterior activity needs to derive from inner stillness and strength and to be a natural consequence of the unfolding and expression of a person's inner potential or life path. Yang and Yin are then working together in harmony.

Many people in the modern world have lost contact with their inner self, so that they experience separation of Yang and Yin. Their external activity does not derive from inner stillness and strength, but from inner restlessness and weakness, as a compensation for the loss of contact with the inner self. Much of their actions result not from their inner unfolding, but as a consequence of trying to escape the tangled consequences of being out of tune with this. Yang has lost its foundations in Yin, so that Yin and Yang become depleted, and individuals experience the inner discomfort of Yin-Yang imbalance.

Men and women each have their male and female aspects, each have their Yang and their Yin. As a generalization, in men the Yang is emphasized and in women the Yin. In women there tends to be a stronger link with the inner-self and with intuition, in men there is a stronger tendency to be active and assertive in the outer world.

PROBLEMS FOR MEN

For men, the problem has always been overemphasis on external activity, Yang, and a loss of contact with the inner world, Yin. This not only results in burnout of Yin but also in loss of contact with the softer Yin qualities of tenderness, compassion and caring. This results in a world of fear, insecurity, hatred, aggression, warfare and cruelty, which affects both men and women.

Since the focus of men is outward, they tend to have difficulty in developing their intuition, and achieving a balance between intuition and analysis. This is aggravated by the modern overemphasis on analysis and the lack of trust or training in intuition, which is the voice of the inner self.

To correct this imbalance, most men need to learn to

direct their attention inward, to create a stronger contact with the inner self, so that they can bring more of the feminine qualities of the inner self out into their lives and into the world around them.

PROBLEMS FOR WOMEN

In most of the societies of the past, the problem for women was exhaustion of Yin through continual childbirth and child care.

In modern society, as women become more active in the external world, they are increasingly suffering from the same problems as men, in overemphasis of Yang, loss of contact with the inner-self and intuition, and the burnout of Yin. This is reflected in a change in disease patterns, for example, an increase in myocardial infarction. In addition, not only do many women have the double load of motherhood and job, but also this is a time of confusion and uncertainty about the nature of femininity, and the balance of the male and female aspects for women.

Whilst women tend to have a naturally stronger contact with the inner-self and intuition, they often find it difficult to trust their intuition, live by it, and bring it into the outer world, especially in the current climate of the worship of analysis and logic. For women with full-time jobs and careers, there is the double danger of the overemphasis of the Yang or male aspect, and of the Stagnation of the Yin, or female energies. Acupuncture and meditation can both help to harmonize the Yin–Yang balance. Points on the Conception channel can be combined with Extra channel Opening points as a basis for treatment. Point combinations for the Yin and Yang Extra channel personality types are discussed in Chapter 10 and summarized in Table 10.5.

CHILDREN AND YIN–YANG

Early childhood is a time of acting out of the inner world, a time of living from the imagination, a time of the development and growth of Yin.

In Western society there is increasing pressure on children to look and behave like teenagers or even like adults. Also, to a large extent, the development of the imagination has been replaced by video-games and television. This devaluation and shortening of childhood is not simply the loss of a magic time in life, it is a weakening of the development of the Yin qualities which form the foundations of adult life.

This situation is made worse by the current weakening of the family and social structure, and by the confusion about the nature and roles of men and women. Ideally,

children need to experience both the Yang and the Yin qualities of the father, and both the Yang and the Yin qualities of the mother. They need to experience the masculine and feminine aspects of both parents, so that their own male–female balance can develop harmoniously.

In reality, many children grow up in one-parent families, whilst the majority develop in families where the parents are neither in balance with themselves nor each other. In these conditions of confusion, conflict, insecurity and uncertainty, arise not only childhood diseases and juvenile crime, but also an unstable foundation for adult life. Acupuncture treatment of children is therefore very often enhanced by acupuncture treatment and counselling of the parents.

YIN–YANG AND THE AGEING PROCESS

In the Western world, the pressure for children and teenagers is to look and act like adults. For adults, there is enormous pressure to maintain a youthful appearance, even in old age. Indeed, due to a loss of contact with the inner self, people identify with their external appearance, and cannot accept the ageing process.

At midlife, between about 40 and 50 years of age, there is an opportunity to gain great strength and wisdom by assimilating the experiences of adult life, and continuing active life with a deeper understanding and awareness. Midlife is a time when the quality of Yang can be increased by a return to Yin, and there can be the establishment of a new balance of Yin–Yang. However, for many, this opportunity is restricted by a feeling of despair at growing old and an attempt to hold on to the past.

In old age, from 65 onwards, there is a decline of Yang, a reduction in outer activity, and a return to Yin. If people accept this, old age can be a time of inner development and contentment, but if they do not, it can be a time of frustration, bitterness and depression.

The Extra channel pairs are particularly useful in treating physical and psychological problems associated with the different major stages of the developmental process, and in re-establishing the Yin–Yang balance at each phase.

TREATMENT OF DEFICIENT YANG

The emphasis of this section has been on the origins and treatment of Deficient Yin. However, there are those who are Deficient Yang, either by constitution, physical overwork and exposure to Cold, or because they were originally healthy or Deficient Yin, but burned out their Yang by stressful activity.

Treatment of Deficient Yang has several aspects:

tonify Qi
tonify Yang
disperse Cold and Damp
relieve depression
prevent future burnout.

TONIFY QI

To provide a solid foundation for Yang, it is necessary to tonify Qi, Blood and Yin. This can be done with combinations like CV.4, ST.36 Rf M; SP.6 Rf.

TONIFY YANG

Yang itself can be strengthened by needle or moxa on such points as GV.1, GV.4, GV.14 and GV.20. The Yang specific organs can be treated with needle and moxa on the Fire point of that organ, e.g. KI.2, LR.2, SP.2, HT.8, PC.8, LU.10; or Governor or Bladder point associated, e.g. GV.11 and BL.15 for the Heart.

DISPERSE COLD AND DAMP

In addition to needle and moxa of the Fire points, Cold and Damp can be dispersed by the use of such points as CV.6, CV.8, CV.9, CV.12, ST.36, ST.40 and SP.9 with Reinforcing method and moxa.

RELIEVE DEPRESSION

Deficient Yang can lead to lack of movement of both mind and emotions, partly due to Deficiency, and partly due to the Stagnation that follows it. Points can be chosen according to the situation and the energy centres affected. For example, CV.3 + CV.6 for depression with infertility, CV.3 + CV.17 for sadness with irregular menstruation, CV.6 + CV.14 for fearful depression with lack of will. All points can be used with Even method and moxa.

PREVENT FUTURE BURNOUT

For those who have become Deficient Yang due to burnout there is a problem that as soon as they gain a little more energy, their restlessness and frustration will tend to the overactivity that will burn out Yang again.

Moxa must be used with great caution with these patients, since they can easily change from Deficient Yang back to Deficient Yin. Points need to be added to calm the mind and to relax the will, such as GV.9, GV.20, yìn táng, BL.7, GB.13, CV.14, KI.1 and KI.7. These points can be used with Even or Reducing method, providing other points are tonified to strengthen Qi and Yang.

YIN-YANG AND THE FOUR IMBALANCES

The next chapter expands the classification of disharmonies into Yin or Yang, by using the concept of the four main imbalances of Qi, Deficiency, Excess, Stagnation and Irregularity.

Deficiency and Stagnation are relatively Yin, and Excess and Irregularity are relatively Yang:

Yin	Yang
Deficiency	Excess
Stagnation	Irregularity

Deficiency, Excess, Stagnation and Irregularity 6

The concept of the four main Qi imbalances was developed by the author as a system of the classification of disharmonies, which could be used to integrate acupuncture, energy work and meditation. Once the disharmony has been classified in this way, the principle of treatment is the same in all three therapies.

THE FOUR MAIN QI IMBALANCES

The four main Qi imbalances are Deficiency, Excess, Stagnation and Irregularity. All Qi disharmonies can be classified in terms of these four main imbalances or their combinations.

DEFINITIONS

Deficiency is a lack of energy, either in the body as a whole, or in specific organs, or body parts. Stagnation is insufficient movement in or between specific channels, organs or parts. It is associated with blocks or obstructions in the flows of energy. There may be Deficiency of energy in front of a block and Excess of energy accumulated behind it. Irregularity is disturbance in the smooth flow of energy within or between channels, organs or parts with associated disturbances in physical functions, emotions and behaviour.

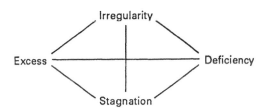

Fig. 6.1 The four main Qi imbalances.

Examples of Irregularity are shown in Table 6.1.

Table 6.1 Examples of irregularity of Qi

Organ syndrome	Ailment
Rebellious Lung	cough, asthma
Kidney fear invades Heart	fearful anxiety
Hyperactive Liver Yang	dizziness, irritability, touchiness
Disturbance of Heart Spirit	mania, hysteria, dream-disturbed sleep
Rebellious Spleen Qi	diarrhoea, borborygmus
Rebellious Stomach Qi	nausea, vomiting, belching, hiccups

PULSES

Each of the four main imbalances can be associated with a group of pulses as shown in Table 6.2.

Table 6.2 Pulses of the four imbalances

Imbalance	Pulse groups
Deficiency	empty, thin, choppy, minute
Excess	full, flooding
Stagnation	wiry, hindered
Irregular	irregular, moving, scattered

In this chapter, the words empty, full, wiry and irregular will be used to indicate their respective pulse groups. If the word 'empty' is used, as in Table 6.4 and Figure 6.2, for example, it can indicate any one of the four pulses in the Deficiency group.

PRINCIPLES OF TREATMENT

For the four basic imbalances, the same principles of treatment apply whether the practitioner uses acupuncture, energy techniques or meditation:

tonify Deficiency
disperse Excess
move Stagnation
calm Irregularity.

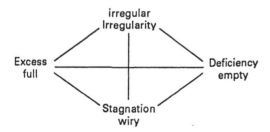

Fig. 6.2 The pulse groups of the four imbalances.

METHODS OF TREATMENT

The methods of treatment using acupuncture can be summarized as follows:

Deficiency	Rf, M
Excess	Rd, El, C, B
Stagnation	Rd, E, El, M, C, B
Irregularity	Rd (for Irregularity with Excess)
	E (for Irregularity with Deficiency).

Methods are shown in more detail in Table 6.4.

OTHER IMBALANCES

WIND, HEAT, DRYNESS, COLD AND DAMP

Besides the four imbalances of Qi, there are the imbalances associated with Wind, Heat, Dryness, Cold and Damp, each of which can be either Exterior or Interior.

• Wind represents movement and change and is Yang. Exterior Wind results in acute Excess in the surface of the body. Interior Wind is Irregularity which can be associated with Excess, e.g. Liver Fire, or Deficiency, e.g. Deficient Liver Blood.

• Heat is Yang and increases movement and is therefore more likely to be associated with Irregularity than Stagnation, although Heat can be associated with Stagnation as in Liver–Gallbladder Damp Heat, or when the Heat is associated with Retention of Phlegm in the Lungs. Heat can be associated with either Deficiency or Excess.

• Dryness may originate from Excess Heat patterns or be associated with Deficient Blood or Deficient Yin. It is itself a Deficiency pattern representing a lack of fluids.

• Cold is Yin and may originate from Exterior Excess of Cold or from Interior Deficient Yang. In itself, it slows movement and tends to cause Stagnation of Qi and Blood.

• Damp is Yin, whether it originates from Exterior Excess of Damp or Interior Deficient Spleen and Kidneys. Damp is heavy and lingering and is associated with Stagnation.

PRINCIPLES OF TREATMENT

• Exterior Wind is dispersed and Interior Wind is calmed. In addition, if the origin of Interior Wind is Excess, this is dispersed; if Deficiency, this is tonified.

• Exterior Heart or Interior Excess Heat are dispersed, and for Interior Deficiency Heat, the Heat is dispersed and the Deficient Yin is tonified.

• For Exterior Wind Dryness, the Wind is dispersed and if necessary, Yin is tonified.

• For Interior Dryness, tonify Yin.

• Exterior Cold, Excess Cold are dispersed, and for Interior Deficiency Cold, the Cold is dispersed and the Deficient Yang is tonified.

• Exterior or Interior Damp must be dispersed and the associated Stagnation moved, and if the Interior Damp is based on Deficiencies of Spleen and Kidneys, these must be tonified.

COMBINATIONS OF THE FOUR MAIN IMBALANCES

There are six combinations of the four main imbalances as shown in Figure 6.3:

PRINCIPLES OF TREATMENT

Which principle of treatment is emphasized will depend on which of the two imbalances in a combination is dominant at a particular time. For example, for the combination of Excess and Deficiency, it is not possible for full Excess and full Deficiency to exist in the same organ at the same time. However, it is common for Excess to dominate in the acute phase during an attack, whilst Deficiency dominates in the chronic phase between attacks. For example, during the acute phase of violent headache, disperse the Excess Liver Fire; and during the chronic phase, tonify the Deficient Liver Yin on which the temporary Excess is based.

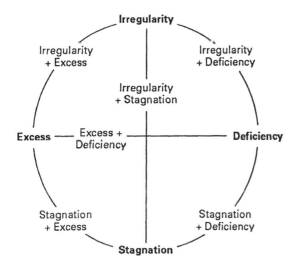

Fig 6.3 Combination of the four main imbalances.

As another example, for a combination of Deficient Lung Qi with Stagnant Lung Qi, it is possible to use some points with Even or Reducing method to move the Stagnant Lung Qi, e.g. CV.17, BL.13, whilst at the same time reinforcing other points to tonify the Lung Deficiency, e.g. LU.9 and ST.36.

CLASSIFICATION OF THE ORGAN SYNDROMES

The organ syndromes can be classified into the 10 categories of Deficiency, Excess, Stagnation and Irregularity and their six combinations as shown in Table 6.3. It can be seen from the table that the Kidneys tend to Deficiency and Irregularity and not so much to Excess. The Liver and the Heart are especially prone to patterns of Irregularity, due to the disturbance associated with Heart Fire, Liver Fire, Hyperactive Liver Yang, or Liver Wind rising up the body, causing Disturbance of Heart Spirit.

SUMMARY OF THE TEN IMBALANCES

The four basic imbalances and their six combinations are summarized in Table 6.4.

CLASSIFICATION OF POINT TYPES

Acupuncture as a therapy has a self-regulating effect on the body, so for any acupuncture point, the insertion of a needle will tend to tonify if there is Deficiency, disperse if there is Excess, move if there is Stagnation, or calm if there is Irregularity. However, some point types tend to have more specific effects. For example, Source points are most used to tonify and Accumulation points are most used to disperse and move. Table 6.5 summarizes the main uses of each point type.

Table 6.6 takes the Conception channel as an example to show how the different points on a channel can be used in different ways.

APPLICATIONS OF THE CONCEPT OF THE FOUR IMBALANCES

The concept of the four main Qi imbalances, Deficiency, Excess, Stagnation and Irregularity, is most useful in understanding the origins of diseases. It is helpful in understanding the clinical applications of the Five Element theory (Chapter 9), and it is essential in extending the range of use of the Extra channels (Chapter 10). It can illuminate an understanding of the treatment of psychological disorders, since the mind and emotions can be seen as Qi-flow phenomena.

Table 6.3 Classification of the organ syndromes

Imbalance	Lungs	Kidneys	Liver	Heart	Spleen–Stomach
Deficiency	Def.LU Qi Def.LU Yin Def.LU Yang	Def.KI Jing Def.KI Qi Def.KI Yin Def.KI Yang	Def.LR Blood Def.LR–GB Qi	Def.HT Qi Def.HT Blood Def.HT Yin Def.HT Yang	Def.SP–ST Qi Def.ST Yin Def.SP Yang
Excess	LU Fire		LR–GB Fire	HT Fire	ST Fire
Stagnation	St.LU Qi	St.KI Qi	St.LR Qi St.LR Blood	St.HT Qi St.HT Blood	St.SP–ST Qi
Irregularity	Reb.LU Qi	KI fear invades HT	Hyp.LR Yang LR Wind	Dist. of HT Spirit	Reb.ST Qi Reb.SP Qi
Deficiency + Excess	Def.LU Yin + LU Fire	Def.KI Yang + Damp	Def.LR Yin + LR Fire	Def.HT Yin + HT Fire	Def.SP Yang + Damp
Irregularity + Excess	Reb.LU Qi + Retention of Phlegm in LU		LR Wind + LR Fire	Dist. of HT Spirit + HT Fire	Reb.ST Qi + ST Fire
Irregularity + Deficiency	Reb.LU Qi + Def.LU Qi	fear disturbs HT + Def.KI Qi	Hyp.LR Yang + Def.LR Blood	Dist. of HT Spirit + Def.HT Qi	Reb.ST Qi + Def.ST Qi
Irregularity + Stagnation	Reb.LU Qi + St.LU Qi		Hyp. LR Yang + St.LR Qi	Dist. of HT Spirit + St.HT Qi	Reb.ST Qi + St.ST Qi
Stagnation + Excess	Retention of Phlegm in LU		LR–GB Damp Heat	Phlegm Cold in HT	Damp Heat in SP
Stagnation + Deficiency	St.Qi + Def.LU Qi	St.KI Qi + Def.KI Qi	St.LR Qi + Def.LR Yang	St.HT Blood + Def.HT Yang	St.SP–ST Qi + Def.SP–ST Qi

Def., Deficiency; St., Stagnation; Reb., Rebellious; Hyp., Hyperactive; Dist., Disturbance.

Table 6.4 Summary of the ten imbalances

Imbalance	Principle of treatment	Pulse group	Method of treatment	Example syndrome	Example ailment	Point combination
Deficiency	tonify	empty	Rf M	Def. KI Qi	impotence	GV.4, GV.20, BL.23, ST.36 Rf M
Excess	disperse	full	Rd, El, C, B	LR Fire	aggression	GV.20, KI.1, LR.3 Rd; PC.9, LR.1B
Stagnation	move	wiry	Rd, E, El, M, C, B	St. LR Qi	depression	CV.6 E M; CV.17, PC.6, LR.3 Rd
Irregularity	calm	irregular	Rd, E	Reb. ST Qi	nausea	CV.14, PC.6, ST.36 E
Deficiency + Excess	tonify + disperse	empty or full	Rf, M Rd, El, C, B	Def. LR Yin + LR Fire	conjunctivitis	SP.6, LR.8 Rf GB.1 E; GB.38 Rd; LR.1B
Irregularity + Excess	calm + disperse	irregular + full	Rd, E Rd, El, C, B	Dist. of HT Spirit + HT Fire	mania and anxiety	CV.14, HT.7, SP.6 E Rd HT.8, KI.1 Rd
Irregularity + Deficiency	calm + tonify	irregular + empty	Rd, E Rf, M	fear disturbs HT + Def.KI Qi	fear and apprehension	CV.14, PC.6, HT.7 Rd CV.4, KI.3, ST.36 Rf M
Stagnation + Excess	move + disperse	wiry + full	Rd, E, El, M, C, B Rd, B	Retention of Phlegm Cold in LU	chronic bronchitis	CV.17, LU.1, LU.6 Rd; BL.13, ST.40 Rd M
Irregularity + Stagnation	calm + move	irregular + wiry	Rd, E Rd, E, El, M, C, B	Hyp. LR Yang + St. LR Qi	premenstrual syndrome	GV.20, GB.20E LR.2, LR.14, SP.6 Rd
Stagnation + Deficiency	move + tonify	wiry + empty	Rd, E, El, M, C, B Rf, M	St. HT Blood Def. HT Yang	angina pectoris	CV.17, SP.4 Rd M; SP.21, PC.6 Rd CV.4, ST.36 Rf M

Pulse names refer to the pulse group, see p. 44, not the individual quality.
Def., Deficiency; St., Stagnation; Reb., Rebellious; Hyp., Hyperactive; Dist., Disturbance.
Rf., Reinforcing; Rd, Reducing; E, Even; M, moxa; B, bleeding; EL, electroacupuncture; C, cupping.

Table 6.5 Classification of point types

Point type	Point use			
	Deficiency	Excess	Stagnation	Irregularity
Source	X			X
Connecting			X	
Accumulation			X	
Alarm	x	X	X	X
Well	x	X	x	x
Back Transporting	X	x	x	x
Five Element	x	x	X	x
Opening	x	x	X	x
Window of Heaven		X		x

X, primary use; x, secondary use.

Table 6.6 Classification of Conception channel points

Point type	Point use			
	Deficiency	Excess	Stagnation	Irregularity
CV.24		x	X	X
CV.22		X	X	X
CV.17	x	x	X	x
CV.14	x	x	x	X
CV.12	X	X	X	X
CV.6	x		X	
CV.4	X			X
CV.3	x	X	X	

CV.4 can be used for Irregularity only when this is based on Deficiency, since CV.4 can tonify the underlying Deficiency.
X, primary use; x, secondary use.

ACUPUNCTURE AND ENERGY WORK

The classification of the Four Imbalances was specifically designed by the author as a system of differentiation to integrate acupuncture, energy work and meditation. The same principle of treatment applies in each case.

For example, for a patient where Irregularity of movement in the head is associated with Deficiency of the Kidneys, the principle of treatment in each of the three therapies is to tonify the Deficiency and to calm the Irregularity. Acupuncture treatment can do this with CV.4, KI.3, ST.36 Rf; GV.20, KI.1 Rd. The practitioner can then enhance the effect of the acupuncture by using energy work (Qi Gong) firstly to strengthen the Dan Tian centre, and then to sink energy down in the body to relieve Irregularity in the head. The patient can then be given specific meditation exercises which strengthen Kidney energy and balance the distribution of energy in the body.

How to make effective 7 combinations

TREATING CAUSE AND EFFECT

Illnesses tend to have one or more underlying cause, Ben, and one or more external manifestation, Biao. For example, a common cold may have underlying Deficiency of Qi, Ben, with outward signs of Exterior Wind, Biao, e.g. sneezing and chills. The underlying Deficiency of Qi, the cause, allows the Invasion of Exterior Wind, the effect.

The question in forming a point combination is when to treat the cause and when to treat the effect. There are various possibilities:

treat effect only
treat cause only
treat cause then effect
treat effect then cause
treat cause and effect simultaneously.

TREAT EFFECT ONLY

This is usually only done when the effect is Exterior *and* is dominant to the cause. For example, when there is Wind Cold invasion with only mild underlying Deficiency of Qi, so that this Deficiency will be corrected by the body itself, without further treatment, once the Exterior Wind Cold has been expelled, e.g. with LU.7 + LI.4 Rd. This is rare in the clinical experience of the author, since most of his patient's have had chronic underlying Deficiencies which needed tonifying, after the Exterior factor was removed.

If both cause and effect are Interior it is more common to treat them successively or simultaneously, rather than treat the effect only. For example, if there is insomnia from Deficient Heart Yin, ān miān for insomnia can be used at the same time as HT.3 for Deficient Heart Yin.

TREAT CAUSE ONLY

This is not used for Exterior conditions, since the Exterior factor must be expelled first.

It may be enough in some internal problems to treat the root only. For example, CV.4, ST.36, KI.3 Rf M for an underlying condition of Deficient Kidney Yang, may relieve the symptoms of tiredness and impotence. However, additional points are often needed to treat the symptoms, especially if these are local, e.g. cold hands and feet. SP.2 and PC.8 Rf M can then be added to the points for the cause.

TREAT CAUSE THEN EFFECT

This is rare in Exterior conditions, since the Exterior factor is usually expelled first. It is also uncommon in Interior conditions, since the Interior cause and Interior effect are often treated together.

TREAT EFFECT THEN CAUSE

This is very common for illnesses when there is a chronic Interior condition, with occasional more severe aggravations, and also for illnesses where the effect is so urgent it must be dealt with immediately.

Chronic Interior plus acute Exterior

For example, a chronic Interior condition of Deficient Qi, with tiredness, may allow periodic Exterior invasion by Wind Cold, with influenza. During the acute phase, the influenza, the effect is treated by expelling the Wind Cold; during the chronic phase, the cause is treated by tonifying the Qi.

chronic phase	acute phase
(between attacks)	(during attacks)
e.g. Deficient Kidney and Lungs with tiredness and reduced resistance to infection	e.g. Wind Cold invasion with influenza
CV.4, CV.17, LU.9, KI.3, ST.36 Rf	GV.14, LU.7, LI.4 Rd

Chronic Interior plus acute Interior

For example, Deficiency of Spleen Qi may result in the Spleen not holding the blood, with severe haemorrhage. The acute effect must be treated first, for example, with points such as SP.1 and SP.10 Rf M. Once the bleeding has stopped, the Deficiency of Qi that caused it, and the Deficiency of Blood resulting from it, can be treated with points such as BL.17, BL.20, BL.43 Rf M.

TREAT CAUSE AND EFFECT SIMULTANEOUSLY

This is not used for Exterior problems, since the Exterior factor must be expelled first. It is, however, the commonest method of treating Interior problems. For example, a

headache associated with Hyperactive Liver Yang may have an underlying cause of Deficient Kidney Qi. CV.4 and KI.3 Rf M for the Deficient Kidney can be used simultaneously with GB.34 and GB.20 Rd for the Hyperactive Liver Yang.

A MATTER OF EMPHASIS

Often, between attacks, a combination is selected that is predominantly for treating the cause, but with a few points to treat the effect. For example, for headaches after menstruation due to Deficient Blood, between attacks, the combination could be:

BL.17, BL.20, BL.23, BL.43 Rf M; GV.20 E

In this combination most points are for Deficient Blood, but the GV.20 is added to harmonize the movement of Qi in the head. During attacks, the combination could be:

GV.20, GB.20, yìn táng, LI.4 E; ST.36 Rf M

Here, the majority of points are for the acute effect, but ST.36 is to treat the underlying cause.

The relative number of points included to treat cause and to treat effect, will depend on the relative dominance of cause and effect at any given time.

GENERAL GUIDELINES

This section includes a discussion of:

Ah Shi, local, adjacent and distal points
chains of points
single points
encircling an area
points on Yin and Yang channels
combining according to the Six Divisions
points on front and back
point and energy centres
points above and below
points right and left
common formulas.

AH SHI, LOCAL, ADJACENT AND DISTAL POINTS

This system is especially useful for local problems and channel problems. The principle is to use Ah Shi points, adjacent points, and local and distal points on the affected channel.

Ah Shi points

These are points in the affected area, which are painful on

pressure, and which may be on or off the channels. Needle or moxa of Ah Shi points can often help to relieve local problems.

Local points

These are points on the channels, which are in or close to the problem area. For example, LI.20 is a local point for rhinitis. As another example, LI.11 was used as the local point in a case of tennis elbow since although it was not in the problem area it was close to it, and was the nearest channel point.

Adjacent points

These are points that are not in the problem area, but are adjacent to it. For example, GB.20 for tinnitus, or ST.36 as the adjacent point for pain at ST.35, the local point.

Distal points

Distal points are points far from the problem area, e.g. LI.4 and LR.3 for headache. They are not necessarily on the same channel as the problem area, for example, PC.6 for pain in the area of ST.21. However, when distal points are on the same channel as the affected area, they may be combined with local points on the same channel. For example, LI.4 and LI.15, for shoulder stiffness around LI.15.

Sometimes it is better to use distal points than local points. For example, some migraines are made worse by the use of local points, such as GB.14 and GB.20, but greatly improved by a distal point such as GB.34.

CHAINS OF POINTS

A chain of points along a channel is often based on the combination of local, adjacent and distal points. For example, GB.1, GB.20 and GB.44 for conjunctivitis; or LI.15, LI.14 and LI.4 for shoulder sprain.

Since the basis of point combination is minimum effective number of needles, chains of points should generally be used only when one or two points on a channel have not given sufficient results. It is often advisable to start with one point on a channel, check the pulse, insert a second point if necessary, check the pulse, and insert a third point if required. For example, CV.6 can be used for depression, CV.17 added if required, and CV.22 used in addition, if the pulse does not sufficiently alter after the insertion of the other two points.

CHAINS OF POINTS ON RELATED CHANNELS

Chains of points on related channels can be used, for example, Lung and Kidney channels are related according to the Extra vessels, so that LU.1, LU.6 and LU.7 can be combined with KI.6, KI.8 and KI.13 for infertility and depression. As another example, Liver and Pericardium channels are related according to the Six Divisions, so that PC.1, PC.4 and PC.6 can be combined with LR.1, LR.3 and LR.14 for poor circulation and emotional frustrations.

SINGLE POINTS

Sometimes a single point can be very effective, for example, KI.1 unilaterally for headache with hypertension, CV.8 for diarrhoea, or GV.26 for fainting. However, single points are not generally as effective as combinations.

ENCIRCLING AN AREA

This is an effective method for local problems, for example, a varicose ulcer, a psoriasis lesion, a herpes zoster lesion, or a painful scar. Needles are inserted at a shallow angle under the skin around the area, at intervals of about 1 unit.

This technique is often combined with distal points on the nearest channels to the area. For example, for varicose ulcer in the SP.6 area, SP.1 and SP.10 can be used in addition to the encircling needles. In the case of herpes zoster lesions, the jiā jǐ points for the affected spinal nerves can also be used.

POINTS ON THE YIN AND YANG CHANNELS

Points on Yin and on Yang channels can be combined to maintain the balance of Yin and Yang in the body. For example, if the Extra channel combination of BL.62 and SI.3 is used for spinal problems, KI.6 may be added to balance an otherwise rather Yang treatment.

Also, points on the Yin and Yang paired channels can be used together to maintain the balance between a Yin–Yang pair. For example, SP.6 may be added to ST.25, ST.37 and ST.44 for constipation, to maintain a harmony between the Yang Stomach and the Yin Spleen. A special case of this, is the combination of Connecting points and Source points. When a Source point is used to strengthen a Deficient organ, the Connecting point of the paired channel can be added as a secondary point to enhance the effect. For example, St.40, the Connecting point of the Stomach can be added to SP.3, the Source point of the Spleen, for Deficient Spleen and Damp.

COMBINING ACCORDING TO THE SIX DIVISIONS

This system has the advantage of combining points on hands and feet.

Greater Yang	BL	SI
Lesser Yang	GB	TE
Bright Yang	ST	LI
Greater Yin	SP	LU
Terminal Yin	LR	PC
Lesser Yin	KI	HT

AREAS OF THE BODY

The Greater Yang channels, BL + SI, control the back of the body, the Lesser Yang channels, GB + TE, the sides, and the Bright Yang, ST + LI, the front. Points such as BL.60 and SI.3 can be combined to treat general stiffness and pain of the back of the body, head and legs. Points such as GB.34 and TE.6 can treat problems of the sides of the body, head and neck; and points like ST.40 and LI.4 can treat problems of anterior legs, abdomen, chest and face.

ORGAN RELATIONSHIPS

The Lesser Yin organs, Heart and Kidney, are also related via the Control cycle of the Five Elements. The Lesser Yin points are therefore especially useful to maintain the balance of Water and Fire, as in insomnia and anxiety. The Terminal Yin organs, Liver and Pericardium are also related via the ability of their points to move Stagnant Qi and Blood; LR.3 and PC.6 are thus often combined for chest pain, depression and poor circulation. The Greater Yin organs are also related via the Promotion cycle of the Five Elements, so that Earth is the mother of Metal. ST.36 and LU.9 are often combined for recurring respiratory infections and low energy.

INJURIES

For acute ankle sprain, for example, points can be selected on the wrist, on the same or opposite side, according to the Six Division relationships. For example, if the main ankle pain is around GB.40, then TE.4 would be chosen. If the pain were more at ST.41, then LI.5 might be used.

POINTS ON FRONT AND BACK

This is done to maintain balance between back and front, Yang and Yin. For example, GB.14 and GB.20 for head-ache, GV.16 and CV.24 for mental confusion, and dìng chuǎn and LU.1 fo asthma. A special case of this is the combination of Back Transporting points and Alarm points; for example, BL.13 and LU.1 for bronchitis, BL.14 and CV.17 for chest pain, and BL.15 and CV.14 for palpitations.

COMBINATION OR ALTERNATION

Throughout this book, combinations on the back of the body are often given as alternatives for combinations on the front. The front and back combinations can be used successively in one treatment, or used in alternate treatments. For example, for prostatitis, a front combination such as CV.3, CV.6, TE.6 and SP.6 can be alternated with a back combination, such as BL.20, BL.23, BL.32 and BL.60.

Sometimes, back and front points are combined at the same time to strengthen the treatment. For example, the basic formula for asthma:

dìng chuǎn, BL.13, CV.17, LU.7, PC.6, ST.40 Rd; KI.3 Rf

POINTS AND ENERGY CENTRES

Points can be combined according to their horizontal level on the body. Such combinations are governed by three overlapping concepts:

Western segmental theory
Chinese point function
energy centre theory.

WESTERN SEGMENTAL THEORY

According to this concept, points on the surface of a particular segment of the body may influence the skin, muscles and viscera associated with the spinal nerves controlling that segment.

For example, jiā jǐ points, GV.9, BL.17 and BL.46 can be combined for problems at the level of the seventh thoracic vertebra, or CV.18, KI.24 and ST.16 can be combined for problems at the level of the third intercostal space. However, this theory is at present concerned mainly with physical problems relating to the affected segment.

CHINESE POINT FUNCTIONS

This concept allows treatment not only of physical problems, both inside and outside of the segment in which the points are located, but also of emotional and mental disorders. For example, BL.18 and BL.47 can be combined not only for pain at the level of the ninth thoracic vertebra, but for dizziness due to Deficient Blood, blurred vision, irritability and poor planning ability, since all these are aspects of Liver imbalance and BL.18 and 48 are the Back Transporting points for the Liver.

ENERGY CENTRE THEORY

There is often a close correspondence between the functions of the Governor, Bladder and Conception points, and the functions of the energy centres. For example, both the Heart organ system and the Heart energy centre are concerned with the energies of love and compassion. Indeed, organ systems and energy centres are overlapping concepts, the difference being that the energy centres are located mainly on the central axis, and are more concerned with the flows of energy and less with the physical body, than are the organ systems.

The energy centres, as represented by the Governor and Conception points, can be used together with the Opening points of the Extra channels, as a basis for point combination.

Example

A woman of 37 had intermittent chest pains and also pain at menstruation. These problems had arisen during the course of an increasingly difficult relationship. The pulse was hindered, especially in the first and third positions on both hands.

The diagnosis was Stagnation of Qi in the Heart and Reproductive energy centres due to continual obstruction and suppression of feelings in the unsatisfactory relationship.

CV.3 and CV.17 were therefore chosen as the basis of treatment, in combination with LU.7 + KI.6.

POINTS ABOVE AND BELOW

It is necessary to maintain a balance of energy in the body between front and back, right and left, and most important, above and below. The upper body corresponds more to the Yang aspect, Heaven, and to movement and energy, and the lower body corresponds more to the Yin aspect, Earth, and to solid matter.

The pathologies of Heat, Interior Wind, Hyperactive Liver Yang and Disturbance of Heart Spirit, tend to affect the upper body more, with Excess or Irregular movement, whilst the lower body is more liable to Deficiency and Stagnation of energy, and therefore to Cold and Damp. This is obviously a generalization, but has important relationship to the polarity of pathology. This is linked to the energy centres.

Under the pressures of modern society, the energy centres of the upper body, and those of the head, Heart and Solar Plexus especially, tend to negative overactivity. For example, the Brow centre is associated with excessive negative mental overactivity, such as worry; the Heart centre with the negative emotions of sadness and passion; and the Solar Plexus centre with excessive fear and anger. In contrast to this, the lower centres, especially those of the Spleen and Dan Tian can become Deficient or obstructed. This results in an overemphasis of energy and attention in the head and chest and an underemphasis of energy and attention in the lower body and the physical body in general.

This is an oversimplified picture, but it is important to point combination according to polarity of energy. For the average person in modern society, acupuncture, Qi Gong or meditation therapies, can often focus initially on the Dan Tian centre and the centres on the soles of the feet, at KI.1. This can have the effects of:

- strengthening the lower body and the physical body in general

- increasing awareness of the physical body and so taking excessive attention away from the head

- sinking excessive irregular energies in the head, such as Heat, Yang and Wind.

For example, in headaches due to mental and emotional pressure, the use of local points such as GB.14, GB.20 and tài yáng sometimes aggravates the condition. Often in such cases KI.1 alone will remove the headache, by sinking the disturbed energies and redistributing the energy in the body. This can often be enhanced by finger pressure by the practitioner on SP.4, with palms on the dorsum of the patient's feet, whilst the patient puts their attention on SP.4, and visualizes the energy of the breath flowing down to this point.

There are exceptions to this, so that disturbed energy in the head is sometimes better treated with head points such as BL.7 and GB.13, and with the practitioner gently holding the head with light massage, to disperse accumulated energy.

For acute Excess in the head and upper body, points can either be on the lower body only, e.g. KI.1, or points at the two extremities can be combined, e.g. GV.20 + KI.1 or GV.20 + LR.3. If points at both extremities are used, then the lower points are inserted first, and removed last at the end of the treatment. This is to focus the attention of the patient in the lower body. The polarity of the treatment may be emphasized by using more needle manipulation or Qi Gong energy work at the lower body than the upper.

SINKING OF QI

Deficiency of Qi and Yang with Sinking of Qi, can have the effect of Deficient energy in the head, which can then lead to Irregularity of movement. In this situation moxa, or needle and moxa, on GV.20, can be combined with moxa and needle on points on the lower body which tonify Deficiency, e.g. CV.4, KI.3 or ST.36. In this case, the head points are inserted first and removed last, to bring energy up to the head. Qi Gong or meditation techniques that sink the attention down the body, towards the feet, are contraindicated.

This account is highly simplified; in practice, treatment would aim at correcting each imbalanced energy centre, and putting the centres in harmony with each other. For example, if there were headache associated with stress and overwork due to the fear of losing control, during the acute headache, KI.1 might be combined with GV.20 with Reducing method. Between headaches, the Dan Tian centre might be strengthened, to give the faith in self that overcomes fear, using CV.4, KI.7 and ST.36 with Reinforcing method and moxa, and CV.14 with Even method to calm the Solar Plexus centre and reduce the effects of fear.

POINTS RIGHT AND LEFT

Using points on the right and left helps to balance Yin and Yang, and can strengthen the effect of the treatment, even if the problem is only on one side. For example, LI.4 can be used bilaterally for unilateral face pain. However, because the right and left sides of the principal channels interconnect, points can be used unilaterally to affect both sides of the body.

Points can be used unilaterally in a variety of situations:

Extra channel treatments
treatment of children
treatment of the affected side only
balancing treatment on the affected side
difficulty in treating the affected side only
after prolonged treatment of the affected side.

EXTRA CHANNEL TREATMENTS

This is discussed in detail in Chapter 10. A popular method for using the Opening points of the Extra channel pairs, is first to needle the Opening point of the primary channel on the dominant side, and then to needle the Opening point of the secondary channel on the opposite side. Traditionally, the dominant side is the left in men and the right in women.

For example, to use the BV + Yang LV pair in a woman to treat premenstrual syndrome, GB.41 is first inserted on the right, and TE.5 is then inserted on the left. The needles are withdrawn in the opposite sequence. If this treatment is seen to be too Yang for a particular woman, or if Hyperactive Yang is based on Deficient Blood, after TE.5 has been inserted SP.6 could be inserted also on the left. If there were also insomnia, then in addition, HT.6 might then be inserted on the right. The needles would be withdrawn in the opposite sequence.

TREATMENT OF CHILDREN

Babies usually only need two needles, and children between 2 and 5 years old, usually only two to six needles. In babies especially, it is usually only necessary to treat unilaterally for systemic problems. If preferred, one needle can be on the right and one on the left. For example, for chronic respiratory catarrh, LU.6 on the right can be combined with ST.40 on the left, or vice versa.

TREATMENT OF THE AFFECTED SIDE ONLY

This is the usual method for treating problems which are on the channel rather than the organ system. For example, for right shoulder sprain, LI.4, LI.10 and LI.15 may be used on the right only. However, especially if there is an underlying organ system problem, the Connecting point of the paired Yin organ may be used on the opposite side to balance the treatment, in this case LU.7.

BALANCING TREATMENT ON THE AFFECTED SIDE

Another example would be needling BL.23 on the right, to balance the use of local back points and distal leg points on the left side, for a left-sided problem. Usually, only one or two points are used on the opposite side to balance the use of three or more points on the affected side.

DIFFICULTY IN TREATING THE AFFECTED SIDE ONLY

In hemiplegia, if the affected side is markedly spastic or atrophied, unilateral treatment may be made on the healthy side, perhaps in alternation with treatments on the affected side.

In varicose ulceration, the ulcer often covers SP.6, which can then be used on the more healthy side, and where it is not possible to use a point because of underlying swollen veins, that point can be used on the opposite side.

In acute ankle sprain, points can be used on the opposite wrist, according to the channel relationship of the Six Divisions. For example, for a right ankle sprain with pain centred around GB.40, TE.4 can be used on the left wrist.

AFTER PROLONGED TREATMENT OF THE AFFECTED SIDE

For example, for facial paralysis, facial tic or trigeminal neuralgia, where there has been prolonged treatment, with decreasing success, it may be effective to treat temporarily on the healthy side. Alternatively, the majority of points can be used on the healthy side with only one or two points on the affected side. For example, for trigeminal neuralgia on the right side, ST.3 could be used on the right, and ST.4 and SI.18 on the left; distal points, such as LI.4 and LU.7 could be used bilaterally.

COMMON FORMULAS

There are many well-known traditional combinations or formulas which can be used symptomatically or incorporated into a fuller treatment. For example, the famous pairs of points:

LI.4	+ KI.7	for excess or deficient sweating
HT.6	+ KI.6	for nightsweats
LI.4	+ ST.36	for Deficient Qi and Blood
ST.36	+ SP.6	for tiredness and debility
LI.4	+ SP.6	for uterine pain or difficult labour
LI.4	+ LI.11	for fevers
LI.4	+ LR.3	for nervous tension.

Classical texts, such as the *Ode to the One Hundred Symptoms* (included in *The Golden Needle*, translated by R. Bertschinger, Churchill Livingstone, UK, 1991), list many other pairs of points, less well used than those just listed. For example, ST.25 + KI.5 for menorrhagia, or CV.10 + ST.43 for borborygmus. An example of incorporation of a famous formula into an energetic treatment is LI.4 + LR.3 added to GV.20 + KI.1 for acute Excess headache due to extreme nervous tension. Another example is HT.6 + KI.6 added to SP.4 + PC.6 for insomnia and nightsweats linked to Deficient Heart Blood and Yin.

TYPES OF POINTS

Combination according to point type, is dealt with in detail in Chapter 8. A brief summary is given here.
The main point types are:

Source points

Connecting points
Accumulation points
Alarm points
Back Transporting points
Window of Heaven points
Lower Sea points
Gathering points
Crossing points
Five Transporting points
Five Element points
Opening points.

Source points

These are mainly used to tonify Deficiency and thus to stabilize the balance of Yin–Yang and the emotions. For example, HT.7 + KI.3 is a Source point combination to stabilize the balance between Five and Water, between overenthusiasm and fear.

Connecting points

These are often used to involve both channels or organs of a Yin-Yang pair. For example, SP.4 the Connecting point of the Spleen can treat problems of both Stomach and Spleen. SP.4 combines with ST.40 the Connecting point of the Stomach to enhance this effect.

Accumulation points

These are mainly used for acute severe painful Excess conditions. For example, LU.6 can treat acute bronchitis with chest pain. Accumulation points can combine with Alarm points, for example, LU.6 can combine with LU.1, the Alarm point of the Lungs, for acute asthma.

Alarm points

These can be used for chronic Deficiency, but are more often used for Excess. For example, the Alarm points of Pericardium and Heart, CV.17 and CV.14, can be combined for chest pain and palpitations, with Reducing method.

Back Transporting points

These points are mainly used for chronic Deficiency conditions, or to balance emotional and mental aspects. For example, BL.20, the Back Transporting point for the Spleen, can be used for debility, emotional insecurity, or for mental congestion. It can be combined with GV.6 or BL.49 at the same level, to enhance these effects.

Window of Heaven points

These points on the upper body are mainly used to disperse Stagnant Qi to treat either depressions and phobias, or local neck problems. For example, BL.10, the Window of Heaven point for the Bladder channel, can treat fearful depression, and can be combined with SI.3 + BL.62 for this.

Lower Sea points

These are used mainly to treat physical problems of their respective organ system. For example, ST.37, the Lower Sea point for the Stomach, can treat diarrhoea, or constipation, and can be combined with ST.25, the Stomach Alarm point.

Gathering points

These are used mainly for Deficiency and Stagnation in their respective systems. For example, BL.11, the Gathering point for the Bones, can be used for joint problems, together with BL.23 and KI.3, the Back Transporting point and Source point of the Kidneys.

Crossing points

These are points where two or more channels meet, and are useful in linking treatment of more than one channel. For example, CV.3 is the Crossing point of Conception and Liver channels, so that it can be used for Damp Heat in the Lower Energizer (for example, vaginitis), especially if combined with LR.5, the Connecting point of the Liver.

Five Transporting points

The most important of these are the Well and Spring points, which are often combined together, either to disperse Heat, or to tonify Fire and Yang. For example, KI.1 and KI.2, the Well and Spring points of the Kidney, can be reduced to drain Kidney Fire as in hypertension; or LR.1 and LR.2, the Well and Spring points of the Liver, can be used with Reinforcing method and moxa to increase Liver Fire, to treat lack of self-confidence and assertion.

Five Element points

These are most effective when used to treat problems of emotional blockage or imbalance. For example, HT.8, the Fire point of the Fire element can be used with Reinforcing method and moxa to control grief and withdrawal associated with the Lungs, the Metal element. HT.8 can be combined with LU.10, the Fire point of the Lungs, to balance grief via the Control cycle.

Opening points

These points control the Extra channel pairs, and are best used when groups of organs are affected. For example, the Opening points of the TV + Yin Link pair, SP.4 + PC.6, can be used to treat problems of the organ group Kidney, Heart and Spleen. Points on the Conception channel can be added; for example, CV.4 for cold hands and feet.

ENERGETIC FUNCTIONS OF THE POINTS

Some points have energetic functions in addition to those of their point type. For example, LI.4 can be used as the Source point to tonify the Bright Yang channels, but in addition has many other uses, for each of which it can be combined with other points. For example:

moves Qi and Blood	+ SP.6
drains Heat in the Blood	+ LI.11
calms Hyperactive Yang	+ LR.3
expels Exterior Wind	+ LU.7
clears the nose	+ LI.20.

These energetic functions are described in great detail in Part II.

HARMONY

An harmonious treatment is based on a thorough understanding of the patient's imbalances and needs, and uses the simplest treatment strategy and the minimum number of needles that are necessary to be effective. The points in an harmonious combination enhance each other's effects, blending well together, without mutual interference.

For example, for cold feet due to Stagnation and Deficiency of Qi, CV.4, PC.6 and SP.4 can be a simple, harmonious and effective combination. The treatment strategy is simple, using the Extra channel pair of TV + Yin LV, which combines harmoniously with CV.4, representing the Dan Tian energy centre. The number of needles is minimal, since for unilateral treatment the total is three.

An example requiring a greater number of points, is multiple sclerosis with visual and urinary problems. The treatment can be based on SI.3, BL.10, BL.23, BL.32, BL.62. Here, the treatment strategy uses the Extra channel pair GV + Yang HV with the points SI.3 and BL.62, and BI.23 is added to tonify the Kidneys, with BL.10 for the eyes and the neck vertebrae and BI.32 for the urinary problems and the lower back.

An inharmonious treatment is one where the practitioner tries to do too much, has a treatment strategy that is too complex, or where he is not sure of the role of each point. For example, in the author's opinion, combining Five Elements with Extra channel strategies can easily lead to an overly complex treatment, where points are being used according to two or more conflicting principles.

Good acupuncture is like Qi Gong, the simpler the image or visualization in the practitioner's mind, the clearer it is and the easier for energy to flow through it. Also, the simpler the idea, the more flexible it is when it has to adapt and change to match the reality of the patient's body.

The combination of Qi Gong and acupuncture is not just directing energy between needles, it is developing a clear analogy of the patient's needs and allowing energy to flow through this mental image. The analogy can be in the language of the Five Elements, the Extra channels or the Stems and Branches, as required. What is important is that it is relevant to the patient's needs, and though it may be detailed, is in essence clear and simple.

EMPIRICISM

As discussed in Chapter 1, good acupuncture is a blend of analysis, intuition and empiricism. Each plays its part. Analysis may organize the details of the case history in the mind of the practitioner, and intuition can create an overall picture from these details and put it in the perspective of the patient's life. Point choice can be based on both analysis and intuition, but it is only when the combination is actually tried out and found to be successful, that we can say the analysis and intuition were accurate. Therefore, during treatment, after insertion of each needle group, it can be helpful to check the pulse to see if it has become more harmonious, and to ask the patient not only if the symptoms are reducing, but also if they feel better or worse in themselves. If a combination is used and after 5 or 10 minutes the patient says they feel worse, disturbed, uncomfortable or very strange, then one or more needles should be removed, the patient allowed to rest for 5 minutes, and if appropriate, different needles inserted.

Example 1

A patient with headache was diagnosed as Hyperactive Liver Yang, and the combination GB.14 and GB.34 used as a basis, but the patient felt no better after 10 minutes. The choice then was either to keep the strategy, and add further points, such as GB.1 and GB.20, or to change the strategy. The patient was asked how she felt and said that she felt hot and restless but exhausted. The strategy was therefore modified to include Deficiency Fire, and KI.6 was reinforced and KI.2 reduced. The pulse improved, the headache declined and the patient felt more comfortable in herself.

Example 2

A man was treated for severe right-sided migraine at GB.14 and tài yáng. The points used were GB.14, tài yáng and GB.34 on the right, with SP.6 on the left to balance the treatment. After 10 minutes there was no improvement, and the man was asked in detail how he felt. He said he had been under enormous business stress which was making him desperate and his head felt like it was bursting. The treatment strategy was changed and sì shén cōng and KI.1 were added with Reducing method to release the pressure in the head and to sink the excess energy, respectively. The pulse became less full and wiry, the headache decreased, and the man experienced a pleasant sensation of lightness and floating.

Example 3

A patient with panic attacks was diagnosed as Kidney fear invading Heart, and the combination of CV.14, SP.4 and PC.6 was used. However, the patient felt more disturbed and restless after the insertion of CV.14 and asked for it to be removed. This was done and after a few minutes, ST.36 was inserted and moxa cones were used on it, and finally moxa stick was used on KI.1. The pulse became less erratic and the patient felt calmer.

MODIFICATIONS OF COMBINATIONS DURING A SERIES OF TREATMENTS

It is possible to use the same combination for many treatments, providing the patient continues to improve, and their general life pattern remains the same. However, there are various situations in which a combination may need to be modified or even completely changed:

patient does not improve
patient has only limited improvement
some symptoms improve but not others
patient develops new illnesses or problems.

PATIENT DOES NOT IMPROVE

As stated in the previous section on empiricism, if a patient feels worse during a treatment, the combination can be changed or modified during that session.

CHANNEL PROBLEMS

If a patient attending for a purely local channel problem, such as tennis elbow, genuinely feels no better by the time they come for the second treatment, then the diagnosis should be reassessed.

Perhaps the wrong channel has been selected; for example, on closer investigation it proves that the problem area is nearer to the Triple Energizer than to the Large Intestine channel. Local and distal points on the Triple Energizer channel can then be substituted for Large Intestine points. Perhaps the Ah Shi points were not quite in the right place or at the right depth. Perhaps the wrong method of treatment was used, for example, electroacupuncture when moxa would have been more effective. Perhaps, it is not purely a local problem, but is linked to an underlying systemic problem, such as rheumatoid arthritis, which requires systemic as well as local treatment.

However, if the diagnosis is correct, then additional Ah Shi, local or distal points can be used, or the distal points can be changed. For example, for the tennis elbow, where LI.4 was used on the affected side as a local point, LI.4 can additionally be used on the healthy side, or LI.4 on the affected side can be changed to LI.7, the Accumulation point.

ORGAN PROBLEMS

If a person with an organ system problem, such as depression and tiredness from Stagnant Liver Qi, genuinely feels no better by the second treatment, and their pulses are unchanged, the combination may need to be modified or changed completely, after the diagnosis has been reassessed. However, if the patient feels no better, but the pulses have improved, the combination may be repeated or slightly modified, and the patient may then improve due to the slow but cumulative effects of treatment.

For example, if the combination CV.6 E M; LR.3, PC.6 Rd had been used for the depression and tiredness, and the pulse had become less wiry and less empty by the second treatment, although the patient felt no better, then LR.1 Rd; ST.36 Rf M could be added. The Well point, LR.1, would help to move Stagnant Liver Qi and ST.36 would help to tonify Qi and help tiredness.

PATIENT HAS ONLY LIMITED IMPROVEMENT

Very frequently, a combination may give continuous improvement up to a certain point, and then no further improvement is gained, or the condition may start to deteriorate. The first step is to check the pulses, reassess the diagnosis, and determine if any new factor is interfering with the treatment, such as a change of medication, diet or lifestyle. If there are none of these, then the combination can either be considerably modified or changed completely.

For example, CV.17, HT.7, PC.6, SP.4 E had been successful for four treatments in a case of palpitation. The condition then started to deteriorate for no apparent

reason. The combination was modified by the addition of CV.14 E; ST.36 Rf, with CV.14 E being added to calm the Spirit and ST.36 Rf added to strengthen Heart Qi and Blood. There was no improvement by the next treatment, so the treatment strategy was changed from one based on the SP.4 + PC.6 Extra channel pair, to GV.20, HT.7, KI.1 E; KI.3 Rf, which is based on the Source points HT.7 and KI.3, and on points at the opposite end of the body, GV.20 and KI.1. Improvement followed.

SOME SYMPTOMS IMPROVE BUT NOT OTHERS

This is a very common situation. Strategy depends on whether the different symptoms have a common cause, or have different causes.

COMMON CAUSE

An example of different symptoms with a common cause could be Hyperactive Liver Yang with symptoms of unilateral headache, dizziness and photophobia for which the combination could be GV.20, GB.20, GB.34, SP.6 E. If the headache and dizziness improved, but not the photophobia, it would be necessary to check that there was not an additional cause for the photophobia, such as Deficient Kidney Qi, or Yin, or alternatively, chronic eyestrain from excessive reading or use of a computer terminal. If the Hyperactive Yang were the only cause, then local points (e.g. GB.1), adjacent points (e.g. BL.10), or distal points (e.g. GB.37) could be added for the eyes.

DIFFERENT CAUSES

An example of a patient with symptoms with different causes, could be dysmenorrhoea due to Stagnant Blood, gastritis due to Deficient Stomach Qi, and cold extremities due to Deficient Heart Qi and Blood. Although the three symptoms have different causes, one combination could be used to treat all three, and could be modified according to which problem was dominant.

CV.6, CV.12 E M; PC.6, SP.4 E; ST.36 M

CV.6 and SP.4 can move Stagnant Blood in the Lower Energizer, and LI.4 and ST.29, with Reducing method could be added for dysmenorrhoea. The whole combination can strengthen Stomach Qi, and CV.12, PC.6, SP.4 and ST.36 are specific for gastritis. ST.21 could be used as an additional point for gastritis. CV.6, PC.6 and SP.4 can improve circulation, and ST.36 can strengthen Heart Qi and Blood. PC.8 and SP.2 can be added with needle and moxa, if the poor circulation is dominant.

PATIENT DEVELOPS NEW ILLNESSES OR PROBLEMS

This can be due to climatic factors, lifestyle changes, or to new developments in the unfolding of the patient's personality.

CLIMATIC FACTORS

For example, a patient was being treated with slow but definite progress, for tiredness due to Deficient Kidney Yang, with the combination CV.4, CV.6, HT.8, KI.2, KI.7 Rf M.

The patient went walking in the mountains in the cold wind and suffered acute lower back ache and stiffness, with feeling of cold in the lower back, but some feverishness and sneezing. The point combination was changed to LU.7, LI.4 Rd; GV.2, GV.3, BL.25, BL.26, BL.62 E M. The LU.7, LI.4 Rd was to disperse Wind Cold in the upper body, and the other points were to disperse Wind Cold and Stagnation in the lower back, whilst at the same time warming and strengthening Yang by using moxa.

After the patient had recovered from the acute problems, the original combination was used but in alternation with GV.3, GV.4, BL.23, BL.26, BL.60 Rf M, to strengthen the back in addition to strengthening Yang.

LIFESTYLE CHANGES

A patient was being treated for stiffness in the neck and upper back, due to Hyperactive Liver Yang and Stagnation of Liver Qi, with the combination GV.12, GV.15, PC.6, GB.20, GB.21, GB.34, LR.3 E. Then the problem began to deteriorate as the patient was given extra work-load and responsibility in her job, due to the illness of her superior.

Although the symptoms were discomfort in the upper back, the origin was stress and exhaustion, and so the following combination was temporarily adopted:

GV.20, yìn táng, LI.4, GB.21, LR.3 E; CV.6,
ST.36 Rf M; KI.1 M

The GV.20, yìn táng, LR.4 and LR.3 were to reduce stress, GB.21 for the neck and upper back, CV.6 and ST.36 for exhaustion, and KI.1 with moxa only was both to reduce tension and to strengthen the Kidneys.

Although the shoulders then improved, sleep became a problem, so that LI.4 and KI.1 were removed from the combination, and SP.1, SP.2 and HT.6 were added with Even method.

INTERNAL CHANGES

Individuals may go on for years in a certain pattern until they slowly become dissatisfied, or else a sequence of events can catalyse a relatively sudden desire for change.

For example, a woman was being treated for nervous anxiety and generalized headaches, with GV.20, PC.6, SP.4, KI.1 E as the basic combination, with variations according to her changing situations. During the course of treatment she became increasingly aware of a need either to change her work or to reorient herself within the existing job. The more she felt the need to change, the greater her lack of confidence, and the greater her uncertainty as to the direction of change.

The treatment strategy was then changed in order to increase her clarity and self-confidence, and the new combination was GV.20, HT.7, TE.4, KI.3, GB.13, GB.40, GB.44 Rf. The Source points of the Lesser Yin, HT.7 and KI.3, and of the Lesser Yang, TE.4 and GB.40, were selected to decrease fear and anxiety and give confidence. GV.20, GB.13 and GB.40, can treat the headache, in addition to calming and clearing the mind. GB.44, the Well point, can be added to assist the other Gallbladder points in treating indecision.

The woman became more clear and more confident and decided to change her role within her existing job. However, she drove herself too hard in her desire for rapid change, and became tense and depressed. GB.44 was removed from the combination, and KI.1 was added with Even method to relax the pressure of her ambition and to calm the tension.

CONTINUITY OF STRATEGY

It is vitally important for practitioners to resist the temptation to keep changing between one strategy and another just to try to get results. It is necessary to formulate a definite treatment strategy on the basis of an accurate differentiation of syndromes and a clear understanding of the patient, and to keep to the strategy as far as possible. This steady focusing of the energies of both practitioner and patient through a consistent framework can produce cumulative results.

It is also necessary, whenever possible, to choose a treatment strategy which has a basic core that can continue through many treatments, but which is flexible and easily modified according to changing conditions. For example, people with the Lesser Yin constitution, i.e. that of Gallbladder–Triple Energizer, can have a variety of symptoms that change from time to time. These can include eczema of the ear, conjunctivitis, migraines, gastritis, cholecystitis, sciatica, vaginitis, irritability, lack of confidence and hasty unwise decisions, in any combination. The common core of the strategy is to harmonize the Lesser Yin and regulate the Belt and Yang Link channels. This can be done with the basic combination TE.5, GB.41, SP.6 E. This flexible combination can then be modified in many ways according to the additional symptoms, for example:

+ TE.17, GB.2 E   for eczema of the ear
+ PC.6, CV.12 E   for gastritis
+ GB.24, GB.34 E   for cholecystitis
+ CV.3, GB.26 E   for leucorrhoea
+ GV.20, LR.2 E   for depression and irritability.

Types of points 8

SOURCE POINTS

Table 8.1 Source points

Yin channels	Yang channels
LU.9	LI.4
PC.7	TE.4
HT.7	SI.4
SP.3	ST.42
LR.3	GB.40
KI.3	BL.64

SOURCE POINT THEORY

The Yuan Qi, or Original or Source Qi, is said to be stored in the Dan Tian and to be linked with the Kidneys. It circulates in the channels and catalyses and activates all the functions of the body.

FUNCTIONS OF THE YIN SOURCE POINTS

The source points of the Yin channels are among the most effective and widely used points in acupuncture, since they have the following important functions: to tonify deficiency; to balance Yin and Yang; to disperse excess or tonify deficiency; to stabilize emotions.

Tonify Deficiency

By tonifying the Source Qi for a particular organ, its Source point can tonify Deficiency. For example, LU.9 can be used for Deficient Lung Qi.

Balance Yin and Yang

The source points of the Yin organs are relatively neutral and can be used to tonify either Deficient Yin or Deficient Yang, or to restore the Yin–Yang balance of an organ. For example, KI.3 can tonify Deficient Kidney Yin or Deficient Kidney Yang, and can be used when there are oscillations in the Yin–Yang balance, as in some menopausal syndromes.

Disperse Excess or tonify Deficiency

Although Source points are mainly used to tonify, they have a balancing or homoeostatic effect, so that they can be reduced for Excess or reinforced for Deficiency. For example, HT.7 can be reinforced to treat Deficient Heart Qi, or reduced to treat Heart Fire or to calm Disturbed Heart Spirit.

Stabilize emotions

The fact that the Yin Source points are also the Earth points, gives them a stabilizing effect on the body, emotions and mind, especially if an organ is unstable because of Deficiency. For example, if a person is feeling hypersensitive and vulnerable due to Deficient Liver Blood, LR.3 can be reinforced to stabilize the personality by tonifying Liver Blood and calming the Hyperactive Liver Yang associated with it.

FUNCTIONS OF THE YANG SOURCE POINTS

The Yang Source points are mainly used to disperse Excess. For example, LI.4 can disperse Wind Heat or Wind Cold for influenza; TE.4 can disperse Wind Heat as in conjunctivitis; SI.4 can move Stagnant Liver Qi for pain in the hypochondrium; ST.42 can disperse Stomach Fire for epigastric pain; GB.40 can disperse Gallbladder Damp Heat as in cholecystitis; and BL.64 can move Stagnant Qi in the Bladder channel as in back pain.

LI.4, GB.40 and BL.64 can be used for tonification. For example, LI.4 can be used to tonify Qi and Blood, but this is usually when LI.4 is combined with ST.36. Also, GB.40 can treat indecision and lack of self-confidence by tonifying Gallbladder Qi; and BL.64 can help to treat fear and depression by tonifying Qi of Kidney and Bladder. However, generally other points, such as ST.36 and GB.34 which are both Earth points and Lower Sea points, are more effective for tonifying the Yang organs.

USING THE SOURCE POINTS

Source points can be used by themselves, or in combination with other point types, as outlined next.

SOURCE POINTS ONLY

Using only the Source points is a good safe method of

acupuncture since they are neutral, self-regulating and stabilizing. However, it is rare to use the Source points of one organ only, and more usual to combine the Source points of two or more organs. This can be according to Yin–Yang pairs, such as KI.3 + BL.64 for urinary problems, HT.7 + SI.4 for insomnia and melancholia, or LU.9 + LI.4 for chronic bronchitis. Or, combination may be according to organ relationships on the Five Elements Control cycle; for example, KI.3 + HT.7 for insomnia, or SP.3 + LR.3 for indigestion due to Liver invading Spleen.

It is often an advantage if one pair of Source points is on the hands and one on the feet, to balance the effects on the upper and lower body; for example, KI.3 and LU.3 for chronic bronchitis due to Deficient Qi of Kidneys and Lungs.

SOURCE POINTS + CV POINTS

Combining Source points with CV points can enhance their effect, since the Conception channel is linked to the Dan Tian, the Kidneys and to Source Qi. Source points can be combined with the CV point that represents the same organ, for example:

KI.3 + CV.4   for exhaustion and impotence
SP.3 + CV.12   for chronic gastritis
HT.7 + CV.17   for palpitations
HT.7 + CV.17   for bronchitis.

SOURCE POINTS + BACK TRANSPORTING POINTS

This is also a good combination since both these types of points are neutral, with the ability to tonify Yin or Yang, to disperse Excess or to tonify Deficiency, or to balance emotions. Although the Back Transporting points can move Stagnation or disperse an external factor, like the Yin Source points their most important function is tonifying chronic Deficiency.

BL.64 + BL.28 for cystits
KI.3 + BL.23 for weak will
GB.40 + BL.48 for uncertainty and indecision.

The points for the Yin and Yang paired organs can be combined for enhanced effect, e.g. BL.64 + BL.28 with KI.3 + BL.23 for urinary incontinence due to Deficiency. The combination of Source points + CV points can be alternated with the combination of Source points + Back Transporting points. For example, for chronic bronchitis due to Deficient Kidney and Lung Qi, alternate:

KI.3, LU.9, BL.23, BL.13 with KI.3, LU.9, CV.4, CV.17.

SOURCE POINTS + TONIFICATION OR SEDATION ON OTHER POINTS

Source points can be used to stabilize another treatment, especially if this treatment tends to be extreme. For example, to reinforce and moxa HT.8, the Fire point, for depression may swing the Yin–Yang balance too far over into mania and hyperactivity. To simultaneously reinforce HT.7, the Source point, may stabilize the treatment and prevent this.

As another example, to reduce KI.2, the Fire point, to disperse Kidney Fire, may drain too much Fire so that the patient becomes cold and hypoactive. Simultaneously reinforcing KI.3, the Source point, may prevent this by stabilizing the Yin–Yang balance.

SOURCE POINTS TO STABILIZE EMOTIONS

Source points can be used alone or in combination with other points to treat emotional lability due to Deficiency. For example:

KI.3 + BL.52 for fear and paranoia
PC.7 + CV.17 for manic depression
LR.3 + GB.40 for hypersensitivity and irritability.

It should be emphasized that Source points are mainly for Deficiency. For Stagnation of Qi, for example, the Yin Source points are not generally appropriate. For example, for blocked grief, LU.7, the Connecting point, is superior to LU.9, the Source point. The exception to this is LR.3 which is more effective at moving Stagnation than at tonifying Deficiency.

SOURCE POINTS + CONNECTING POINTS

This is discussed in the next section.

CONNECTING POINTS

Table 8.2 Connecting points

Yin channels	Yang channels
LU.7	LI.6
PC.6	TE.5
HT.5	SI.7
SP.4	ST.40
LR.5	GB.37
KI.4	BL.58

The Connecting points for the Yin and Yang channels are listed in Table 8.2. In addition, GV.1 is the Connecting point of the Governor channel, CV.15 of the Conception channel and SP.21 of the Great Spleen Connecting channel.

CONNECTING POINT THEORY

Each of the 12 main channels has a Connecting channel which starts from the Connecting point on the main channel and splits into two branches. These are the Transverse Connecting channel, which connects with the Yin–Yang paired channel, and the Longitudinal Connecting channel which has its own pathway. Although some Longitudinal channels connect internally with the organs, they are generally relatively superficial branching pathways, linking the main channel with the body tissues.

USING THE CONNECTING POINTS

The Connecting points, sometimes called Luo or Junction points, can be used to treat Excess or Deficiency conditions of the Longitudinal Connecting channels. However, since the author does not use this technique it is not discussed here.

CONNECTING POINTS ONLY

Connecting points can be used to treat both channels in a Yin–Yang pair. For example, ST.40 can be used to treat conditions involving disharmonies of both Spleen and Stomach, e.g. gastritis and abdominal distension. SP.4 can be used in the same way, e.g. for Deficient Blood due to Deficient Spleen with indigestion due to Rebellious Stomach Qi.

In certain circumstances, ST.40 and SP.4 can be combined together for enhanced effect, e.g. for epigastric and abdominal pain and distension. As another example, LR.5 can move Stagnant Liver Qi and disperse Damp Heat in the Liver and Gallbladder but predominantly in Liver, whilst GB.37 has a similar function, but predominantly for Gallbladder. Again the two points can be combined for enhanced effects.

In addition, pairs like ST.40 and SP.4, and GB.37 and LR.5, can improve the balance between the two organs of the Yin–Yang pair. For example, ST.40 + SP.4 can be used for Deficient Spleen with Excess Stomach.

CONNECTING POINTS USED UNILATERALLY

In certain cases, Yin Connecting points can be used to balance the use of many points on the Yang paired channel. For example, for a patient with right-sided headache and eye inflammation, where GB.1,14,20 and 34 have been used on the right side, LR.5 can be used on the left side as a Yin point, to balance this otherwise rather Yang treatment, and to balance the right and left sides of the body. LU.7 could similarly be added on the right side to balance the use of Large Intestine points on the left side for left-sided headache, neck and shoulder pain.

FREQUENTLY USED CONNECTING POINTS

It is a matter of opinion, which Connecting points are more important, but LU.7, PC.6, SP.4 and TE.5 are especially popular because they are not only Connecting points, but also the Opening points of Extra channels (see Chapter 10). ST.40 is popular because of its symptomatic use to clear Damp and Phlegm, and LR.5 because it clears Damp Heat, especially for genital problems. HT.5, although not so frequently used as the abovementioned points, is important because it links Heart and Small Intestine to treat Heart Fire in the lower body, and because it is specific for speech problems. KI.4, LI.6, SI.7, GB.37 and BL.58 are not so frequently used as Connecting points.

CONNECTING POINTS OF GOVERNOR, CONCEPTION AND GREAT SPLEEN CHANNELS

GV.1 regulates the back and head; CV.15 regulates the abdomen, especially the skin; and SP.21 regulates the chest and ribs. These points are often combined according to the principle of polarity, with points at the other end of the channel. For example:

GV 1 + GV.20 for haemorrhoids
CV.15 + CV.3 for abdominal rash
SP.21 + SP.4 for chest pain.

CONNECTING POINTS + SOURCE POINTS

When a Source point is used to tonify an organ, the Connecting point of the paired channel can be added as a secondary point, to enhance the effect. For example, for chronic bronchitis, LU.9 the Source point of the Lungs, and LI.6, the Connecting point of Large Intestine can be combined with Reinforcing method.

However, a much more common combination is LI.4, the Source point of Large Intestine, with LU.7, the Connecting point of Lungs, both with Reducing method, for Excess conditions of Wind Cold or Wind Heat, such as influenza or allergic rhinitis.

ACCUMULATION POINTS

Table 8.3 Accumulation points

Yin channels	Yang channels
LU.6	LI.7
PC.4	TE.7
HT.6	SI.6
SP.8	ST.35
LR.6	GB.36
KI.5	BL.63
Yin HV KI.8	BL.59 Yang HV
Yin LV KI.9	GB.35 Yang LV

ACCUMULATION POINT THEORY

The Accumulation points, sometimes known as Xi–Cleft points, are points where the Qi channel accumulates, and so are used with Reducing method in acute Excess painful conditions. They are usually used in combination with other points for example:

LU.6 + LU.1, CV.17, ST.40   for acute painful cough
PC.4 + HT.6, CV.17, BL.17   for angina pectoris
SP.8 + CV.3, LI.4   for dysmenorrhoea
KI.8 + KI.13, CV.3, LU.7   for dysmenorrhoea.

In the opinion of the author, LU.6, PC.4, SP.8 and HT.6 are the most effective of these points. LU.6 in particular, can have a more immediate effect on asthma than any other point. The use of strong Reducing method is essential.

ALARM POINTS

Table 8.4 Alarm points

Yin organs		Yang organs	
LU	LU.I	LI	ST.25
PC	CV.17	TE	CV.5
HT	CV.14	SI	CV.4
SP	LR.13	ST	CV.12
LR	LR.14	GB	GB.24
KI	GB.25	BL	CV.3

ALARM POINT THEORY

The Alarm points, sometimes called Mu or Front Collecting Points, are all on the front or sides of the chest or abdomen. They are points where the energy of the organ gathers, and hence can be used for diagnosis or treatment.

DIAGNOSIS

These points may be tender either spontaneously or on palpitation when the organ is disordered. However, in the experience of the author, this form of diagnosis is not always reliable. When CV.14 is spontaneously tender it is just as likely to signify problems of the Stomach as problems of the Heart. Similarly, pain or lack of sensation around CV.4 is just as likely to relate to problems of the uterus or Deficiency of Kidney Qi as it is to problems of Small Intestine.

TREATMENT

While both Back Transporting and Alarm points can treat both Excess and Deficiency conditions, the Back Transporting points are relatively more for chronic Deficiency, and the Alarm points relatively more for acute Excess. However, Back Transporting and Alarm points can be combined together in one treatment, or alternated. For severe acute conditions such as asthma or bronchitis, the two types of points are often best combined; for example, with the patient sitting, BL.13, CV.17, LU.1 and LU.6 can be inserted at the same time.

If the patient is not seen frequently, the points can either be combined, or the alternation can be in the same treatment session. For example, for prostatitis, CV.3, GB.25, BL.64 can be used, the needles are removed, the patient's position changed and then BL.23, BL.28 and BL.32 can be used in the same treatment session. If the patient is being treated more frequently, at least once per week, then it is better to use the alternate treatments in different sessions.

Using the Alarm points as local points, distal points on the same channel can be combined, in certain cases. For example, LR.1 can be combined with LR.14 for hypochondriac pain, LU.7 can be combined with LU.1 for asthma, or ST.37 can be combined with ST.25 for diarrhoea with abdominal pain.

BACK TRANSPORTING POINTS

Table 8.5 Back Transporting points

Associated Yin organs		Associated Yang organs	
LU	BL.13	LI	BL.25
PC	BL.14	TE	BL.22
HT	BL.15	SI	BL.27
SP	BL.20	ST	BL.21
LR	BL.18	GB	BL.19
KI	BL.23	BL	BL.28

BACK TRANSPORTING POINT THEORY

These are sometimes called the Associated points, since each of these points (see Table 8.5) is specifically associated with one of the organ systems of Chinese medicine, for example BL.13 is associated with all the functions of the Lungs system, whether physical, emotional or mental.

These points are also called the Back–Shu points, since shu means to transport, and these points are said to transport Qi to the organs, so that they have a direct communication with them and a direct effect upon them. In Western medicine, this can be explained in terms of the neural organization of the spinal segments; and in the theory of energy circulation, it can be explained in the terms of the areas controlled by the main energy centres or chakras.

DEFICIENCY, EXCESS, STAGNATION AND IRREGULARITY

As seen from Table 8.6, the Back Transporting points can treat conditions of Deficiency, Excess, Stagnation and Irregularity, whether they are acute or chronic, Cold or Hot, Interior or Exterior. However, the Back Transporting points are especially useful for chronic Deficiency disorders.

Table 8.6 Back Transporting points and the four Qi disharmonies

Disharmony	Syndrome	Methods
Deficiency	Deficiency of Qi, Jing, Blood, Yin or Yang	Rf M(unless Deficient Yin)
Excess	Wind Cold, Wind Heat, Cold, Damp	Rd M(for Wind Cold, Cold and Damp) C(for Wind Cold, Cold, Damp)
	Interior Heat, Interior Wind	Rd
Stagnation	Stagnant Qi and Blood (due to Deficiency, trauma, lack of exercise, emotion, Cold, Damp, etc.)	Rd E M(unless signs of Heat)
Irregularity	Disturbance of Heart Spirit, Hyperactive Liver Yang, Rebellious Stomach Qi, Rebellious Lung Qi	Rd(or E, if there is Deficiency)

Rf, Reinforcing method; M, moxa; Rd, Reducing method; C, cupping; E, Even method.

TREATING THE ORGAN SYSTEMS

Treating an organ system not only affects the physical functions of that organ, but its emotional and mental aspects as well. Also, it can treat the tissue and sense organ associated with the organ system. For example, BL.18 can treat physiological problems of the Liver, such as headaches, digestive and menstrual problems; emotional conditions relating to anger, frustration and depression; mental problems associated with planning and intuition; disorders of the muscles, the associated tissue, and the eyes, the associated sense organ. Further examples are:

BL.13   for skin conditions associated with Lungs
BL.15   for nervous anxiety associated with Heart
BL.19   for indecision associated with Gallbladder
BL.20   for tiredness from Deficient Blood, associated with Spleen
BL.23   for bone problems associated with Kidneys.

OUTER AND INNER BACK TRANSPORTING POINTS

The Bladder channel on the back has an inner line, comprising points BL.11–BL.30, and an outer line of points BL.41–BL.54. Both outer and inner line Bladder points of the Five Yin organs can be used for both physiological and psychological problems. However, the outer Bladder line points are seen to be especially appropriate for psychological problems.

COMBINING THE BACK TRANSPORTING POINTS WITH OTHER POINT TYPES

Combination depends on the type of imbalance, whether Deficiency, Excess, Stagnation or Irregularity, as shown in Table 8.7. There are obvious overlaps between the categories in the table; for example, overlap between Excess and Deficiency, as in the syndromes Retention of Phlegm in the Lungs, or Stagnation of Heart Blood.

WINDOW OF HEAVEN POINTS

The 10 Window of Heaven points, often called Window of the Sky points, are:

LU.3   tiān fǔ
LI.18   fú tū
PC.1   tiān chí
TE.16   tiān yǒu
SI.16   tiān chuāng
SI.17   tiān róng
ST.9   rén yíng
BL.10   tiān zhù
CV.22   tiān tū
GV.16   fēng fǔ

Table 8.7 Combining Back Transporting points with other point types

Disharmony	Point		Example
Deficiency	Source	BL.15, BL.20, HT.7, KI.3	insomnia with Deficient HT and SP Blood
	Five Element	BL.44, BL.52, HT.8, KI.2	depression with Deficient HT and KI Fire
	Opening	BL.23, SI.3, BL.62	arthritis in the elderly with Deficient KI Jing and Yin
	Lower Sea	BL.20, ST.36	tiredness with Deficient SP Qi
	Gathering	BL.18, GB.34	weak muscles with Deficient LR Blood
Excess	Accumulation	BL.13, LU.6	asthma with Retention of Phlegm in LU
	Alarm	BL.13, LU.1	bronchitis with Retention of Phlegm in LU
	Opening	BL.13, LU.7, KI.6	depression with Stagnant LU Qi
	Well	BL.17, PC.9	acne and boils with Heat in the Blood
	Five Element	BL.44, HT.8	mania with HT Fire
	Opening	BL.10, BL.11, SI.3, BL.62	stiff neck with Wind Cold invasion
Stagnation	Connecting	BL.15, SP.21	chest pain with Stagnant HT Qi
	Accumulation	BL.14, PC.4	angina pectoris with Stagnant HT Blood
	Alarm	BL.23, GB.25	renal colic with Stagnant KI Qi
	Opening	BL.13, LU.7, KI.6	depression with Stagnant LU Qi
	Lower Sea	BL.25, ST.37	constipation with Stagnant Intestine Qi
	Gathering	BL.47, GB.34	frustration and tight muscles with Stagnant LR Qi
	Window of Heaven	BL.13, LU.3	inability to express grief with Stagnant LU Qi
Irregularity	Source	BL.13, BL.23, LU.9, KI.3	asthma and cough with Deficient LU and KI Qi
	Connecting	BL.44, PC.6	anxiety with Disturbance of HT Spirit
	Alarm	BL.14, CV.17	palpitations with Disturbance of HT Spirit
	Five Element	BL.18, LR.2	headache with Hyperactive LR Yang
	Opening	BL.15, BL.23, SP.4, PC.6	panic attacks with HT anxiety and KI fear
	Lower Sea	BL.18, BL.23, GB.34	dizziness with Hyperactive LR Yang and Deficient KI Qi
	Gathering	BL.17, BL.20, GB.34	muscle tics and tremors with Deficient Blood
	Window of Heaven	BL.44, BL.52, BL.10	anxiety and depression with Disturbance of HT Spirit

LOCATION

Eight of these points are on the neck. The exceptions are LU.3 on the upper arms and PC.1 on the chest.

POINT NAMES

Seven of these 10 points include the element tiān as a part of their name. Tiān can be translated as heaven or sky. For example, BL.10 is tiān zhù, which can be translated as Heaven's Pillar, the neck being the pillar which supports the head (heaven). Tiān may in some cases refer to the upper third of the body, especially the head.

INTERPRETATION

There is very little discussion of the Window of Heaven points in the Chinese classics. However, in the last 25 years an interpretation of the Window of Heaven points has developed in the West to include the treatment of psychological disorders, such as depression and phobias. The general idea being that when a patient is locked in the dark prison of their own negative patterns, the Window of Heaven points can be used to open a window to hope and to the light and illumination of Heaven. This can create a 'window of opportunity', so that the patient is encouraged to change their patterns of thought and behaviour, to let go of the chains of the ego and to begin to create a world of light within and around themselves.

Obviously, the Window of Heaven points are not the only points that can assist in this process, but eight of the Window of Heaven points are located on the neck, an area which is most susceptible to blockage in the flow of energy.

WINDOW OF HEAVEN POINTS AND THE CIRCULATION OF QI

Blockage of energy circulation in the neck, the pathway between head and body, has four main aspects:

circulation through the joints
circulation through the Governor and Conception channels
circulation between the energy centres
circulation through the other neck channels.

CIRCULATION THROUGH THE JOINTS

Any joint between bones is an area of potential energy block. The intervertebral joints of the neck and the joint between the skull and the atlas vertebra are examples of this. BL.10 and GV.16 can therefore be used for problems of Stagnation of Qi and Blood around the skull–atlas–axis junctions. These energy blocks can not only cause pain and stiffness in the back and neck and occipital or frontal headache, but also depression and disorientation.

In such cases, BL.10 and GV.16, can be combined with points on the Bladder or Governor channels above or below the block, such as BL.11, BL.9 or BL.1, or GV.1, GV.14, GV.15, or GV.20. These points can be combined with the Opening points SI.3 and BL.62, which can move Stagnation of Qi in the Governor, Bladder and Small Intestine channels; and thus in the joints of the neck vertebrae SI.16 and SI.18 may be added.

CIRCULATION THROUGH THE GOVERNOR AND CONCEPTION CHANNELS

The Governor and Conception channels comprise the central axis for energy circulation in the body. If their circulation through the neck region becomes blocked, there can be signs of Deficiency, Excess, Stagnation or Irregularity not just in the head or neck, but in the body as a whole, with generalized tiredness and depression.

Specifically, the Governor channel regulates the Yang of the body, so that BL.10 and GV.16 can be used for patterns of Excess and Irregularity associated with upward-moving Fire of Kidneys, Heart or Liver, with Disturbance of Heart Spirit, and with Hyperactive Liver Yang or Interior Wind. There may then be signs such as fever, headache, dizziness, mania, restless anxiety or aggressive behaviour. The Window of Heaven points BL.10 and GV.16 can then be combined with such points as SI.3, BL.62, GV.14, GV.20 and KI.1.

The Conception and Thoroughfare channels circulate through the throat and blockage of their pathways may be associated with Stagnant or Rebellious Qi of Lungs or Stomach, and signs such as cough, asthma, nausea, vomiting or hiccup, in addition to psychological problems such as depression or anxiety. CV.22 can be combined with SP.4 and PC.6 for oesophageal spasm, nausea, vomiting or hiccup, linked to anxiety; or CV.22 can be combined with LU.7 and KI.6 for cough, asthma or dyspnoea linked to fear and suppressed grief.

CIRCULATION BETWEEN THE ENERGY CENTRES

GV.16 and CV.22 both relate to the throat energy centre, which links the energy centres of the body to those of the head, and which has the specific function of regulating speech and the expression and communication of love, feelings and ideas. Stagnation and irregularity of Qi flowing through the throat centre can be associated with problems of speech and communication, with depression, frustration, loneliness and alienation.

For problems of suppressed grief, CV.22 can be combined with LU.3, LU.7 and BL.13. For inability to express feelings in a love relationship, CV.22 may be combined with PC.1, PC.6 and BL.15. In both these examples, CV.17 can be added to help communication between the Throat and Heart energy centres. If there is difficulty in expressing ideas due to mental confusion and a block between Throat and Brow energy centres, then GV.16 may be combined with HT.5 and yìn táng.

If communication is blocked by fear and stress, this may be eased by combining CV.14 with CV.22 or CV.23, to relax the stresses originating from the Solar Plexus energy centre which are creating tensions in the throat and mind.

CIRCULATION THROUGH THE OTHER NECK CHANNELS

Since the Bladder channel is linked to the Kidney organ, BL.10 can be used to treat fearfulness, phobias, panic attacks and paranoia. It is then often combined with BL.23 to strengthen the Kidney, and with BL.1 to regulate the mind and the endocrine system.

LU.3 can be combined with such points as BL.13, LU.1 and LU.7 to release suppressed grief and to assist the process of letting go. If the person is holding on to the past due to fear of letting go, the BL.10 and BL.23 can be added to BL.13 and LU.3.

LI.18 can be combined with LU.3 to open a window on to the light for those locked in the prison of their own negative beliefs, or LI.18 can be combined with LI.4 and LI.11 for skin diseases of the upper body and face, such as acne and boils, that are linked to difficulties of self-expression.

TE.16 can be combined with TE.5 and TE.17 for problems of neck, throat and ear, and SI.2 and SI.3 can be added.

ST.9 is a useful local point for difficulty in swallowing, when it can be combined with LI.4 and LI.18 for painful sore throat, or with PC.6 and ST.36 for nausea and vomiting. It can be combined with ST.36 and KI.1 for hypertension with headache, dizziness and feelings of heat in the head and face.

ST.9 can be combined with ST.40 and with SP.4, PC.6 and CV.14 for mental disorders associated with Heart Phlegm and Disturbance of Heart Spirit.

PC.1 can be combined with PC.6, CV.17 and LR.3 for depression, loneliness and frustration coming from difficulties in self-expression.

COMBINATION OF WINDOW OF HEAVEN POINTS WITH OTHER POINT TYPES

As shown in the previous discussion, Window of Heaven points can be combined with Connecting points such as LU.7, Alarm points such as LU.1, and Opening points such as SP.4 and PC.6, all of which regulate Stagnation and Irregularity of Qi. They can also be combined with Back Transporting points such as BL.23, which will regulate Irregularity by strengthening Deficient Kidney Qi.

In Five Element treatments where there is a block between successive organs on the Promotion cycle, e.g. when Lungs are + and Kidneys -, the Window of Heaven point, LU.3 can be added to the Five Element treatment LU.5 plus KI.7.

LOWER SEA POINTS

The arm Yang channels each have a Lower Sea Point on the legs which can be used to treat their respective organs since they have a direct connection with them.

Large Intestine	ST.37	diarrhoea, constipation, abdominal pain and distension
Triple Energizer	BL.39	enuresis, urinary retention, incontinence, dysuria
Small Intestine	ST.39	diarrhoea, lower abdominal pain, acute intestinal obstruction.

ST.37 and ST.39 have overlapping function in that both will treat diarrhoea due to Damp Heat, but ST.37 is more for Large Intestine problems and ST.39 more for Small Intestine disorders.

COMBINATION OF LOWER SEA POINTS WITH OTHER POINT TYPES

The Lower Sea points are mainly combined with Back Transporting points or with points on the abdomen. For example:

ST.37 + BL.25	for constipation
ST.39 + BL.27	for intestinal pain
BL.39 + BL.22, BL.28, BL.32	for urinary retention.

BL.22 represents the Triple Energizer, BL.25 the Large Intestine, BL.27 the Small Intestine, BL.28 the Bladder, and BL.32 is a sacral point for urinary problems.

ST.37 + SP.15, GB.28, GB.24, CV.6, TE.6	for constipation
ST.39 + ST.27, ST.29, CV.6, GB.34	for pain from Stagnant Qi in Small Intestines
ST.39 + ST.25, LI.11, SP.6, SP.9	for diarrhoea with Damp Heat in intestines
BL.39 + ST.28, CV.3, CV.6, TE.6, SP.6	for urinary retention.

GB.27 and GB.28 are local points for constipation, SP.15 is a local point for the ascending and descending loops of the Large Intestine, ST.28 regulates the Bladder.

POINTS OF THE SEA OF BLOOD

Classically the Thoroughfare channel is considered to be the Sea of the Main channels, reaching BL.11 in the upper body and ST.37 and ST.39 below. The Thoroughfare channel is specifically concerned with the Blood, and BL.11, ST.37 and ST.39 can be used together to tonify the Sea of Blood, for conditions of Blood Deficiency.

Professor Mei Jianghan of Nanjing College of TCM (*Journal of Chinese Medicine* 1993, **43**, 27–31) has also used these points for Excess conditions of the Thoroughfare channel, such as vertigo and dizziness or cough and asthma, bleeding BL.11 and reducing ST.37 and ST.39.

GATHERING POINTS

The eight Gathering points are:

Yin organs	LR.13
Yang organs	CV.12
Qi	CV.17
Blood	BL.17
sinews	GB.34
arteries	LU.9
bones	BL.11
marrow	GB.39

These points, bā huì xué, sometimes called the Eight Influential points, are said to have specific effect on their respective organs, Substance or tissue. The most widely used of these are BL.17, GB.34, BL.11 and GB.39. CV.17 is more used to regulate the Qi of the chest, than the Qi of the entire body, although in regulating breathing and heart beat, it has this effect in theory.

BL.17 may be combined with BL.18, BL.20, BL.43, ST.36 and SP.6 to tonify the Blood. It can be combined with BL.14, BL.18, SP.4, PC.6 or SP.8 to move Stagnant Blood. It can also be combined with BL.40, LI.4, LI.11, SP.6 and SP.10 for Heat in the Blood.

GB.34 can be combined with BL.18 and LR.8 with Reinforcing method to strengthen the sinews and muscles by strengthening Liver Blood. GB.34 can also be used with GB.21, GV.9 and SP.6 with Reducing method to relieve tension and spasm of sinews and muscles due to Hyperactive Liver Yang and Stagnant Liver Qi.

BL.11 and GB.39 can be used together and combined with BL.23 and KI.3 to strengthen bones, or combined with SI.3 and BL.62 for spinal problems due to Deficient Kidney Jing and Stagnation of Qi and Blood.

To treat a joint deficiency of Kidney Jing and Liver Blood, with weak joints and sinews, GB.34, GB.39 and BL.11 can be combined with BL.18 and BL.23.

CROSSING POINTS

These are points where two or more channels meet. Crossing points can be useful in the clinic, since one point can be used to treat disharmonies of more than one organ. SP.6 is an excellent example, since it is the Crossing point of the Spleen, Liver and Kidney channels. It can be used to treat the syndromes of Deficient Spleen Blood, Stagnant Liver Qi and Deficient Kidney Yin, either singly or in combination. CV.3 is similarly a Crossing point of Spleen, Liver and Kidney channels with the Conception channel. It can be used to treat problems of the Small Intestine (regulated by the Spleen), and Damp Heat in the Liver channel, or to tonify Kidney Yang.

A special case of this is Extra channels which have no points of their own but borrow points from the main channels. Each of these borrowed points can be said to be a Crossing point of the Extra channel with the main channel. Table 8.8 shows the main Crossing points on the Yang and Yin channels. It includes the Governor and Conception points, but not the Extra channels that borrow points from other channels, since these have been listed in Chapter 10.

FIVE TRANSPORTING POINTS

The Five Transporting points of the Yin and Yang channels are shown in Tables 8.9 and 8.10 respectively.

CHINESE NAMES AND LOCATIONS

The Chinese names for the five transporting points are:

Well—jǐng   Spring—yíng   Stream—shū

River—jīng   Sea—hé

• The Well points are the nail points, with the exception of KI.1 on the sole of the foot, and PC.9 which is sometimes listed as a nail point and sometimes as at the tip of the middle finger.

• The Spring points are either on the fingers or toes, just distal to the foot or hand respectively, or are on the distal half of the hand or foot.

• The Stream points of the Yin channels of the hand are at the wrist crease, and the other Stream points are between the Spring points and the wrist or ankle. SP.5,

Table 8.8 The Crossing points

Point	Yang channels							Yin channels							Point	Yang cross
	LI	TE	SI	ST	GB	BL	GV	LU	PC	HT	SP	LR	KI	CV		
LI.20				X							X				LU.1	
TE.17					X							X			PC.1	GB
TE.20	X				X							X	X		SP.6	
TE.22			X		X							X			SP.12	
SI.12	X	X			X							X			SP.13	
SI.18		X													LR.13	GB
SI.19		X			X						X				LR.14	
ST.4	X											X			CV.2	
ST.7					X						X	X	X		CV.3	
ST.8					X						X	X	X		CV.4	
GB.1		X	X								X				CV.10	
GB.3		X		X											CV.12	SI, TE, ST
GB.4		X		X											CV.13	SI, ST
GB.6		X		X											CV.24	LI, ST, GV
GB.7						X										
GB.8						X										
GB.10						X										
GB.11						X										
GB.12						X										
GB.15						X										
GB.21		X														
GB.30						X										
BL.1			X	X												
BL.11			X													
BL.12							X									
GV.13						X										
GV.14				X	X	X										
GV.17						X										
GV.20						X										
GV.24				X												
GV.26	X			X												

Table 8.9 The Five Transporting points of the Yin channels

Transporting point Element	Well Wood	Spring Fire	Stream Earth	River Metal	Sea Water
LU	LU.11	LU.10	LU.9	LU.8	LU.5
PC	PC.9	PC.8	PC.7	PC.5	PC.3
HT	HT.9	HT.8	HT.7	HT.4	HT.3
SP	SP.1	SP.2	SP.3	SP.5	SP.9
LR	LR.1	LR.2	LR.3	LR.4	LR.8
KI	KI.1	KI.2	KI.3	KI.7	KI.10

Table 8.10 The Five Transporting points of the Yang channels

Transporting point Element	Well Metal	Spring Water	Stream Wood	River Fire	Sea Earth
LI	LI.1	LI.2	LI.3	LI.5	LI.11
TE	TE.1	TE.2	TE.3	TE.6	TE.10
SI	SI.1	SI.2	SI.3	SI.5	SI.8
ST	ST.45	ST.44	ST.43	ST.41	ST.36
GB	GB.44	GB.43	GB.41	GB.38	GB.34
BL	BL.67	BL.66	BL.65	BL.60	BL.40

LR.4, LI.5, SI.5, ST.41 and BL.60 are located between wrist and elbow or between ankle and knee.

• The Sea points are all located at or near the elbows or knees.

THEORY OF THE FIVE TRANSPORTING POINTS

The points between finger tip and elbow or toe tip and knee are among the most energetically powerful points of the body. They include not only the Five Transporting points, but also the Connecting points and the Accumulation points. This is said to be because between fingers and elbows, or between toes and knees, the polarity of the energy is changing, from Yin to Yang, or Yang to Yin, and it is where the polarity is changing that the greatest therapeutic effects can be made.

In the system of the Five Transporting points, wǔ shū xué, each type of point has its own energetic quality, and its own therapeutic effect. The Chinese classics are somewhat confusing and contradictory in their descriptions of the Five Transporting points, and since a good discussion of the classical material is given in 'The Foundations of Chinese Medicine' by Giovanni Maciocia (Churchill Livingstone, Edinburgh, 1989), it will be omitted here. The discussion is this section is limited to modern clinical use of the Five Transporting points.

CLINICAL USE OF THE FIVE TRANSPORTING POINTS

Of the five types of points, Well, Spring, Stream, River and Sea, by far the most clinically important are the Well points. The Spring points have some clinical importance, but the functions of Stream, River and Sea points are overshadowed by the functions of these same points according to their Five Element or Source point qualities.

WELL POINTS

The Well points are mostly the nail points on the fingers and toes. They share with the shí xuān points at the tips of the fingers the functions of treating acute severe fevers, convulsions and loss of consciousness.

In addition, the Well points can be used to treat:

severe Excess Heat syndromes of specific organs (bleed)
Stagnant Qi in specific channels and organs (reduce)
Deficient Yang and Fire of specific organs (moxa).

The Well points of the Yin organs are more important for removing Excess Heat from the organs, and the Well points of the Yang organs are more effective in removing Wind Heat. ST.45 is the exception, in that it is more for

Excess Heat in the Stomach than for Wind Heat. See Table 8.11.

Some Well points are more important than others in moving Stagnation and invigorating the channel and the organ and are listed in Table 8.12. Well points that are especially good in warming their corresponding organs are given in Table 8.13.

Well points have important psychological effects mainly based on their ability to remove Heat and move Stagnation. While all Well points calm the Spirit by reducing Heat, more specific effects are given in Table 8.14.

Table 8.11 Use of Yin Well points to remove Excess acute Heat

Well point	Ailment
LU.11	acute tonsillitis, acute skin or respiratory disorder with Lung Heat
PC.9	acute sunburn or sunstroke, severe hot skin rashes, loss of consciousness
HT.9	severe hot skin rashes or bleeding due to Heart Fire, mania, loss of consciousness
SP.1	Heat in Spleen or Stomach with cracked lips, blood in the stool, abnormal uterine bleeding
LR.1	Liver Fire with hypertension, aggression, epistaxis, abnormal menstrual bleeding
KI.1	acute severe Fire of Kidneys, Liver or Heart with severe hypertension, restlessness, aggression or mania, loss of consciousness

Table 8.12 Use of certain Well points to move Stagnant Qi

Well point	Ailment
PC.9	chest or epigastric pain, poor circulation in hands
SP.1	abdominal distension, poor circulation in legs and feet
LR.1	irregular menstruation, genital pain
LI.1	hangover, mental congestion
SI.1	mastitis, insufficient lactation, chest pain
ST.4	hangover, epigastric pain and indigestion
BL.67	malposition of fetus, eye pain, headache

Table 8.13 Use of certain Well points to tonify Yang and Fire

Well point	Ailment
PC.9	poor circulation in the hands
HT.9	depression, lack of joy or interest in life
SP.1	oedema or abdominal distension from Deficient Spleen Yang, poor circulation in the feet
LR.1	lack of self-assertion
KI.1	exhaustion, fainting, impotence, lack of drive
ST.4	poor concentration, slow thinking
BL.6	mental dullness, lack of perseverance

Table 8.14 Psychological effects of Well points from removing Heat and moving Qi

Well point	Ailment
PC.9	frustration and depression with Stagnant Heart and Liver Qi
HT.9	overexcitement, mania, hysteria with Heart Fire
SP.1	depression, melancholy, overconcern with Stagnant Spleen Qi
LR.1	aggression and anger with Liver Fire, depression and frustration with Stagnant Liver Qi
KI.1	hyperactivity, fearful anxiety, hysteria, anger, aggression with Kidney, Heart and Liver Fire
ST.45	mental dullness, depression, disorientation, dream-disturbed sleep with Phlegm or Stomach Fire disturbing Heart Spirit
GB.44	hypertension, restlessness, dream-disturbed sleep with Gallbladder Fire
BL.67	mental dullness, disorientation and depression with Stagnation and Deficiency of Kidney and Bladder Qi

COMBINING WELL POINTS WITH OTHER POINT TYPES

Well points + Spring points

This combination can be used with Reducing method or bleeding to remove Heat, or with Reinforcing method and moxa to tonify Yang:

e.g. KI.1 + KI.2 Rf + M   for impotence from Deficient Kidney Yang
e.g. HT.9 + HT.8 Rd   for mania with Heart Fire.

The combination of Well points and Spring points is discussed in more detail on pages 42–43, in the section on Skin disorders.

Well points + Water points of Yin Hand Channels

e.g. PC.9 + PC.3 B   for sunburn with Heat in the Blood
e.g. HT.9 + HT.3 B   for severe acute hyperactivity and insomnia with Heart Fire.

Well point + point at opposite end of the channel

This combination can be effective for Stagnant Qi:

e.g. PC.9 + PC.1   for melancholy from Stagnant Heart Qi
e.g. SP.1 + SP.21   for chest pain from Stagnant Blood
e.g. LR.1 + LR.14   for frustration from Stagnant Liver Qi
e.g. BL.67 + BL.1   for mental congestion.

SPRING POINTS

Like the Well points, the Spring points can clear Heat, but the Well points are better for more severe acute fevers, convulsions and loss of consciousness. The Spring points are for less severe acute Heat, for example Wind Heat, or for less severe acute Heat of specific organs.

For example, KI.2 is for less severe cases of Kidney Fire than KI.1, and can also be used in situations involving chronic Deficiency Fire of Kidneys. For acute Heat in specific organs, the difference is sometimes not so great, and LR.2 can be used in preference to LR.1, or HT.8 in preference to HT.9.

The Spring points of the Yin channels are Fire points and the Spring points of the Yang channels are Water points, but both types of Spring points are reduced to remove Heat. For example, ST.44 is reduced to remove Stomach Fire, even though it is a Water point, which logically should be tonified to strengthen Water to cool Fire.

All the Well points can be used with moxa to tonify Yang and Fire, but this only applies to the Spring points of the Yin organs, which are Fire points, and not to the Spring points of the Yang organs, which are Water points. Also, although the Well points can be used to move Stagnant Qi and Blood, the Spring points are not so effective for this.

Table 8.15 Use of Spring points

Spring point	Point	Ailments
LU.10	Fire	sore throat with Wind Heat, haemoptysis, fever, chest pain with acute or chronic Lung Heat
PC.8	Fire	fungal infections of hands with Damp Heat, epistaxis or skin rash with Heat in the Blood
HT.8	Fire	pruritus with Damp Heat, boils with Heat in the Blood; mania or insomnia with Heart Fire
SP.2	Fire	restlessness with insomnia or excessive appetite with acute or chronic Spleen and Stomach Fire
LR.2	Fire	anger and restlessness with acute or chronic Liver Fire
KI.2	Fire	sore throat or cystitis with Excess or Deficiency Kidney Fire
LI.2	Water	
TE.2	Water	fever, sore throat, dry mouth with Wind Heat
SI.2	Water	
ST.44	Water	gastritis, gingivitis, conjunctivitis with acute Stomach Fire or chronic Deficient Stomach Yin
GB.43	Water	hypertension, anxiety, restlessness, conjunctivitis with Gallbladder Fire
BL.66	Water	headache with Wind Heat, cystitis from Kidney Fire, fearful insanity with Kidney and Heart Fire

STREAM POINTS

In the case of the Stream points, there is wide variation in the functions given in the classical texts.

THE YIN STREAM POINTS

The Stream points of the Yin channel are also the Source points and Earth points of those channels. In the opinion of the author, the Source point function is dominant, and the Stream point function the least important of the three.

THE YANG STREAM POINTS

The Stream points of the Yang channels are also the Wood points. Some of the Yang Stream points can treat malaria, 'the disease manifesting intermittently', for example, TE.3, but TE.1, TE.2 and TE.4 can also treat malaria.

The Stream points of the Yang channels can be used for joint pain, such as arthritis, for example LI.3, but LI.1, LI.2, LI.4, LI.5 can also treat joint pain.

In the opinion of the author, the main use of the Yang Stream points is as local points, and in addition, SI.3 and GB.41 have enormous importance as the Opening points of the Governor and Belt channels respectively.

RIVER POINTS

The classics state that the River points can be used for cough, asthma, problems of the voice and problems of the sinus and bones. It is the opinion of the author that the River points are no more appropriate to these problems than the Stream points or Sea points. Of the Yin River points, KI.7 is the most important, as the Tonification point of the Kidneys, and as a point to tonify Kidney Yang and firm Kidney Qi. The other Yin River points are among the least-used points on their respective channels. The Yang River points are mainly used as Fire points, to reduce or to strengthen Fire. For example, BL.60 can be used with moxa to warm and strengthen Cold and Deficiency in the Bladder channel, and GB.38 can be used with Reducing method to remove Fire in the Gallbladder channel.

SEA POINTS

According to the classics, the Sea points can treat diseases of the Yang organs, diseases of the skin, stomach problems, Rebellious Qi and diarrhoea. The Yang Sea points can treat diseases of the Yang organs, but then so can the Well, Spring, Stream or River points. The theory is that at the Sea points the energy is flowing deeper, in a more inward direction, and more slowly. Therefore, Sea points should be appropriate for chronic diseases of the organs. In the opinion of the author, they are no appropri-

ate for this than the Yin Stream points, since these are also the Source points, which are specific for chronic Deficiency. However, the Yin Sea points can all be used for skin problems, since they are the Water points with cooling effect on hot skin rashes. Also, most of the Yang Sea points have specific indications for skin rashes due to Damp Heat or Heat in the Blood, specifically, LI.11, TE.10, GB.34 and BL.40.

PC.3, SP.9, LI.11, ST.36 and GB.34 are the Sea points most used to treat stomach problems or diarrhoea, often in combination with ST.37 and ST.39, the Lower Sea points for the Large Intestine and Small Intestine respectively.

SUMMARY

The Well points have by far the most important functions of the Five Transporting points in clinical practice. The Well point function dominates the other functions of these points as Wood or Metal points.

The Spring points can be used with Reducing method to clear Heat, whether they are Fire points or Water points, but the Stream, River and Sea points are more important for their other functions, such as local points or Opening points, than for their Transporting point function. One clear exception to this is the use of Sea points for skin problems.

FIVE ELEMENT POINTS

The Five Transporting points can also be classified according to the Five Elements, as shown in Tables 8.9 and 8.10. Five Element treatments are discussed in detail in Chapter 9. In addition, the Element points can be used according to the seasons, or the time of day.

TREATMENT ACCORDING TO THE SEASON

Theoretically, Fire points can be chosen in the summer, Earth points in late summer, Metal points in autumn, Water points in winter and Wood points in spring, if this fits in with the patient's needs. For example, Wood points such as LR.1 and PC.9 could be chosen for a depression occurring in spring, and Fire points such as HT.8 and LU.10 could be chosen for a bereavement occurring in summer.

TREATMENT ACCORDING TO THE TIME

Points can be selected according to the current hour, day,

month and year, regardless of the patient's ailment or needs. The author does not practice this system, and he feels that unless it is also related to the hour, day, month and year of the patient's birth, it is generally too unspecific to be effective.

A small part of the system of treatment according to time is the so-called Chinese Clock, treatment according to the hour. The idea is that there is a circulation of energy through the 12 channels, so that each of the channels has a 2-hour period in the 24 hours, when its energy is at maximum.

The Element point of each channel is sometimes called the Horary point in this context, and can be used in the peak 2-hour period to strengthen its channel, as shown in Table 8.16. For example, for bronchitis from Lung Deficiency, LU.8 could be reinforced between 3 and 5 a.m. The author lost interest in this system, many years ago, after treating a patient at 3 a.m. for poor planning and decisions. Both patient and practitioner expressed a desire for uninterrupted sleep, and a more user-friendly system of point choice was adopted.

OPENING POINTS

The Opening points are discussed in detail in Chapter 10 on the Extra channels.

Table 8.16 Treatment according to the hour

Channel	Peak time	Element point
HT	1100–1300	HT.8
SI	1300–1500	SI.5
BL	1500–1700	BL.66
KI	1700–1900	KI.10
PC	1900–2100	PC.8
TE	2100–2300	TE.6
GB	2300–0100	GB.41
LR	0100–0300	LR.1
LU	0300–0500	LU.8
LI	0500–0700	LI.1
ST	0700–0900	ST.36
SP	0900–1100	SP.3

Five Element treatments 9

The Basic Theory

THE SIMPLEST LEVEL: TONIFICATION AND SEDATION POINTS

The simplest level of treatment using the Five Element system, is to tonify Deficiency and to sedate Excess, using Reinforcing and Reducing needling methods respectively.

THE PROMOTION CYCLE

According to the rule of Mother–Child, classically called the rule of Mother–Son, each element promotes the growth of the next element in the sequence. For example, Fire promotes the growth of Earth, or we can say that Fire is the mother who nourishes Earth, the child.

Each channel has on it the Five Element points, the five so-called Transporting points. For example, the Spleen channel has a Fire point, an Earth point, a Metal point,

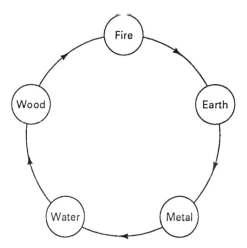

Fig. 9.1 The Promotion cycle.

a Water point and a Wood point. If the Spleen organ or channel is Deficient, then SP.2, the Fire point, can be reinforced, since it is the point of the mother element on the Spleen channel.

USING THE TONIFICATION POINTS FOR DEFICIENCY

The mother point on a channel is called the Tonification point, which can be used to tonify Deficiency of that channel. The 12 Tonification points are shown in Table 9.1.

For example, a patient has a cough, weak voice and frequent colds, associated with Deficient Lungs. Since the Lungs are associated with the Metal element, and since Earth is the mother of Metal, the Mother point, or Tonification point of the Lung channel is LU.9, the Earth point, which can be used with Reinforcing method to treat this patient.

Table 9.1 Tonification points

Channel	Element of channel	Tonification point	Element of Tonification point
KI	Water	KI.7	Metal
BL	Water	BL.67	Metal
HT	Fire	HT.9	Wood
SI	Fire	SI.3	Wood
PC	Fire	PC.9	Wood
TE	Fire	TE.3	Wood
LR	Wood	LR.8	Water
GB	Wood	GB.43	Water
SP	Earth	SP.2	Fire
ST	Earth	ST.41	Fire
LU	Metal	LU.9	Earth
LI	Metal	LI.11	Earth

USING THE SEDATION POINTS FOR EXCESS

According to the rule of Mother–Child, an Element in Excess can be treated by draining the excess energy in the affected element into the next element in the sequence of the Promotion cycle. For example, if Earth is in Excess, then the excess energy can be drained into Metal, the child of Earth.

This can be done by reducing the Child point on the channel, which is known as the Sedation point. For example, for an Excess Spleen, we reduce SP.5, since the Spleen corresponds to Earth, and SP.5 is the Metal point on the Spleen channel, and therefore the Child point or Sedation point. Take, for example, a patient who has a heavy cough with much phlegm and a full and obstructed feeling in the chest, associated with Excess in the Lungs. Since the Lungs relate to the Metal element and since Water is the child of Metal, the Child point or Sedation

point of the Lung channel is LU.5, the Water point, which can be used with Reducing method to treat this patient.

Table 9.2 Sedation points

Channel	Element of channel	Sedation point	Element of Sedation point
KI	Water	KI.1	Wood
BL	Water	BL.65	Wood
HT	Fire	HT.7	Earth
SI	Fire	SI.8	Earth
PC	Fire	PC.7	Earth
TE	Fire	TE.10	Earth
LR	Wood	LR.2	Fire
GB	Wood	GB.38	Fire
SP	Earth	SP.5	Metal
ST	Earth	ST.45	Metal
LU	Metal	LU.5	Water
LI	Metal	LI.2	Water

SUMMARY OF THE SIMPLEST LEVEL

The simplest level of Five Element treatment is to reinforce the Tonification point for Deficiency of a channel or organ, and to reduce the Sedation point for Excess. The Tonification and Sedation points are summarized in Table 9.3.

Table 9.3 Tonification and Sedation points

Channel point	Tonification point	Sedation
KI	KI.7	KI.1
BL	BL.67	BL.65
HT	HT.9	HT.7
SI	SI.3	SI.8
PC	PC.9	PC.7
TE	TE.3	TE.10
LR	LR.8	LR.2
GB	GB.43	GB.38
SP	SP.2	SP.5
ST	ST.41	ST.45
LU	LU.9	LU.5
LI	LI.11	LI.2

WHEN MORE THAN ONE ORGAN IS AFFECTED

In the clinic it is common for more than one organ to be affected at the same time. If the different organ problems are not related to each other, then it will be necessary to treat each affected organ separately, using its Tonification or Sedation point as appropriate. If the different organ problems are related to each other, it is necessary to determine which organ is the primary cause. It may then be possible to treat all the affected organs just by using the Tonification or Sedation point of the primarily affected organ.

There are three main possibilities:

two or more organs Deficient
two or more organs Excess
some organs Deficient and some organs Excess.

TWO OR MORE ORGANS DEFICIENT

For example, if Heart and Lungs are both Deficient, and there is no obvious link between these problems, it may be necessary to reinforce both HT.9 and LU.9, the Tonification points of the Heart and the Lung channels.

If for example, Liver, Heart and Spleen are all Deficient, and it is clear that the Deficiencies of Heart and Spleen are dependent on the Deficiency of the Liver, it may be possible to resolve all three deficiencies by reinforcing LR.8 only, the Tonification point of the Liver.

However, if there is doubt, it may be better to use the Tonification points of all the affected organs. Sometimes, even if one organ, for example the Liver, is the primary cause, the dependent organs, in this case the Heart and the Spleen, may in a long chronic ailment become so disordered, that they need separate treatment to ensure full recovery.

TWO OR MORE ORGANS EXCESS

For example, if both Heart and Lungs are Excess, and there is no obvious link between their problems, it may be necessary to reduce both HT.7 and LU.5, the Sedation points of the Heart and Lung channels. If for example, Liver, Heart and Spleen are all Excess, and it is clear that the Excess in Heart and Spleen relates to a hyperactive Liver, it may be possible to balance all three organs simply by reducing LR.2, the Sedation point of the Liver. Again, if there is doubt, it may be better to reduce the Sedation points of all organs affected.

SOME ORGANS DEFICIENT AND SOME ORGANS EXCESS

It is very common in the clinic to have one or more organ Excess at the same time as one or more organ Deficient.

In a particular patient, it is possible for some organ imbalances to be related to each other, while some imbalances are separate. For example, a patient has Deficient Lungs, Deficient Kidneys and Excess Liver. The Kidneys may be Deficient because they, the mother, are being exhausted by the demands of the Liver, the child, which is in Excess. If the Deficiency of the Lungs is here a separate problem, unrelated to the imbalances of Kidneys and Liver, it may need separate treatment. For this patient, reducing LR.2 the Sedation point of the

Liver, may be enough to resolve the problems of both Liver and Kidneys, but it may be necessary to reinforce LU.9, the Tonification point, to treat the separate problem of the Lungs.

Again, if there is doubt, it may be better to use the Tonification or Sedation points for all affected organs.

WITHIN ELEMENT AND BETWEEN ELEMENTS TREATMENTS

WITHIN ELEMENT TREATMENTS

So far we have been discussing Within Element treatments, that is when the points used for each affected organ are on the channel of that organ only. For example, if the Kidneys are Deficient or Excess, we use the Tonification point KI.7 or the Sedation point KI.1, respectively, and not the points of any other channels. Figure 9.2, shows the 12 organs as they are linked by the Promotion and Control cycles. In fact, each organ system has within it each of the Five Elements, linked by its own *internal* Promotion and Control cycles. Each of the Five Elements within an organ system is represented by the five Transporting points on the channel of the organ. This is shown in Figure 9.3, where for simplicity only the five main Yin organs are included, although the same principle applies to each of the 12 organs.

THE ELEMENT POINTS

In Figure 9.3, the Tonification, Sedation, Element and Control points have been marked. The Element point for an organ is the point of the same Element as that organ. For example, SP.3, the Earth point, is the Element point of the Spleen which is an Earth organ. Also, KI.10 the Water point, is the Element point of the Kidneys which are a Water organ.

Table 9.4 shows the Element points for each channel.

Table 9.4 The Element points

Channel	Element point	Element
KI	Water	KI.10
BL	Water	BL.66
HT	Fire	HT.8
SI	Fire	SI.5
PC	Fire	PC.8
TE	Fire	TE.6
LR	Wood	LR.1
GB	Wood	GB.41
SP	Earth	SP.3
ST	Earth	ST.36
LU	Metal	LU.8
LI	Metal	LI.1

BETWEEN ELEMENTS TREATMENT

In a Within Element treatment we use points on the channel of the affected organ. If the organ is Deficient, we reinforce the Tonification point of the channel, and if the organ is Excess we reduce the Sedation point of the channel. For example, for Heart Deficiency, we reinforce HT.9, the Tonification point, and for Heart Excess we reduce HT.7, the Sedation point.

In a Between Elements treatment, we use the Element point of the organ preceding or succeeding the affected organ in the Promotion cycle. If an organ is Deficient, we reinforce the Element point of the preceding or mother organ. If an organ is Excess, we reduce the Element point of the succeeding or child organ. For example, for Heart Deficiency, we reinforce LR.1, the Wood point since it is the Element point of the Liver, which is a Wood organ and the mother of the Heart. For Heart Excess we reduce SP.3, the Earth point, since it is the Element point of the Spleen, which is an Earth organ and the child of the Heart.

Tables 9.5 and 9.6 explain the Between Elements treatments for Deficiency and Excess respectively, and Table 9.7 is a summary.

WITHIN ELEMENT OR BETWEEN ELEMENTS?

Both Within Element and Between Elements treatments are methods based on the Five Element rule of Mother–Child on the Promotion cycle. The question is when it is better to use a Within Element treatment and when it is better to use a Between Elements treatment.

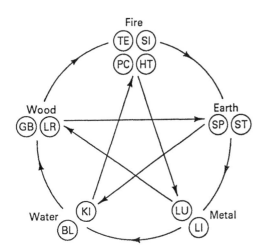

Fig. 9.2 The Five Elements and the 12 organs.

Table 9.5 Between Elements treatments: Deficiency

Channel	Element of channel	Preceding element	Element point of preceding channel
KI	Water	Metal	LU.8
BL	Water	Metal	LI.1
HT	Fire	Wood	LR.1
SI	Fire	Wood	GB.41
PC	Fire	Wood	LR.1
TE	Fire	Wood	GB.41
LR	Wood	Water	KI.10
GB	Wood	Water	BL.66
SP	Earth	Fire	HT.8
ST	Earth	Fire	SI.5
LU	Metal	Earth	SP.3
LI	Metal	Earth	ST.36

Table 9.6 Between Elements treatments: Excess

Channel	Element of channel	Succeeding element	Element point of succeeding channel
KI	Water	Wood	LR.1
BL	Water	Wood	GB.41
HT	Fire	Earth	SP.3
SI	Fire	Earth	ST.36
PC	Fire	Earth	SP.3
TE	Fire	Earth	ST.36
LR	Wood	Fire	HT.8
GB	Wood	Fire	SI.5
SP	Earth	Metal	LU.8
ST	Earth	Metal	LI.1
LU	Metal	Water	KI.10
LI	Metal	Water	BL.66

Table 9.7 Between Elements treatments: Summary

Channel	For Deficiency reinforce	For Excess reduce
KI	LU.8	LR.1
BL	LI.1	GB.41
HT	LR.1	SP.3
SI	GB.41	ST.36
PC	LR.1	SP.3
TE	GB.41	ST.36
LR	KI.10	HT.8
GB	BL.66	SI.5
SP	HT.8	LU.8
ST	SI.5	LI.1
LU	SP.3	KI.10
LI	ST.36	BL.66

WITHIN ELEMENT TREATMENTS PREFERRED

When only one or two organs are affected and the practitioner prefers not to disturb healthy organs, a Within Element treatment is better, since only points on the affected channels are used.

If an organ is Excess, but its child is Deficient, it is not wise to use the Between Elements treatment to sedate the mother, since this involves reducing the Element point of the child, which is already Deficient. It is better to use the Sedate Mother–Tonify Child method as shown on page 81.

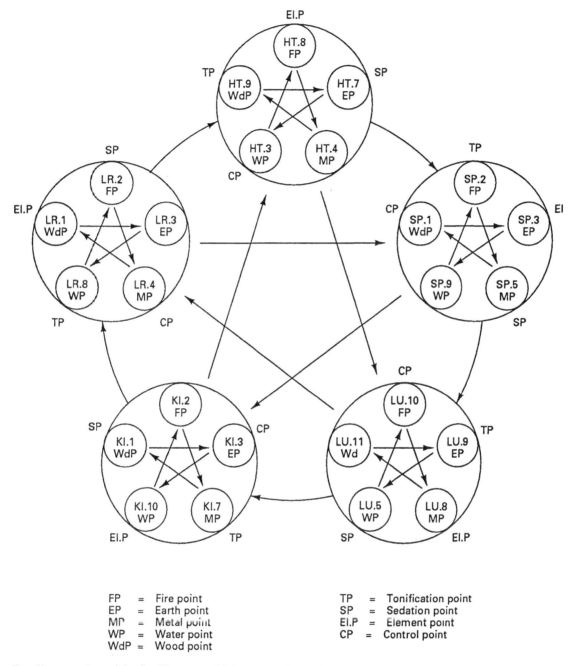

FP = Fire point
EP = Earth point
MP = Metal point
WP = Water point
WdP = Wood point

TP   = Tonification point
SP   = Sedation point
El.P = Element point
CP   = Control point

Fig. 9.3 The Five Element points of the five Yin organs. FP, Fire point; EP, Earth point; MP Metal point; WP, Water point; WdP, Wood point; TP, Tonification point; SP, Sedation point; ElP, Element point; CP, Control point.

BETWEEN ELEMENTS TREATMENTS PREFERRED

If the preceding or succeeding organs are also affected, or are involved in the disharmony, then a Between Elements treatment may be better. For example, if both Spleen and Lung are Deficient, then it may be most effective to reinforce the Element point of the Spleen, SP.3, to tonify the Lungs and decrease the strain on the mother in supplying an exhausted child.

COMBINING WITHIN ELEMENT AND BETWEEN ELEMENT TREATMENTS

If an organ is Deficient, for example Deficient Lungs, it may be best to combine the two types of treatment to tonify the organ:

Within Elements	reinforce LU.9	Tonification point of Lungs
Between Elements	reinforce SP.3	Element point of preceding organ.

THE FOUR NEEDLE METHOD

The combination of Within Element and Between Elements treatments is here called the Four Needle method, since it uses two points bilaterally, for example LU.9 on the left and right and SP.3 on the left and right. It is a useful method which combines the advantage of each form of treatment.

The Four Needle method can also be used for Excess, for example, Excess Lungs:

Within Element	reduce LU.5	Sedation point of Lungs
Between Elements	reduce KI.10	Element point of succeeding organ.

Table 9.8 summarizes the Four Needle method for each channel.

Table 9.8 The Four Needle method: combining the Within and Between Elements treatments

Channel	Deficiency		Excess	
	Within Reinforce Tonification pt	**Between** Reinforce Element pt	**Within** Reduce Sedation pt	**Between** Reduce Element pt
KI	KI.7	LU.8	KI.1	LR.1
BL	BL.67	LI.1	BL.65	GB.41
HT	HT.9	LR.1	HT.7	SP.3
SI	SI.3	GB.41	SI.8	ST.36
PC	PC.9	LR.1	PC.7	SP.3
TE	TE.3	GB.41	TE.10	ST.36
LR	LR.8	KI.10	LR.2	HT.8
GB	GB.43	BL.66	GB.38	SI.5
SP	SP.2	HT.8	SP.5	LU.8
ST	ST.41	SI.5	ST.45	LI.1
LU	LU.9	SP.3	LU.5	KI.10
LI	LI.11	ST.36	LI.2	BL.66

Caution

For treating Excess, the Between Elements method, and the Four Needle method, which includes the Between Elements method, both involve reducing the Element point of the succeeding organ. This can be done when the succeeding organ is also in Excess, but should not be done when the succeeding organ is Deficient.

In the example of Excess Lungs above, KI.10 should not be reduced if the Kidneys are Deficient.

TWO EXAMPLES OF THE FOUR NEEDLE METHOD

A patient comes with a severe headache and periodic outbursts of anger. The diagnosis was Liver Excess. According to the Four Needle method the practitioner reduced LR.2 and HT.8.

Another patient complained of ache and coldness in the lower back which was worse with tiredness. The diagno-sis was Kidney Deficiency. According to the Four Needle method the practitioner reinforced KI.7 and LU.8.

COMBINATIONS OF EXCESS AND DEFICIENCY AND THE PROMOTION CYCLE

ORGAN AND PULSE

Simple Five Element treatments are based on whether an organ is Deficient or Excess. This may be reflected in pulse volumes of Empty and Full respectively, and indicated by – or +, as shown:

Organ	Deficiency	Excess	Health
Pulse	Empty	Full	Normal
Symbol	–	+	✓

TWO-ORGAN RELATIONSHIPS

There are various possible relationships between two adjacent organs on the Promotion cycle, with respect to Deficiency, Excess and Normality, as indicated by –, + and ✓. Six of the main possibilities, which are illustrated in Figure 9.4, will be discussed.

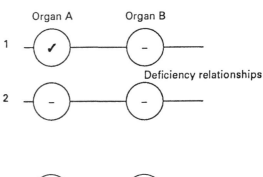
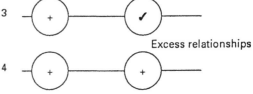
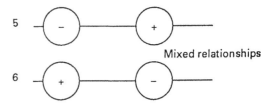

Fig. 9.4 Two-organ relationships.

DEFICIENCY RELATIONSHIPS

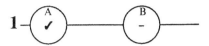

This is a situation where only one organ, the child, is affected, and the mother organ is healthy. Therefore the best treatment may be a Within Element treatment to reinforce the Tonification point of organ B, since this does not directly interfere with the healthy organ A.

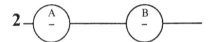

In this situation, where both mother and child are Deficient, it may be enough to reinforce the Tonification point of organ A, the mother, which will then nourish the child. However, this may not be enough, and it may be better to use a Four Needle treatment, reinforcing the Element point of A and the Tonification point of B. Another possibility would be to reinforce the Tonification points of both organs.

EXCESS RELATIONSHIPS

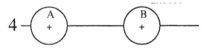

This situation resembles **1** above, since only one organ is affected. This time it is the mother which is in Excess, while the child is healthy. Therefore the best treatment may be a Within Element treatment to reduce the Sedation point of organ A, since this does not directly interfere with the healthy organ B.

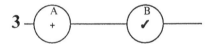

In this situation, where both mother and child are in Excess, the best treatment may be a Four Needle treatment, reducing the Sedation point of organ A and the Element point of organ B.

MIXED RELATIONSHIPS

Here, the mother is Deficient and the child is Excess. This

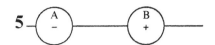

may be because the child is hyperactive and is draining the mother. The first step must be to sedate the child. To tonify the mother whilst the child is hyperactive may not correct the situation but simply add fuel to the fire. So first reduce the Sedation point of the child. When the child is healthy, the mother can be tonified, if necessary, by reinforcing the Tonification point of the mother organ.

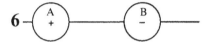

Here the mother is Excess and the child is Deficient. This is often due to an energy block between the two organs in the Promotion cycle, where energy builds up in the mother without moving on to the child. For example, energy accumulates in the Liver as anger, and does not progress round the cycle to manifest as joy, the emotion of the Heart.

SEDATE MOTHER–TONIFY CHILD METHOD

In the opinion of the author, it would be incorrect to use the Between Elements or the Four Needle methods here, since these involve reducing the Element point of the child, which is already Deficient. It would be better to use the method of Sedate Mother–Tonify Child. In this method, the Sedation point of the mother is reduced, as in the Four Needle Method, but then the Tonification point of the child is reinforced. This treatment will draw energy from the mother into the child by opening both ends of the energy block.

For example, a patient has great worry and overconcern about her family, she has abdominal distension and cough, associated with Excess Spleen and Deficient Lungs. According to the method of Sedate Mother–Tonify Child, SP.5 is reduced and LU.9 reinforced (see Fig. 9.5).

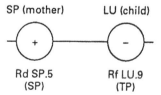

Fig. 9.5

The Between Elements method, and the Four Needle system, which combines the Within Element and Be-

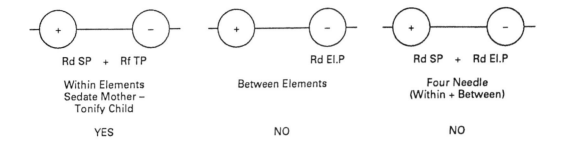

Rd SP + Rf TP

Within Elements
Sedate Mother –
Tonify Child

YES

Rd El.P

Between Elements

NO

Rd SP + Rd El.P

Four Needle
(Within + Between)

NO

Fig. 9.6

tween Elements systems, both involve reducing the Element point of the child. This is best in situation **4** (see Fig. 9.4), when both mother and child are Excess. It can also be used in situation **3**, but with caution since it involves reducing the Element point of a healthy child. As stated it is not suitable for situation **6**.

The same caution applies to the Eight Needle method on page 84.

THE CONTROL CYCLE

Classically, the mother nourishes and the grandmother controls. These opposite influences create a natural balance. Two main imbalances can occur, Under Control and Over Control.

UNDER CONTROL

Each organ controls the next-but-one in the Promotion cycle, i.e. the grandmother controls the grandchild. For example, Liver controls Spleen, and is controlled by the Lungs.

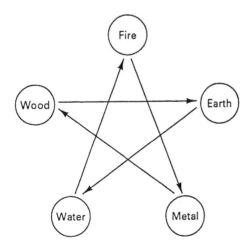

Fig. 9.7 The Control cycle.

If the Liver becomes Deficient, then it may not be able to control the Spleen, which then becomes Excess. The patient may then irritate others by sweet, sugary niceness and overconcerned, intrusive behaviour.

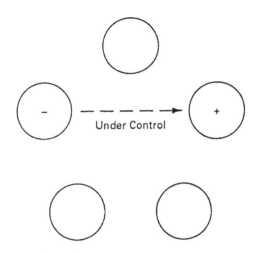

Fig. 9.8 Under Control.

Alternatively, the Spleen may become Excess and create imbalance and Deficiency in the Liver, For example, the patient may become lazy and lethargic, ignoring the need for careful planning and organization.

OVER CONTROL

Here we have the opposite situation of grandmother Excess and child Deficient, of which the Liver–Spleen relationship is an excellent example. The Liver naturally tends to Hyperactivity and Excess, and the Spleen tends to Deficiency. It is very common for an Excess Liver to invade a Deficient Spleen, with signs such as headache, loss of appetite and lethargy.

CONTROL POINTS

Each organ has an internal Promotion cycle and an

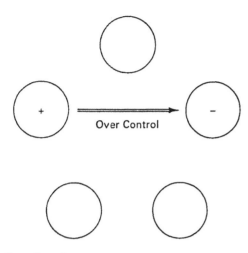

Fig. 9.9 Over Control.

internal Control cycle (see Fig. 9.2) For example, the Heart is a Fire organ, and on the Heart's internal Control cycle, Water is the controlling element, so that the Control point of the Heart is HT.3, the Water point on the Heart channel. The Control points are summarized in Table 9.9.

Table 9.9 The Control points

Channel	Element of channel	Controlling Element	Control point
KI	Water	Earth	KI.3
BL	Water	Earth	BL.40
HT	Fire	Water	HT.3
SI	Fire	Water	SI.2
PC	Fire	Water	PC.3
TE	Fire	Water	TE.2
LR	Wood	Metal	LR.4
GB	Wood	Metal	GB.44
SP	Earth	Wood	SP.1
ST	Earth	Wood	ST.43
LU	Metal	Fire	LU.10
LI	Metal	Fire	LI.5

UNDER CONTROL: THE BASIC TREATMENT

The basic treatment is to reinforce the Control point of the grandchild and to reinforce the element point of the grandmother. For example, Water, the Kidneys, is not controlling Fire, the Heart. The patient is hot, overexcitable, but tired. The principle is to strengthen Water to control Fire. This is done by reinforcing HT.3, the Control point of the Heart, and by reinforcing KI.10, the Element point of the Kidneys.

Reinforcing HT.3 is the Within Element part of the treatment, since HT.3 is the Water point of the Heart, the Control point on the Heart's internal Control cycle. Reinforcing KI.10 is the Between Elements part of the treatment, since KI.10 is the Water point of the Kidneys, the Element point, that can strengthen the Kidneys so that it can control its grandchild, the Heart.

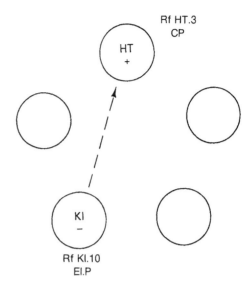

Fig. 9.10 Under Control: the basic treatment.

OVER CONTROL: THE BASIC TREATMENT

The basic treatment is to reduce the Control point of the grandchild and to reduce the Element point of the grandmother.

For example, Water, the Kidneys, is overcontrolling fire, the Heart. The patient is cold and apathetic. The principle is to sedate Water, to normalize the control of Fire. This is done by reducing HT.3, the Control point of the Heart, and by reducing KI.10, the Element point of the Kidneys.

Reducing HT.3 is the Within Element part of the treatment since HT.3 is the Water point of the Heart, the Control point on the Heart's internal Control cycle. Reducing KI.10 is the Between Elements part of the treatment since KI.10 is the Water point of the Kidneys,

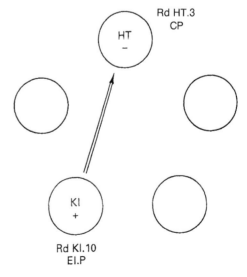

Fig. 9.11 Over Control: the basic treatment.

the Element point, and reducing it will reduce the overcontrol of Fire by Water.

COMPARISON OF UNDER AND OVER CONTROL

In both Under and Over Control, we use the Control point of the grandchild and the Element point of the grandmother. In Under Control we reinforce these points to increase the control of the grandchild by the grandmother, and in Over Control we reduce these points to decrease this control.

For example, if the Kidney is being undercontrolled by the Spleen, with the Kidney in Excess and the Spleen Deficient, we reinforce KI.3, the Control point of the Kidney, and SP.3, the Element point of the Spleen. If the Kidney is being overcontrolled by the Spleen, with the Kidney Deficient and the Spleen in Excess, we reduce these same points.

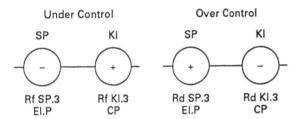

Fig. 9.12 Comparison of Under and Over Control.

UNDER CONTROL: EIGHT NEEDLE METHOD

The Eight Needle treatment for Under Control is simply the Four Needle treatment plus the basic treatment for Under Control described earlier.

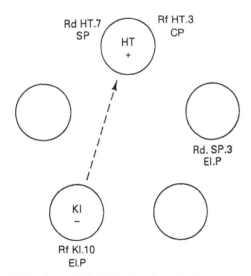

Fig. 9.13 Under Control: the Eight Needle method.

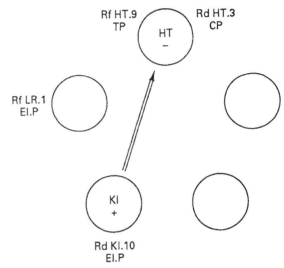

Fig. 9.14 Over Control: the Eight Needle method.

For the example of Kidney not controlling Heart, we reinforce HT.3 and KI.10 as in the basic Under Control treatment. Also, we reduce HT.7 and SP.3, as in a Four Needle treatment for Excess where we reduce the Sedation point of the affected organ, and reduce the Element point of the child.

OVER CONTROL: EIGHT NEEDLE METHOD

The Eight Needle treatment for Over Control is the Four Needle treatment plus the basic treatment for Over Control described earlier.

For the example of Kidney overcontrolling Heart, we reduce HT.3 and KI.10, as in the basic Over Control treatment. Also, we reinforce HT.9 and LR.1, as in a Four Needle treatment for Deficiency, where we reinforce the Tonification point of the affected organ and reinforce the Element point of the mother.

The Eight Needle method is so called because it uses four points bilaterally. As discussed, it is a progression of the Four Needle method described on page 80. Table 9.10 summarizes the Eight Needle combinations for Deficiency and Excess.

WHEN TO USE THE EIGHT NEEDLE METHOD

This method has already been described for Over Control and Under Control, and the examples of Heart Deficiency and Heart Excess have been given.

Simple Excess or Deficiency

It is possible to use this complex method for Deficiency or

Table 9.10 The Eight Needle method

Channel	Deficiency (Over Control)				Excess (Under Control)			
	Reinforce		Reduce		Reduce		Reinforce	
	TP g'child (WE)	ElP of mother (BE)	CP g'child (WE)	ElP of g'mother (BE)	SP g'child (WE)	ElP of child (BE)	CP g'child (WE)	ElP of g'mother (BE)
KI	KI.7	LU.8	KI.3	SP.3	KI.1	LR.1	KI.3	SP.3
BL	BL.67	LI.1	BL.40	ST.36	BL.65	GB.41	BL.40	ST.36
HT	HT.9	LR.1	HT.3	KI.10	HT.7	SP.3	HT.3	KI.10
SI	SI.3	GB.41	SI.2	BL.66	SI.8	ST.36	SI.2	BL.66
PC	PC.9	LR.1	PC.3	KI.10	PC.7	SP.3	PC.3	KI.10
TE	TE.3	GB.41	TE.2	BL.66	TE.10	ST.36	TE.2	BL.66
LR	LR.8	KI.10	LR.4	LU.8	LR.2	HT.8	LR.4	LU.8
GB	GB.43	BL.66	GB.44	LI.1	GB.38	SI.5	GB.44	LI.1
SP	SP.2	HT.8	SP.1	LR.1	SP.5	LU.8	SP.1	LR.1
ST	ST.41	SI.5	ST.43	GB.41	ST.45	LI.1	ST.43	GB.41
LU	LU.9	SP.3	LU.10	HT.8	LU.5	KI.10	LU.10	HT.8
LI	LI.11	ST.36	LI.5	SI.5	LI.2	BL.66	LI.5	SI.5

TP, Tonification point; SP, Sedation point; WE, Within Element; CP, Control point; ElP, Element point; BE, Between Elements.

Excess of a single organ, e.g. Deficiency or Excess of Heart, but this would only be done if simpler methods, e.g. Within Element, Between Elements, or Four Needle method, were unsuccessful.

Control cycle imbalances

The Eight Needle method is best used when there is an imbalance on the Control cycle, of either Under or Over Control. In this case, two organs, the grandmother and grandchild are imbalanced. For example, the Kidney–Heart situations discussed earlier.

Complex Promotion and Control cycle imbalances

The Eight Needle method can be effective when there are complex imbalances of the organs.

EIGHT NEEDLE METHOD FOR DEFICIENCY

This is appropriate if it is a problem of Kidney overcontrolling Heart. It is not so appropriate if it is an energy block between Kidney and Liver, so that Liver and Heart are starved of energy. In this case, it would be better to reduce the Sedation point of Kidney and reinforce the Tonification point of Liver.

EIGHT NEEDLE METHOD FOR EXCESS

This may be appropriate if Spleen is Excess, but if Spleen is Deficient, then it might be unwise to reduce an already Deficient organ. This is the same caution as for the use of Between Elements and Four Needle techniques on page 80.

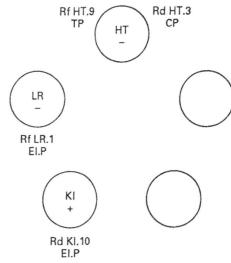

Rf HT.9
TP

Rd HT.3
CP

HT
−

LR
−

Rf LR.1
El.P

KI
+

Rd KI.10
El.P

Fig. 9.15 The Eight Needle method for Deficiency.

COMBINING POINTS ON THE UPPER AND LOWER LIMBS

Acupuncture treatments can often be made more effective by combining points on the arms and legs. The exception to this is when the treatment aims to direct energy to the upper or lower body specifically, and then points on arms or legs only may be used.

The majority of point selections in the Four Needle method combine points on the arms with points on the legs (see Table 9.8). For example, the points for Lung Deficiency are LU.9 and SP.3, and the points for Lung Excess are LU.5 and KI.10.

Even if the Four Needle or Eight Needle methods are not used, simple Five Element treatments can be enhanced if Tonification or Sedation points are used from channels on both arms and legs. For example, the

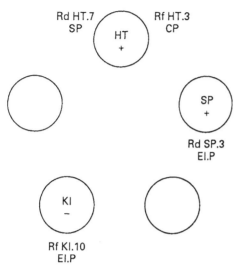

Fig 9.16 The Eight Needle method for Excess.

Tonification points SP.2 and LU.9, to tonify Spleen and Lungs, or the Sedation points LR.2 and HT.7, to sedate Liver and Heart.

FIVE ELEMENTS AND THE SIX DIVISIONS

A more sophisticated method of combining Five Element points on arms and legs, is to combine points according to their relationships not only on the Five Element cycles but also according to the Six Divisions (see Table 9.11).

For example, we can reduce the Sedation points TE.10 and GB.38, for Gallbladder Fire associated with ear inflammation, since Gallbladder and Triple Energizer are related by the Six Divisions and their channels surround the ear.

As another example, we can reinforce the Tonification

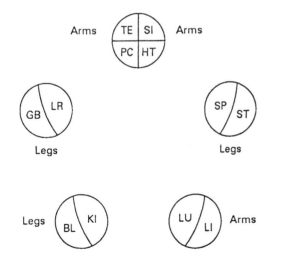

Fig. 9.17 Treatment on arms and legs.

Table 9.11 Five Elements and Six Divisions

Division	Legs	Arms	Type of Five Element relationship
Yang channels			
Greater Yang	BL (Water)	SI (Fire)	control
Bright Yang	ST (Earth)	LI (Metal)	mother–child
Lesser Yang	GB (Wood)	TE (Fire)	mother–child
Yin channels			
Greater Yin	SP (Earth)	LU (Metal)	mother–child
Lesser Yin	KI (Water)	HT (Fire)	control
Terminal Yin	LR (Wood)	PC (Fire)	mother–child

points BL.67 and SI.3 for neck stiffness associated with deficient Bladder channel, since we have points on both arms and legs that are related by the Six Divisions, and also SI.3 is specific for neck problems.

CRITICAL ASSESSMENT OF TONIFICATION AND SEDATION POINTS

In most cases, the use of the Five Element points of Tonification and Sedation does not correspond with the traditional functions and indications of these points, as listed in textbooks.

TONIFICATION POINTS

As shown in Table 9.12, of the 12 Tonification points, only three have the listed function of tonifying their respective organ, and the other nine are mainly listed for sedation. In the table, the column 'Yes/No' indicates whether or not the Tonification point has the listed function of tonifying its respective organ, and the column 'Main points' gives the points that are generally used to tonify this organ. For example, ST.36 is generally considered a far more powerful point to tonify the Spleen than SP.2, which outside the Five Element system is generally used with reducing method to cool Heat in the Blood.

SEDATION POINTS

Of the 12 sedation points, six have the listed main function of sedating their respective organs: KI.1, PC.7, LR.2, GB.38, ST.45, LU.5. However, LI.1, LR.2, GB.38 and ST.45 can also be used with Reinforcing method and moxa to tonify the Fire and Yang of their respective organs, and LU.5 can also be used with Reinforcing method to tonify Lung Yin.

SUMMARY

This does not mean that the Five Element system of

Table 9.12 Assessment of Tonification points

Tonification point	Element of point	Other point function	Indications for Tonification		Assessment
			Yes/No	Main points	
KI.7	Metal		Yes	KI.3, BL.23	Not so much to tonify Kidney Qi, more with Rf M to tonify Kidney Yang and firm Kidney Qi. Also Rd to drain Damp Heat
BL.67	Metal		No	BL.64, CV.4	Not much used to tonify Bladder Qi, mainly Rd for Excess Wind and Heat, or E M to clear mental stagnation
HT.9	Wood	Well	No	HT.7, BL.15	Mainly Rd or B as Well point to remove acute Heart Fire. Can be Rf M for Deficient Heart Fire
SI.3	Wood	Opening point Governor	No	ST.36, ST.25	Mainly Rd for Excess Governor conditions, or for hand or neck problems
PC.9	Wood	Well	No	PC.7, HT.7	Mainly Rd or B as Well point to remove acute Fire and Wind. Can be Rf M for Deficient Heart Fire
TE.3	Wood		No	TE.4, BL.22	Mainly Rd to clear Wind, Heat and Damp Heat from ears and eyes
LR.8	Water		Yes	LR.8, BL.18	Main point to tonify Liver Blood and Yin and cool Liver Deficiency Fire, since it is the Water point, but not to tonify Liver Qi
GB.43	Water		No	GB.40, BL.19	Mainly Rd for Liver Yang or Damp Heat
SP.2	Fire	Spring	No	SP.3, ST.36	Mainly Rd for Heat in the Blood, or Rf to tonify Spleen Yang. Not to tonify Spleen Qi
ST.41	Fire		No	ST.36, CV.12	Mainly Rd for Stomach Fire or for ankle arthritis
LU.9	Earth	Source	Yes	LU.9, BL.13	Much used to tonify Deficient Lung Qi, since it is the Source point
LI.11	Earth		No	ST.36, LI.4	Can be Rf to tonify Large Intestine, but mostly Rd for Heat in the Blood, or E M to clear mental stagnation

Rd, Reducing method; Rf, Reinforcing method; E, Even method; M, moxa; B, bleeding.

Table 9.13 Assessment of Sedation points

Sedation point	Element of point	Other point function	Indications for Sedation		Assessment
			Yes/No	Main points	
KI.1	Wood	Well	Yes	KI.1, KI.2	Main point to drain Excess Fire from Kidney, Liver and Heart, since it is a Well point. Can Rf M to tonify Kidney Fire
BL.65	Wood		not a main point	BL.60, BL.62	Can be Rd for Wind Heat, but not a main point to sedate Bladder
HT.7	Earth	Source	sometimes	HT.5, HT.6	Mainly Rf as a Source point to tonify Heart Qi and Blood. Also Rd to calm the mind
SI.8	Earth		sometimes	ST.25, ST.39	Mainly Rd for local elbow problems
PC.7	Earth	Source	sometimes	PC.8, PC.9	Rd to calm the mind like HT.7, but not for acute Excess, when PC.3, 4, 5, 6, 8 and 9 are better
TE.10	Earth		not a main point	TE.5, TE.6	Can be Rd for Wind Heat, but mainly local point for elbow problems
LR.2	Fire	Spring	Yes	LR.2, LR.3	The main point to disperse Liver Fire, since it is a Spring and a Fire point. LR.3 is better for Hyperactive Liver Yang and Wind
GB.38	Fire		Yes	GB.34, GB.41	Rd for Gallbladder Fire. GB.34 and GB.41 are better for Damp Heat or Hyperactive Liver Yang
SP.5	Metal		No	SP.4, SP.6	Not much used, apart from ankle problems
ST.45	Metal	Well	Yes	ST.40, ST.44	Can be Rd as a Well point, to calm and clear the mind
LU.5	Water		Yes	LU.6, LU.7	Rd for Lung Heat. Also Rf to tonify Lung Yin to cool Lung Fire
LI.2	Water	Spring	not a main point	LI.11, ST.37	Can be Rd for Wind Heat, but not a main point to sedate Large Intestine

Rd, Reducing method; Rf, Reinforcing method; M, Moxa.

Tonification and Sedation points is incorrect, but it does mean that it can be used selectively for best effect. For example, for Deficient Lungs, the Five Element system may be a good choice, since LU.9 is a Source point and is listed for strengthening the Lungs. However, for Deficient Stomach, the Five Element system may not be such a good choice, since ST.41, as the Fire point of the Stomach, is mainly used for sedating Stomach Fire, and ST.36 is a more powerful point to strengthen the Stomach.

The question of when and when not to use the Five Element system is discussed in more detail in the next section.

When to use the Five Element system

INTRODUCTION

DEFINITION

The Five Element system is here defined as the specific system of point choice based on the theory of the Promotion and Control cycles, involving use of the Tonification, Sedation, Element and Control points.

GENERAL

In the past, the Five Element system has often been used in the West with inflexibility and fanaticism combined with an ignorance of other systems. A more tolerant and informed atmosphere is now developing, where the different systems of acupuncture are each seen to be useful alternative treatment strategies and not exclusive divine law. For example, the systems of Five Elements, Eight Principles and Eight Extra channels each have their strengths and weaknesses, and each have their areas of application.

This section examines the situations in which the Five Element system is most suitable. What follows is the opinion of the author based on his experience. It can be used as a guideline, or as a starting point to provoke thought or discussion; it is not meant to represent unassailable fact.

THE KEY

The two main guidelines for use of the Five element system are:

  energy blocks between two or more organs
  correspondence with the traditional functions of the points.

ENERGY BLOCKS BETWEEN TWO OR MORE ORGANS

The basis of Five Element physiology is the energy communication between organs. Five Element pathology deals with energy blocks between the organs on the Promotion and Control cycles. Five Element treatments are most applicable when there is a block in the flow of energy between two or more organs.

Tonification points link the affected organ and the preceding organ on the Promotion cycle, and Sedation points link the affected organ with the succeeding organ on the cycle. For example, use of the Tonification point HT.9, links the Heart, the child, with the mother organ, the Liver.

CORRESPONDENCE WITH THE TRADITIONAL FUNCTIONS OF THE POINTS

In the past, the Tonification and Sedation points of the Five Element system have usually been used in Five Element treatments without regard for the traditional functions of the individual points. For example, HT.9 is often used as the Tonification point to tonify Heart Deficiency, without regard for either the type of Deficiency or the traditional functions of HT.9 outside of the Five Element system. The main traditional function of HT.9 is as a Well point, to disperse severe acute conditions of Excess Heart Fire, not as a point to strengthen Heart Qi. HT.9 can be used to tonify, but mainly in two specific ways, relating to its functions as a Well point. Firstly, it can be used with moxa, or Reinforcing method and moxa, to tonify Heart Yang and Heart Fire. Second, it can be used with Even method to move Stagnation of Heart Qi associated with Deficient Heart Qi.

This means that the Five Element system can be used selectively. HT.9 can be used as a Tonification point when either there is Deficient Heart Fire or Stagnation of Heart Qi. However, HT.9 may not be appropriate as a Tonification point for Deficient Heart Qi, Deficient Heart Blood or Deficient Heart Yin. In these three cases, it may be better not to use the Five Element system, but to select points according to more specific criteria, e.g. HT.7 for Deficient Heart Qi and Blood or HT.6 or HT.3 for Deficient Heart Yin.

THE FIVE ELEMENT SYSTEM AND EXTERIOR CONDITIONS

The Five Element system is for Interior conditions, and is not appropriate for Exterior conditions such as Wind Cold, Wind Heat or Summer Heat.

THE FIVE ELEMENT SYSTEM AND CHANNEL PROBLEMS

Illnesses can be divided into:

organ problems
channel problems
channel and organ problems.

ORGAN PROBLEMS

These are problems where the main imbalance and symptoms are of the organ not the channel. The main use of the Five Element system is for organ problems, especially those with a strong psychological component, where the problem arises, not so much from single Excess or Deficiency, but from an energy block between two or more organs.

CHANNEL PROBLEMS

These are problems of pain or difficulty along the course of the channel in which there is no organic involvement. In the opinion of the author the Five Element system is not so effective for channel problems, which are more successfully treated by a combination of Ah Shi points and local and distal points on the channel affected.

The first step is correctly to identify the channel or channels affected. The second step is to use distal empirical points where appropriate, for example ST.38 for 'frozen shoulder'. The third step is then to use Ah Shi points plus local and distal points on the affected channel.

For the distal points, some practitioners use the Well points while other practitioners use the Tonification or Sedation points. However, the author uses those distal points on the affected channel that have specific effect on the problem area of the body. For example, for toothache around LI.19, LI.4 would be chosen as the distal point, since of all the distal Large Intestine points, LI.4 has greatest effect on the teeth and jaw. For chest pain around SP.21, SP.4 would be chosen as the distal point, since it is the distal Spleen point with greatest effect on the chest.

CHANNEL AND ORGAN PROBLEMS

These are of two types:

channel and organ problems unrelated
channel and organ problems related.

Where channel and organ problems are unrelated, the Five Element system is inappropriate for the channel problem, although it may be used for the problem of the organ. The channel problem can be treated by the system above. Where channel and organ problems are related, the Five Element system can be used, if appropriate, as a basis for treatment of both channel and organ, but in most cases, Ah Shi points and local points on the affected channel, will also be required.

For Example, a patient has chronic back pain at the level of BL.24, associated with Deficient Kidney. KI.7, the Tonification point could be used with Reinforcing method. However, the treatment is generally far more effective when BL.24 and Ah Shi points are added to KI.7, and even better when a distal point such as BL.59, 60 or 64 is also used on the affected channel.

THE FIVE ELEMENTS AND DEFICIENCY, EXCESS, STAGNATION AND IRREGULARITY

THE FIVE ELEMENT SYSTEM AND DEFICIENCY

Two main situations will be discussed:

moderate Deficiency of one or two organs
severe Deficiency of most or all organs.

MODERATE DEFICIENCY OF ONE OR TWO ORGANS

In this situation, the Within Element, Between Elements or Four Needle methods can be used, as appropriate. However, there is a variety of other systems for treating Deficiency, for example:

Source points
Back Transporting points
CV or GV points, at the anatomical level of the organ
Well points
Element points according to the season or to the Chinese clock
Eight Extra channel combinations
Specific point functions, e.g. ST.36 for general Deficiency
Specific point combinations e.g. ST.36 + LI.4 for Deficient Qi and Blood.

The Five Element system is best used for Deficiency, when the Deficiency relates to a lack of flow between two adjacent organs on the Promotion cycle e.g. Lungs and Kidneys. In this case, the Tonification point, KI.7, may be the most effective treatment.

SEVERE DEFICIENCY OF MOST OR ALL ORGANS

In this situation the author would not use the Five Element system. He would use either the combination of Source points and Back Transporting points, or the combination of Eight Extra channels and Conception channel points.

For example, for severe combined Deficiencies of Kidneys, Spleen and Lungs, either of the combinations below can be used, or they can be alternated:

Source points + Back Transporting points
KI.3, SP.3, LU.9 + BL.23, BL.20, BL.13

or:

Eight Extra points + CV points
SP.4, PC.6 + CV.4, CV.12, CV.17

In the author's opinion, these combinations are more powerful than the Five Element system in treating severe Deficiency.

THE FIVE ELEMENT SYSTEM AND EXCESS

Two main situations are discussed here:

chronic Excess of one or more organs
severe, acute Excess.

CHRONIC EXCESS OF ONE OR MORE ORGANS

In this situation the Within Element, Between Elements or Four Needle methods can be used as appropriate. However, there are other systems for treating Excess for example:

Accumulation points
Back Transporting points
Alarm points
CV or GV points at the anatomical level of the organ
Well points
Spring points
Eight Extra channel combinations
Specific point functions, e.g. LI.11 to clear Heat in the Blood
Specific point combinations, e.g. SP.6 + SP.9 to clear Damp.

The comparative functions of these different systems are shown in Table 9.14. The Five Element system is best used for Excess, when the Excess relates to a block in the flow between two adjacent organs on the Promotion cycle, for example, Liver and Heart. In this case, the Sedation point, LR.2, may be the most effective treatment.

SEVERE, ACUTE EXCESS

In this situation, the author would not use the Five Element system being of the opinion that reducing either the Well points or the Accumulation points would have a more rapid and powerful effect.

THE FIVE ELEMENT SYSTEM FOR MIXED EXCESS AND DEFICIENCY

This refers to situations where some organs are Deficient and other organs are Excess. It does not refer to situations where Yin–Yang pairs are in disharmony, e.g. Liver in Excess and Gallbladder Deficient, since these would be better treated by using the Connecting points. It does not refer to situations where one organ alternates between Excess and Deficiency, e.g. the Heart in manic depression, since these would be better treated by using the Source or the Back Transporting points. It does refer to Promotion cycle relationships of the type:

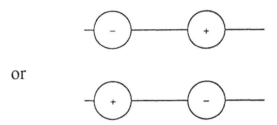

or

and it also refers to Control cycle problems.

PROMOTION CYCLE -/ +

Here the mother is Deficient and the child is Excess. If a hyperactive child is draining the mother, reduction of the Sedation point of the child is a suitable treatment. For example, KI -/ LR +, where there is tiredness and back pain in combination with aggressive hyperactivity; reduce LR.2 the Sedation point of the Liver.

PROMOTION CYCLE + /-

This is the classic situation for use of the Five Element system, an obvious energy block between adjacent organs on the Promotion cycle.

It is incorrect to use the Four Needle method, as discussed on page 80. The ideal treatment is to reduce the Sedation point of the mother and reinforce the Tonification point of the child, to open both ends of the energy block. For example, Lungs Excess and Kidney Deficient, with unexpressed grief accumulating and lack of will power; reduce LU.5 and reinforce KI.7.

CONTROL CYCLE PROBLEMS

If the Liver, Wood, is overcontrolling the Spleen, Earth, and the patient has headache, nausea and loss of appetite, then the basic Five Element treatment is to reduce the Control point of the Spleen, SP.1, and reduce the Element point of the Liver, LR.1. However, this situation could also be treated by reducing LR.3 and reinforcing ST.36, or even better by the combination LR.3, LR.13, PC.6 Rd; ST.36, CV.12 Rf.

In the author's opinion, if the situation was chronic with a moderate headache and moderate nausea, SP.1 and LR.1 is a viable treatment. This is because these are Well points which by moving Stagnation in their respective organs will tend to balance the Liver–Spleen relationship.

If, however, there were severe Stagnation of Liver Qi and Hyperactive Liver Yang, LR.1 alone probably would be insufficient and it probably would also be necessary to reduce LR.3. If these Liver factors invaded the Spleen and Stomach with severe nausea, then LR.13 might need to be added and probably PC.6 also. If there were severe Deficiency of Spleen and Stomach, then it might be better to change SP.1 to ST.36.

In any event, the basic Five Element Control Cycle treatment of LR.1, SP.1 Rd, or even the Eight Needle treatment of LR.1, SP.1 Rd; HT.8, SP.2 Rf might be inadequate in most cases of severe acute headache and nausea, where the alternative combination of LR.3, LR.13, PC.6 Rd; ST.36; CV.12 Rf would be preferable.

THE FIVE ELEMENT SYSTEM AND STAGNATION

Acupuncture is based on the movement of energy and is an effective therapy for removing energy blocks. The Five Element system has its greatest strength in moving energy blocks, but these blocks are specifically between adjacent organs on the Promotion cycle. The Five Element system therefore does not have direct effect on energy blocks at specific joints such as ankles, knees, hips, shoulders, elbows and wrists or between spinal vertebrae. It does not have direct effect on blocks at or between the chakras, or on blocks between the front and back of the body at a specific spinal level.

The Five Element system can have direct effect on blocks between the 12 organs, but its effect on blocks of other kinds is indirect. For example, for a patient with insomnia and loss of appetite, where there is a block between Heart and Spleen, and energy is in Excess in the Heart, the Five Element treatment of HT.7 Rd + SP.2 Rf may be the most effective.

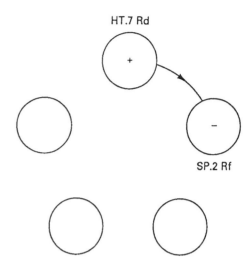

Fig. 9.18 Five Elements and Stagnation.

BLOCK BETWEEN ENERGY CENTRES

However, for a patient with fullness and pain in the chest and obstruction and pain in the throat, associated with the inability to express feelings in a close relationship, HT.7 Rd + SP.2 Rf might be inappropriate. It might be necessary to use CV.17 and CV.23 to work directly on the blocked energy centres and to use points such as HT.5 and LU.7 which have specific effect to release the blocked emotions and free the vocal chords and speech. Here, the block is not between two organs on the Promotion cycle, but at and between two energy centres on the vertical energy axis of the body.

THE FIVE ELEMENT SYSTEM AND IRREGULARITY

Irregularity means a disturbed and irregular movement of Qi, for which the principle of treatment is to calm. If the Irregularity is combined with Deficiency, Excess or Stagnation, then in addition to calming, there must also be strengthening, dispersing or moving respectively as discussed in Chapter 6.

If we look at the combination of Irregularity and Deficiency, we can use the example of disturbance of Heart Spirit associated with Deficient Kidney. In the Five Element system, this would be seen as a case of Under Control, and could be treated by reinforcing the Water points KI.10 and HT.3 (the Element point of the Kidney and the Control point of the Heart).

According to the traditional functions of the points, this Five Element treatment would be especially appropriate for Deficient Yin of the Heart and Kidney, since KI.10 and HT.3 are the Water points. However, this treatment would not be so suitable for Deficient Qi of the Heart and

Kidney, since in this case the Source points, KI.3 and HT.7 might be more effective.

This emphasizes that the Five Element system can be used selectively, and that it may be most effective when the points chosen according to the Five Elements are also indicated according to the traditional functions of the points.

SUMMARY

The Five Element system is most effective when there are energy blocks between two or more organs, and when there is a correspondence between Five Element theory and traditional point functions for each of the points chosen.

A study of Table 9.14 which outlines when to use the Five Element system, shows that in the opinion of the author, the Five Element system may not be appropriate in the following situations: Exterior syndromes, channel problems, severe Deficiency, severe acute Excess, Yin–Yang pair imbalances, mixed Deficiency and Excess in one organ, Stagnation in the joints, Stagnation at and between energy centres. In the opinion of the author the Five Element system can be effective where there are energy blocks between two or more organs, whether associated with moderate Deficiency, moderate Excess, mixed Deficiency and Excess, Stagnation or Irregularity.

COMBINING THE FIVE ELEMENT SYSTEM WITH OTHER METHODS

The Five Element system can be used either alone or in combination with other methods of point choice. However, if it is so combined, *the other methods of point choice used must be secondary to the Five Elements and in harmony with it.* The essence of a good point combination is simplicity and harmony. If the point choice logic becomes too complicated, the practitioner will lose the clear visualization of the treatment and so restrict the flow of energies through practitioner and patient. In the opinion of the author, some systems combine well with the Five Elements, and some do not, as discussed next.

SOURCE POINTS

This is seen as an alternative system to the Five Elements, and the author does not use these two systems in combinations.

CONNECTION POINTS

Connection points can be incorporated into a Five Ele-

ment energy rebalancing, when the problem includes imbalance between a Yin–Yang pair, such as Liver and Gallbladder. For example, where Liver is Excess and Heart and Gallbladder are Deficient, the treatment could be to reduce LR.2, the Sedation point, and to reduce LR.5, the Connecting point of the Liver. If necessary, HT.9, the Tonification point of the Heart, and GB.37, the Connecting point of the Gallbladder, can also be used with Reinforcing method.

ACCUMULATION POINTS

This is an alternative system to the Five Elements, mainly used for severe, acute Excess, and the author does not combine these two systems. The Accumulation points can be used in an early stage of treatment or during an acute phase of the treatment, whilst the Five Element system is more appropriate for more gradual balancing of chronic problems.

WELL POINTS

Because of their powerful effect, the author does not generally combine Well points with Five Element treatments, feeling that the Well points would override the more subtle and gradual effects of the Five Element combinations. The Well points are appropriate not only in acute, severe conditions, but also to powerfully tonify Fire and to move Stagnation.

BACK TRANSPORTING POINTS

The Back Transporting points can be seen as an alternative system, which is superior to the Five Elements for treating severe Excess, severe Deficiency, Exterior Invasion, and mixed conditions of excess and Deficiency of Yin and Yang in one organ. However, the Back Transporting points can also be used as a secondary system to reinforce a Five Element treatment, as in the following examples:

• Reinforce LU.9 the Tonification point of Lungs, and BL.13 the Back Transporting point for the Lungs, to treat Deficient Lungs with grief and withdrawal.

• Reduce LR.2 the Sedation point of Liver and BL.18 the Back Transporting point of the Liver, to treat Excess Liver with anger and generalized muscle tension.

• Reinforce KI.10, the Element point of the Kidney, HT.3, the Control point of the Heart, and BL.23 the Back

Transporting point of the Kidneys, for Under Control of Heart by Kidney, with fear and insomnia.

If preferred, the inner Bladder line can be used for more physical problems and the outer Bladder line for more psychological problems.

WINDOW OF HEAVEN POINTS

These form an ideal combination with Five Element treatments, since both systems are dealing with energy blocks, and with chronic problems with a strong psychological component. Five Element treatments for a particular organ can simply be combined with the Window of Heaven point for that organ, and/or its Yin–Yang pair.

For example, for an Excess Heart condition with frustration in relationships, HT.7, the Sedation point, can be combined with PC.1 or SI.16 and SI.17, the Window of Heaven points for Pericardium and Small Intestine respectively. Both Pericardium and Small Intestine can have close links to the Heart.

As another example, LU.5, the Sedation point for the Lung, can be combined with LU.3 and LI.18, the Window of Heaven points for Lung and Large Intestine, to treat bereavement and unexpressed grief. BL.42, the outer Bladder line point for the Lungs, can also be combined in this treatment. Alternatively, CV.17 can be reduced to assist the Lungs in the process of letting go.

CONCEPTION AND GOVERNOR CHANNEL POINTS

The author does not use the Five Element system when working on the energy centres, since he uses a more flexible and specific system based on the traditional functions of the points, and the classification of disharmonies into Deficiency, Excess, Stagnation, Irregularity and their combinations.

However, a Five Element treatment can be enhanced by adding the GV or CV point at the anatomical level of organs to be treated. For example:

CV.17 or GV.11 for Heart
CV.17 or GV.12 for Lungs
CV.14 or GV.8 for Liver
CV.12 or GV.6 for Spleen
CV.4 or GV.4 for Kidneys.

In these situations, the Five Element treatment is dominant and the use of GV or CV points is secondary. This can be combined with Back Transporting points and/or Window of Heaven points as required. For example, for a patient locked in an internal world of

Table 9.14 When to use the Five Element system

Situation	Yes/No	Comments
Exterior problems	no	Five Element System is not appropriate for Exterior syndromes, it is better for Interior conditions
Channel problems	no	better treated with Ah Shi, local and distal points on affected channel
Deficiency		
moderate	yes	when Deficiency relates to energy block between two or more organs
severe	no	better treated with Source points and Back Transporting points
Excess		
moderate	yes	when Excess relates to energy block between two or more organs
severe, acute	no	better treated with Well points or Accumulation points
Mixed Excess and Deficiency		
Yin–Yang pairs	no	better treated with Connecting points
mixed conditions in one organ	no	better treated with Source or Back Transporting points
in Promotion or Control cycles	yes	but with awareness of other possibilities which may be preferable in some cases
Stagnation		
blocks between joints	no	better treated with local points
blocks between energy centres	no	better treated with GV and CV points
blocks between organs	yes	but with awareness of other possibilites
Irregularity	yes	but points chosen according to Five Elements are more effective if appropriate according to their traditional functions

worry and obsessive thought:

reduce ST.45, the Sedation point of the Stomach
reduce ST.9, the Window of Heaven point of the Stomach
reduce CV.12, the GV point for the Spleen and Stomach.

ALARM POINTS

Alarm points are superior to Five Element combinations for severe acute conditions. However, in chronic conditions, especially of Excess, they can be used as secondary points to enhance a Five Element treatment. For example, Excess Lungs, with asthma and bronchitis, can be treated by reducing LU.5 the Sedation point and LU.1 the Alarm point.

EIGHT EXTRA CHANNEL OPENING POINTS

The author never combines Five Element system with Eight Extra channel treatments, since he believes that each of these systems must be used as the dominant, with the other points added as secondaries. He feels that each system is unique in itself, and that the two systems are very different, involving different systems of visualization, which would become confused if they were used together.

LOCAL AND DISTAL POINTS

As discussed earlier in this chapter, Five Element Sedation or Tonification points can be used as the distal points in a mixed organ and channel condition, provided the organ and channel problems are related. The local points could then be selected on the same (affected) channel.

For example, a patient has trapezius muscle spasm associated with emotional tension and Excess Gallbladder. GB.38, the Sedation point of the Gallbladder can be reduced, and also GB.21 as a local point. However, if the Five Element treatment is designed to regulate the organ, the number of local points should be kept to a minimum, or the effect of the Five Element points will be swamped by the group effect of the local points. In the example given, GB.38 and GB.21 is a balanced treatment, but if GB.20 and TE.15 and TE.16 were added, the Five Element emphasis of the treatment could be lost.

TRADITIONAL FUNCTIONS OF THE POINTS

As has been discussed, an excellent way of both enhancing the Five Element treatments, and making them more specific, is only to use the Tonification and Sedation points when their Five Element indications correspond with the traditional functions of the points.

SUMMARY

While certain Five Element systems, such as the Four Needle and the Eight Needle methods are sufficiently complex and balanced to be used by themselves, the simpler systems of Tonification or Sedation points are often greatly enhanced by combination with other systems, as discussed earlier. These combinations are summarized in Table 9.15.

Table 9.15 Combining the Fire Element system (FES) with other methods

Combination	Yes/No	Comment
Traditional functions of the points	yes	excellent combination, enables FES to be used selectively for more specific situations
Ah Shi, local and distal points	yes	Tonification points or Sedation points can be used as distal points in this system, providing only one or two local points are used
Source points	no	used as an alternative to FES; superior to FES for severe Deficiency
Connection points	yes	useful in FES treatments involving imbalance of a Yin–Yang pair
Accumulation points	no	an alternative to FES; superior to FES for acute Excess
Well points	no	too powerful, would swamp FES, and superior to it for acute Excess
Back Transporting points	yes	can be used as alternative to FES, or as excellent secondary to it
Window of Heaven points	yes	excellent addition to FES, especially for psychological problems
CV and GV points	yes	useful addition to FES, but only as secondary to it. If it is desired to concentrate on energy centres, FES is not appropriate
Alarm points	yes	can be used as alternative to FES and superior to it for acute Excess, but can also be used as secondary additions to FES treatments
Eight Extra channel Opening Points	no	best not mixed with FES

EXAMPLES OF FIVE ELEMENT TREATMENTS

The following are examples of situations in which the author might use the Five Element system. There are, of course, alternative treatment strategies in each case.

Example 1 Four Needle method for Deficiency: Deficient Kidney Yin and Deficient Liver Blood

The patient was tired and restless with a weak back, dull headache, insomnia and feelings of lack of confidence.

The Four Needle method for Deficiency was selected in this case, since the Five Element points had traditional functions that matched the syndrome. KI.10, the Element point of the Kidney and LR.8 the Tonification point of the Liver were reinforced. Since KI.10 is the Water point, it can tonify Kidney Yin and cool Kidney Deficiency Fire. LR.8 as the Water point can tonify Liver Yin and it is also indicated to tonify Deficient Liver Blood.

In this example, the choice of points according to the Five Elements corresponds with the choice of points according to their traditional functions. BL.23 and BL.18 were also reinforced to strengthen the Five Element treatment and to tonify Kidney Yin and Liver Blood.

Example 2 Four Needle method for Excess: Chronic Liver and Heart Fire

---

The patient was restless, irritable and easily overexcited. She suffered from insomnia and occasional palpitations, associated with chronic Liver and Heart Excess Fire of moderate degree.

The Four Needle method for Excess was selected in this case, since the traditional functions of the points chosen complemented their Five Element status. LR.2, the Sedation point of the Liver, and HT.8, the Element point of the Heart, were reduced. Since both these points are Fire points and Spring points, they are specific for Excess Fire of their respective organs. Later in the course of treatments, yìn táng and ān mián were added to calm the mind and ease the insomnia. This is an example of enhancing a Fire Element treatment with Extra points.

Example 3 Sedate Mother–Tonify Child method: Stagnant Lung Qi and Deficient Kidney

---

The patient came with insomnia, depression and lack of drive. This was associated with holding on to accumulated unexpressed grief.

The Lung pulse was + and the Kidney pulse –. Both ends of this block between Lung and Kidney were treated by reducing LU.5, the Sedation point, and reinforcing KI.7, the Tonification point. KI.7 is especially good in this case since it will firm the will, increase the inner strength and so reduce the fear of letting go. CV.17 and CV.22 were also reduced to loosen blocked grief and allow tears to flow.

Example 4 Basic Under Control treatment: Deficient Heart Fire and Stagnant Lung Qi

---

The patient came with depression and lack of interest in life. She seemed withdrawn, joyless, and cut-off within herself. She had cold hands and a feeling of fullness in the chest with occasional sighing.

The Element point of the Heart, HT.8, and the Control point of the Lungs LU.10, were reinforced to allow Fire to regain control over Metal. Since there was no sign of either manic depression or of Deficient Yin, moxa cones were used on both Fire points HT.8 and LU.10 to allow the warmth of Fire to melt the bars of the Metal prison in which the patient had enclosed herself.

Later in the treatment, BL.42, the outer BL line point for the Lungs was reduced, and BL.44 the outer BL line point for the Heart was reinforced. At a further treatment, instead of BL.42 and BL.44, Even method and moxa cones were used on CV.17, and Reducing method on LU.3, the Window of the Sky point for the Lungs.

Example 5 Eight Needle method for Over Control: Stagnant Liver Qi Invades Cold, Deficient Spleen

---

The patient had loss of appetite, abdominal distension, depression and lethargy. His abdomen was cold and he had a preference for warm food and drink.

The basic Over Control treatment was to reduce LR.1, the Element point of the Liver, and SP.1, the Control point of the Spleen. SP.2, the Tonification point of the Spleen, and HT.8, the Element point of the Heart, were added to tonify the Spleen and to complete the Eight Needle treatment.

Since it was felt that LR.1 was not enough to clear the Stagnation in the Liver, LR.14, the Alarm point of the Liver, was added with Reducing method. This is the system of using the points at the two extremes of the channel. Since the Spleen was Deficient in Fire and Yang, moxa cones were used on SP.2, since this is the Fire point of the Spleen and ideal for tonifying Spleen Yang.

This is another example of how a Five Element treatment has been selected because the traditional functions of the points used match the detailed organ syndromes. If the Deficiency of the Spleen had been of Qi and Blood, rather than Yang, then SP.2 might not have been so effective, and a Five Element treatment might not have been used.

Example 6 Eight Needle method for Under Control: Deficient Spleen Qi and Excess on Kidney and Liver

---

The patient came with generalized headache and nervous tension. He was ruthless and impatient with himself and others, with lack of sympathy or consideration for other people, and with deep inner insecurity. It was felt that the Deficient Spleen was resulting both in insecurity and in a lack of the natural control of ruthless ambition by kindliness and concern. The lack of control of Kidney Will was also resulting in impatience by putting pressure on the Wood element to effect goals and plans.

The basic Under Control treatment was to reinforce SP.3, the Element point of the Spleen, and KI.3, the Control point of the Kidneys. KI.1, the Sedation point of the Kidneys, and LR.1, the Element point of the Liver, were reduced to disperse the Excess in Kidneys and Liver, and to complete the Eight Needle method.

Once again, this Five Element treatment was selected because the traditional functions of the points used match this specific situation. For example, KI.1 has the traditional functions of sedating Kidneys and Liver and relieving associated nervous tension and headache. SP.3 is excellent to strengthen the Spleen to give security, and to control fear with kindliness, since it is both the Source point and the Earth point. The Back Transporting points for Kidneys, Liver and Spleen could be added to this treatment, either on the inner or outer Bladder line.

Qualitative use of the Points of the Elements

GENERAL

The points of the Five Elements may be used in various ways:

according to the hours of the day
according to the seasons
according to the Five Element systems
according to the physical and psychological qualities

associated with the Five Elements and the five Yin organs.

USE ACCORDING TO THE FIVE ELEMENT SYSTEM

In the basic Five Element system, the points of the elements are used as Tonification, Sedation, Control and Element points, according to *quantity* of energy only. That is, according to whether an organ is showing signs of Deficiency or Excess. This Five Element system can be extended to include use of the points of the elements in a qualitative way.

USE ACCORDING TO THE QUALITIES OF THE FIVE ELEMENTS

We can say that, especially for the Yin organs, all the points of a particular element have shared qualities relating to the characteristics of that element. For example, all the Earth points of the Yin organs can be reinforced to strengthen the Earth quality of security, and therefore to reduce worry, insecurity and overconcern. By strengthening the Earth quality of rooting the spirit more firmly in the physical body, the Earth points of the Yin organs can be used to stabilize extreme oscillations of the other emotions, e.g. fear, anger, joy and grief.

The qualities of the points of the elements of the Yin organs are outlined in Table 9.16, and the qualities of Fire and Water are also discussed in the next section.

SOURCE OF INFORMATION

The author has not seen detailed discussion of the psychological qualities of the points of the elements in Chinese textbooks. In the opinion of the author, most of the interpretations in the West of the psychology of the Five Elements, have originated with Western practitioners as extrapolations of the scanty Chinese material. What follows here is the author's personal interpretation, which is coloured by his own background and experience. Practitioners are free to develop their own schemes — the only important criterion being whether the scheme is clinically effective.

MODIFICATION OF ELEMENT QUALITIES ACCORDING TO OTHER POINT FUNCTIONS

In many cases, the Element quality of a point is enhanced or altered by the other functions of the point. For example, for the Yin organs, the function of the Wood

Table 9.16 Qualities of the Element points of the Yin organs

Point type	Functions
Fire points	give the expansive, uplifting qualities of vitality, warmth and light, to bring the person out of withdrawal, sadness and depression to a lively enjoyment and participation in life
Earth points	give nourishment, solidity, security and stability, and by grounding the spirit in the physical body, give a rootedness and pleasure in the physical world without overattachment to it
Metal points	give wisdom by giving a balance in the taking in and letting go of information and experience and in the forming and breaking of personal bonds: can give a firmness and clarity by reducing things to their essentials
Water points	can moisten, cool and calm, to give peace and rest, at the same time as maintaining fluidity of movement; where the Fire points can help to bring the excitement and energy of the spirit into daily living, the Water points can help to bring the deep inner peace of the spirit into every aspect of life
Wood points	can be used to move stagnation of energy to release emotional blocks, or to disperse Excess to calm extreme emotions

points to move Stagnation is enhanced by the fact that they are also Well points, which can have this same function. However, since Well points can also disperse acute severe Fire conditions, the Wood points of the Yin organs can be used especially to move Stagnation of Heat and Fire in the body. This is not the case for the Wood points of the Yang organs, since they are Stream points not Well points.

ELEMENT POINTS OF THE YIN AND YANG ORGANS

For the Yin organs, the Fire, Earth and Water points especially, have a powerful function associated with their respective Elements. For the Yang organs, the points of the elements do not have such a clear and strong effect. For example, the Fire points of the Yang organs are not so much used to tonify Yang, and the Water points of the Yang organs are not so much used to tonify Yin, as their counterparts of the Yin organs.

FIRE POINTS OF THE YIN ORGANS

Table 9.17 shows how the element of Fire manifests through each of the five Yin organs, and lists the Fire points that can be used to regulate each organ. The Fire points of the Yin organs are also the Spring points of these organs. The functions of Fire points and Spring points overlap in that Spring points can be used to drain Fire in their respective organs.

Table 9.17 Fire points of the five Yin Organs

Fire point	Functions
HT.8	regulates the degree of excitement, interest, pleasure, warmth and love in life and in relationships
SP.2	regulates the degree of interest in food, the physical body, and material possessions, and regulates the degree of thoughtfulness, care and concern about self and others; mainly used with Reinforcing method and moxa
LU.10	to increase interest in living in the present, participating in life and in forming close bonds in relationships
KI.2	regulates the degree of personal ambition and sexual drive; regulates the balance between activity and rest, regulates the force and intensity of the focused directed will
LR.2	regulates the drive to expand and develop the personality, to expand personal boundaries, to manifest personal uniqueness and creativity, and to assert the ego

FIRE POINTS OF THE YANG ORGANS

The Fire points of the Yang organs are the River points, and with the exception of GB.38, are not as much used as the Fire points of the Yin organs to disperse Fire. Nor do they have such a strong effect as the Fire points of the Yin organs to tonify Yang, when used with Reinforcing method and moxa.

EARTH POINTS OF THE YIN ORGANS

The Earth points of the Yin organs can each be used to nourish and tonify their respective organ. Strengthening the Qi of the organ can stabilize extremes and fluctuations of its corresponding emotions. Earth points can give stability and balance to the organs. This effect is enhanced by the fact that the Earth points of the Yin organs are also the Source points.

For example, HT.7 can be used with Reinforcing method to nourish Heart Qi and Blood, and to balance oscillations between apathy and overenthusiasm. Similarly, KI.3 can nourish both the Yin and the Yang of the Kidney, to create a balance between fearfulness and risk-taking, dare-devil behaviour.

EARTH POINTS OF THE YANG ORGANS

LI.11, ST.36, GB.34 and GB.40 are four of the most widely used points of acupuncture, but with the exception of ST.36, they are not mainly used as Earth points, to nourish and stabilize, but are used to disperse Excess.

METAL POINTS OF THE YIN ORGANS

The Fire, Earth and Water points of the Yin organs have clearly defined element effects, and are in constant clinical use. The Metal points do not have such a marked element function, they are the least used of the points of the Five Elements, and indeed LU.8, HT.4, SP.5 and LR.4 are among the most unpopular points on their respective channels.

The exception is KI.7, which can be used as a Metal point to give the strength, courage, firmness and clarity needed to let go of attachments. People tend to hold on to the past, because they feel that if they let go they will be left small, alone and exposed to face the enormity of the present. This is frightening, so people tend to hold on tight to outworn situations and relationships, even if these are painful to them. KI.7 can help to overcome this.

METAL POINTS OF THE YANG ORGANS

The Metal points of the Yang organs are also the Well points, and the Well point functions of clearing acute Excess Fire, or moving Stagnant Qi, are dominant. However, LI.1, ST.45 and BL.67 can each be used as Metal points to clear and firm the mind, to let go of the irrelevant and concentrate on the essentials. They can be used for mental congestion, confusion and vagueness, just as they can be used to relieve the effects of a hangover.

WATER POINTS OF THE YIN ORGANS

Table 9.18 shows how the element of Water manifests through each of the five Yin organs, so that each Water point has its special character. KI.10, LR.8 and HT.3 are the Water points that are most important in controlling the Fire element in their respective organs, and SP.9 is the Water point that is reduced to drain Excess Water, rather than reinforced to help Water to cool excess Fire.

WATER POINTS OF THE YANG ORGANS

The Water points of the Yang organs are more commonly used as Spring points, so that they are reduced to disperse Fire, rather than reinforced to tonify Water and Yin, as in the case of the Water points of the Yin organs. For example, ST.44 is generally reduced to disperse Stomach Excess or Deficiency Fire, rather than reinforced to strengthen Water to cool Fire.

Table 9.18 The Water points of the five Yin organs

Water point	Functions
HT.3	can give a quiet serenity and pleasure in just being, to balance the fiery tendency of the Heart Spirit to overenthusiasm and overexcitement
SP.9	mainly used to drain Exess Damp, which can counteract a feeling of mental dullness, heaviness and lethargy
LU.5	can give a greater peace and flexibility in relationships to create more enduring and long-lasting bonds
KI.10	can calm and moderate an overintense and fiery will, to give peace, rest and a sense of proportion, to prevent physical and mental exhaustion
LR.8	can balance the quick, restless, egotistical tendency of Liver Fire, to give through peace and serenity a deeper intuitive understanding of self and others, and an increased patience and tolerance

WOOD POINTS OF THE YIN ORGANS

The Wood points of the Yin organs are also Well points, and the Well point functions are dominant. All the Yin Well points can be bled or reduced to drain acute Excess, and all the Yin Well points can be used with moxa and Reinforcing method to tonify Yang and Fire. HT.9, LR.1 and SP.1 can also be reduced to move Stagnation of Qi in the channel and relieve emotional stagnation. This is a shared property of Wood points and Well points. PC.9, LU.11 and KI.1 are reduced mainly to disperse Heat, and if they are used for Stagnation, it is more for Stagnation of Heat and Fire.

WOOD POINTS OF THE YANG ORGANS

These are SI.3, TE.3, ST.43, LI.3, BL.65 and GB.41. They can all be reduced to clear Wind Heat, and none of them has a marked function as a Wood point. TE.3 is widely used for eye and ear problems and SI.3 and GB.41 are the Opening points of the Governor and Belt channels respectively.

SUMMARY

The points of the Five Elements may be used according to the qualities of their respective elements, but this is mainly important for Fire, Earth and Water points, and much less so for Metal and Wood points.

Balancing Fire and Water

GENERAL

The Yin–Yang polarity of Fire and Water is an older and simpler system than the Five Elements. The simplest treatment aims at restoring balance between Fire and Water by needling the Fire or Water point on the channel of the affected organ. Balancing Fire and Water is a separate system from the Five Elements, but one which sometimes coincides with it.

Table 9.19 Fire and Water points

Channel	Fire point	Water point
KI	KI.2	KI.10
BL	BL.60	BL.66
HT	HT.8	HT.3
SI	SI.5	SI.2
PC	PC.8	PC.3
TE	TE.6	TE.2
LR	LR.2	LR.8
GB	GB.38	GB.43
SP	SP.2	SP.9
ST	ST.41	ST.44
LU	LU.10	LU.5
LI	LI.5	LI.2

EXCESS FIRE/DEFICIENT WATER

If there is excess Fire, we can reduce the Fire point of the affected organ, e.g. HT.8 Rd for insomnia. If there is also Deficient Water, we can reinforce the Water point of the affected organ, e.g. HT.3 Rf for Deficient Heart Yin. The treatment is then reduce the Fire point and reinforce the Water point: HT.8 Rd; HT.3 Rf.

Since the Kidneys, the Water element, supply Water and Yin for the other organs, we can also reduce KI.2, the Fire point of the Kidneys, and reinforce KI.10, the Water point of the Kidneys, if required. The treatment is then HT.8, KI.2 Rd; HT.3, KI.10 Rf. This principle can also be used for Excess Fire and Deficient Water in Lungs or Liver:

LU.10, KI.2 Rd; LU.5, KI.10 Rf e.g. for haemoptysis
LR.2, KI.2 Rd; LR.8, KI.10 Rf e.g. for impatience.

It is not so much used for the Spleen, since this organ tends to Cold and Damp.

DEFICIENT FIRE / EXCESS WATER

If there is Deficient Fire, we can reinforce and moxa the Fire point of the affected organ, e.g. HT.8 Rf M for depression. If there is also Excess Water, we can reduce the Water point of the affected organ, e.g. HT.3 Rd for cold extremities and ankle oedema from Deficient Heart Yang. The treatment is then reinforce and moxa the Fire point and reduce the Water point.

Since the Kidneys, the Water element, govern the balance of Fire and Water in the body, it may also be necessary to reinforce and moxa KI.2, the Fire point of the Kidneys, and reduce KI.10, the Water point. The treatment is then HT.8, KI.2 Rf M; HT.3, KI.10 Rd, the opposite of the treatment for Excess Fire / Deficient Water. This principle can also be used for Deficient Fire / Excess Water in Spleen or Lungs:

SP.2, KI.2 Rf M; SP.9, KI.10 Rd   e.g. for oedema
LU.10, KI.2 Rf M; LU.5, KI.10 Rd   e.g. for watery cough.

It is not much used for the Liver, since this organ tends to Heat and Dryness.

Eight Extra channels 10

Introduction

GENERAL

There is relatively little information on the Eight Extra channels in translation, and while the account that follows is based on Chinese material, the greater part of it is based on the personal interpretation and clinical experience of the author, for example, the section classifying the Extra channels according to Deficiency, Excess, Stagnation and Irregularity.

NOMENCLATURE

The nomenclature adopted here is according to the 1991 WHO proposal.

Pinyin name	English name	Abbreviation
dū mài	Governor channel	GV
rèn mài	Conception channel	CV
chōng mài	Thoroughfare channel	TV
dài mài	Belt channel	BV
yīn qiāo mài	Yin Heel channel	Yin HV
yáng qiāo mài	Yang Heel channel	Yang HV
yīn wéi mài	Yin Link channel	Yin LV
yáng wéi mài	Yang Link channel	Yang LV

Note that the word 'channel' replaces 'vessel'.

CLASSIFICATION

The Extra channels can be classified in various ways, according to:

possession of their own or borrowed points
location
Six Divisions
Yin–Yang pairs
special pairs.

Table 10.1 The eight Extra channels

Extra channel	Main associated channels	Main associated organs	Borrowed points	Opening points
GV	GV,BL,SI	KI,LR,HT	–	SI.3
Yang HV	BL	–	BL.62, BL.61, BL.59, GB.29, SI.10, LI.15, LI.16, ST.4, ST.3, BL.1, GB.20, GV.16	BL.62
CV	CV	KI,LU	–	LU.7
Yin HV	KI	–	KI.2, KI.6, KI.8, ST.12, BL.1	KI.6
BV	GB,LR	GB,LR	LR.13, GB.26, GB.27, GB.28	GB.41
Yang LV	GB, TE	–	BL.63, GB.35, SI.10, TE.15, GB.21, ST.8, GB.13, GB.14, GB.15, GB.16, GB.17, GB.18, GB.19, GB.20, GV.16, GV.15	TE.5
TV	KI, SP	KI,SP	CV.1, ST.30, KI.11, KI.12, KI.13, KI.14, KI.15, CV.7, KI.16, KI.17, KI.18, KI.19, KI.20, KI.21	SP.4
Yin LV	KI, PC, SP	KI,HT	KI.9, SP.13, SP.15, SP.16, LR.14, CV.22, CV.23	PC.6

The heading 'Main associated channels' includes both the more important main channels from which the channel borrows points, and the main channel of its Opening point.

For an account of the Extra channel pathways, see *Acupuncture: a Comprehensive Text* translated and edited by J. O'Connor and D. Bensky, Eastland Press, Chicago, 1981.

OWN OR BORROWED POINTS

Governor and Conception have their own points, but the other six channels do not have their own points, and borrow points from the main channels. For example, the Thoroughfare channel (TV), crosses the Conception channel at CV.1 and CV.7, the Stomach channel at ST.30 and the Kidney channel at KI.11 to KI.21.

LOCATION

All the Extra channels run vertically on the body, except the Belt channel (BV), which runs horizontally around the waist. The vertical channels can be divided according to whether their pathways are on the front, sides or back of the body:

Front: CV, TV, Yin HV, Yin LV
Sides: Yang HV, Yang LV
Back: GV

SIX DIVISIONS

Two of the special pairs of Extra channels relate to paired channels of the Six Divisions classification: see Figure 10.1. The GV + Yang HV pair has the Opening points SI.3 and BL.62. The SI and BL channels are paired in the Six Divisions classification as Greater Yang, which rules the back of the legs, body, neck and head. The BV + Yang LV pair has the Opening points GB.41 and TE.5. The GB and TE channels are paired as Lesser Yang, according to the Six Divisions, which governs the sides of the legs, body, neck and head.

YIN–YANG PAIRS

Whilst GV and CV, Yang HV and Yin HV, Yang LV and Yin LV can be arranged in Yin–Yang pairs, there is not such an obvious relationship between BV and TV.

SPECIAL PAIRS

Each Extra channel can be activated by its Opening point; for example, LU.7 is the Opening point for CV. The most important clinical use of the Extra channels is when the channels are used in special pairs, as shown in Table 10.2. Each pair is activated by using the Opening points of its two channels; for example the CV + Yin HV pair is activated by using LU.7 with KI.6, the Opening points of CV and Yin HV respectively.

FUNCTIONS

GENERAL FUNCTIONS OF THE EXTRA CHANNEL SYSTEM

The Extra channel system is complementary to the main channel system, and is specifically related to the ability of the Kidneys to store and distribute Qi and Jing, as shown

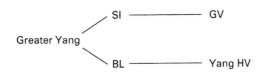
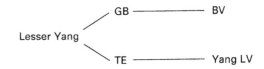

Fig. 10.1 Extra channel pairs and Six Divisions.

Table 10.2 The special pairs of Extra channels.

Extra channel pair	Main associated channels	Main associated organs	Opening points
GV + Yang HV	GV,BL,SI	KI,HT,LR	SI.3 + BL.62
CV + Yin HV	CV,KI,LU	KI,LU	LU.7 + KI.6
BV + Yang LV	GB,TE,LR	GB,LR	GB.41 + TE.5
TV + Yin LV	KI,SP,PC	KI,SP,HT	SP.4 + PC.6

in Figure 10.2. The Extra channels are closely related to the Kidneys. GV, CV and TV originate in the Kidneys and TV borrows mainly KI points. Yin HV and Yang HV are extensions of the KI and BL channels, respectively; and Yin LV and Yang LV originate in KI and BL points, respectively.

EXTRA CHANNEL SYSTEM AS A RESERVOIR FOR ENERGY

Classically in Excess conditions, the Extra channel system was seen as a safety reservoir that could take overflow from the main channel system. In Deficiency conditions, the Extra channel system could act as a reserve of energy.

EXTRA CHANNEL SYSTEM AND THE CIRCULATION OF JING AND QI

The Extra channel system can act as an intermediary between the Kidneys and the main channels, to integrate the Qi and Jing stored in the Kidneys into the main energy circulation system. Because the Extra channels can represent the final reserves of energy, and because one of the energies they store, Jing, is more precious and less easy to replace than Qi, the Extra channels should be used with caution, especially in cases of Deficiency of Qi and Jing—see notes on CV.4 on page 132.

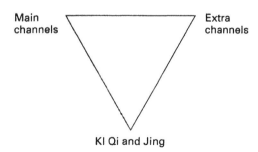

Fig. 10.2

EXTRA CHANNEL SYSTEM REGULATES 7- AND 8-YEAR CYCLES

Kidney Jing, the Extra channel system in general, and CV and TV in particular, regulate the 7- and 8-year cycles in the lives of women and men respectively. This is not only the physiological and reproductive changes of puberty, pregnancy, motherhood, menopause and old age, but also the psychological reactions to these changes.

Table 10.3 Functions of individual Extra channels

GV
Tonifies Yang
    tonifies KI Yang
    tonifies HT Yang
    helps SP hold up organs
    disperses Interior Cold and
    Damp
 	
Tonifies KI, Brain and Spine
    tonifies KI Jing
    strengthens mind
    strengthens spine
 	
Expels Exterior Wind
 	
Moves Stagnation of Qi and
Blood in back, neck and head
 	
Calms Irregularity and
Disperses
    calms Hyperactive Yang
    disperses Excess Fire
    calms Interior Wind
    calms HT Spirit
	BV
	Calms Hyperactive LR Yang
	Disperses LR–GB Fire
	Moves Stagnant LR Qi
	Disperses LR–GB Damp Heat
	Regulates menstrual cycle
	
	TV
	Tonifies Qi of KI and SP–ST
	Tonifies Blood of SP and HT
	Moves Stagnant Qi and Blood
	    in HT and chest
	    in epigastrium
	    in uterus
	    in arms and legs
	
	Calms emotions
	    calms KI fear
	    calms SP worry
	    calms HT anxiety

CV
Tonifies KI
    tonifies KI Jing
    tonifies KI Qi
    tonifies KI Yin
    tonifies KI Yang
 	
Removes Damp in Lower
Abdomen
Moves Stagnant Qi
    of HT, LU and breasts
    of LR, SP and ST
    in uterus and lower
    abdomen
 	
Regulates emotions
    calms fear
    disperses grief
    relieves depression
 	
Regulates female
reproductive cycle and
associated psychological
changes
	Yang HV
	Expels Exterior Wind
	Moves Stagnant Qi in BL
	channel for back, hip and leg
	pain
	
	Disperses Hyperactive Yang in
	the head
	
	Yin HV
	Regulates uterus
	Strengthens legs
	Regulates sleep
	
	Yang LV
	Wind Heat
	Regulates sides of the body,
	ears and head
	Calms Hyperactive LR Yang
	Disperses LR–GB Damp Heat
	
	Yin LV
	Moves Stagnant Qi and Blood
	in throat, HT, chest and
	epigastrium
	
	Regulates balance of HT and
	KI and calms the mind

EXTRA CHANNEL SYSTEM ASSISTS CIRCULATION OF DEFENSIVE QI

The strength of the resistance of the body to disease, not only to Exterior invasion but also to Interior factors, depends on the strength of the stored energy in the kidneys. As an extension of the Kidney system, the Eight Extra channels, especially GV, CV and TV, assist the circulation of Defensive Qi throughout the body, and so contribute to prevention of illness.

SPECIFIC FUNCTIONS OF THE INDIVIDUAL EXTRA CHANNELS

These are summarized in Table 10.3.

FUNCTIONS OF THE EXTRA CHANNEL PAIRS

The physiological and psychological functions of the

Extra channel pairs are summarized in Tables 10.4 and 10.5.

OVERLAPPING FUNCTIONS OF THE EXTRA CHANNEL PAIRS

GENERAL

There are clear differences in the clinical functions of the pairs: see Figure 10.3. However, there are some important overlaps in function which need to be clarified.

GV + YANG HV AND CV + YIN HV

Both these pairs can be used to tonify Kidney Jing, but fertility and sexual problems in women are usually treated on the Conception and not the Governor channel. Problems of fertility or impotence in men can be treated

Table 10.4 Comparison of the Extra channel pairs

GV + **Yang HV**	CV + **Yin HV**	BV + **Yang LV**	TV + **Yin LV**
Governs back of body, relating to areas supplied by GV, BL and SI channels. For problems of back of head and neck; of bones, joints, tendons and muscles of spine; of spinal nerves, brain, eyes and ears, of backs of legs. Deficiency patterns relate to Deficient KI Jing and Qi, e.g. degeneration of spinal nerves as in multiple sclerosis (MS), degeneration of the bones as in osteoporosis, and ageing problems, e.g. impotence, blurred vision, deafness, dizziness and poor circulation.	Governs front of throat, chest and abdomen, especially LU, KI and uterus. Can treat LU problems, e.g. cough, asthma and dyspnoea; KI problems, e.g. oedema and urinary retention; and problems of emotional balance, e.g. panic attacks, phobias, depression and withdrawal, based on KI fear and LU grief.	Governs sides of body, relating to areas supplied by LR, GB and TE channels. For problems of ears, eyes, sides of head, neck, trunk areas, hips, legs and external genitals.	Governs front of throat, chest and abdomen, especially HT, SP, KI and uterus. Deficiency patterns can have constitutionally weak KI and SP, with weak digestion, weak muscles, exhaustion and depression, with no energy reserves.
Excess patterns relate to Exterior Wind, e.g. influenza, or to Excess Heat, e.g. high fevers. Stagnation patterns include Stagnation of Qi and Blood in GV, BL and SI channels with pain and stiffness in spine, e.g. neck arthritis or back sprain. Irregularity patterns include panic attacks, mania, disorientation and depression.	Regulates the cycles of female sexual development, e.g. menstruation, pregnancy, motherhood and menopause, and psychological adaptation to these role changes.	Treats ear and eye infections, dizziness, lateral headaches and migraines, especially related to premenstrual tension, muscular aches, pains and stiffness down sides of body, sciatica, indigestion and GB disorders and skin rashes and external genitals problems due to Damp Heat.	Both Deficiency and Stagnation patterns can have cold hands and feet, and Stagnation patterns can have pain in chest, epigastrium, uterus or legs.
Psychological problems are based on fear. Yin type fails to take control of life from fear of failure, and Yang type tries to overcontrol life from fear of losing control, resulting in stiffness and rigidity.	Can treat suppressed grief and problems of letting go, e.g. separation, divorce, children leaving home, bereavement, rejection of femininity or fear of loss of femininity, associated with the changes in women's life cycle. Can treat physical signs of Stagnant Qi from fear and grief, e.g. breast lumps and uterine fibroids, also amenorrhoea and infertility.	For menstrual problems with Hyperactive LR Yang and Stagnant LR Qi, with irritability and depression, especially side-effects of birth control pill.	Irregularity patterns can be digestive problems of nausea, vomiting or oesophageal spasms or emotional problems, e.g. KI fear, SP worry or HT anxiety, with palpitations and insomnia.
		Constitutional type tends to be impatient, irritable, snappy, tense and stressful. Yin type is more meek, uncertain, indecisive, lacking self-confidence, touchy and hypersensitive. Yang type is more forceful, aggressive, angry, domineering, intolerant and inflexible, bitter and resentful.	Yin type can be depressed and lonely, lost in an internal world of worry and nervous tensions, unable to feel peace or pleasure in life and relationships. Yang types can feel blocked in expressing affection or communication in relationships. Fears of loss of control, or fear of surrender in sex or relationships, may cause Stagnation of Blood and Qi.

Table 10.5 Yin and Yang psychological types of the Extra channel pairs

Yin type	Yang type
GV + Yang HV have let go of their control of life, and are oversurrendered, spineless and weak-willed; lacking determination to start tasks and to persevere despite difficulties or dangers; have given up on life, do not fully participate in life from fear of failure; lacking clarity, courage and strength of character; needing firmness and backbone	are tense and pressured from trying to overcontrol life, and attempting to restrict reality; fearful of letting go and flowing with life, and afraid of loss of control; are stiff, rigid, inflexible, blinkered, angular, awkward, narrow-minded; needing to relax and gain fluidity and flexible adaptability
CV + Yin HV are weak and depressed, lacking interest in life or sex, lacking drive and ambition, withdrawn due to fear of participation in life, with fear of forming bonds due to fear of loss, and difficulty in forming strong or lasting relationships; nostalgic, daydreaming, living in an inner world of past memories	actively participating in some aspects of life, but tending to hold in and suppress grief, and failing to let go completely of outworn attachments; holding on to relationships and situations due to fear of the pain of loss and of being alone, perhaps with resulting Stagnation of Qi and associated breast lumps and carcinomas and uterine fibroids and carcinomas
BV + Yang LV seeming weak, ineffectual and indecisive, lacking self-confidence, being touchy, hypersensitive, snappy and irritable	tending to be angry, frustrated, intolerant, aggressive, domineering, inflexible, vindictive, vengeful, bitter, resentful, selfish and self-opinionated people
TV and Yin LV physically and emotionally weak and easily exhausted or depressed; easily disturbed by emotions and slow to regain balance; fearful, anxious and jumpy; lacking inner peace and contentment, living in a lonely inner world of worry and nervous tension, often fail to participate in the outer world or to gain pleasure from life and relationships	having the strength and interest to participate actively in life, but tending to Stagnation of Qi and Blood in chest, epigastrium and uterus, related to fear, worry, anxiety, sadness or to difficulties and obstructions in expressing affection and communicating in relationships; fear may be of loss of control, and also of fear of surrender and loss of ego in sex and relationships

For each Extra channel pair, people may have aspects of both the Yin and Yang type, they may oscillate from one type to another, depending on the situation, or they may change type with age.

on either Governor or Conception channels, depending on the overall pattern. For example, impotence with lower back weakness would be treated on the Governor channel, while impotence with grief and depression might be treated on the Conception channel. For men, Governor and Conception treatments can often be alternated, for example, impotence with prostatitis, where the treatment can be alternated between SI.3, BL.62, GV.4, BL.32 and LU.7, KI.6, CV.3, CV.6, ST.29.

PERSONALITY TYPES

Both the GV + Yang HV and the CV + Yin HV Yin personality types have reduced participation in life. The Yin GV + Yang HV type because they do not take control from fear of failure (Kidneys), and the Yin CV + Yin HV type because they withdraw into themselves or into their past from fear of or difficulty in forming bonds (Lungs and Kidneys).

The Yang types of both pairs create Stagnation of Qi by blocking the flow of their lives, and hence the flow of Qi through their bodies. The Yang GV + Yang HV type try to overcontrol life because of the fear of losing control (Kidneys and Heart), and the Yang CV + Yin HV type try to hold on to outworn attachments, from the fear of letting go (Lungs and Kidneys).

Some point combinations for these four personality types are shown in Figure 10.4.

GV + YANG HV AND BV + YANG LV

GV + Yang HV is mainly concerned with the back of the body and BV + Yang LV with the sides. The areas of overlap are in problems of head and neck, ears and eyes, and hips and legs.

HEAD AND NECK

Both pairs can treat headaches and neck problems from Hyperactive Yang and muscle tension, or from Exterior Wind Invasion. GV + Yang HV is used for problems in the areas of the GV and BL channels, for injury or deterioration of the vertebrae or the spinal nerves, and for muscular tension generated by fear of losing control. BV + Yang LV is used for problems in the areas of the GB and TE channels, and for muscular tension generated by frustration, uncertainty and suppressed anger.

EARS AND EYES

Both pairs can treat problems of the eyes due to Exterior Wind, but GV + Yang HV is slightly more for Wind Heat. The local points GB.1 and BL.1 can be combined with either pair. GV + Yang HV is used more for deterioration of vision and hearing due to declining Kidney Jing, and

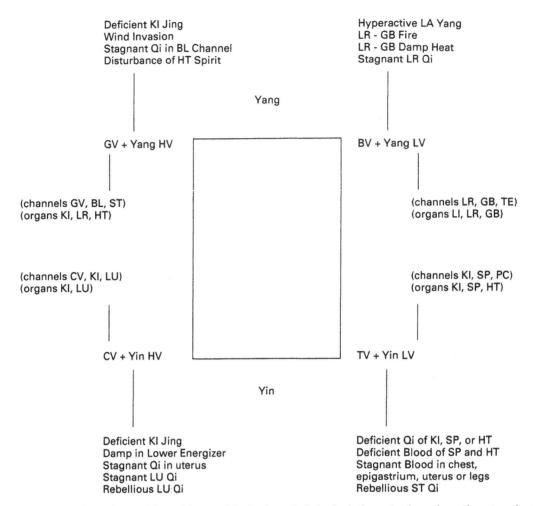

Fig 10.3 Functions of the Extra channel pairs ('channels' as used in the figure includes both the main channels on the external pathway of the Extra channel and the channels of the Opening points).

BV + Yang LV is used more for Excess conditions of Liver –Gallbladder Fire or Damp Heat.

HIPS AND LEGS

GV + Yang HV is more for problems of weakness in hips and legs due to Deficient Kidney Jing, Qi or Yang; and especially down the backs of the legs, and where there is an associated weakness of the lower back and spine. BV + Yang LV is more for problems of sides of hips and legs, involving generalized muscular tension associated with nervous tension, frustration and anger.

Both pairs may be associated with Deficient Kidney Qi or Yin, and the points KI.3, KI.6 or SP.6 may be added to the Opening point combinations SI.3 + BL.62 and GB.41 + TE.5.

CV + YIN HV AND TV + YIN LV

These pairs are compared in Table 10.8 later.

CV + YIN HV AND BV + YANG LV

Both pairs can be used to treat Stagnation of Qi or Damp Heat, as in headaches, chest pain, breast and menstrual problems.

STAGNATION OF QI

CV + Yin HV is mainly used to treat Stagnation of Qi originating from Lung grief or Kidney fear, while BV + Yang LV treats Stagnation mainly due to Stagnant Liver Qi.

LU.7 + KI.6 can be used for headaches, breast problems, chest pain, dysmenorrhoea, amenorrhoea or irregular menstruation when these problems are linked to

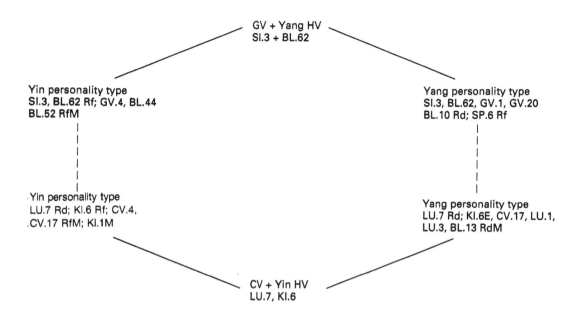

Fig 10.4 Comparison of GV + Yang HV and CV + Yin HV.

Stagnant Lung or Kidney Qi. LU.7 + KI.6 is more for chronic breast lumps, due to long Stagnation of Qi due to grief, whilst GB.41 + TE.5 is more for the temporary swelling of breasts during menstruation due to temporary rise of Stagnant Liver Qi or Hyperactive Liver Yang.

GB.41 + TE.5 can be used for lateral headaches, pain in the chest or hypochondrium, and breast swelling during menstruation, due to a combination of Stagnant Liver Qi and Hyperactive Liver Yang. These Opening points can also treat irregular menstruation or dysmenorrhoea due to Stagnant Liver Qi, Stagnant Blood or Damp Heat.

DAMP HEAT

CV + Yin HV can treat leucorrhoea or pruritus due to Damp Cold or Damp Heat, whilst BV + Yang LV is mainly for leucorrhoea, pruritus, or pelvic inflammation due to Damp Heat.

Also, LU.7 + KI.6 is used more for skin rash due to Damp Heat on the front of the abdomen or chest, while GB.41 + TE.5 is more for Damp Heat rashes on the sides of the body, arms and legs, or including the ears.

CV + YIN HV AND DEFICIENT YIN/DEFICIENT YANG

LU.7 + KI.6 may be used to treat patterns of both Deficient Yin or Deficient Yang, for example:

Deficient Yang of Kidney and Lung	e.g. asthma LU.7, KI.6 Rf; CV.4, CV.17 Rf M
Deficient Yin of Kidney and Lung	e.g. laryngitis LU.7, KI.6, CV.4 Rf, CV.23 Rd.

LU.7 + KI.6 may also be used to treat patterns where there is an oscillation between Deficient Yin and Deficient Yang, as in some patients with menopausal neurosis, who are sometimes cold and depressed, and sometimes hot and agitated:

Deficient Yin/Deficient Yang of Kidney and Heat	LU.7, KI.6, CV.4, C.17, HT.6, ST.36 Rf.

EXTRA CHANNELS AND THE ENERGY CENTRES

As seen from Figures 10.5 and 10.6, the Kidney–Dan Tian system is the basis for the GV–CV circulation system, and the Extra channel system radiating from it. The Extra channels, other than GV and CV, do have relationship with the energy centre system, but their main link is to the Dan Tian centre and to the Kidneys.

The relationship of the Extra channel pairs with the energy centres on the front of the body is shown: detail in Table 10.10 later.

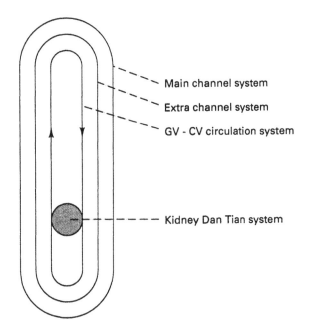

Fig. 10.5 Extra channel relationships.

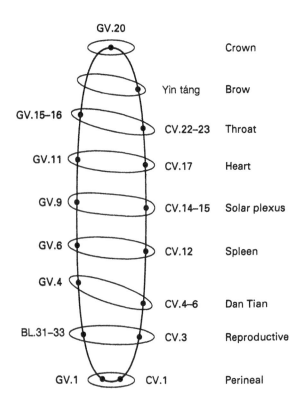

Fig. 10.6 Energy centres on the GV and CV system.

Classification of Extra channel syndromes according to Deficiency, Excess, Stagnation and Irregularity

INTRODUCTION

The imbalances of each of the Extra channel pairs can be classified into four types: Deficiency, Excess, Stagnation and Irregularity (see Fig. 10.7). This gives 16 possible combinations, of which some are clinically more important than others as shown in Table 10.6.

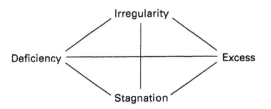

Fig. 10.7

Table 10.6 Main uses of the Extra channel pairs

	Deficiency	Excess	Stagnation	Irregularity
GV + Yang HV	X	X	X	X
CV + Yin HV	X	x	X	X
BV + Yang LV	x	X	X	X
TV + Yin LV	X	x	X	X

X, primary use; x, secondary use.

DEFICIENCY

In the context of the Extra channel pairs, Deficiency often involves Deficiency of Kidney Jing and Qi. This may affect the reproductive system, the spine and joints, the eyes and ears, mental functions, or the strength of will, depending on the pair. Stagnation and Irregularity may arise secondarily to the Deficiency. Stagnation may be associated with poor circulation or depression, and Irregularity with palpitations or emotional instability, for example.

EXCESS

True Excess patterns are more associated with the two Yang pairs, and not so much with the two Yin pairs. GV + Yang HV can be used for Excess patterns of Wind Cold, Wind Heat or Excess Heat. BV + Yang LV can be used for Excess patterns of Liver–Gallbladder Fire and Damp Heat. CV + Yin HV and TV + Yin LV are not often used to treat pure Excess, and are more frequently used when local Excess is associated with Stagnation.

STAGNATION

The effects of Stagnation in the Extra channel pairs depends on the areas of the body controlled by each pair. For example, GV + Yang HV controls the spine and the back of the body; BV + Yang LV controls the sides of the body; CV + Yin HV and TV + Yin LV control the uterus and the front of the body.

The effects of Stagnation also depend on the functions of the organs associated with each pair. For example, CV + Yin HV is associated with Lungs and with respiratory stagnation; TV + Yin LV is associated with Heart and with circulatory stagnation, and BV + Yang LV is associated with Liver and with Stagnation of Qi in the muscles and tendons.

IRREGULARITY

Whilst Irregularity may be associated with Excess in the case of the two Yang pairs, it is more usually associated with Deficiency or Stagnation for the two Yin pairs. GV + Yang HV may have Irregularity associated with Excess patterns such as Kidney, Liver or Heart Fire and Hyperactive Liver Yang or Liver Wind. BV + Yang LV may have Irregularity associated with Liver–Gallbladder Fire or Hyperactive Liver Yang. CV + Yin HV and TV + Yin LV may have Irregularity patterns such as Disturbance of Heart Spirit associated with Deficiency patterns, e.g. Deficient Kidney Qi. Alternatively, the Yin pairs may

have Irregularity patterns associated with Stagnation, such as dyspnoea or nausea and vomiting.

GV + YANG HV

GENERAL

The GV + Yang HV pair controls the GV, Bladder, Small Intestine and Yang HV channels and therefore the spine and the back of the body, arms and legs. The main organs associated with GV + Yang HV are Kidneys, Heart and Liver.

DEFICIENCY

Deficiency symptoms of GV + Yang HV can include: weakness and deterioration of the spinal nerves and the areas or organs they control; weakness of the bones, joints and muscles of the neck, back and knees; deterioration of vision, hearing, memory and mental clarity; deterioration of mental, physical or sexual energy. The basic treatment for GV + Yang HV Deficiency patterns involves SI.3 + BL.62 with Reinforcing method, and with moxa, unless there is concurrent Deficient Yin.

When there is deterioration at a particular spinal segment, as in multiple sclerosis, for example, then the huá tuó, GV and BL points in that segment may be added to SI.3 + BL.62, with Reinforcing method and moxa if appropriate.

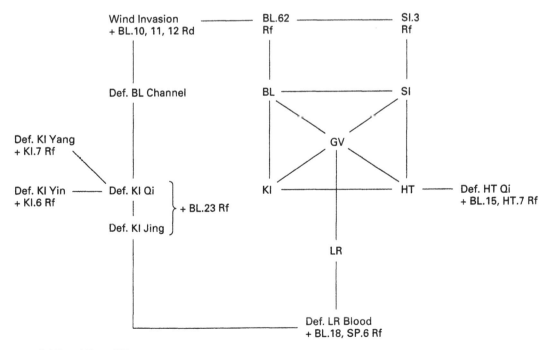

Fig. 10.8 Deficiency of GV and Yang HV.

Table 10.7 Combinations with SI.3 + BL.62 for GV + Yang HV Deficiency

Syndrome	Example	Combinations
Def. KI Jing	bone deterioration	BL.11, BL.23, GB.39 Rf M
Def. LR Blood	weak tendons	BL.18, SP.6, GB.34 Rf M
Def. HT Qi	palpitations	BL.15, HT.7 Rf
Def. KI Yang	impotence	BL.23, GV.4, KI.7 Rf M
Def. KI Yin	inflamed joints	BL.23, KI.6 Rf M
Def. KI Jing and	visual weakness	BL.1, GB.1, GB.20 Rf; BL.18,
Def. LR Blood		BL.23, GB.37 Rf M
Def. KI Qi	poor concentration	BL.1, BL.10 Rf; BL.23, BL.67,
		GV.4, GV.20 Rf M

If combination SI.3 + BL.62 is used for women, KI.6 may be added.

EXCESS

The combination of SI.3 and BL.62 can be used with Reducing method for acute Excess conditions such as Wind Cold or Wind Heat, as in common cold or influenza, or Excess Heat as in severe fevers.

In the case of Wind Cold, points such as BL.1,2,10,11,12,13; SI.9,10,11,12,13,14,15; GV.14,15,16 and GB.20 can be added with Reducing method, moxa or cupping as appropriate. If the temporary Excess due to Wind Cold is a result of Deficient Kidney and Bladder Qi allowing the invasion, then the underlying Deficiency can be treated after the temporary acute Excess has been removed.

In the case of Wind Heat, for example, with feverishness and inflammation of eyes and nose, BL.2,10, GV.14 and LI.20 can be added with Reducing method.

For extreme Heat with fever and delirium, GV.13 or GV.14 can be added with Reducing method and SI.1 can be bled. This category is often associated with Interior Wind as in meningitis, and the categories of Excess and Irregularity are combined.

STAGNATION

Stagnation of Qi and Blood on the pathways of GV, BL and upper SI channels, may be due to trauma, lack of exercise, Cold Invasion or to the Deficiency of Qi. However, the most typical for the GV–Yang LV pair, is the Stagnation associated with the rigidity and restriction that comes with the blocking of energy flows due to fear of loss of control. The stress and pressure of trying to hold on to control, or in attempting to extend control over an ever-expanding area of life, can result in spinal stiffness, in mental and emotional inflexibility, and also in serious heart conditions.

The principle of treatment is to move Stagnation to relieve the local or general stiffness and pain, and also to regulate Kidneys, Heart and Solar Plexus centre to reduce the pressure of the fear of loss of control. When the fear is reduced, the person does not hold on so hard, freeing the energies which were blocked and stagnant, and allowing the muscles and tendons to relax.

As in the treatment for Deficiency, when there is a local problem at a particular spinal segment, then the huá tuó, GV and BL points in that segment may be added to SI.3 and BL.62. In this case all points are reduced. In addition, the points KI.3 and HT.7 or KI.6 and HT.6 can be added to SI.3 and BL.62, to strengthen Kidneys and Heart to reduce fear and anxiety. This can be done either unilaterally or bilaterally.

Fear may be combined with mania, hysteria, thoughts of suicide, depression and disorientation. BL.9 or BL.10 and GV.15 or GV.16 can then be added to SI.3 and BL.62, especially if there is a neck stiffness and headache or confusion of speech. BL.1 can be added for spinal stiffness or mental confusion.

IRREGULARITY

The main three organ relationships of the GV–Yang HV pair are with Kidneys, Heart and Liver. Kidney fear, Hyperactive Liver Yang, Liver Fire and Liver Wind resulting from anger, and overstimulation of the Heart itself by excitement or anxiety, can disturb the Heart Spirit leading to Irregularity of mind and emotions. Signs may be extreme restlessness, insomnia, convulsions, panic attacks, mania, delirium, mental confusion, dizziness, disorientation, feelings of alienation and unreality and violent uncontrollable mood swings.

Treatment depends on the Zang Fu syndromes. The basic combination is SI.3 + BL.62 with Reducing method. In addition:

for Deficient Kidney and Heart Yin	add KI.6, HT.6 Rf
for Deficient Kidney and Liver Yin	add KI.6, LR.8 Rf
for Deficient Kidney and Heart Yin	add LR.8, HT.6 Rf
for Hyperactive Liver Yang	add GB.20, GV.20 Rd
for Kidney and Heart Fire	add KI.1, HT.8, GV.1, GV.11 Rd
for Kidney and Liver Fire	add KI.1, LR.2 Rd
for Liver Wind	add KI.1, GV.16, GV.20 Rd.

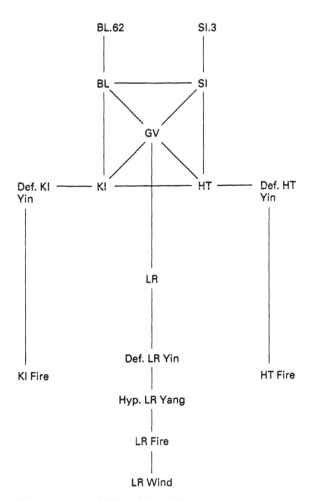

Fig. 10.9 Irregularity of GV and Yang HV.

CV + YIN HV

GENERAL

The CV + Yin HV pair controls the front of the body, the abdomen and chest, especially the uterus, Kidneys and Lungs, and can be used to treat four main areas:

reproduction
water metabolism
respiration
emotional balance.

DEFICIENCY

For deficiency of CV + Yin HV, the basic combinations of LU.7 and KI.6 can be reinforced often in combinations with CV.4, which can be used with Reinforcing method and moxa, unless there is Deficient Yin. The precautions in using CV.4 are discussed on page 132.

REPRODUCTION

LU.7 and KI.6 can be used for amenorrhoea, infertility, habitual miscarriage and lack of sexual interest, especially when these problems are associated with exhaustion and depression. For infertility, CV.4 and KI.13 can be added to the basic combination.

WATER METABOLISM

LU.7 and KI.6 can be used for oedema, urinary incontinence, and the incomplete urination associated with prostatitis, if these problems are linked to energy deficiency. For oedema, CV.4 and CV.9 can be added to the basic combination and moxa can be used unless there is deficient Yin. For prostatitis, a balance between Yin and Yang treatments can be achieved by alternating combinations based on LU.7, KI.6 and CV.4 with combinations based on GV.4 and BL.31.

RESPIRATION

LU.7 and KI.6 can be reinforced to treat shortness of breath, weak cough and asthma, when these problems are linked to Deficient Lungs with Deficient Kidneys and there are other signs indicating a CV + Yin HV pattern. CV.4 and CV.17 are often added to LU.7 and KI.6 to strengthen Kidneys and Lungs together. For asthma of this type, other points, e.g. LI.1, BL.13 and dìng chuǎn, may be added to CV.4 and CV.17.

EMOTIONAL BALANCE

The Extra channels are linked to the cycles of change in the lives of men and women. The Conception channel is particularly important in the changes in the lives of women that accompany puberty, motherhood and menopause. If there is a deficiency of energy of the Conception channel, there may be the physical signs of amenorrhoea, infertility, miscarriage, postnatal exhaustion and menopausal syndrome.

In addition to the physical signs, there may not be enough energy for the woman to make a psychological transformation at the key times and she may be unable to adapt to her new role and suffer great depression and loss of self-esteem.

For example, for menopausal depression based on deficiency of the Conception channel, CV.4, CV.17, LU.3 and yìn táng, can be added to the basic combination, to give the strength and clarity to adjust to the changes of the menopause.

EXCESS

This Extra channel pair is not often used to treat pure Excess. There may be situations where local Excess is associated with a basic Deficiency, such as in asthma or oedema, and here the principle of treatment is to tonify the Deficiency, so that the Excess resolves without further treatment. Similarly, local Excess can be associated with a basic Stagnation of Qi, as in dysmenorrhoea of fibroids, and here the principle of treatment is to move the Stagnation as the primary problem.

STAGNATION

The two main problems of CV + Yin HV are Deficiency and Stagnation, as these factors affect reproduction, water metabolism, respiration and emotional balance. Often Deficiency and Stagnation may occur together, but in this section the emphasis is on the Yang aspects of Stagnation.

People of the Yang type CV + Yin HV personality (summarized in Table 10.5), have the energy and the strength of character to participate actively in life, but because they fear the pain of loss and being alone, they may suppress grief and hold on to outworn attachments, instead of letting go and following the flow of life. This suppression and this holding, may stagnate the flow of energy in the chest and reproductive centres, producing not only such illnesses as asthma and dysmenorrhoea, but also benign tissue accumulations such as breast lumps and uterine fibroids, as well as carcinomas of the breast, uterus and cervix.

Also, fear and resentment at the main changes in the female cycle may stagnate the energy. Pain in menstruation or in pregnancy may be associated with fear of loss of control, fear of the unknown, fear of surrendering to one's own femininity, or resentment at surrendering a part of oneself to another being, whether child or partner. Fear and resentment at getting old, fear and grief at apparent loss of femininity, fear of being unattractive and of being alone, may stagnate the energies and produce irregularities at menopause. This is exaggerated by the emphasis in modern society on youth and beauty in women. Menopausal symptoms are less in cultures where status increases for women after menopause.

CV.6 and CV.17 can be added to LU.7 and KI.6, since Stagnation in the lower abdomen can be regulated by CV.6 and Stagnation in the chest area by CV.17. If there are specific uterine problems, CV.3, KI.8, KI.13, or zǐ gōng may be added. For depression with problems of respiration or breasts, LU.1, LU.3, LU.6, KI.24–27 or CV.22 may be added. All points are used with Reducing method, unless there is underlying Deficiency, in which case CV.6 and CV.17 are used with Even method. For oedema linked to depression and to Stagnation in the Lower Energizer, CV.3, CV.6 and CV.9 can be combined with LU.7 and KI.6, and if necessary ST.28 can be added.

For impotence and prostatitis linked to fear and depression an effective combination can be LU.7 and KI.6, with LU.1, CV.2, CV.6, CV.14, CV.17 all with Even method, and moxa an KI.1.

IRREGULARITY

The main patterns of CV + Yin HV are Deficiency and Stagnation. Rebellious Lung Qi may be associated with breathing irregularities such as cough, asthma, dyspnoea and panic attacks. However, although CV + Yin HV can involve Heart signs, this is more the domain of TV + Yin LV, which is associated with the Kidneys, Spleen, Heart relationship.

Irregularity of Lung Qi, as in panic attacks linked to Lungs and Kidneys, can be treated with LU.7, CV.14, CV.17 Rd; KI.6, CV.4 Rf; KI.1 M. LU.1 and LU.6 may be added with Reducing method if there is accumulation of Phlegm.

BV + YANG LV

GENERAL

The BV + Yang LV pair controls the sides of the body, head, arms and legs, and also the external genitals, through its connections with the Liver, Gallbladder and Triple Energizer channels. It is linked to the Liver and Gallbladder organs and can regulate physiological and emotional aspects of the menstrual cycle.

DEFICIENCY

This Extra channel pair is more usually associated with Excess Liver–Gallbladder Yang and Fire, and with Stagnation of Liver–Gallbladder Damp Heat, than it is with Deficiency. However, the Yin constitutional type of this pair, is associated with Deficient Kidney Qi or Yin, as a basis for the Hyperactive Yang or Fire of Liver and Gallbladder: a combination of Deficiency and Irregularity.

In this situation, while the basic combination of GB.41 and TE.5 is used with Even or Reducing method to calm and or disperse Fire, other points must be reinforced to correct the Kidney Deficiency. For example, for a patient with migraine, dizziness, lack of confidence and timidity associated with Hyperactive Liver Yang and Deficient Kidney Qi, KI.3 and CV.4 can be added with Reinforcing method. Or, for a patient with eye inflammation, headache, restlessness, hypersensitivity and irritability associated with Deficient Kidney Yin and Deficiency Fire of Liver and Gallbladder, KI.6 and LR.8 can be added with Reinforcing method.

EXCESS

The main use of BV + Yang LV is to treat Excess patterns of Liver–Gallbladder Fire and Stagnation patterns of Stagnant Liver Qi with Liver–Gallbladder Damp Heat. In fact, the Excess patterns usually have some element of Stagnation and the Stagnation patterns usually are of the Excess type. Where Excess is the dominant pattern, there may be such Liver–Gallbladder Fire signs as severe lateral headache, high blood pressure, pains down the side of the body, and aggressive or vindictive behaviour.

The basic combination of GB.41 + TE.5 may be used with KI.1 and GV.20 with Reducing method, and tài yáng may be bled.

STAGNATION

The basic combination of GB.41 and TE.5 can be used with Reducing method for Stagnation of Damp Heat in the Liver and Gallbladder channels, and combined with other points depending on the problems:

+ GB.1, TE.23	for Damp Heat eye problems
+ GB.2, TE.17	for Damp Heat ear problems
+ LR.13, GB.2	for Damp Heat affecting Gallbladder and Stomach
+ CV.4, GB.26	for Damp Heat leucorrhoea
+ CV.3, LR.5	for Damp Heat vaginitis
+ GB.20, GB.31	for Damp Heat eczema.

GB.41 and TE.5 can also be used with Reducing method for Stagnant Qi in the Liver and Gallbladder channels, and combined:

+ GB.14, GB.20	for headaches and depression
+ GB.20, GB.21	for headaches and trapezius muscle spasms from suppressed anger
+ TE.16, TE.17	for frustration with tense neck and jaw
+ GB.22, GB.24	for hypochondriac stiffness and pain
+ GB.29, GB.30	for hip problems
+ GB.31, GB.35	for leg problems.

Stagnation in the BV + Yang LV pair can be associated with frustration, depression and suppressed anger. When there is the additional factor of Damp Heat, the emotions of bitterness and lingering hatreds and resentments may be added. For Stagnation with Damp Heat in Liver–Gallbladder, LR.5 or SP.6 may be added. When this Damp Heat expresses in a skin rash, LR.1 and PC.9 may be bled.

IRREGULARITY

For this pair, the main pattern of Irregularity is that of Hyperactive Liver Yang, with symptoms of dizziness, headache or moving sensation in the head; irritability, hypersensitivity, confusion and disorientation. This pattern of Irregularity may be combined with Deficiency, Excess or Stagnation.

For example, three patterns of lateral headache:

- **Irregularity + Deficiency** – Hyperactive Liver Yang + Deficient Kidney Qi
  GB.41, TE.5 Rd + GV.20, GB.1, GB.14 Rd; CV.4, KI.3 Rf
- **Irregularity + Excess** – Hyperactive Liver Yang + Liver–Gallbladder Fire
  GB.41, TE.5 Rd + GV.20, GB.1, GB.14, KI.1 Rd; LR.1B
- **Irregularity + Stagnation** – Hyperactive Liver Yang + Stagnant Liver Qi
  GB.41, TE.5 Rd + GV.20, GB.1, GB.14, GB.21, SP.6 Rd

TV + YIN LV

GENERAL

While the Conception channel relates more to Deficiency and Stagnation of Qi, the Thoroughfare channel relates more to Deficiency and Stagnation of Blood. While the CV + Yin HV pair relates more to the Kidney–Lung relationship and the emotions of fear and grief, the TV + Yin LV pair relates more to the relationship between Kidneys, Spleen and Heart, and the emotions of fear, worry and anxiety.

DEFICIENCY

Both Yin Extra channel pairs can treat female reproductive problems associated with exhaustion and depression, but where the CV + Yin HV pair pattern includes asthma and oedema, the TV + Yin LV pair pattern can include poor peripheral circulation, weak digestion, and muscular weakness or atrophy.

The combination of SP.4 and PC.6 can be used for Deficiency situations especially in five areas:

reproduction
circulation
digestion
muscle strength
emotional balance.

REPRODUCTION

For example, amenorrhoea, infertility and postnatal problems associated with signs of Deficient Blood, and with exhaustion, depression and poor circulation. CV.4 is added to the basic combination with Reinforcing method and moxa if appropriate. KI.13 or zǐ gōng can be added if necessary.

CIRCULATION

Coldness of lower abdomen, back and extremities, associated with Deficiency of TV + Yin LV can be treated by adding CV.4 to the combination of SP.4 and PC.6. For cold feet, SP.1 and SP.2 can be added and for cold fingers, PC.7, 8 and 9. All points can be used with Reinforcing method, and moxa if appropriate.

CV.12 and CV.17 can be added if there are Deficiencies in Spleen and Heart that are contributing to the circulation problem. In men especially, this treatment on the front of the body can be alternated with BL.20, BL.23, ST.36 and LI.4.

DIGESTION AND MUSCLE STRENGTH

The Thoroughfare channel links the production of energy by the Spleen with the storage of energies by the Kidneys. SP.4 and PC.6 can be used for exhaustion associated with weak constitution and especially weak digestion. This can be associated with emaciation, muscle atrophy, muscle weakness, or poor muscle tone in a person who is generally physically weak, easily tired, and who has difficulty in absorbing the necessary nourishment from their food. Such a person may have a pulse that is thin and choppy or empty and choppy, and a tongue that is pale and thin or pale and flabby.

The basic combination is SP.4, PC.6, CV.4, CV.12 and ST.36 with Reinforcing method and moxa as appropriate. In men especially, this can be alternated with GV.4, GV.6, BL.20, BL.23, ST.36 and LI.4.

EMOTIONAL BALANCE

For the TV + Yin LV pair, Deficiency is often associated with Irregularity. For example, if the Qi of Kidneys, Spleen and Heart, and the Blood of Spleen and Heart are Deficient, then the emotions of Kidneys, Spleen and Heart will not be stable and the person will experience a feeling of weakness, vulnerability and depression, in addition to the insecurity of fear, worry and anxiety.

The combination of SP.4 and PC.6 can be used to treat this pattern. CV.4 can be added for worry due to Deficient

Spleen Qi and Blood, and CV.17 can be added for depression and anxiety due to Deficient Qi and Blood of Heart. This treatment can be alternated with BL.15, 20, 23, 44, 49 and 52.

EXCESS

For this Extra channel pair, Deficiency is often associated with Irregularity, and Excess is usually associated with Stagnation. Patterns of pure Excess, such as Cold, Heat, Fluid or Phlegm are not common. Mixed patterns of Stagnation and Excess can occur.

STAGNATION

Together, SP.4 and PC.6 can move Stagnation in the arms and legs and the front of the body. SP.4 can move stagnation in the chest, epigastrium, lower abdomen and legs, and PC.6 can move stagnation in the throat, chest, epigastrium and arms. Although TV + Yin LV and CV + Yin HV can both move Qi and Blood, TV + Yin LV and the points SP.4 and PC.6 are more for Stagnant Blood, and CV + Yin HV and the points LU.7 and KI.6 are more for Stagnant Qi.

Both pairs are linked to the Kidneys and the stagnating effect of fear, but CV + Yin HV is associated with the combinations of fear and grief and their effect on the Lungs and the flow of Qi, whilst TV + Yin LV is

Table 10.8 Comparison of Stagnation in CV + Yin HV and TV + Yin LV

	CV + Yin HV	TV + Yin LV
Opening points	LU.7 + KI.6	SP.4 + PC.6
Related organs	KI, LU	KI, SP, HT
Related emotions	fear, grief	fear, worry, anxiety and sadness
Stagnation	Stagnant Qi, Damp	Stagnant Blood, Stagnant Qi
Pathology	respiration, water metabolism, reproduction	circulation, digestion, reproduction
	respiration + CV.17, LU.1, LU.3 or LU.6 Rd	**coronary circulation** + CV.17, PC.1, SP.21, HT.6 Rd
	breast problems + CV.17, CV.22, LU.1, LU.3, BL.13 Rd	**peripheral circulation** + CV.6, CV.17, PC.9, SP.1 Rd
	water metabolism + CV.6, CV.9, SP.9 Rd	**digestion** + CV.12, ST.21, ST.40, LI.10 Rd
	reproduction + CV.3, CV.6, KI.8, KI.13 Rd	**reproduction** + CV.3, CV.6, ST.29 Rd

associated with the combination of fear, worry and sadness and its effect on the Heart and the flow of Blood.

It can be seen from Table 10.8 that both pairs can combine with CV points. However, a basic difference is that CV + Yin HV tends to combine with Lung points, while TV + Yin LV combines with points on the Heart and Pericardium channels. Both pairs may have chest and uterine problems associated with Stagnation of the emotions, but CV + Yin HV relates to the Lungs, and to grief and problems of letting go or to withdrawal from relationships.

TV + Yin LV relates to problems of sharing or communication of affection in relationships, and to the Heart.

IRREGULARITY

Irregularity in TV + Yin LV can be associated with Stagnation and Excess; for example, Rebellious Stomach Qi, with belching, nausea and vomiting. However, for this Extra channel pair, Irregularity is mainly associated with Deficiency.

The basic combination is SP.4 + PC.6 with Even method, and points can be added according to the pattern. CV points can be used to regulate the Heart, Solar Plexus, Spleen and Dan Tian energy centres especially:

+ CV.4 Rf	to tonify Kidney Qi or Yang, to calm fear and stabilize emotions
+ CV.12 E	to regulate Spleen and calm worry
+ CV.14 Rd	to calm fear, anxiety and worry
+ CV.17 E	to calm heart beat and breathing
+ CV.24 E	to calm fear and anxiety
+ GV.20 M	to tonify Spleen Qi, to raise energy and to reduce depression
+ yìn táng	to calm worry and clear the mind
+ ST.36	to tonify Qi and Blood to stabilize the emotions.

Table 10.9 Summary of Extra channel pair syndromes

Channel pair	Syndrome	Ailment	Combination
GV + Yang HV			
Deficiency	Deficient KI Jing + Deficient LR Blood	weak back in the elderly	SI.3 + BL.62 Rf; BL.11, BL.18, BL.23, GV.4 Rf M
Excess	Wind Cold	influenza with aching neck	SI.3 + BL.62 Rd; BL.10, BL.11, BL.13, GV.14 Rd M
Stagnation	Stagnant Qi in BL channel	stiff spine	SI.3 + BL.62; GV.1, GV.12, GV.20 E; KI.6 Rf
Irregularity	Disturbance of HT Spirit	panic attacks mental confusion	SI.3 + BL.62; BL.10, GV.16, GV.20 E; KI.6 Rf
CV + Yin HV			
Deficiency	Deficient KI Qi	oedema	LU.7 + KI.6 Rf; CV.4, CV.9 Rf M
Excess	-		
Stagnation	Stagnant LU Qi	depression	LU.7 Rd + KI.6 E; LU.1, CV.6, CV.17 Rd M
Irregularity	Rebellious LU Qi	cough and asthma	LU.7 Rd + KI.6 E; CV.17, CV.22, BL.13 E
BV + Yang LV			
Deficiency	(see Irregularity)		
Excess	LR–GB Fire	migraine	GB.41 + TE.5; KI.1, GV.20 Rd; tài yáng B
Stagnation	LR–GB Damp Heat	otitis media	GB.41 + TE.5; GB.2, TE.17, SP.6 Rd
Irregularity	Deficient KI Qi + Hyperactive LR Yang	headache	GB.41 + TE.5; GB.1, GB.14, GB.20 Rd; CV.4, KI.3 Rf
TV + Yin LV			
Deficiency	Deficient SP Qi + Deficient KI Qi	weak digestion weak muscles	SP.4 Rf M + PC.6 Rf; CV.4, CV.12, ST.36 Rf M
Excess	-		
Stagnation	Stagnant Blood in the uterus	dysmenorrhoea	SP.4 + PC.6; CV.3, ST.29 Rd
Irregularity	Disturbance of HT Spirit	panic attacks	SP.4 + PC.6; CV.14, CV.24, GV.20 Rd; KI.1 M

Only one example of syndrome, ailment and combination has been given for each category; different examples could be presented.
Rd, Reducing method; Rf, Reinforcing method; E, even method; M, moxa.

Table 10.10 Combination of Extra channel Opening points with CV points, GV.20 and yìn táng

Point	Channel pair	Syndrome	Example	Combination
CV.1	CV + Yin HV	Damp Heat in Lower Energizer	genital and abdominal itching	LU.7, KI.6, CV.1, CV.6 Rd
	BV + Yang HV	LR–GB Damp Heat	leucorrhoea and hypochondriac pain	GB.41, TE.5, CV.1, CV.3, GB.24, GB.26 Rd
CV.3	CV + Yin HV	Stagnant Qi in Lower Energizer	amenorrhoea	LU.7, KI.6, CV.3, CV.6, KI.8, KI.13 Rd
	BV + Yang HV	LR–GB Damp Heat	pelvic inflammatory disease	GB.41, TE.5, CV.3, CV.6, SP.6, GB.26 Rd
	TV + Yin LV	Stagnant Blood in the uterus	dysmenorrhoea	SP.4, PC.6, CV.3, ST.29 Rd
CV.4	CV + Yin HV	Deficient KI Yang	impotence and depression	LU.7, KI.6 Rf; CV.4, CV.17, GV.20, KI.1 Rf M
		Deficient KI Qi and Damp	urinary retention	LU.7, KI.6 Rf; CV.4 Rf M; CV.3 Rd
	BV + Yang HV	Hyperactive LR Yang and Deficient KI Qi	headache	GB.41, TE.5, GB.1, GB.14, CV.4, KI.3 Rf
	TV + Yin LV	Deficient KI Qi	exhaustion, cold extremities	SP.4, PC.6 Rf; CV.4, ST.36 Rf M
		Deficient KI Yin	tired but restless	SP.4, PC.6, CV.4, HT.6, yìn táng Rf
CV.6	CV + Yin HV	Stagnant Qi and Damp	abdominal distension and oedema	LU.7, KI.6, ST.28, ST.40 Rd
	BV + Yang LV	Stagnant LR Qi	abdominal and hypochondriac pain	GB.41, TE.5, CV.6, GB.24, GB.28 Rd
	TV + Yin LV	Stagnant Blood	Buerger's disease	SP.4, PC.6, CV.6, ST.30, ST.31, ST.41 Rd
CV.9	CV + Yin HV	Stagnant Qi and Damp	oedema	LU.7, KI.6, CV.3 Rd; CV.6, CV.9, SP.9 Rd M
CV.12	TV + Yin LV	Deficient SP Qi	tiredness, poor appetite	SP.4, PC.6 E; CV.12, ST.25, SP.1 Rf M
CV.13	TV + Yin LV	Rebellious ST Qi	nausea and belching	SP.4, PC.6, CV.13, ST.21 Rd
CV.14	CV + Yin HV	KI invades LU	panic attacks and phobias	LU.7, KI.6, CV.14, CV.17, LU.3 E
	BV + Yin LV	Deficient KI Qi and Hyperactive LR Yang	fear, lack of confidence, muscle tension	GB.41, TE.5, CV.14, GB.21 Rd; CV.4, SP.6 Rf
	TV + Yin LV	Deficient KI Qi and Deficient SP Qi	fear, worry and insecurity	SP.4, PC.6, CV.14 E; CV.4, CV.12 Rf M
		Deficient KI Qi and Deficient HT Qi	insomnia	SP.4, PC.6, CV.14, ān mián Rd; CV.4, SP.10 Rf
		Stagnant ST Qi	epigastric pain and pain	SP.4, PC.6, CV.14, ST.21 Rd; ST.36 Rf
CV.17	CV + Yin HV	Stagnant LU Qi	grief and depression	LU.7, KI.6 Rd; CV.17, LI.1 Rd M
	TV + Yin LV	Deficient HT Blood	palpitations	SP.4, PC.6, CV.17 E; SP.10, ST.36, HT.7 Rf
		Stagnant HT Blood	angina pectoris	SP.4, PC.6, CV.17, SP.21, PC.1 Rd
CV.22	CV + Yin HV	Phlegm in LU	cough	LU.7, KI.6, CV.17, CV.22, ST.40 Rd
	TV + Yin LV	Stagnant Qi	oesophageal spasm	SP.4, PC.6, CV.14, CV.17, CV.22 Rd; KI.1 M
CV.23	CV + Yin HV	Deficient Qi and LU Yin	sore throat	LU.7, KI.6, CV.22, CV.23 E
CV.24	TV + Yin LV	Deficient Qi and Yin	fearful anxiety	SP.4, PC.6, CV.14, CV.24 Rd; CV.4, ST.36 Rf
yìn táng	GV + Yang HV	Deficient KI Qi and Jing	poor concentration	SL.3, BL.22, yìn táng, BL.67, KI.6 Rf
	TV + Yin LV	Deficient SP Qi and Phlegm	mental dullness and confusion	SP.4, PC.6, CV.12, yìn táng, ST.40 Rd
		Deficient SP and HT Blood	poor memory	SP.4, PC.6, yìn táng, GV.20, ST.36 Rf
GV.20	GV + Yang HV	Hyperactive LR Yang and Deficient KI Qi	headache and spinal stiffness	SI.3, BL.62, GV.12, GV.20 Rd; SP.6 Rf
		Disturbance of HT Spirit	depression and mental confusion	SI.3, BL.62, GV.16, GV.20, BL.10 E; KI.6, HT.6 Rf
		Deficient KI Yang	impotence, weak lower back	SI.3, BL.62, SP.6, HT.7 Rf; GV.4, GV.20, BL.23 Rf M
	BV + Yang LV	Hyperactive LR Yang	migraine	GB.41, TE.5, GV.20, GB.1, GB.20 Rd; SP.6 Rf
	TV + Yin LV	Deficient SP and KI Qi	mental exhausion and worry	SP.4, PC.6 E; GV.20, ST.36, ST.45, SP.1 Rf

Rd, Reducing method; Rf, Reinforcing method; E, Even method; M, moxa.

Clinical use of Extra channels

INTRODUCTION

USE OF INDIVIDUAL CHANNELS

The Governor and Conception channels have their own points, which can be used:

to treat a specific energy centre
to treat a specific spinal segment
according to the traditional energetic functions of the points.

GV and CV points are discussed in detail in Chapters 11 and 12. Each of the Eight Extra channels can be used individually, by using the Opening point, to treat failure of any of the functions listed in Table 10.3. For example, GB.41, the Opening point for the Belt channel can be used for vaginitis due to Liver–Gallbladder Damp Heat.

USE OF EXTRA CHANNEL PAIRS

The Extra channels are normally used in pairs, and by using just the Opening points of a pair, it is possible to treat complex conditions with minimum needles to obtain powerful results.

GROUPS OF CHANNELS

Each pair can treat a group of channels. For example, SI.3 + BL.62 can treat pain and stiffness occurring simultaneously in the Governor, Bladder and Small Intestine channels on the back, shoulders and neck.

GROUPS OF ORGANS

Each pair can treat a group of organs. For example, SP.4 + PC.6 can treat patterns involving Kidneys, Spleen and Heart together, e.g. a patient with fear, worry, anxiety, palpitations, weak digestion and no energy reserves.

CONSTITUTIONAL AND PERSONALITY TYPES

Each pair is associated with a particular constitutional and personality type, as shown in Tables 10.4 and 10.5. For example, a woman with depression, lack of energy, lack of sexual interest, and amenorrhoea could be treated with LU.7 and KI.6; or a man with spinal stiffness, mental and emotional inflexibility, and fear of losing control in life could be treated with SI.3 and BL.62.

Use of the Opening points of the Extra channel pairs is considered in detail in the next section.

COMBINING OPENING POINTS WITH OTHER POINT TYPES

The Opening point pairs can be used by themselves, or act as the basis for more complex combinations. However, the basic advantage of using the Extra channel pairs is that a small number of needles can treat complex conditions involving two or more organs. As with all acupuncture treatments, the principles are simplicity and harmony. Simplicity, in using the minimum number of needles to produce the desired result, and harmony, in creating a balanced point combination in which the points enhance, rather than interfere with, each other's effectiveness.

The author does not combine Extra channel Opening points and Five Element techniques, because he feels that the two systems are quite different, and using them together would introduce excessive theoretical complexity into the treatment.

OPENING POINTS ONLY

Occasionally the opening point pair is sufficient by itself,

e.g. SP.4 + PC.6 for a patient with fearful nervous anxiety and insomnia. Often an Extra channel treatment starts with the insertion of the Opening points, then the practitioner checks to see if the pulse has changed sufficiently, or whether the insertion of further needles is necessary.

COMBINATION WITH CV AND GV POINTS

Perhaps the most powerful combination of the Opening points is with points on the Conception or Governor channels. This enhances the power of the treatment by targeting a specific organ, energy centre or spinal segment. For example, for a patient with cold hands and feet due to Deficient Qi in Kidneys and Dan Tian energy centre, SP.4 + PC.6 can be combined with Reinforcing method and moxa on CV.4. As another example, if SI.3 and BL.62 are used for stiffness and sensation in the upper back and neck, GV.12 and GV.14 can be added with needle and moxa. If the problem is in both lower back and neck, then GV.4 and GV.14 can be added to SI.3 and BL.62.

Table 10.10 shows combinations with CV points.

USING BORROWED POINTS AS LOCAL POINTS

For the Extra channels that do not have their own points, but borrow points from other channels (see Table 10.1), borrowed points can be used as local points in combination with the Opening point pair. For example, for a patient with headache due to Hyperactive Liver Yang, GB.14 and GB.20 can be added to GB.41 + TE.5.

USING POINTS ON THE CHANNELS OF THE OPENING POINTS

For example, the Opening points of TV + Yin LV are SP.4 + PC.6. For a patient of the TV + Yin LV constitutional type, with Stagnant Heart Qi and Blood with chest pain, SP.21 can be added since it is on the same channel as SP.4, the Opening point for TV, and PC.1 can be added since it is on the same channel as PC.6, the Opening point for Yin LV. Similarly, LU.1 and KI.13 can be added to LU.7 + KI.6, for a patient with infertility linked to depression.

The two examples just given use additional points on the Opening point channels as local points. However, in the last example, KI.8 could be added as a distal point on the Kidney channel, since it is the Accumulation point of Yin HV.

USING POINTS OF ASSOCIATED ORGANS

For example, TV + Yin LV is linked to the organs of Kidneys, Heart and Spleen, so that points on these channels could be combined with SP.4 + PC.6. For a patient with palpitations and insomnia due to Deficient Heart Qi and Blood, HT.7 could be added to SP.4 + PC.6. Alternatively, if the patient had Deficient Heart Yin, HT.6 could be added to SP.4 + PC.6. As another example, LR.5, the Connecting point of the Liver could be added to GB.41 + TE.5, for Damp Heat in Liver–Gallbladder.

COMBINATION WITH APPARENTLY UNRELATED POINTS

Some of the points shown in Table 10.11 have no obvious relationship to the Extra channel pair with which they are combined; for example, SP.6 in combination with GV + Yang HV.

However, SP.6 can tonify Yin of Kidneys, Heart and Liver, and so balance the GV + Yang HV treatment, which is otherwise rather Yang. Also, SP.6 can be combined with BV + Yang LV for any one of three reasons: it tonifies Yin of Kidneys and Liver; it moves Stagnant Liver Qi; and it disperses Damp Heat.

SP.9 and ST.40 can combine with CV + Yin HV, because they are points which drain damp and relieve abdominal distension, and ST.40 is a point on a Yang channel which balances the rather Yin combination of CV + Yin HV.

HT.6 can be combined with CV + Yin HV, where this pair is being used for menopausal neurosis with Deficient Heart Yin, since HT.6 and KI.6 are an effective pair to treat this situation and to control sweating.

COMBINATION WITH BACK TRANSPORTING POINTS

The Extra channel pairs can be combined or alternated with Back Transporting points.

GV + Yang HV

This pair can be combined with:

BL.11	to strengthen the bone
BL.15	to tonify Heart Qi and Yang
	to disperse Heart Fire

Table 10.11 Combination of Opening points with single points on arms or legs

	Point	Syndrome	Example
GV + Yang HV (SI.3 + BL.62)	KI.1	Deficiency KI Qi and Yang	mental and physical exhaustion with difficulty in concentration fear, disorientation and paranoia
	KI.6	Deficiency KI Yin	arthritis with stiff hot inflamed joints
	KI.7	Deficiency KI Yang with Kidney Qi not firm	impotence with weak will and no determination
	SP.6	Deficiency KI, HT or LR Yin	headache, irritability and mental confusion
	HT.7	Disturbance of HT Spirit	impotence with depression and nervous tension
CV + Yin HV (LU.7 + KI.6)	KI.1	Deficiency KI Yang and Qi	asthma with much fear
	KI.8	Stagnant Qi in lower abdomen	infertility
	HT.6	Deficiency KI and HT Yin	menopausal neurosis with perspiration
	SP.9	Damp	oedema
	ST.40	Stagnant Qi, Damp and Phlegm in lower abdomen	abdominal pain and distension
BV + Yang HV (GB.41 + TE.5)	KI.3	Deficiency KI Qi	headaches worse with tiredness and with weak lower back
	KI.6	Deficiency KI Yin	headaches with tiredness and restlessness
	SP.6	Deficiency KI and LR Yin	headaches with insomnia, impatience and dry eyes
	LR.3	Stagnant LR Qi	sore breasts before menstruation
	LR.5	Damp Heat Damp Heat in LR–GB	red skin rashes with fluid-filled blisters genital itching with yellow discharge
TV + Yin LV (SP.4 + PC.6)	KI.1	Disturbance of HT Spirit	insomnia
	LR.1	Heat in the Blood, Damp Heat	varicose veins with itching
	SP.1	Deficiency Yang Heat in the Blood	cold feet inflamed varicose veins
	SP.10	Deficiency Blood	palpitations and insomnia
	ST.36	Deficiency Qi in Blood	exhaustion and depression and emotional lability
	PC.9	Deficiency HT Yang	cold hands
	HT.6	Deficiency HT Yin Stagnant HT Blood	restless anxiety angina pectoris
	HT.7	Deficiency HT Qi and Blood	emotional lability and tiredness

BL.17   to relax the diaphragm and calm fear
         to tonify Liver Blood
BL.18   to calm Hyperactive Liver Yang and Wind
         to disperse Liver Fire
BL.23   to tonify Kidney Jing, Qi, Yin or Yang
         to disperse Cold and Damp
BL.31–33 to regulate sex and reproduction.

CV + Yin HV

This pair can be combined with BL.13 for asthma; or alternated with, for example, BL.13, BL.17 and BL.23 to tonify Lungs and Kidneys and calm fear.

BV + Yang LV

This pair can be alternated with, for example, BL.23 to tonify Kidney Yin plus BL.18 to move Stagnant Liver Qi and BL.32 to disperse Damp Heat in the vagina, to treat a combination of hypochondriac pain, leucorrhoea and cystitis.

TV + Yin LV

Some examples of alternation of Back Transporting points with this pair are:

BL.15, BL.17   chest pain from stagnant Blood
BL.15, BL.20, BL.43   for palpitations from Deficient
                      Blood of Heart and Spleen
BL.15, BL.23   for fearful anxiety from Deficient
                      Qi of Kidney and Heart
BL.17, BL.21   epigastric pain from Stagnant
                      Blood
BL.20, BL.23   exhaustion from Deficient Qi of
                      Kidney and Spleen
BL.24, BL.32   dysmenorrhoea from Stagnant
                      Blood.

METHODS OF USING THE OPENING POINTS

There are various methods of using Opening points, and in the opinion of the author, it is merely a matter of personal preference, and an intuitive assessment of the needs of a particular patient and situation. The Opening points of both channels of the pair can be used bilaterally or unilaterally.

Table 10.12 Governor and Yang heel channels: point combinations with SI.3 + BL.62

Point	Problems
GV.1	spinal stiffness, agitation, depression
GV.4	back problems, exhaustion, coldness, impotence, agitation, lack of determination and ambition
GV.8	muscle spasm of back, shoulders and neck with frustration, anger and inability to concentrate
GV.9	fearful agitation, oversensitivity to environment, fear of loss of control, emotional rigidity
GV.11	depression, anxiety, poor memory, restlessness, inability to concentrate, palpitations
GV.12	spasm or weakness of the muscles of upper back and neck
GV.14	stiffness and pain in the neck, depression, mania, common cold and influenza
GV.15 & 16	neck problems, occipital headaches, cerebral problems, depression, mania, fear, dizziness, speech problems
GV.20	vertex headaches, dizziness, confusion, mental dullness, agitation, depression, exhaustion, insomnia
GV.23 & 24	confusion, agitation, frontal headaches, eye problems
BL.1 & 2	eye problems, frontal headaches, mental dullness, depression, insomnia
BL.9 & 10	occipital headaches, neck problems, depression, mental confusion
BL.11	problems of the bones, neck and spinal problems, influenza
BL.15	depression, anxiety, disorientation, stress in relationships, dream-disturbed sleep, chest pain
BL.18	muscle tremors and spasms, spinal stiffness, headache, dizziness, anger, frustration, depression
BL.23	weak spine, lower back problems, exhaustion, lack of drive, lack of sexual interest, easily frightened and discouraged, fear of loss of control
BL.31–34	sacral problems, sexual problems, faecal and urinary incontinence
BL.40	knee, leg and lumbar problems
BL.59	leg problems (Accumulating point of Yang HV)
SI.9–12	shoulder problems
SI.14–15	neck problems
SI.16–17	depression, the feeling of being stuck in a role, difficulty in a relationship
GB.20	eye problems, influenza
GB.29–30	hip problems, especially in old people with degeneration of the bones
GB.38	bone problems

Table 10.13 Conception and Yin heel channels: point combinations with LU.7 + KI.6

Point	Problems
CV.1	genital pain and irritation, prolapses
CV.3	urinary, genital and reproductive disorders
CV.4	asthma, shortness of breath, oedema, exhaustion, lack of will and drive, depression, fearfulness, infertility, impotence, fear and withdrawal in sexual relationships
CV.6	depression, oedema, abdominal pain and distension, abdominal masses
CV.9	oedema and abdominal distension
CV.14	fear of loss of control, asthma with fear and nervous tension
CV.17	asthma, depression, suppressed grief, withdrawal, menopausal anxiety, fear of letting go, fear of loneliness
CV.22	asthma, cough, tension of vocal cords with fear
CV.24	fear and panic
KI.1	exhaustion, depression, infertility, impotence, fear in sexual relationships, fear restricting breathing. depression and anxiety with out-of-the-body sensation
KI.8	urinary retention, dysmenorrhoea (Accumulation point of Yin HV)
KI.13–14	infertility, amenorrhoea
KI.24–25	asthma
KI.27	asthma, mental tiredness, disorientation
LU.1	depression, suppressed grief, feeling of fullness in the chest, asthma
LU.3	depression, withdrawal, fear of participating in life
BL.1–2	insomnia, depression, mental dullness
yìn táng	mental congestion, mental confusion, the need to let go and see reality clearly

Table 10.14 Belt and Yang link channels: point combinations with GB.41 + TE.5

Point	Problem
GB.1	eye problems
GB.2	ear problems
GB.13	indecision, uncertainty and irritability combined with will weak or not firm
GB.14	eye problems, frontal headaches
GB.20	headaches, dizziness, neck and shoulder problems, ear problems, eye problems
GB.21	trapezius muscle spasm associated with frustration, suppressed anger, and nervous tension
GB.22–24	chest and side problems
GB.25	side and lumbar problems
GB.26–28	vaginal discharge and irritation, irritable bowel syndrome
GB.29–30	hip problems
GB.31	skin problems, thigh problems
GB.32	thigh problems
GB.33	knee problems
GB.35	calf problems (Accumulation point of Yang HV)
TE.15	shoulder and neck problems
TE.16	frustration, depression (Window of Heaven point)
TE.17	all ear problems, tension in jaw muscles
TE.23	eye problems
CV.1	genital inflammation
CV.3	leucorrhoea, genital problems, irregular menstruation
CV.4	headaches, dizziness, ear or eye infections associated with Hyperactive Liver Yang or Fire based on Deficient Kidney Qi or Yin
CV.6	Damp Heat urogenital problems associated with Stagnant Qi in the lower abdomen
CV.14	Hyperactive Liver Yang headaches or muscle tension associated with fear, anger and oversensitivty
LR.5	LR–GB Damp Heat urinary or genital problems
LR.8	LR–GB Yang and Fire based on Deficient Liver Yin with eye or ear problems, headache or irritability
LR.12	local point for genital problems
KI.3	Hyperactive Liver Yang based on Deficient Kidney Qi, e.g. headaches, dizziness, emotional lability
KI.6	LR–GB Hyperactive Yang and Fire based on Deficient Kidney Yin, e.g. restless irritability, eye and ear inflammations, headaches
SP.6	Hyperactive Liver Yang associated with Stagnant Liver Qi, or with Deficient Yin of Kidney, Liver, Stomach or Heart, e.g. eye, ear, head, digestive, urinary, gynaecological, psychological and leg problems

Table 10.15 Thoroughfare and Yin link channels: point combinations with SP.4 + PC.6

Point	Problems
SP.1	poor circulation (with moxa) or inflammation (bleed) in toes, feet or legs
SP.5–9	local leg problems, e.g. varicose veins
SP.10	Deficient Blood
SP.12–13	local points for groin problems
SP.15	irritable bowel syndrome with nervous anxiety, abdominal distension and pain
SP.21	lethargy, depression, chest pain
ST.21	epigastric distension and pain
ST.25	abdominal distension and pain
ST.29	dysmenorrhoea
ST.30	dysmenorrhoea, impotence, infertility, genital pain, poor circulation in legs
ST.31	leg pain, poor circulation in legs
ST.36	Deficient Qi and Blood
ST.40	abdominal distension and pain
PC.1	loneliness, depression, chest pain
PC.8–9	depression, poor circulation in hands
KI.9	mania, anxiety, depression, feeling of tightness in the chest, palpitations (Accumulation point of Yin Link)
KI.13	infertility
CV.3	dysmenorrhoea associated with Stagnant Blood
CV.4	exhaustion, depression, poor circulation, anxiety associated with Deficient Qi and Yang, and infertility or impotence associated with Deficient Jing
CV.6	abdominal pain or depression associated with Stagnant Qi
CV.12	poor appetite, exhaustion, emaciation associated with Deficient Qi, epigastric pain associated with Stagnant Qi and Blood, or nausea and hiccups associated with Rebellious Stomach Qi
CV.13	nausea, vomiting, hiccup, belching associated with stress
CV.14	digestive, circulatory or reproductive problems associated with fear and anger
CV.17	heart and circulatory problems of Deficiency, Excess, Stagnation or Irregularity
CV.22	nervous swallowing or spasm of the oesophagus
CV.23	problems of speech and communication of feelings associated with anxiety, fear or depression
CV.24	panic, fear, terror and anxiety
yìn táng	excessive worry and mental preoccupation associated with fear and insecurity

BILATERAL USE

Needles are inserted on both right and left for each of the two Opening points. If additional points are used then these can also be used bilaterally. An example would be using GV + Yang HV and inserting SI.3 and BL.62 bilaterally as Opening points, and then adding HT.6 and KI.6 bilaterally as additional points for panic attacks due to Deficient HT and KI Yin.

UNILATERAL USE FOR MEN AND WOMEN

It is generally agreed that in each Extra channel pair, one channel is of primary and the other channel of secondary importance:

Primary	Secondary
GV	Yang HV
CV	Yin HV
BV	Yang LV
TV	Yin LV

Also, traditionally, the left side of the body is dominant on a man and the right side on a woman. Therefore, a popular unilateral method is to needle first the Opening point of the primary channel on the dominant side, and then the Opening point of the secondary channel on the opposite side.

For example in the use of GV + Yang HV on a man, insert first SI.3 on the left, then BL.62 on the right. To use GV + Yang HV on a woman, insert first SI.3 on the right, then BL.62 on the left. Needles are removed in reverse order to insertion. However, some practitioners feel that GV + Yang HV is too Yang a treatment for women, and that it should be combined with CV + Yin HV. So SI.3 is first inserted on the right, then BL.62 on the left, followed by LU.7 on the left and KI.6 on the right. Again the needles are removed in reverse order (see Fig. 10.11).

Figure 10.12 shows the unilateral use of HT.6 and KI.6 as additional points to GV + Yang HV for panic attack due to Deficient Heart and Kidney Yin.

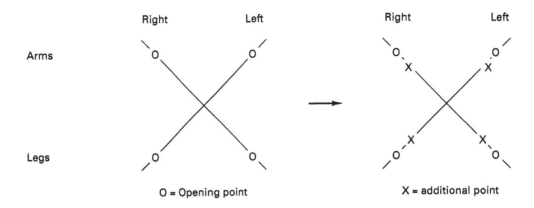

Fig. 10.10

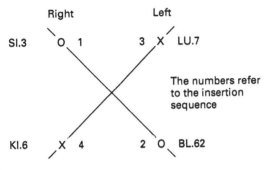

Fig. 10.11

However, this may be considered too Yang a treatment for a woman, and indeed for a man it will need to be modified if there is Deficient Yin of Kidneys or Liver. SP.6 could be used as an additional point, and in this case it would be used on the opposite side, i.e. on the left. The additional point is used on the opposite side to give a treatment which has a better right–left balance.

SEQUENCE OF INSERTION

First needle the Opening point of the primary channel, bilaterally or unilaterally as preferred. Then needle the Opening point of the secondary channel. If a second pair of Extra channels is being combined with the first, as in the example of combining GV + Yang HV with CV + Yin HV, next needle first the Opening point of the primary and the Opening point of the secondary channels in this second pair. Alternatively, if additional points with energetic effect are being used on the arms and legs, as in the example of adding HT.6 and KI.6, these would be inserted next. Following these would be the insertions of

UNILATERAL USE OF THE AFFECTED SIDE

If there is a problem that is solely or predominantly on one side of the body, then the Opening points of both channels can be used on the affected side only. For example, a patient with headache and hypochondriac pain on the right side of the body can be treated with GB.41 and TE.5 on the right side only.

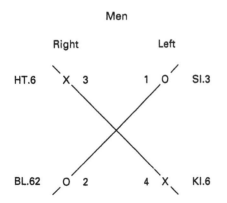

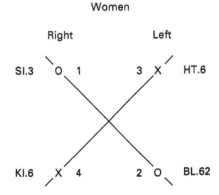

Fig. 10.12

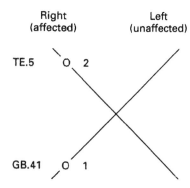 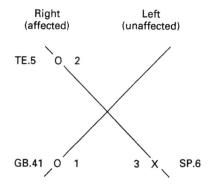

Fig. 10.13

CV or GV points, then Back Transporting points, and finally points with local effect, such as GB.1 and GB.14 for a headache. Needles are removed in reverse order to insertion.

Point combinations for the main acupuncture points

Each of the 14 main channels is given a chapter in Part II. Each chapter is divided into three sections: Channel, Points, Point comparisons and combinations.

CHANNEL

This section discusses the Main channel and Connecting channel pathways and connections, the relationships of the channel to other channels, organs and energy centres, and the general functions of the channel points. A summary table is given of the point combinations for the main organ syndromes, where appropriate.

POINTS

This is the main section of each chapter. Each of the commonly used points on the channel is discussed in detail. Where appropriate, the different syndromes for a point are listed, and then, for each syndrome, the following are given: pulse, indications, example, combination. For example, for SP.6, nine syndromes are given, each with details of pulse, indications, example and combination.

POINT COMPARISONS AND COMBINATIONS

The functions of the main points of the channel are compared in a table, and the most important functions are underlined. Some common combinations of the channel points with each other are summarized in a table, which where appropriate gives combinations of two, three or even four points. For some channels there are further tables of combination of the channel points with points from other channels, for example, combinations of Conception with Liver points.

Conception 11

CHANNEL CONNECTIONS

MAIN CHANNEL PATHWAY

The Conception channel is connected with the Kidney and starts inside the lower abdomen, descending, through the uterus in women, and emerging at the perineum. It ascends the front midline of the body, to surround the mouth, meeting the Governor channel at GV.28, and continuing up to the eyes to meet the Stomach channel at ST.1.

CONNECTING CHANNEL PATHWAY

This channel starts from CV.15 and spreads over the abdomen.

Table 11.1 Crossing points on the Conception channel

Point	Crossing	Other function
CV.24	CV, GV, LI, ST	
CV.23	CV, Yin Link	
CV.22	CV, Yin Link	
CV.17		Alarm point of Pericardium, Gathering point of Qi, Sea of Qi point
CV.15		Connecting point of Conception
CV.14		Alarm point of Heart
CV.13	CV, SI, ST	
CV.12	CV, SI, ST, TE	Alarm point of Stomach, Gathering point of Yang Organs
CV.10	CV, Thoroughfare	
CV.6		
CV.5		Alarm point of Triple Energizer
CV.4	CV, KI, SP, LR	Alarm point of Small Intestine
CV.3	CV, KI, SP, LR	Alarm point of Bladder
CV.2	CV, LR	
CV.1	CV, GV, Thoroughfare	

THE CONCEPTION CHANNEL AND THE ENERGY CENTRES

THE CONCEPTION AND GOVERNOR ENERGY CYCLE

The Governor channel runs up the spine from GV.1, over the head, to meet the Conception channel at CV.24. The Conception channel flows between the head and the perineum, where it links again with the Governor channel at CV.1, completing the cycle.

Together, these two channels form the vertical axis of the energy circulation within the body. The energy centres are the major foci, or crossroads, of energy flows upon this vertical axis.

THE ENERGY CENTRES ON THE CONCEPTION CHANNEL

Centres 1–7 in Table 11.2, are the main energy centres on the Conception channel. There are also centres on the Governor channel on the back of the body, roughly corresponding to these centres on the Conception channel on the front. The function of these energy centres is discussed in Chapter 2.

Table 11.2 Conception energy centres

No.	Centre	Point
9	Crown	GV.20
8	Brow	yin táng
7	Throat	CV.22–23
6	Heart	CV.17
5	Solar Plexus	CV.14–15
4	Spleen	CV.12
3	Dan Tian	CV.4–6
2	Reproduction	CV.2–3
1	Perineal	CV.1

The Qi flow at an energy centre can be Deficient, Excess, Stagnant or Irregular, and in addition the centres may not be in balance with each other. Acupuncture and Qi Gong can be used together to regulate individual centres and to harmonize the balance between the centres.

THE USE OF CV POINTS ACCORDING TO DERMATOME THEORY

The relationship of the CV, Stomach and Kidney points on the chest and abdomen to the segmental arrangement of spinal nerves is briefly discussed in Chapter 1.

FUNCTIONS OF CONCEPTION POINTS

TONIFY JING

As part of the Eight Extra channel system which is closely associated with the Kidneys, the Conception channel is involved in the storage of Jing and with its distribution through the body. This means that the Opening points of the Conception channel, LU.7 and KI.6, and also especially CV.4, can be used to tonify Jing and treat problems of conception, of physical, mental and sexual development, and of premature ageing.

TONIFY YUAN QI AND KIDNEY QI

Yuan Qi is stored in the area of the Dan Tian in the lower abdomen and is available to catalyse the functions of all the organs. It is an especially dynamic energy, intermediate between Jing and Kidney Qi. CV.4 especially can be used to tonify Yuan Qi and Kidney Qi to tonify the other organs and to firm and stabilize their associated emotions and mental functions.

TONIFY YIN

The Conception channel is said to coordinate all the Yin channels of the body. Again, CV.4 especially, because it can tonify Kidney Yin which is the basis of the Yin of the other organs, can be used to tonify the Yin of any organ in the body.

Since Yin is the basis for the Blood, in certain cases, for example, where Deficient Yin is associated with Deficient Blood, CV.4 can be used to tonify Blood. Examples of this would be insomnia with restlessness and poor memory, or menopausal flushes with dizziness and tiredness.

MOVE STAGNANT QI

One of the most useful functions of the Conception channel in the clinic is that it not only moves Stagnant Qi, but also conditions that derive from Stagnant Qi, such as Stagnant Blood, Stagnant food, Stagnant Fluids, accumulation of Phlegm and Stagnant emotions.

CV points are often used segmentally to remove Stagnation in their local area, e.g. CV.3 or CV.6 in the Lower Energizer, CV.12 or CV.13 in the Middle Energizer, CV.17 in the Upper Energizer and CV.22 or CV.23 in the throat.

CALM IRREGULARITY OF QI

CV.12 or CV.10 can be used to calm Rebellious Qi of

Stomach and CV.17 or CV.22 can be used to calm Rebellious Qi of the Lungs. However, in addition to this CV.14, 15 and 24 can be used to calm the Heart Spirit when it is disturbed by fear or anxiety. CV.4 is often combined with these points, since by tonifying Kidney Qi and the Yuan Qi of the appropriate organs, it can stabilize emotions which are labile due to Deficiency.

REGULATE WATER

Either by means of its Opening points, LU.7 and KI.6, or by means of its channel points, such as CV.4, 6, 9 and 12 especially, the Conception channel can be used to tonify Spleen, Kidneys and Lungs to transform Stagnant Fluids and to disperse the Stagnation of Qi associated with their accumulation.

REGULATE THE UTERUS

Firstly, the CV points in the Lower Energizer are local to the area of the female reproductive system. Then, by tonifying and regulating Jing, the Conception channel plays a part in regulating the development, functioning and decline of sex and reproduction. Also, by tonifying Kidney Qi and Yin, the Conception channel provides the energy and the materials for menstruation and conception. By moving Stagnant Qi, the Conception can assist dispersal of Stagnant Blood in the uterus, e.g. dysmenorrhoea, Stagnant Fluids, e.g. premenstrual oedema, and accumulation of Phlegm in the Lower Energizer, e.g. fibroid.

Most important, the Conception channel points can help to balance many of the emotional problems associated with reproductive problems. For example, depression due to Stagnant Qi or Deficient Qi or emotional instability due to Deficient Qi or emotional instability due to Deficient Qi or Deficient Yin with Hyperactive Liver Yang or Heart and Liver Fire.

COMPARISONS OF CONCEPTION WITH OTHER SYSTEMS

CONCEPTION AND GOVERNOR CHANNELS

The Conception channel controls the Yin and the Governor channel the Yang, and between them balance the Yin–Yang of the body. Both can be used to tonify Kidney Jing, Yuan Qi, Qi and Yang, for example, CV.4 and GV.4. While GV.4 is more for controlling and tonifying Yang and treating back and spinal problems, CV.4 is also for tonifying Yin and regulating the uterus. However, the

segmentally corresponding points, such as CV.4 and GV.4, can be used in combination or alternation to treat the organs controlled by a particular spinal segment, and also the emotions and mental capacities controlled by these organs.

CONCEPTION AND THOROUGHFARE CHANNELS

Although Conception is Yin relative to Governor, it is Yang relative to the Thoroughfare channel. All three channels originate in the Kidney area, and have a Crossing point at CV.1. The Conception and Thoroughfare channels have overlapping functions in regulating the uterus in menstruation and conception. However, the Conception channel is more to tonify Yin and move Stagnant Qi, while the Thoroughfare channel is more to tonify Blood and move Stagnant Blood. The uses of the pairs of Opening points of LU.7 and KI.6 for CV and SP.4 and PC.6, reflect these differences. The CV pair is more for depression, asthma and oedema relating to gynaecological problems, while the Thoroughfare pair is more for pain in Lower, Middle or Upper Energizer, with nervous anxiety and weak digestion, associated with reproductive problems.

CONCEPTION AND BELT CHANNELS

The Conception and Belt channels also overlap in their reproductive indications and indeed both can be used for Damp Heat conditions in the Lower Energizer. Also, since Belt relates to Gallbladder and Liver, and since the Conception channel resembles the Liver channel in preventing Stagnation of Qi, the Conception and Belt have some similar functions. However, the Belt is specifically related to Liver–Gallbladder problems with involvement of the Triple Energizer and Gallbladder channels, and in gynaecology is especially for Liver–Gallbladder-type problems related to the birth control pill. The Conception channel is also concerned with conditions of Deficient Kidney Jing, Qi, Yin or Yang, such as impotence, infertility and amenorrhoea.

CONCEPTION AND LIVER CHANNELS

As stated above, both Conception and Liver control the free flow of Qi. In problems of digestion and menstruation, CV and Liver points can be used in a similar way, e.g. CV.6 and LR.3 for dysmenorrhoea or CV.12 and LR.13 for Liver invading Spleen. However, the CV points are more related to a segmental arrangement and also to the Kidneys so that they can be used more for tonification than the Liver points.

CONCEPTION AND KIDNEY CHANNELS

Although the point CV.4 is very similar to KI.3 in its tonifying effects and its effects on stabilizing the emotions, the CV points have a more powerful effect in moving Stagnant Qi than do the Kidney points. On the leg, only KI.8 has significant Qi-moving functions. However, on the body, the Kidney points can be used in a segmental system, combined with the CV point in the same segment, and here they can have local effect to move the Qi. For example, KI.14 and CV.5 for infertility, or KI.23 and CV.17 for asthma.

CAUTION ON THE USE OF CONCEPTION POINTS WITH REDUCING METHOD

Reducing method of needling should be used with caution on the Conception channel points, since this channel is an important reservoir for the energies of the body. This is especially so for CV.4, 5 and 6, which represent the Dan Tian energy centre.

CV.4

Never reduce CV.4 is the safest rule.

CV.6

Only reduce CV.6 in a purely Excess acute condition, and never repeatedly, in a chronic situation. If the condition is a mixture of Excess and Deficiency, then either use CV.6 with Even method, or tonify CV.6 and use points on the other channels with Reducing method.

CV.3

It is safer to reduce CV.3 than to reduce CV.4 or CV.6. However, like CV.6, even CV.3 should not be reduced repeatedly in chronic situations. Either other points should be alternated with CV.3, like BL.31, or points should be added to tonify Deficiency, like KI.6.

CONCEPTION SYNDROMES

Conception channel syndromes are discussed in detail in Chapter 10.

Conception points

CV.1 huĭ yìn

Meeting point of the Conception, Governor and Thoroughfare channels.

General

As a local point, CV.1 can be used for local anal and urogenital problems. As an energy centre of the body, the Perineal centre, CV.1 is concerned with survival of the individual, hence its use to restore consciousness. It is also involved in reproduction, the survival of the species. However, the Reproduction centre at CV.3 is more used to treat reproductive problems with a more than local involvement, for example involving hormonal and emotional imbalance.

As an energy centre on the GV–CV energy circulation system, CV.1 is important in advanced Qi Gong exercises, having its own special functions. It is indicated in acupuncture to calm the mind, but is seldom used for this function. In summary, this point is seldom used, and when it is, the main indication is for local anal and urogenital problems.

Syndrome

Damp Heat and/or Deficiency Heat affecting local anogenital region

Pulse. Slippery, rapid, maybe thin or wiry.

Indications. Anal or genital itching swelling or pain, dysuria, prostates, haemorrhoids.

Example. Orchitis with red sore itchy scrotum.

Combination. CV.1, CV.3, LR.5, LR.12, ST.30, SP.6, KI.2, Rd.

CV.2 qū gŭ

Meeting point of the Conception and Liver channels.

General

CV.2 and CV.3 are included in the energy centre of the body termed the Reproduction centre, and of the two points, CV.3 is more widely used. CV.2 can be used like CV.1 for the local urogenital problems due to Damp Heat or Deficiency Fire, but in addition, can also be used to raise the Qi and to warm and tonify the Yang of Bladder and uterus.

Syndromes

Damp Heat in Lower Energizer
Deficient Yang and Cold in Lower Energizer
Sinking of Qi in Lower Energizer

Damp Heat in Lower Energizer

See **CV.1**.

Deficient Yang and Cold in Lower Energizer

Pulse. Empty, deep, slow, maybe tight.

Indications. Infertility, amenorrhoea, impotence, pain and sensataion of cold in uterus or genital, urinary problems.

Example. Impotence with feelings of tiredness and cold.

Combination. CV.2, CV.4, GV.20, KI.7, BL.60, ST.36, Rf M; KI.1, M.

Sinking of Qi in Lower Energizer

Pulse. Empty, deep, maybe choppy.

Indications. Uterine bleeding, uterine prolapse.

Example. Uterine bleeding after childbirth with feelings of exhaustion and depression.

Combination. CV.2, CV.6, CV.12, GV.20, KI.3, ST.36, Rf M; HT.7 Rf.

CV.3 zhōng jí

Alarm point of the Bladder, Crossing point of Conception, Liver, Spleen and Kidney channels

General

CV.3 is the main point representing the Reproduction energy centre of the body. There is some overlap in function and location between the Reproduction centre and the centre above it, the Dan Tian, which is a focal point in the body for the storage and distribution of energy. Thus CV.4 can be used for reproduction problems and CV.3 can be used to warm and tonify the kidneys. However, the main indication of CV.3 is to use it with Reducing method for Excess Damp Heat conditions of the Lower Energizer, and the main indication of CV.4 is to use it with Reinforcing method to tonify the Kidney.

CV.3 and the bā liáo points

The bā liáo points, the points within the eight sacral foramina, BL.31, BL.32, BL.33 and BL.34, represent an energy centre on the Governor channel on the back of the body, that closely corresponds with the Reproduction centre on the front of the body, represented by CV.2 and CV.3.

Both sets of points treat urogenital problems, especially due to Damp Heat in the Lower Energizer, but also due to Deficient Yang and Sinking of Qi in the Lower Energizer. One significant difference between them is due to their physical location: the bā liáo points are indicated for local back pain, whilst CV.2 or CV.3 are for local abdominal pain or itching. In additon, the bā liáo are more used for difficult or delayed childbirth, whilst CV.3 is more used for stones in the lower urinary tract.

Syndromes

Damp Heat in the Lower Energizer
    Damp Heat in the Lower Energizer with Stagnant Liver Qi
    Damp Heat in the Lower Energizer with Deficient Fire of Kidneys and/or Heart

Stagnant Qi in the Lower Energizer with Heat in the Blood
Stagnant Qi in the Lower Energizer with Deficient Kidney Qi
Deficient Qi and Yang of Bladder and Kidneys

Damp Heat in the Lower Energizer with Stagnant Liver Qi

Pulse. Wiry, slippery, rapid.

Indications. Pelvic inflammatory disease, irregular menstruation, genital pain or itching, dysuria.

Example. Irregular menstruation with depression, frustration and yellow leucorrhoea.

Combination. CV.3, LR.5, SP.6, PC.6, Rd.

Damp Heat in the Lower Energizer with Deficiency Fire of Kidneys and/or Heart

Pulse. Thin, slippery, rapid, maybe irregular.

Indications. Genital pain or itching, dysuria, premature ejaculation.

Example. Cystitis with restlessness, insomnia and anxiety.

Combination. CV.3, SP.6, KI.2, HT.8, Rd; KI.10, HT.3, Rf.

Stagnant Qi in the Lower Energizer with Heat in the Blood

Pulse. Wiry, rapid, maybe full or flooding.

Indications. Menorrhagia, leucorrhoea with bleeding, genital rashes.

Example. Menorrhagia restlessness, irritability and anger.

Combination. CV.3, SP.1, SP.6, SP.10, LR.2, LR.1, Rd; PC.9 B.

Stagnant Qi in the Lower Energizer with Deficient Kidney Qi

Pulse. Wiry, empty.

Indications. Amenorrhoea, prostatitis, urinary retention, oedema, stones in lower urinary tract.

Example. Prostates, worse with tiredness and depression.

Combination. CV.3, ST.29, SP.6, KI.8, TE.6 E M; ST.36 Rf M.

Deficient Qi and Yang of Bladder and Kidneys

Pulse. Empty, deep, maybe slow or slippery.

Indications. Infertility, white leucorrhoea, oedema, urinary incontinence, impotence.

Example. Impotence with unresolved grief.

Combination. CV.3, KI.2, KI.7, ST.29, ST.36 Rf M; LU.7 Rd.

CV.4 guān yuán

Alarm point of Small Intestine, Crossing point of the Conception, Liver, Spleen and Kidney channels.

General

Dan Tian

The area around CV.4 to CV.6, is called the Dan Tian. This is an energy centre of the body, which is concerned with the storage and distribution of energy, both Qi and Jing. CV.4 is used mainly to strengthen the storage aspect of the Dan Tian, so it is usually used with Reinforcing method to tonify Kidney Qi, Jing, Yin or Yang. CV. 6 corresponds more to the distribution aspect of the Dan Tian, so it is mostly used with Reducing or Even method to disperse Stagnation of Qi.

Kidney Jing

CV.4 tonifies Kidney Jing, which controls the process of conception, birth, development and ageing. CV.4 can therefore be used as a basis for point combinations to treat infertility, retarded physical, mental or sexual development, menstrual problems, premature ageing and the problems of old age such as poor hearing and vision and weak joints and muscles.

Source Qi

Classically, the Source Qi (Yuan Qi) is stored in the area between the Kidneys, corresponding to the Dan Tian (see *Nan-Ching: The Classic of Difficult Issues*, translated by Paul U. Unschuld, University of California Press, Berkeley, 1986). The Yuan Qi, intermediate in function between Jing and Qi, catalyses all the activities of the body. CV.4 can therefore be combined with the Source points (Yuan points) of specific organs, to tonify their Yuan Qi.

Precautions in using CV.4

Since CV.4 represents the storage aspect of the Dan Tian, involving the body reserves of Qi, Yuan Qi and Jing, needling with Reducing method is contradicted. Since CV.4 deals with Jing and Yuan Qi, it can make available deeper and less easily replaceable energies than ordinary Qi. Therefore, it should not be used for merely day-to-day tiredness, but for chronic deep-seated exhaustion. If the patient, on feeling more energy available from the treatment, is simply going to use up that energy for more hectic living, and not conserve it to allow healing to take place, this point should not be used. This point calls up the deeper reserve energies of the body, which if frittered away are difficult to replace.

CV.4 tonifies Yin and Yang of all organs

This is because CV.4 tonifies Kidney Yin and Yang, and Kidney Yin and Yang is the source of the Yin and Yang of the other organs. Therefore CV.4 can be used to tonify Lung Yang or Heart Yin, in combination with the appropriate points.

CV.4 and Qi Gong

The action of CV.4 to tonify Qi Yuan and Jing can be increased by combining acupuncture with Qi Gong exercises that increase and conserve the store of Qi at the Dan Tian, and that increase the efficiency with which this energy is made available to other organs. In addition, the Qi Gong exercises can reduce Kidney fear and also strengthen the will.

CV.4 and the treatment of mind and emotions

As was discussed in Chapter 8, CV.4 can be combined with the Source points to strengthen the five mental aspects, to stabilize the five emotional types and also to treat depression due to Deficiency.

CV.4 and GV.4

GV.4, represents an energy centre on the Governor channel on the back that corresponds to the Dan Tian in the front of the body. Both points tonify Kidney Jing, Qi and Yang, but GV.4 is more specifically to tonify Yang, to regulate the GV channel and to treat the back, while CV.4 can also tonify Yin and Blood and regulate the uterus.

Syndromes

  Deficient Kidney Jing
      Deficient Kidney Jing and Deficient Kidney Yang
      Deficient Kidney Jing and Deficient Blood

  Deficient Kidney Qi
      Kidney Qi not Firm
      Kidney fails to receive Qi (Deficient Kidney Qi and Deficient Lung Qi)
      Spirit not stable (Deficient Kidney Qi and Deficient Heart Qi)
      Deficient Kidney Qi and Deficient Spleen Qi
      Deficient Kidney Qi and Hyperactive Liver Yang

  Deficient Kidney Yang
      Deficient Kidney Yang and Interior Cold
      Deficient Kidney Yang and Water Overflowing
      Deficient Kidney Yang and Deficient Spleen Yang (Sinking of Spleen Qi)

  Deficient Kidney Yin and Deficient Qi and Blood

Deficient Kidney Jing

Deficient Kidney Jing and Deficient Kidney Yang

Pulse. Thin to minute, deep, slow, maybe choppy, maybe weak.

Indications. Premature ageing, infertility, impotence, inability to focus the mind.

Example. Impotence.

Combination. CV.4, KI.2, KI.3, ST.30, Rf M: yín táng Rf.

Alternation. GV.4, BL.23, BL.60, BL.64, Rf M; GV. 20 Rf.

Deficient Kidney Jing and Deficient Blood

Pulse. Thin, choppy, maybe weak–floating.

Indications. Premature ageing, infertility, amenorrhoea, hair loss, greying of hair, dry wrinkled skin, weak muscles and joints, poor memory.

Example. Weak legs in the elderly.

Combination. CV.4, KI.3, SP.6, ST.36, LI.4, Rf.

Alternation: GV.4, BL.11, BL.17, BL.23, GB.34, GB.39, Rf.

Deficient Kidney Qi

Kidney Qi Not Firm

Pulse. Empty, deep.

Indications. Enuresis, urinary frequency, dribbling or incontinence, spermatorrhoea, lack of will.

Example. Enuresis with lack of energy and frightening dreams.

Combination. CV.4, KI.7, KI.10, ST.36, GV.20, Rf.

Alternation. GV.4, BL.23, BL.28, BL.64, GV.20 Rf.

Kidney fails to receive Qi (Deficient Kidney Qi and Deficient Lung Qi)

Pulse. Empty.

Indications. Cough, asthma, shortness of breath on exertion, difficulty in inhalation, easily tired on exertion, easy sweating on exertion.

Example. Asthma especially when tired, with weak cough and shortness of breath.

Combination. Between attacks CV.4, CV.17, KI.6, LU.7; Rf.

Alternation. BL.23, BL.13 Rf; dìng chuǎn Rd.

Spirit not stable (Deficient Kidney Qi and Deficient Heart Qi)

Pulse. Empty, maybe changing, in extreme cases may be scattered or moving.

Indications. Emotions instability, easily fearful or anxious, jumpy, palpitations, easily tired.

Example. Easily disturbed and easily tired by emotions; feeling shaky, weak and insecure.

Combination. CV.4, CV.14, CV.17, KI.3, HT.7, ST.36 Rf.

Alternation. GV.4, GV.11, GV.20, BL.52, BL.44, BL.64 Rf.

Deficient Kidney Qi and Deficient Spleen Qi

Pulse. Empty, choppy, changing.

Indications. Weak constitution, no reserves of energy, weak digestion, weak back.

Example. Easily tired, worried, insecure, poor appetite.

Combination. CV.4, CV.12, SP.4, PC.6 Rf M.

Alternation. BL.23, BL.20 Rf M.

Deficient Kidney Qi and Hyperactive Liver Yang

Pulse. Empty, wiry, maybe deep or changing.

Indications. Tiredness, emotional hypersensitivity, irritability, dizziness, migraine, hypertension.

Example. Headache, photophobia, weak lower back, tense shoulders and neck.

Combination. CV.4, KI.3 Rf; LR.3, GB.14, GB.20, GB.21, GV.20 Rd.

Deficient Kidney Yang

Deficient Kidney Yang and Interior Cold

Pulse. Empty, deep, slow, maybe tight.

Indications. Exhaustion, extremities and whole body cold.

Example. Depression, lack of energy and will, poor circulation.

Combination. CV.4, KI.1, KI.2, KI.7, HT.7 Rf M.

Alternation: GV.4, GV.14, BL.23, BL.60 Rf M.

Deficient Kidney Yang and Water Overflowing

Pulse Empty, deep, slow, maybe slippery.

Indications. Feelings of cold, urinary retention, oedema.

Example. Oedema, abdominal distension, depression.

Combination. CV.4, CV.9, KI.7, SP.9, ST.28 Rf M.

Alternation: GV.4, GV.14, BL.23, BL.22, BL.39 Rf M.

Deficient Kidney Yang and Deficient Spleen Yang (Sinking of Qi)

Pulse. Empty, deep.

Indications. Prolapse, haemorrhage, loose stools.

Example. Stomach prolapse, exhaustion, feelings of cold.

Combination. CV.4, CV.12, ST.21, ST.36, KI.7, GV.20 Rf M.

Deficient Kidney Yin and Deficient Qi and Blood

Pulse. Thin, rapid, choppy.

Indications. Tiredness, restlessness, insomnia, palpitations, amenorrhoea, infertility.

Example. Tiredness and insomnia with feelings of heat in the chest.

Combination. CV.4, SP.6, ST.36, KI.6, HT.7, HT.3 Rf; ān mián E.

CV. 6 qì hǎi

General

CV.6 and CV.4

CV.6 and CV.4 represent the Dan Tian, the energy centre of the body responsible for energy storage and distribution. The two points have overlapping functions; both tonify Deficiency and both can move Stagnant Qi. However, CV.4, like CV.12 is more for treating Deficiency, and CV.6, like CV.17, is better for dispersing Stagnation.

CV.6 and CV.3

CV.6 and CV.3 can both regulate the uterus and disperse Damp Heat. However, CV.3 is mainly used for Excess Damp Heat problems in the lower Energizer, whilst CV.6 can treat Stagnant Qi in the whole body.

CV.6 and CV.9

Both points treat the accumulation of Damp by tonifying Qi and by moving Stagnant Fluids. However, while CV.9 is limited to this use only, CV.6 can move Stagnant Qi and Stagnant Blood, so that CV.9 is mostly for oedema, whilst CV.6 is also for depression and dysmenorrhoea for example.

CV.6 and LR 3

The CV and Liver channels are both involved with maintaining a free flow of Qi throughout the body. CV.6 and LR.3 can both treat problems arising from Stagnant Qi, such as Stagnant Fluids or Stagnant Blood, and can both regulate the uterus. However, LR.3 is specific for

Wood disorders such as headaches and anger, while CV.6 is more for tonifying Yang and Qi, and LR.3 is more to tonify Blood, or remove Excess Fire and calm the mind. CV.6 can treat depression due to Deficiency or Stagnation but is not much use to treat irregularity of Qi for calming.

Syndromes

Stagnant Qi
Stagnant Qi and Blood in the Lower Energizer
Stagnant Liver Qi invades the Intestines
Stagnation of Damp Heat in the Lower Energizer
Stagnation of Cold Damp in the Lower Energizer
Stagnation of Qi of the chest
Stagnant Qi and Deficient Qi of Kidneys and Heart

Deficient Kidney Qi and Yang

Stagnant Qi

Stagnant Qi and Blood in the Lower Energizer

Pulse. Wiry, maybe choppy, maybe full.

Indications. Lower abdominal pain, sequelae of trauma or surgery in lower abdomen, irregular menstruation, dysmenorrhoea.

Example. Dysmenorrhoea with frustration and depression.

Combination. CV.6, LR.3, LR.14, SP.6, PC.6, Rd.

Stagnant Liver Qi invades the Intestines

Pulse. Wiry, maybe flooding.

Indications. Constipation, lower abdominal distension and pain, flatulence, colitis, irregular defecation.

Example. Constipation with stress and depression.

Combination. CV.6, SP.15, ST.25, ST.37, LR.3, LR.13, PC.6 Rd.

Stagnation of Damp Heat in the Lower Energizer

Pulse. Wiry, slippery, rapid.

Indications. Dysuria, menorrhagia, genital pain and itching.

Example. Cystitis, frustration in relationships.

Combination. CV.6, CV.3, SP.6, SP.9, LR.3, PC.6 Rd.

Stagnation of Cold Damp in the Lower Energizer

Pulse. Wiry or tight, slippery, maybe empty and deep.

Indications. Orchitis, oedema, urinary retention, abdominal distension.

Example. Oedema in lower abdomen and legs.

Combination. CV.6, SP.6, SP.9, ST.28, ST.40 Rd M; LI.4 Rd.

Stagnation of Qi of the chest

Pulse. Wiry, maybe irregular.

Indications. Asthma, palpitations, obstructed feeling in the chest, menopausal depression, premenstrual syndrome.

Example. Unresolved grief with depression and withdrawal.

Combination. CV.6, CV.17 E M; CV. 22, KI.6, LU.7, LU.1 E.

Stagnant Qi and Deficient Qi of Kidney and Heart

Pulse. Wiry, empty.

Indications. Depression, tiredness.

Example. Cold extremities with depression and loss of appetite.

Combination. CV.6, ST.36 E M; SP.4, PC.6 E; HT.9, SP.1 M.

Deficient Kidney Qi and Yang

See CV.4. CV.6 can be used, like CV.4, to tonify Deficient Qi and Yang of the Kidney, to help the Qi and Yang of the other organs and of the entire body. However, when CV.6 is used for Deficiency, it is mainly used to treat a mixture of Deficiency and Stagnation.

CV.9 shuĭ fēn

General

Regulates the Water passages

By improving the transformation, transportation and excretion of fluids, CV.9 can treat problems due to accumulation of Damp, such as oedema.

CV.9 and BL.22

CV.9 is very similar to BL.22 the Back Transporting point for the Energizer. Both points are located on the body around the division between the Lower and Middle Energizer. On the front, CV.9 is between CV.4 which tonifies the Kidneys and CV.12 which tonifies the Spleen. On the back, BL.22 is between BL.23 the Back Transporting point for the Kidneys and BL.21 the Back Transporting point for the Stomach. Both CV.9 and BL.22 remove Damp, partly by tonifying the Kidneys and partly by tonifying the Spleen. Both points are more for Damp associated with Deficiency and Cold, than for Damp Heat. Both points can treat such problems as indigestion and lower back pain, but are especially for fluid problems such as abdominal oedema, and for problems involving the Small Intestine and fluid balance such as dysentery and diarrhoea.

There is not much difference in use between the two points; BL.22 is more used for local back problems and CV.9 with oedema involving Conception channel dysfunctions.

Damp in Lower Energizer

Pulse. Slippery, empty, maybe deep and slow, maybe wiry.

Indications. Abdominal oedema, abdominal distension and pain, borborygmus, diarrhoea, urinary retention, dysuria.

Example. Oedema with loss of appetite and lower backache.

Combination. CV.9, SP.6, LI.4 M; CV.4, CV.12, SP.9, ST.36 M.

Alternation. BL.22, BL.39 M; TE.4, BL.64 M.

CV.10 xià wǎn

Crossing point of Conception and Spleen channels.

General

The main function of CV.10 is, by controlling the cardiac sphincter, to link the Stomach and Intestines. The relationship of CV.10 to CV.12 and CV.13 is discussed on p. 138. CV.12, by tonifying and regulating Spleen and Stomach, allows the unobstructed passage of food from stomach to intestines.

Syndromes

Retention of food in the stomach
Damp Heat in Intestines

Retention of food in the stomach

Pulse. Full or flooding, slippery, maybe wiry.

Indications. Epigastric distension and pain, bad breath, sour regurgitation, nausea, vomiting, loss of appetite, insomnia.

Example. Food retained in stomach with belching, abdominal distension and borborygmus.

Combination. CV.10, CV.13, ST.21, ST.37, PC.6 Rd.

Damp Heat in Intestines

Pulse. Flooding, slippery, rapid.

Indications. Diarrhoea, dysentery.

Example. Diarrhoea with borborygmus and abdominal distension.

Combination. CV.10, SP.15, ST.25, ST.39 Rd, CV.6 E.

CV.12 zhōng wǎn

General

The Spleen centre

CV.12 corresponds to the energy centre known as the Spleen centre, which on the physical level, is responsible for the organs and processes of digestion, from mouth to intestines.

On the emotional level, the function of the Spleen centre is to harmonize the emotional group of worry, insecurity, overconcern and sympathy. At the mental level, it regulates the processes of memory and analytical thought, in other words the processes of obtaining, digesting, assimilating and storing information.

CV.12 for Deficiency

The main use of CV.12 is to tonify Deficient Qi and Yang of Spleen and Stomach and by warming the Middle Energizer to disperse Cold and Damp. CV.12 and CV.4 are similar in that both points are chiefly used to tonify Deficiency, but CV.12 has a wider use than CV.4 in that it can also treat Stagnation and Excess.

CV.12 for Stagnation

CV.12 resembles CV.6 and CV.17 in that it can be used to move Stagnation, but CV.6 and CV.17 are primarily for Stagnation, while CV.12 is especially used to tonify Deficiency.

Both CV.12 and LR.13, the Alarm point of the Spleen, are used to regulate the balance of Liver and Spleen, but although LR.13 can be used to tonify the Spleen, its main function is to treat Stagnation, and it has a greater effect on the Liver than CV.12 does.

CV.12 for Irregularity

While CV.12 can be used to treat Upward Rebellion of Stomach Qi, CV.13 or CV.14 are often better points for this. Also CV.12 does not have a strong calming effect. It can be used to treat chronic worry, since it tonifies and regulates the Spleen, but if an immediate calming effect is required, it is better to add LR.3, PC.6 or yìn táng to the prescription.

Syndromes

Deficient Spleen and Stomach Qi
    Deficient Spleen Qi with Deficient Kidney Qi
    Deficient Spleen Qi with Sinking of Spleen Qi
    Deficient Spleen Qi with Deficient Blood
    Deficient Spleen Qi with Damp
    Deficient Spleen Qi with Liver invading Spleen

Cold Damp in the Middle Energizer
    Cold Damp invading the Spleen
    Cold Invading the Stomach

Retention of food in the stomach
Stomach Qi Rebelling Upward
Heat in the Middle Energizer
    Damp Heat invades the Spleen
    Deficient Stomach Yin with Deficiency Stomach Fire
    Stomach Fire

Deficient Spleen and Stomach Qi

Deficient Spleen Qi with Deficient Kidney Qi

Pulse. Empty, deep.

Indications. Weak constitution, easily tired, weak muscles, weak back, poor appetite.

Example. Tiredness, weakness, worry and insecurity.

Combination. CV.12, CV.4, SP.4 Rf.

Deficient Spleen Qi with Sinking of Spleen Qi

Pulse. Empty, maybe deep.

Indications. Prolapse of organs, flaccid skin and muscles, haemorrhages, person feels tired and wants to lie down.

Example. Stomach prolapse with loss of appetite, epigastric discomfort and feelings of cold.

Combination. CV.12, CV.13, CV.4, ST.21, ST.36 Rf M; GV.20 Rf.

Alternation. BL.20, BL.21, ST.36 Rf M; GV.20 Rf.

Deficient Spleen Qi with Deficient Blood

Pulse. Empty, choppy.

Indications. Anaemia, blurred vision, tiredness, dull headaches, faintness on standing, loss of appetite.

Example. Tiredness with weak muscles and dry skin.

Combination. CV.12, ST.36, SP.6, SP.10, LI.4 Rf.

Alternation. BL.23, BL.20, BL.17, ST.36, LI.4 Rf.

Deficient Spleen Qi with Damp

Pulse. Empty, slippery.

Indications. Abdominal distension, oedema, heavy feeling in the head, mental dullness, lethargy, fluid-filled skin eruptions.

Example. Rheumatoid arthritis aggravated by Damp.

Combination. CV.12, CV.9, SP.6, ST.36, ST.40 Rf; Ah Shi Rd.

Deficient Spleen Qi with Liver invading Spleen

Pulse. Wiry, empty.

Indications. Gastritis, loss of appetite, irregular defecation, borborygmus, tiredness.

Example. Abdominal pain and distension with depression and irritability.

Combination. CV.12, CV.6, LR.3, LR.13, GV.20 E; ST.36 Rf.

Cold Damp in the Middle Energizer

Cold Damp invading the Spleen

Pulse. Slippery, maybe slow.

Indications. Heavy feeling in head, chest or epigastrium, loss of appetite, no thirst, loss of sense of taste, lassitude, loose stools, white leucorrhoea.

Example. Feeling of cold, heaviness and discomfort in epigastrium with sweet taste in mouth and thirst with no desire to drink.

Combination. CV.12, SP.6, SP.9 ST.8 E; SP.3, ST.36 Rf M.

Cold invading the Stomach

Pulse. Tight, maybe deep and slow, maybe full and slippery.

Indications. Acute epigastric pain with feeling of cold, aversion to cold drinks, maybe vomiting clear fluid.

Example. Acute epigastric pain following excessive consumption of cold fluids.

Combination. CV.12, ST.21, ST.40, LI.10, SP.4 Rd M.

Retention of Food in the stomach

CV.12 can be used for this syndrome, but CV.10 is often better to move obstruction from the lower stomach, so that the retained food moves down into the intestines.

Stomach Qi Rebelling Upward

CV.12 can be used for this syndrome, but CV.13 is often better to calm and regulate the upper stomach and lower oesophagus to control nausea, vomiting, belching and hiccup.

Heat in the Middle Energizer

Damp Heat invades the Spleen

Pulse. Slippery, rapid.

Indications. Diarrhoea or loose stools with bad smell, burning sensation of anus on defecation, loss of appetite, nausea, feeling of heaviness.

Example. Diarrhoea with low-grade fever and feeling of heaviness.

Combination. CV.12, SP.15, SP.9, GB.34, LI.11 Rd.

Deficient Stomach Yin with Deficiency Stomach Fire

Pulse. Thin, rapid, maybe wiry.

Indications. Empty sensation in stomach, burning sensation in stomach, epigastric discomfort or pain, thirst, hunger, restless but tired.

Example. Gastritis with thirst and tiredness.

Combination. CV.12, ST.36, SP.6, KI.6 Rf; ST.21, ST.44 Rd.

Stomach Fire

Pulse. Full or flooding, rapid, maybe slippery, maybe wiry.

Indications. Severe burning sensation and pain in the epigrastrium, desire for cold drinks, constant hunger, bad breath, sour regurgitation, bleeding gums.

Example. Severe gastritis with constant hunger, restlessness.

Combination. CV.12, ST.21, ST.44, LI.4, LI.11, PC.6 Rd.

CV.13 shàng wǎn

Meeting point of CV, Small Intestine and Stomach Channels.

General

CV.13 is intermediate in location and function between CV.12 and CV.14. It is closer in function to CV.12 in that it is more used for stomach problems than for disorders of the heart or diaphragm. However, whilst CV.12 is especially useful for deficiency syndromes of Spleen and Stomach, CV.13 is more for acute Excess conditions, where Stomach Qi is rebelling upward.

CV.13 is more for spasms of the lower oesophagus, whilst CV.14 can treat upper oesophageal problems also, such as difficulty in swallowing.

Syndrome

Stomach Qi Rebelling Upward

Pulse. Wiry.

Indications. Nausea, vomiting, belching, hiccup.

Example. Nausea and belching with worry and insecurity.

Combination. CV.13, CV.24, yìn táng, SP.4, PC.6 Rf; ST.36 Rf.

CV.14 jù què

Alarm point of the Heart.

General

The area around CV.14 and CV.15 corresponds to the energy centre called the Solar Plexus. If this centre is overactive and not balanced, the person is too sensitive to impressions from the environment, and their emotional responses to these impressions are too strong, too vivid and too disturbing. In time this can wear down the person's energy, physical health and mental stability. The basic emotion here is fear, associated with the Kidneys, which can invade Liver, Spleen, Heart or Lungs, via the Solar Plexus, which can be a focal point for fear.

The key to understanding CV.14 is that it calms. It can be used to calm the Spirit when this is agitated by Heart Fire or obstructed by Heart Phlegm.

Syndromes

Kidney fear invades Spleen and Stomach
    Kidney fear with Deficient Spleen Qi
    Kidney fear with Stomach Qi Rebelling Upward

Kidney fear invades the Liver
Kidney fear invades Heart
    Deficient Kidney Qi and Deficient Heart Qi
    Deficient Kidney Yin and Deficient Heart Yin

Heart Fire
Heart Phlegm Fire

Kidney fear invades Spleen and Stomach

Kidney fear with Deficient Spleen Qi

Pulse. Empty, maybe changing.

Indications. Tiredness, weak constitution, fear, worry, loose stools, loss of appetite, insomnia, obsession.

Example. Indigestion, abdominal distension, urinary frequency, insecurity.

Combination. CV.14, yìn táng; CV.4, CV.12, KI.3, ST.36 Rf.

Kidney fear with Stomach Qi Rebelling Upward

Pulse. Wiry.

Indications. Nausea, vomiting, belching, hiccup, worry.

Example. Nausea, loss of appetite, indigestion, worry, agitation, fear.

Combination. CV.14, SP.4, PC.6 Rd; CV. 4, KI.3, ST.36 Rf.

Kidney fear invades the Liver

Pulse. Empty, wiry, maybe changing.

Indications. Tense muscles, headache, indigestion, uncertainty, lack of self-confidence, anger and aggression through insecurity, fear, hypersensitivity.

Example. Irritability, touchiness, dizziness and headache.

Combination. CV.14, LR.3, GV.20; CV.4, KI.3, GB.40, GB.13 Rf.

Kidney fear invades the Heart

Deficient Kidney Qi and Deficient Heart Qi

Pulse. Changing, maybe deep.

Indications. Tiredness, palpitations, emotional liability, insomnia, lower back pain.

Example. Paranoia with panic attacks and claustrophobia.

Combination. CV.14, CV.17, CV.24, GV.20, KI.1 E; CV.4, KI.3, HT.7 Rf.

Deficient Kidney Yin and Deficient Heart Yin

Pulse. Thin, rapid, maybe irregular.

Indications. Nervous anxiety, fear agitation, restlessness, insomnia and dream-disturbed sleep, feverish sensation in chest.

Example. Nervous exhaustion with overenthusiasm and anxiety.

Combination. CV.14, CV.17; CV.4, SP.6, KI.6, HT.6 Rf.

Heart Fire

Pulse. Full, rapid, maybe wiry, maybe irregular.

Indications. Manic excitement, extreme restlessness, insomnia, hypertension, palpitations.

Example. Menopausal flushes, agitation and hyperactivity, dizziness and headache.

Combination. CV.14, KI.1, GV.20 Rd; PC.9, ear apex B; KI.3 Rf.

Heart Phlegm Fire

Pulse. Slippery, full, rapid, maybe wiry or irregular.

Indications. Mental confusion, confused speech, dizziness, palpitations, oppressive feeling or pain in chest, headache, nausea.

Example. Manic-depression and mental confusion.

Combination. CV.14, CV.17, PC.6, HT.6, LR.3, ST.40, GV.20 Rd; PC.9 B; SP.6 Rf.

CV.15 jiū wěi

Connecting point of Conception channel, Source point of all Yin organs.

General

CV.14 and CV.15 are both within the area of the Solar Plexus centre and are very similar in function. CV.15 can be used for all the syndromes listed for CV.14. The decision of which of the two points to use can sometimes be made according to which point is more spontaneously tender or tender on palpitation. This can reflect which of the two points has a greater accumulation or disturbance of energy.

CV.17 tàn zhōng

Alarm point of Pericardium, Alarm point of Upper Burner, Sea of Qi point, Gathering point of the Qi.

General

Points in general can be used to reduce Excess, reinforce Deficiency, disperse Stagnation, or to calm Irregularity, and this is especially important for those points that represent major energy centres of the Conception channel.

The main function of CV.17 is to disperse Stagnation of Qi. Since its effect is mainly local to the chest, its main function is to disperse Zong Qi, the Qi of the chest, associated with the functions of the Heart and Lungs. Zong Qi is associated with the Heart Centre, which is not only linked to the physical functions of breathing and circulation, but to the role of the Heart Spirit in speech, communication of feelings and ideas, the sharing of joys and pleasures, social behaviour and relationships.

The Heart Spirit is extremely active and especially susceptible to either obstruction or agitation of its movement. CV.17 can be used to calm the Spirit and CV.14 and CV.15 can be used to remove obstructions to its movement, but generally CV.17 is more used to disperse Stagnation and CV.14 and CV.15 are used to calm agitation of the Spirit. Similarly, although CV.17 can be used to tonify Lung Qi or Heart Qi, its tonifying action is limited, and relates especially to mixed conditions of Deficiency and Stagnation, for example, the Deficiency of the Lungs in their dispensing and descending actions.

If the Deficiency of Heart or Lung Qi is linked to Deficiency of Kidneys or Spleen then these Deficiencies must also be treated, e.g. with CV.4 + KI.3 or CV.12 + SP.3, respectively. CV.17 in the Upper Energizer, does not have such a strong tonic effect as CV.12 in the Middle Energizer, or CV.4 in the Lower Energizer. The function of CV.17 is more like that of CV.6, since both these points are primarily for Stagnation of Qi.

Syndromes

Deficiency of Qi in the Upper Energizer
  Deficient Heart Qi and Yang
  Deficient Lung Qi

Stagnation in the Upper Energizer
  Stagnant Heart Qi
  Stagnant Heart Blood
  Stagnant Lung Qi
  Accumulation of Phlegm in the Lungs
  Stagnation of Qi in the Breasts

Rebellious Qi of Lungs and Stomach

Deficiency of Qi in the Upper Energizer

Deficient Heart Qi and Yang

Pulse. Empty, slow, deep, maybe irregular.

Indications. Poor peripheral circulation, palpitation, lack of joy, apathy.

Example. Depression, worse with tiredness, lack of interest in life.

Combination. CV.17, CV.4, KI.3, ST.36 Rf M; HT.7 Rf.

Deficient Lung Qi

Pulse. Empty.

Indications. Weak cough, weak voice, tendency to catch colds.

Example. Cough and shortness of breath with tiredness.

Combination. CV.17, CV.4, KI.3, ST.36, LU.9 Rf.

Stagnation in the Upper Energizer

Stagnant Heart Qi

Pulse. Wiry, maybe irregular.

Indications. Depression or cold hands and feet, better with exercise or with social activity, chest pain or feeling of fullness in the chest.

Example. Chest pain better with exercise.

Combination. CV.17, PC.6, LR.3, LR.14 Rd.

Stagnant Heart Blood

Pulse. Wiry, knotted.

Indications. Pain in the chest or the heart area radiating to shoulder or inner left arm, cold hands and feet.

Example. Pain and feeling of constriction in the chest.

Combination. CV.17, PC.4, PC.6, SP.4, SP.21 Rd.

Stagnant Lung Qi

Pulse. Wiry, maybe full or deep.

Indications. Retained grief, restricted breathing.

Example. Grief, sadness and depression.

Combination. CV.17, CV.22, KU.1, LU.7, KI.6. E.

Accumulation of Phlegm in the Lungs

Pulse. Slippery, full.

Indications. Asthma or bronchitis with much phlegm in the chest.

Example. Severe cough with white phlegm which is sticky and difficult to expectorate.

Combination. CV.17, LU.1, LU.6, ST.40, PC.6, BL.13 Rd; KI.6 Rf.

Stagnation of Qi in the Breasts

Pulse. Wiry, maybe empty or slippery.

Indications. Insufficient lactation, mastitis, sore breasts before menstruation.

Example. Mastitis.

Combination. CV.17, ST.18, ST.40, SI.1, SI.9, PC.6, LR.3 Rd.

Rebellious Qi of Lungs and Stomach

Pulse. Wiry

Indications. Cough, hiccups, oesophageal spasm.

Example. Hiccups with emotional stress.

Combination. CV.17, CV.14, PC.6, SP.4, GV.20 Rd.

CV.22 tiān tū

Crossing point of Conception and Yin Link channels.

General

CV.22 and CV.23 are associated with the Throat centre, which is responsible for communication, the outward expression of feeling and ideas. The Lungs rule the throat and the strength and quality of the voice and the Heart governs the tongue and speech.

Although the functions of CV.22 and CV.23 overlap, CV.22 is somewhat more concerned with the Lungs, chest and voice, and CV.23 with the upper throat, tongue and speech. CV.22 regulates the dispersing and descending functions of the Lungs to prevent Stagnation or Rebellion of Lung Qi. Stagnation of Lung Qi can further lead to Accumulation of Phlegm in the chest or throat.

Syndromes

Stagnation of Lung and Heart Qi
Accumulation of Phlegm in the Lungs
Rebellious Qi of Lungs or Stomach
Local throat problems

Stagnation of Lung and Heart Qi

Pulse. Wiry.

Indications. Emotions stuck inside, difficulty in expressing feelings to others, communication problems in relationships, fear of showing or sharing affection.

Example. Depression made better by communicating feelings.

Combination. CV.22, CV.17, PC.6, TE.5, TE.16 Rd.

Accumulation of Phlegm in the Lungs

Pulse. Slippery, maybe full.

Indications. Bronchitis or asthma with phlegm in throat and chest.

Example. Cough with yellow phlegm and dry throat.

Combination. CV.22, CV.17, ST.40, LU.6 Rd; LU.5 Rf.

Rebellious Qi of Lungs or Stomach

Pulse. Maybe wiry.

Indications. Cough, asthma, hiccup, oesophageal spasm, vomiting, inability to swallow food.

Example. Oesophageal spasm and soreness.

Combination. CV.22, CV.15, PC.6, SP.4, KI.4, KI.22, KI.27 Rd.

Local throat problems

Pulse. Various possibilities.

Indications. Dryness, inflammation, pain or obstruction in lower throat.

Example. 'Plum seed Qi sensation in throat', worse with depression.

Combination. CV.22, CV.17, PC.6, LR.3, LR.14 Rd.

CV.23 lián quán

Crossing point of Conception and Yin Link channels.

General

CV.23 can be used for the syndromes listed above for CV.22, but CV.23 is especially for problems of voice and speech involving the vocal chords, larynx and tongue.

Speech problems

Pulse. Various.

Indications. Hypersalivation, mouth and tongue ulcers, tonsillitis, hysteria with voice loss, hoarse voice, loss of speech or slurred speech following Windstroke, spasm of the larynx.

Example. Speech problems following cerebrovascular accident (Windstroke) or cerebral trauma.

Combination. CV.23, GV.15, HT.5, PC.6, ST.40, LR.3 Rd.

CV.24 chéng jiāng

Crossing point of Conception, Governor, Stomach and Large Intestine channels.

General

This point is most useful in calming Kidney fear and Heart anxiety, and for this purpose is often combined with CV.4 and CV.14. CV.4 tonifies Qi and Yin of Kidneys and Heart, thus helping to stabilize the Heart Spirit, and CV.14, like CV.24 has a direct effect in calming agitation.

Syndromes

Deficient Qi or Yin of Kidneys and Heart
Wind Cold invasion of the face
Face and mouth problems

Deficient Qi or Yin of Kidneys and Heart

Pulse. Empty or thin, maybe rapid or irregular.

Indications. Fear and anxiety, palpitations, insomnia, emotional lability, tiredness, lower back pain, urinary problems.

Example. Panic attacks and fear of meeting people.

Combination. CV.24, CV.14, PC.6 Rd; CV. 4, KI.3, HT.7, GV.20 Rf.

Wind Cold invasion of the face

Pulse. Tight, maybe deep and empty.

Indications. Facial paralysis.

Combination. CV.23, GV.26, ST.4, ST.36, LI.20, LI.4, local points.

Mouth and face problems

Pulse. Various

Indications. Excessive salivation, mouth and tongue ulcers, gingivitis, facial swelling, tooth pain.

Example. Cracking of lips aggravated by Exterior Wind Cold or warming spices (Stomach Fire).

Combination. CV.24, ST.4, ST.44, ST.45, LI.4, LI.11 Rd.

Conception points comparisons and combinations

The functions of the main CV points are listed in Table 11.3.

Table 11.3 CV points comparison

Point	Syndrome
CV.1	loss of consciousness anal and urogenital problems
CV.2	urogenital problems due to: 　Damp Heat in Lower Energizer 　Deficiency and Cold in Lower Energizer 　Sinking of Qi in Lower Energizer
CV.3	urogenital problems due to: 　Damp Heat in Lower Energizer 　Deficiency and Cold in Lower Energizer 　Stagnant Qi and Blood in uterus
CV.4	uterine problems Deficient Kidney Jing Deficient Qi and Yuan Qi of Kidneys and other organs Deficient Yin and Yang of Kidneys and other organs depression due to Deficiency unstable emotions due to Deficient Qi and Deficient Yin
CV.6	Stagnant Qi and Blood in Lower Energizer Stagnant Qi in Intestines Stagnation of Cold Damp in Lower Energizer Stagnation of Damp Heat in Lower Energizer Stagnation of Qi of chest, with depression Deficient Qi and Yang of Kidneys
CV.9	Damp in Lower Energizer
CV.10	Retention of food in stomach
CV.12	Deficient Spleen and Stomach Qi 　Sinking of Spleen Qi 　Damp in Middle Energizer 　Cold in Middle Energizer 　Liver invading Middle Energizer 　Retention of food in stomach 　Stomach Qi Rebelling Upward 　Heat in Middle Energizer
CV.13	Stomach Qi Rebelling upward
CV.14	Kidney fear invades Liver, Heart, 　Spleen or Lungs 　Stomach Qi Rebelling Upward 　Heart Fire or Heart Phlegm Fire disturbs Spirit
CV.17	Stagnant Qi of Heart or Lungs 　Stagnant Heart Blood 　Accumulation of Phlegm in Lungs 　Stagnation of Qi in breasts 　Rebellious Lung Qi 　Deficient Qi of Heart or Lungs
CV.22	Stagnant Qi of Heart or Lungs Accumulation of Phlegm in Lungs Rebellious Qi of Lungs or Stomach local throat problems
CV.23	speech problems 　local throat problems
CV.24	Deficient Qi or Yin of Kidneys and Heart 　Wind Cold invasion of face 　Face and mouth problems

Some common combinations of CV channel points are summarized in Table 11.4.

Table 11.4 Combinations of CV points

Point	Combination	Syndrome	Example
CV.3	CV.6	Stagnant Qi and Damp Heat in Lower Energizer	prostatitis with dysuria
CV.3	CV.9	Damp Heat in Lower Energizer	nephritis
CV.4	CV.2	Deficient Yang in Lower Energizer	impotence
CV.4	CV.6	Deficient Qi and Stagnant Qi	depression
CV.4	CV.9	Deficient Kidney Qi and Damp	urinary retention
CV.4	CV.12	Deficient Kidney and Spleen Qi with Sinking of Qi	stomach prolapse
CV.4	CV.14	Deficient Kidney and Heart Qi	overexcitability
CV.4	CV.17	Deficient Heart Qi	loneliness
CV.4	CV.24	Deficient Heart Qi	panic and anxiety
CV.6	CV.9	Stagnant Qi in Lower Energizer with Accumulation of Cold Damp	oedema of legs and abdomen
CV.6	CV.10	Stagnation of Qi in Stomach and Intestines	indigestion with constipation
CV.6	CV.12	Liver invading Spleen	indigestion and nausea
CV.6	CV.17	Stagnant Qi of Chest	angina pectoris
CV.6	CV.22	Accumulation of Phlegm in Lungs	asthma
CV.9	CV.12	Deficient Spleen Qi with Damp	abdominal distension and diarrhoea
CV.12	CV.17	Deficient Spleen and Lung Qi	bronchitis with phlegm
CV.13	CV.10	Retention of food in stomach with Rebellious Stomach Qi	nausea and belching
CV.14	CV.17	Heart Phlegm Fire	manic depression
CV.14	CV.24	Deficiency of Heart Qi	fear of people
CV.17	CV.22	Accumulation of Phlegm in Lungs	asthma and cough
CV.17	CV.24	Stagnation of Heart Qi and Disturbance of Spirit	anxiety and depression
CV.22	CV.23	Stagnation of Qi in throat	hoarse voice with phlegm
CV.24	CV.23	Phlegm obstructs Heart	speech defects
CV.3	CV.6, 9	Stagnation of Qi with Damp and Heat in Lower Energizer	urinary retention and dysuria
CV.4	CV.6, 9	Deficiency and Stagnation of Qi with Damp in Lower Energizer	depression with oedema
CV.4	CV.9, 12	Deficient Kidney and Spleen Qi with Damp	oedema, weakness and cold in legs
CV.4	CV.12, 14	Deficient Qi and Blood of Heart with disturbed Spirit	tiredness with palpitations
CV.4	CV.12, 17	Deficient Qi of Kidneys, Lungs and Spleen	easy to get colds
CV.4	CV.17, 24	Deficient Qi of Heart and Kidneys with disturbed Spirit	paranoia and anxiety
CV.6	CV.9, 12	Phlegm Damp disturbs head	mental dullness and lethargy
CV.6	CV.10, 13	Stagnation of Qi in Stomach and Intestines	nausea and abdominal distension
CV.6	CV.12, 17	Cold Phlegm obstructs Heart	depression and confusion
CV.6	CV.12, 22	Deficient Spleen Qi with Phlegm in throat	nausea and catarrh in throat
CV.6	CV.17, 22	Stagnation of Qi of Chest and Throat centres	difficulty in communicating feelings
CV.12	CV.17, 22	Stagnation of Qi in Throat centre	worry and anxiety with loss of voice
CV.14	CV.17, 24	Stagnation of Heart Qi with Heart Fire	hypertension with extreme anxiety
CV.17	CV.23, 23	Deficient Lung Yin and Qi	dry cough with sore, swollen throat
CV.4	CF.14, 17, 24	Deficient Qi of Heart and Kidneys with disturbed Spirit	exhaustion and panic attacks
CV.6	CV.12, 17, 22	Stagnation and Deficiency of Lung Qi with Phlegm	asthma and bronchitis

Combinations of Conception channel points with Kidney, Stomach, Spleen and Liver points are given in Tables 11.5, 11.6, 11.7 and 11.8 respectively.

Table 11.5 Combinations of CV and Kidney points

CV points	KI points	Syndrome	Example
CV.1	KI.1	Collapse of Yang	fainting
CV.3	KI.2	Deficient Kidney Yang	frigidity
CV.3	KI.6	Deficient Kidney Yin	vaginitis
CV.3	KI.7	Damp Heat in Lower Energizer	cystitis
CV.3	KI.8	Stagnation of Qi in uterus	amenorrhoea
CV.3	KI.10	Damp Heat in Bladder	urethritis
CV.3	KI.12	Stagnation of Qi in uterus	fibroid
CV.4	KI.2	Deficient Kidney Yang	lack of ambition
CV.4	KI.3	Deficient Kidney Jing	deafness
CV.4	KI.6	Deficient Kidney Jing and Yin	arthritis in the elderly
CV.4	KI.7	Deficient Kidney Qi	spontaneous sweating
CV.4	KI.10	Damp due to Deficiency	oedema
CV.4	KI.13	Deficient Kidney Qi	tiredness and lack of sexual interest
CV.4	KI.27	Deficient Kidney Qi	asthma
CV.6	KI.3	Deficiency and Stagnation of Qi	depression and tiredness
CV.6	KI.8	Stagnation of Qi in Lower Energizer	abdominal pain and swelling
CV.6	KI.7	Damp Heat in Lower Energizer	leucorrhoea
CV.6	KI.14	Stagnation in Lower Energizer	irregular menstruation
CV.9	KI.2	Damp Cold in Lower Energizer	nephritis
CV.9	KI.3	Deficient Kidney Qi and Accumulation of Damp	urinary retention
CV.9	KI.7	Damp in Lower Energizer	diarrhoea
CV.12	KI.3	Deficient Qi of Kidneys and Spleen	muscle weakness
CV.12	KI.6	Deficient Yin of Kidneys and Stomach	gastritis
CV.14	KI.1	Excess Fire of Kidneys and Heart	extreme anxiety
CV.14	KI.2	Deficiency Fire of Kidneys and Heart	restless agitation
CV.14	KI.3	Deficient Qi of Kidneys and Heart	emotional lability
CV.14	KI.6	Deficient Yin of Kidneys and Heart	palpitations
CV.14	KI.9	Disharmony of Yin Link channel	heat and discomfort in the chest
CV.17	KI.3	Deficient Qi of Kidneys and Heart	heart and chest pain
CV.17	KI.6	Deficient Yin of Kidneys and Heart	insomnia
CV.17	KI.7	Deficient Yang of Kidneys and Heart	poor circulation
CV.17	KI.9	Stagnation of Heart Qi	angina pectoris
CV.17	KI.24	Stagnation of Heart Qi	sadness and depression
CV.22	KI.3	Deficient Qi of Kidneys and Lungs	bronchitis
CV.22	KI.27	Stagnation of Qi in chest	asthma
CV.23	KI.6	Deficient Yin of Kidneys and Lungs	sore throat
CV.24	KI.1	Disturbance of Spirit	panic attacks
CV.24	KI.3	Deficient Kidney Qi	chronic fear
CV.24	KI.6	Deficient Kidney and Heart Yin	overexcitability
CV.24	KI.27	Deficient Kidney and Heart Qi and Yin	anxiety and depression

Table 11.6 Combinations of CV and Stomach points

CV points	ST points	Syndrome	Example
CV.1	ST.30	Sinking of Qi	inguinal hernia
		Damp Heat	penile pain
CV.2	ST.30	Deficient Kidney Qi and Jing	impotence
		Blood not held in	uterine haemorrhage
		Sinking of Qi	uterine prolapse
		Damp Heat	vaginitis
		Cold in uterus	dysmenorrhoea
CV.3	ST.29	Stagnant Blood in uterus	endometriosis
		Deficient Kidney and Bladder Qi	prostatitis
		Damp Heat	leucorrhoea
CV.4	ST.8	Deficient Kidney Qi and Hyperactive Liver Yang	headache
CV.4	ST.28	Deficient Kidney Qi and Damp	oedema
CV.4	ST.30	Deficient Kidney Qi and Jing	impotence and depression
CV.4	ST.36	Deficient Qi and Blood	exhaustion
		Deficient Defensive Qi	recurring infections
		Deficient Kidney Qi and Jing	infertility
		Deficient Bladder Qi and Yang	urinary incontinence
		Deficient Qi and Yang of Spleen and Kidneys	feeling of coldness and pain in the lower abdomen
		Deficient Lung and Kidney Qi	asthma
CV.4	ST.40	Deficient Heart Qi and Heart Phlegm	depression and confusion
CV.4	ST.45	Stagnant and Deficient Stomach Qi	mental exhaustion and congestion
CV.6	ST.8	Stagnant Liver Qi and Hyperactive Liver Yang	headache and depression
CV.6	ST.25	Stagnant Intestinal Qi	constipation
CV.6	ST.28	Stagnant Qi and Damp in Lower Energizer	abdominal distension
CV.6	ST.36	Stagnant Qi and Deficient Qi and Blood	depression and tiredness
CV.6	ST.40	Stagnant Qi and Phlegm Damp	lethargy, head and limbs feel heavy
		Stagnant Heart Qi and Heart Phlegm	confused speech and behaviour
		Stagnant Lung Qi and Lung Phlegm	bronchial asthma
CV.6	ST.45	Stagnant Qi in head	mental stagnation and loss of concentration
CV.8	ST.36	Deficient Qi and Blood	complete exhaustion
CV.9	ST.36	Deficient Spleen and Kidney Qi	oedema
CV.10	ST.37	Stagnation in Stomach and Intestines	epigastric distension and constipation
CV.12	ST.21	Stomach Fire	gastric ulcer
		Liver invades Stomach	vomiting
CV.12	ST.25	Deficient Qi of Stomach and Intestines	constipation in the elderly
CV.12	ST.36	Deficient Qi and Blood	tiredness and depression
		Deficient Spleen Qi	borborygmus and flatulence
		Cold and Damp in Stomach	indigestion and feelings of cold in the epigastrium
CV.12	ST.40	Damp and Phlegm in Stomach	nausea and vomiting
		Damp and Phlegm in head	poor memory and concentration
CV.12	ST.44	Deficient Stomach Yin	restlessness and weight loss
		Stomach Fire	voracious appetite and gastritis
CV.12	ST.45	Stagnant Qi of Liver and Stomach	headache and nausea after excess food and alcohol
CV.14	ST.21	Rebellious Stomach Qi	nausea with extreme worry
		Liver invades Stomach	anger and indigestion
		Kidney fear invades Stomach	fearful insecurity and indigestion
		Stomach and Heart Fire	hyperactivity and gastric ulcer
CV.14	ST.39	Heart and Kidneys invade intestines	fearful anxiety and irritable bowel syndrome
CV.14	ST.40	Phlegm Fire of Stomach and Fire	nausea and gastritis with palpitations and confusion
CV.14	ST.44	Stomach and Heart Fire	insomnia and gastritis
CV.17	ST.15	Stagnant Lung Qi	bronchitis
CV.17	ST.18	Stagnant Liver Qi	insufficient lactation
CV.17	ST.36	Deficient Lung Qi	recurring colds and bronchitis
		Deficient Heart Qi	emotional lability
		Deficient Spleen and Heart Blood	palpitations and insomnia
CV.17	ST.40	Lung Phlegm	bronchiectasis
		Heart Phlegm	depression
		Stagnant Blood in chest	chest injury
CV.17	ST.45	Heart Phlegm	mental dullness and disorientation
CV.22	ST.40	Lung Phlegm	catarrh in the throat
CV.23	ST.40	Damp in throat	hypersalivation
		Lung Phlegm	pharyngitis
		Heart Phlegm	hypertension
CV.23	ST.44	Deficient Stomach Yin	dry mouth and throat
		Stomach and Heart Fire	mouth and tongue ulcers
CV.24	ST.4	Fire Poison and Damp Heat	acne
CV.24	ST.36	Deficient Heart Blood and Yin	anxiety and depression
CV.24	ST.40	Heart Phlegm Fire	hysteria and panic
CV.24	ST.44	Deficient Heart Yin and Heart Fire	fear of people

Table 11.7 Combinations of CV and Spleen points

CV points	SP points	Syndromes	Example
CV.3	SP.1	Heat in Blood	genital itching
CV.3	SP.4	Stagnant Blood in uterus	endometriosis
CV.3	SP.6	Stagnant Blood in uterus	fibroid
		Damp Heat in Lower Energizer	leucorrhoea
		Deficient Kidney Yin and Damp Heat in Bladder	cystitis
CV.3	SP.8	Stagnant Blood in uterus	retained placenta
CV.3	SP.9	Damp Heat in Lower Energizer	prostatitis
CV.3	SP.10	Heat in Blood	menorrhagia
CV.3	SP.12	Stagnant Qi and Blood	groin sprain
CV.4	SP.1	Spleen not holding the Blood	blood in the stool
CV.4	SP.2	Cold and Deficient Spleen	abdominal distension
CV.4	SP.3	Deficient Spleen and Kidney Qi	exhaustion
		Cold and Damp in Lower Energizer	oedema
CV.4	SP.4	Deficient Kidney Qi and Jing	infertility
		Stagnant and Deficient Qi and Blood	cold hands and feet
CV.4	SP.6	Deficient Kidney Yin	weak back, restlessness
		Deficient Kidney and Heart Yin	palpitations and insomnia
		Deficient Kidney Yin and Hyperactive Liver Yang	migraines
		Deficient Qi and Blood	tiredness and depression
		Sinking of Spleen Qi	rectal prolapse
		Deficient Qi and Damp	urinary retention
CV.4	SP.9	Deficient Qi and Damp	leucorrhoea
CV.4	SP.10	Deficient Blood	dizziness and headache
CV.6	SP.1	Stagnant Qi and Blood	depression and melancholia
CV.6	SP.2	Stagnant Qi and Blood	feeling of fullness in chest and abdomen
CV.6	SP.4	Stagnant and Deficient Qi and Blood in Lower Energizer	postpartum haemorrhage
		Stagnant Qi in chest	depression and chest pain
		Stagnant Qi in Lower Energizer	abdominal distension and pain
		Stagnant Blood in uterus	irregular menstruation
CV.6	SP.6	Damp Heat in Lower Energizer	urinary infections
		Stagnant Qi and Cold in Lower Energizer	dysmenorrhoea
		Stagnant Qi and Blood in uterus	postpartum abdominal pain
		Deficient Blood and Stagnant Liver Qi	postnatal depression
		Stagnant Liver Qi and Hyperactive Liver Yang	depression and headache
		Stagnant Heart Qi and Deficient Heart Yin	menopausal syndrome
CV.6	SP.8	Stagnant Blood in legs	cold legs and feet
CV.6	SP.9	Stagnant Qi and Damp in Lower Energizer	chronic diarrhoea
CV.6	SP.15	Stagnant Qi in Intestines	constipation
CV.9	SP.6	Stagnant Qi in Kidneys	urinary retention and lower back pain
CV.9	SP.9	Damp heat in Bladder	urethritis
CV.10	SP.4	Stagnant Food in Stomach	nausea and constipation
CV.12	SP.1	Deficient and Stagnant Qi of Middle Energizer	lack of appetite
CV.12	SP.2	Deficient Spleen Yang	exhaustion and muscular weakness
CV.12	SP.3	Deficient Qi and Blood	mental exhaustion and poor memory
		Deficient Spleen Qi	slow digestion
		Deficient Spleen Qi and Damp	nausea and indigestion
		Damp and Phlegm in head	feelings of heaviness and lethargy
CV.12	SP.4	Stagnant Qi and Blood in Middle Energizer	severe epigastric pain
CV.12	SP.6	Deficient Stomach Yin	worry and insomnia
		Deficient Qi and Blood	insecurity and depression
		Liver invades Stomach	irritability and gastritis
CV.12	SP.9	Deficient Spleen and Damp	abdominal distension and pain
CV.12	SP.15	Deficient Spleen Qi	pain and cold in abdomen and legs
CV.14	SP.4	Deficient Heart Yin and Blood	anxiety, restlessness and insomnia
CV.14	SP.6	Deficient Heart Qi and Blood	emotional lability and palpitations
CV.17	SP.1	Stagnant Heart Qi and Blood	depression and dream-disturbed sleep
CV.17	SP.3	Deficient Blood of Heart and Spleen	emotional vulnerability
CV.17	SP.4	Stagnant Heart Blood	angina pectoris
		Stagnant Blood in chest	chest injury
		Deficient Heart Blood and Yin	overenthusiasm and exhaustion
CV.17	SP.6	Deficient Heart and Kidney Yin	fear and paranoia
		Deficient Heart Yin and Heart Fire	hypertension
		Deficient Heart Qi and Blood	heart arrhythmia
CV.17	SP.21	Stagnant Qi and Blood	chest pain
CV.22	SP.3	Lung Phlegm	throat catarrh
CV.22	SP.6	Deficient Heart Yin	hysteria and voice loss
CV.23	SP.6	Stomach and Heart Fire	mouth and tongue ulcers
CV.24	SP.4	Deficient Heart Blood and Yin	anxiety and depression
CV.24	SP.6	Deficient Heart Yin and Heart Fire	panic attack

Table 11.8 Combinations of CV and Liver points

CV points	LR points	Syndromes	Example
CV.1	LR.5	Damp Heat in Lower Energizer	bleeding haemorrhoids
CV.3	LR.1	Heat in Blood	abnormal menstrual bleeding
	LR.3	Stagnant in Lower Energizer	urinary stones and pain
	LR.5	Damp Heat in Lower Energizer	cystitis
	LR.8	Damp Heat in Lower Energizer	pelvic inflammatory disease
CV.4	LR.1	Reduced muscle tone	uterine prolapse
CV.6	LR.1	Stagnant in Lower Energizer	lower abdominal pain
	LR.3	Stagnant Liver Qi	depression and tiredness
	LR.13	Liver invades Spleen and Intestines	irritable bowel syndrome
	LR.14	Stagnant Heart and Lung Qi	depression and loneliness
CV.9	LR.8	Damp Cold in Lower Energizer	oedema and leucorrhoea
CV.10	LR.3	Stagnant Qi in Stomach and Intestines	epigastric and abdominal distension from food stagnation
CV.12	LR.3	Liver invades Spleen	worry and depression
	LR.13	Deficient Spleen Yang	exhaustion and diarrhoea
CV.13	LR.3	Liver invades Stomach	nausea and vomiting
CV.14	LR.2	Liver Fire invades Heart	anger, anxiety and agitation
CV.15	LR.3	Liver invades diaphragm	tense, restricted breathing
CV.17	LR.1	Stagnant Liver Qi	intercostal pain
	LR.3	Stagnant Liver Qi	sore breasts at menstruation
	LR.14	Stagnant Blood	chest injury
CV.22	LR.3	Stagnant Liver and Lung Qi	sensation of lump in the throat
	LR.14	Stagnant Liver Qi and Lung Phlegm	painful cough
CV.23	LR.2	Liver Fire	dry mouth and dry sore throat
CV.24	LR.3	Disturbance of Spirit	severe anxiety

Governor 12

Governor channel

CHANNEL CONNECTIONS

MAIN CHANNEL PATHWAY

Like the internal Conception channel, the internal Governor pathway is connected with the Kidney and starts inside the lower abdomen, descending, through the uterus in women to emerge at the perineum. The superficial Governor pathway then ascends the midline of the back and neck, passes over the vertex and down the midline of the face, to end at GV.28 on the upper gum.

The internal Governor channel is said to connect with Kidney, Heart and brain, also meeting the CV channel at CV.1 and the Liver internal channel at GV.20.

CONNECTING CHANNEL PATHWAY

This separates from GV.1 and flows up both sides of the spine to the occiput whence it spreads over the top of the head. At the level of the scapulae, a branch meets the BL channel and spreads through the spine.

Table 12.1 Crossing points on the Governor channel

Point	Crossing	Other function
GV.26	SI, LI	
GV.24	ST, BL	
GV.20	BL	Sea of Marrow point
GV.17	BL	
GV.16	Yang Link	Sea of Marrow point
GV.15	Yang Link	Sea of Qi point
GV.14	BL, GB, ST	Sea of Qi point, Gathering point of Yang
GV.13	BL	
GV.12	BL	

THE GOVERNOR CHANNEL AND THE ENERGY CENTRES

THE ENERGY CENTRES ON THE GOVERNOR CHANNEL

The Conception and Governor channels together form a circle of energy circulation on the vertical axis of the body. There are centres on the Governor channel that are approximately equivalent in function to those on the Conception channel, as shown in Table 12.2, and discussed in Chapter 2.

Table 12.2 Governor energy centres

Centre	CV point	GV point	Below vertebra
Crown	–	GV.20	–
Brow	–	yìn táng	–
Throat	22–23	15, 16	C.1, occiput
Heart	17	11	T.5
Solar Plexus	14	9	T.7
Spleen	12	6	T.11
Dan Tian	4–6	4	L.2
Reproduction	2–3	2–3	approx. mid-sacrum
Perineal	1	1	tip of coccyx

FUNCTIONS OF GOVERNOR POINTS

TONIFY KIDNEY JING

The Conception and Governor channels, connecting with the Kidneys, form the core of the Eight Extra channel system. The Jing is stored in the Kidneys and the Eight Extra channels, and through the Jing, the Kidneys rule bones, brain and the reproductive and developmental cycles. However, while CV points, like CV.4, can tonify both the Yin and Yang aspects of Jing, GV points like GV.4, are more used to strengthen its Yang aspects.

JING AND REPRODUCTION

Reproductive problems relating to Jing, e.g. impotence and infertility, are mainly treated, on the Governor channel, by tonifying GV.4.

BONES AND SPINE

The Kidneys rule the marrow and the bones and the Governor channel permeates both spine and brain. Spinal problems can be treated with the GV point in the affected segment, or by GV.1, GV.4, GV.9, GV.12 which have general effects on the spine and the tonus of the spinal muscles.

BRAIN

GV.16 and CV.20 are Sea of Marrow points and are specifically to strengthen the brain, for example in cases of Deficient Kidney, developmental problems, or recovery from cerebral injury.

TONIFY YANG

In general, the GV points are either for tonifying Yang or for controlling it, to achieve a balance of Yang energy on the body.

TONIFY YANG OF THE ORGANS

GV.14 can tonify the Yang of the body in general, GV.4 can do this by tonifying the Yang of the Kidneys. Other GV points can tonify the Yang of the organ associated with a particular spinal segment, e.g. GV.11 can tonify the Yang of the Heart.

DISPERSE INTERIOR COLD AND DAMP

GV.3 and GV.4, by tonifying the Kidneys, can disperse Interior Cold and GV.6, by tonifying SP Yang can remove Interior Damp.

PREVENT EXTERIOR INVASION

By tonifying Yang and Qi, especially of Kidneys, Lungs and Spleen, GV points, such as GV.4, 6 and 12 can prevent the easy invasion of Exterior Wind, Cold and Damp that often follows Deficiency.

DISPERSE EXTERIOR WIND INVASION

Wind, Cold and Damp can invade any exposed area of the back, neck or head, especially if there is either a general Deficiency of Qi and Yang, or a local area of Deficiency and Stagnation of Qi. GV points such as GV.14, 15 and 16 can be used to treat early Greater Yang stage invasion, with either needle, moxa or cupping.

REGULATE LOCAL SEGMENTED PROBLEMS

GV points can be used to regulate Deficiency, Excess, Stagnation or Irregularity of Qi relating to a specific spinal segment. The imbalance may be associated with physical problems such as arthritis at the T.1–T.2 joint, or emotional problems, such as the inability to express oneself in a personal relationship. Where appropriate the GV point may be combined with jiǎ jǐ and/or Back Transporting points in the same segment.

CONTROL FIRE, YANG AND INTERIOR WIND

GV points can both tonify deficient Yang and control its manifestation of Excess and Irregularity: Fire, Hyperactive Yang and Interior Wind.

CONTROL FIRE

GV points such as GV.13 and GV.14 can be used to control acute fevers and GV.11, 14 and 15 can be used to control the effects of Heart Fire.

CONTROL HYPERACTIVE LIVER YANG

GV.8 and GV.9 can regulate all the syndromes of the Liver, but GV.20 is especially for controlling the effects of Hyperactive Yang in the head.

CONTROL INTERIOR WIND

GV points can control Wind arising from fever, e.g. GV.14 and GV.16, or arising from Liver Fire and Hyperactive Liver Yang, GV.8, 9, 15, 16, 20. GV.1 and GV.2 can be used for seizures and convulsions, as can GV.26 at the other end of the channel.

CALM THE SPIRIT

The GV channel is much used for mental and emotional problems because of its connections with the brain and the Heart. The Spirit can be disturbed by Heat, Hyperactive Yang and Wind as described in the previous section, and by reducing these factors, points like GV.8, 9, 13, 14, 15, 20, 24 and 26 can calm the Spirit.

However, GV points are not so effective when the disturbance of the Spirit is due to Deficient Qi, Yin or Blood. Then other points should be used. GV.6, 20 and 24 can also be used when the Spirit, brain and senses are dulled by Damp and Phlegm, with resulting poor memory, loss of concentration and confused thinking and speech.

PRECAUTIONS WHEN USING GV POINTS WITH MOXA

Since the Governor channel is the main one on the body for tonifying Yang, it is relatively easy to use excessive moxa and aggravate an existing Heat condition or originate a new one. It is wisest to use small amounts of moxa on the first treatment and increase them on the next treatment, if pulse, tongue and behaviour are free of Heat signs.

In the following situations, moxa on Governor channel points should be used with great caution or not at all:

• Raised blood pressure: especially avoid moxa on GV.20.

• Deficient Kidney Yang with Deficient Kidney Yin: ensure that some Deficient Yin does not coexist with Deficient Yang for which moxa is required on GV.4.

• Deficient Heart Yang with Deficient Heart Yin: before using moxa on GV.4, 11, 14 and 20 for depression, the case history should be checked very carefully to ensure there is no alternation between depression and mania.

• Deficient Yang with Interior Heat: Deficient Yang may coexist with an Interior Heat pattern such as Damp Heat in the Intestines, in which case moxa on GV.3 and GV.4 is contraindicated while the Damp Heat remains.

GOVERNOR SYNDROMES

Governor channel syndromes are discussed in detail in Chapter 10.

Governor points

GV.1 cháng qiáng

Connecting point of Governor channel.

General

In the circulation of energy, the Governor channel links with the Conception channel at the perineum. From GV.1, energy circulates up the spine to the head. For this reason GV.1 can be used for both spinal and mental problems. GV.1 functions with CV.1 in the Perineal energy centre.

The commonest use of GV.1 is for anal problems such as prolapse or haemorrhoids.

Syndromes

Anal problems
  Damp Heat
  Sinking and Deficiency of Qi
Coccyx and sacral problems
Spinal problems
Mental problems

Anal problems

Damp Heat

Pulse. Slippery, rapid,

Indications. Internal or external haemorrhoids, pain, swelling, pruritis, discharge or bleeding of anus.

Example. External, bleeding haemorrhoids.

Combination. GV.1, BL.32, BL.35, BL.57, SP.10 Rd.

Sinking and Deficiency of Qi

Pulse. Deep, empty.

Indications. External haemorrhoids, anal prolapse, heavy sensation in anus, haemorrhage, exhaustion.

Example. External haemorrhoids with chronic bleeding.

Combination. GV.1, BL.26 E; GV.20, BL.46, CV.4, ST.36 Rf M.

Coccyx and sacral problems

Pulse. Various – often wiry.

Indications. Sacral or coccygeal pain.

Example. Coccyx painful on sitting, after injury.

Combination. GV.1, GV.2, BL.35, BL.60 E.

Spinal problems

Pulse. Maybe empty or wiry.

Indications. Spinal pain, spasm and stiffness, convulsions.

Example. Spinal stiffness.

Combination. SI.3, BL.62, GV.1, GV.8, GV.14 E.

Mental problems

Pulse. Various – from empty and choppy to wiry and rapid.

Indications. Depression, hysteria, mental instability.

Example. Spinal problems aggravated by nervous anxiety.

Combination. GV.1, GV.11, GV.20, BL.62, HT.7, KI.6 E.

GV.2 yāo shū

GV.2 has similar functions to GV.1, except that GV.1 is better for anal problems and GV.2 is more used for epilepsy. Whilst GV.1 is especially for Damp Heat anal problems, GV.2 is more for problems of the lower back and sacrum involving Deficient Kidney Yang, Cold and Damp. GV.2 is therefore intermediate in function between GV.1 and GV.3, because of its location on the spine.

GV.2 does not have the wide urogenital application of CV.2 or CV.3, these points are more similar in function to the bā liáo points on the Bladder channel. GV.2 is more for spinal problems involving the sacrum, lower back and perhaps even leg weakness and for the characteristic Governor function of controlling Interior Wind.

GV.3 yāo yáng guān

GV.3 is similar to GV.4, in that it tonifies Kidney Yang and strengthens the lower back and legs. However, GV.4 has wider applications than GV.3 and is stronger in tonifying Kidney Yang. GV.3 is especially used for local back pain, for back pain radiating to the legs and for pain and weakness in the legs and knees.

GV.3 is closer in function to CV.4 than to CV.3, but like GV.2, is mainly used for local spine and back problems.

GV.4 mìng mén

GV.4 and CV.4

GV.4 relates to the Dan Tian and the storage and movement of Kidney Jing and Qi, as does CV.4, but CV.4 is of wider application than mìng mén. CV.4 can tonify not only Jing, Qi and Yang, but also Yin and Blood. GV.4 is most effective for tonifying Yang and Fire, with the associated functions of warming and drying Cold and Damp. Mìng mén is very much a point of the Governor channel, and can be used for local and general spinal problems, and for regulating Yang and thus strengthening and clearing the brain and calming the spirit. However, its main use is to tonify Yang rather than to regulate it.

Syndromes

Spinal problems
Cold and Damp

Acute Exterior Invasion of Wind Cold Damp
Chronic accumulation of Interior Cold and Damp
Deficient Kidney Yang
Deficient Kidney and Spleen Yang and Sinking of Qi
Deficient Kidney Jing and Yang and Deficient Liver
Blood
Deficient Kidney and Heart Yang

Spinal problems

Local spinal problems

Pulse. Various, maybe wiry.

Indications. Local problems of second and third lumbar vertebrae and associated spinal nerves.

Example. Acute back sprain with pain in left lumbar area radiating down left leg.

Combination. GV.4, jiā jǐ, BL.23, BL.50, BL.40, BL.60 on left side, E M.

General spinal problems

Pulse. Maybe empty, choppy, deep, slow, maybe wiry.

Indications. Pain and stiffness of spine associated with both Deficiency and Stagnation of Qi.

Example. Ankylosing spondylitis with especial stiffness at lumbar and cervical areas.

Combination. SI.3, BL.62, BL.10, GV.2, GV.4, GV.14, GV.15 E M.

Cold and Damp

Acute Exterior Invasion of Wind Cold Damp

Pulse. Superficial, tight.

Indications. Local or general spinal stiffness and discomfort due to Exterior Invasion.

Example. Stiffness and ache in lumbosacral region.

Combination. GV.3, GV.4, BL.23, BL.25, BL.60 E M.

Chronic accumulation of Interior Cold Damp

Pulse. Empty, deep, slow, maybe tight or wiry.

Indications. Lumbar stiffness and discomfort, aversion to cold, tiredness, maybe oedema.

Example. Exhaustion, whole body feels cold, especially lower abdomen and back, lumbar discomfort and stiffness.

Combination. GV.4, BL.23, BL.52, BL.60 KI.2, ST.36 Rf M.

Deficient Kidney Yang

Pulse. Empty to minute, deep, slow.

Indications. Urinary frequency, incontinence or pain, frigidity, impotence, infertility, exhaustion, depression.

Example. Exhaustion, emotional withdrawal, somnolence.

Combination. GV.4, Rf M; GV.20, BL.62, KI.6.

Alternation. CV.4 Rf M; GV.20, BL.62, KI.6.

Deficient Kidney and Spleen Yang and Sinking of Qi

Pulse. Empty, deep, slow, maybe choppy.

Indications. Prolapses, haemorrhage, flaccid skin and muscles, exhaustion, depression.

Example. Prolapsed bleeding haemorrhoids.

Combination. GV.1 E; GV.4, GV.20, BL.23, BL.25, SP.10 Rf M.

Deficient Kidney Jing and Yang and Deficient Liver Blood

Pulse. Empty or thin to minute, deep, choppy, maybe wiry.

Indications. Premature ageing, for example deterioration in eyesight and hearing; stiffness and weakness of muscles and joints; weak back, knees and legs; impotence, infertility.

Example. Timidity, indecision, forgetfulness and unsteadiness of gait.

Combination. CV.4, CV.8, BL.18, BL.23, KI.3, LR.3, GB.34, LR.8 Rf M.

Deficient Kidney and Heart Yang

Pulse. Empty, deep, slow, maybe wiry, maybe scattered.

Indications. Cold body, cold extremities, exhaustion, depression, fearfulness, disorientation, forgetfulness, somnolence.

Example. Exhaustion with paranoia and loneliness, forgetfulness and difficulty in concentration.

Combination. GV.4, GV.11, GV.20, BL.44, BL.52, BL.60, KI.7 Rf M.

Alternation. CV.4, CV.17, GV.20, KI.3, ST.36 Rf M; GV.24, GB.13, HT.5 E.

GV.6 jī zhōng

GV.5 below the first lumbar and GV.6 below the eleventh thoracic vertebra, can both be used to treat digestive problems. The author has chosen GV.6 to represent the Spleen energy centre on the spine because it is level with BL.20 and BL.49 which control the Spleen organ. As discussed on page 150, the GV points representing the five Yin organs, can be used in combination with the inner or outer Bladder channel points at the same spinal level, to treat physical or psychological problems of the associated organ.

Syndromes

 Deficient Spleen Yang
 Stagnation of Spleen Qi

Deficient Spleen Yang

Pulse. Empty, deep, slow, maybe slippery.

Indications. Weak muscles, easily tired, prolapses, bleeding, diarrhoea, loss of appetite, coldness especially of the abdomen, oedema, poor memory, slow dull thinking.

Example. Poor concentration, desire to lie down and sleep, abdominal distension.

Combination. GV.4, GV.6, GV.20, SP.4, ST.36, LI.4 Rf M.

Stagnation of Spleen Qi

Pulse. Maybe empty or maybe full, slippery, slightly wiry.

Indications. Worry with thoughts stuck on one topic, inability to digest and assimilate ideas, indigestion with abdominal discomfort and distension.

Example. Worry, feelings of insecurity, mental congestion from excessive study.

Combination. GV.20 E; GV.6, BL.49, BL.67, KI.1 Rf M.

Alternation. yìn táng, LI.5, ST.40, SP.6 E; ST.45 E M.

GV.8 jīn suō

GV.8 is on the same spinal level as BL.18 and BL.47 relating to the physical, emotional and mental functions of the Liver. Both GV.8 and GV.9 can be used to treat Liver problems. Because of their relative locations, GV.8 is more used for abdominal and GV.9 for chest problems. Both points can be used to regulate the Stagnant Qi, Hyperactive Yang and Interior Wind that can produce stiffness and spasm of the back and spinal muscles.

The Solar Plexus energy centre is located between GV.8 and GV.9 in the spine, roughly equivalent to the centre between CV.14 and CV.15 on the front of the body. GV.8 or GV.9 can therefore be used, like CV.14, to treat emotional tensions and pressures affecting Lower, Middle and Upper Energizers whether due to anger, fear or other emotions.

Syndromes

 Spinal problems
 Stagnant Liver Qi
 Hyperactive Liver Yang
 Internal Liver Wind
 Liver–Gallbladder Fire and Damp Heat
 Nervous tension affecting Lower and Middle Energizers

Spinal problems

Pulse. Wiry.

Indications. Stiffness in spine, neck stiffness, headache, emotional and mental rigidity.

Example. Stiff spine, general muscular tightness, headache, irritability.

Combination. GV.8, GV.14, GV.20, GB.34, GB.21, GB.20 Rd; SP.6 Rf.

Stagnant Liver Qi

Pulse. Wiry, slippery.

Indications. Depression, frustration, gastritis, abdominal distension, rib pain.

Example. Indigestion with abdominal distension, depression and tiredness.

Combination. GV.6, GV.8, BL.18, BL.20, SP.6 E; ST.36 Rf M.

Hyperactive Liver Yang

Pulse. Empty, wiry.

Indications. Headache, irritability, faintness and gastritis if meals are too far apart; symptoms improving after eating.

Example. Tiredness, restlessness and irritability before meals.

Combination. GV.8, BL.18 E; BL.20, ST.36, SP.6 Rf.

Internal Liver Wind

Pulse. Wiry, empty or full, maybe rapid, maybe choppy.

Indications. Muscle spasms, tremors, epilepsy or other convulsions.

Example. Muscle tremor due to Interior Liver Wind associated with Deficient Kidney Yin and Deficient Blood.

Combination. GV.8, GV.17 LR.3, BL.18, BL.20, BL.23, SP.6, KI.6 Rf.

Liver–Gallbladder Fire and Damp Heat

Pulse. Wiry, rapid, maybe slippery.

Indications. Cholecystitis, hepatitis.

Example. Cholecystitis, hypochondriac pain.

Combination. GV.8, BL.18, GB.25, dǎn náng, TE.6 E.

Nervous tension affecting Lower and Middle Energizers

Pulse. Maybe wiry, maybe empty, maybe changing.

Indications. Tension and stress aggravating conditions such as irritable bowel syndrome, diarrhoea, gastritis.

Example. Oversensitivity to environmental stress, greatly disturbed by emotions of anger or fear, nausea, diarrhoea.

Combination. GV.8, BL.18, BL.23, PC.6, SP.4 E; SP.6, ST.36 Rf.

GV.9 zhì yáng

GV.9 is more use for problems of Upper and Middle Energizers while GV.8 is better for Middle and Lower Energizers. GV.9 can therefore be used for the same syndromes as GV.8, with the exception of gastric problems and with the addition of Lung and diaphragm problems.

Syndromes

Spinal problems
Stagnant Liver Qi
Hyperactive Liver Yang } see GV.8
Internal Liver Wind
Liver–Gallbladder Fire and Damp Heat
Nervous tension affecting Middle and Upper Energizers

Nervous tension affecting Middle and Upper Energizers

Pulse. Wiry.

Indications. Feeling of fullness or oppression in chest, cough, asthma, bronchiectasis, sighing, hiccup, dyspnoea.

Example. Restricted breathing aggravated by stress.

Combination. GV.9, BL.13, BL.17, BL.47, KI.6, LU.7, PC.6 E.

GV.11 shén dào

GV.11 is below the spinous process of the fifth thoracic vertebra and is associated with BL.15 and BL.44 in regulating the functions of the Heart organ. It can also be used as the equivalent spinal centre to the Heart centre represented by CV.17 on the front of the body. GV.11 can therefore be used to treat not only physical problems such as heart disease and poor circulation, but psychological problems of speech, communication, the sharing of ideas and feelings and the ability to give and receive love in relationships.

Syndromes

Deficient Heart Yang and Fire
Stagnation of Heart Qi
Disturbance of Spirit by Yang, Fire or Wind

Deficient Heart Yang and Fire

Pulse. Empty, maybe deep and slow, maybe irregular.

Indications. Apathy, depression, sadness, loneliness, exhaustion, cold extremities.

Example. Difficulty in forming and continuing relationships, apparent coldness and lack of affection.

Combination. GV.4, GV.11, GV.14, PC.8 Rf M; KI.3, SP.6, HT.7 Rf.

Stagnation of Heart Qi

Pulse. Maybe wiry, maybe empty, maybe irregular.

Indications. Oppressive feeling in the chest, insomnia, palpitations, occasional pain or aching in chest, difficulty in expressing feelings, depression.

Example. Difficulty in expressing feelings in speech.

Combination. GV.11, BL.44, HT.5, KI.4, PC.7 E.

Alternation. CV.17, CV.23, HT.5, KI.4, PC.7 E.

Disturbance of Spirit by Heart Fire

Pulse. Rapid, full, maybe irregular.

Indications. Feverish or hot, hyperactivity, manic behaviour, hysteria, agitation.

Example. Rushed, overenthusiastic tense activity with severe insomnia.

Combination. GV.1, GV.11, GV.20, KI.1 Rd; HT.7, SP.6 Rf.

Disturbance of Spirit by Hyperactive Liver Yang

Pulse. Wiry, choppy, maybe irregular.

Indications. Dizziness, headache or unpleasant moving or distending feeling in the head or chest, irritability, agitation, palpitations.

Example. Occasional faintness, mental confusion, difficulty in concentration.

Combination. GV.11, GV.20, LR.3, GB.34 E; KI.3, SP.6 Rf.

GV.12 shén zhù

GV.12 is level with BL.13 and BL.42 and is mainly used for Lung problems or to relieve spasms, tremors and convulsions.

Syndromes

Spinal problems
Deficient Lung Qi and Yang
Stagnant Lung Qi

Spinal problems

Pulse. Wiry.

Indications. Spasms, stiffness and pain of lower back or of upper back and neck, tremors or convulsions.

Example. Arthritis and stiffness of upper back and shoulders.

Combination. GV.12, BL.42, BL.62, SI.3, SI.13, SI.15 E.

Deficient Lung Qi and Yang

Pulse. Big, empty, deep, slow, maybe slippery.

Indications. Tiredness, cough with watery sputum, weak breathing, shortness of breath, easy to catch colds.

Example. Bronchitis with feelings of tiredness and cold.

Combination. GV.4, GV.12, BL.13, BL.23, KI.7, ST.36 Rf M; LU.9 Rf.

Stagnant Lung Qi

Pulse. Maybe empty or full and flooding, maybe wiry, maybe slippery.

Indications. Suppressed grief, chronic bronchitis, dyspnoea, oppressive feeling in chest.

Example. Sadness, depression and withdrawal

Combination. GV.11, GV.12, BL.42, BL.44, LU.7, KI.6 E.

GV.13 táo dào

GV.13 can calm the Spirit like GV.11 and GV.14. It can strengthen the Defensive Qi like GV.12 and it can relieve upper spinal stiffness like most of the other GV points. However, the characteristic function of GV.13 is to remove Wind Heat and Interior Heat. It has the traditional indication of Lesser Yang stage fevers with alternation of chills and fever. In practice, GV.13 is mainly used for local spinal problems.

GV.14 dà zhuī

Meeting point of Yang channels, Influential point of Yang, Sea of Qi point.

General

The characteristic functions of GV.14 derive from the fact that it is a GV point and from its specific location.

General GV channel functions of GV.14

As a GV point, dà zhuī can be used to reduce Yang, Heat and Interior Wind, and conversely tonify Deficient Yang or Deficient Fire.

Specific functions of GV.14 resulting from its location

Clears Exterior Wind Invasion. Other GV points can be used for this, but GV.14, 15 and 16 are especially important due to their location on the back of the neck, an area regarded as especially vulnerable to Wind Invasion. GV.14 not only expels Exterior Wind, but can also be used to prevent entry of Exterior Wind since it tonifies Defensive and Nutrient Qi.

A Crossing point of the six Yang channels. This connection between the flows of the six Yang channels with the GV channel makes GV.14 especially important as a means of coordinating and regulating Yang, whether Yang is Hyperactive or Deficient.

A gate between neck, body and arms. GV.14 can be used to regulate the flows of energy in the meridian between not only the body and the neck, but also the arms, shoulders and neck.

Strengthens Dispersing functions of the Lungs. Not only can GV.14 relieve Exterior Wind invading the Lungs, but also it can aid the Dispersing function to treat asthma and cough.

Regulates Heart Yang and Fire. GV.14 can tonify the Yang of the body in general, but, because of its location, it is most effective in tonifying Heart Yang, and also in regulating disturbance of the Spirit due to Heat.

Comparison of GV.14 with other GV points

With GV.4. Both points can tonify Yang of the whole body, and by doing so relieve Interior Cold and Damp and prevent Invasion by Exterior Wind. Both points can tonify and regulate Yang of Kidney and Heart, but GV.4 is relatively more for Kidneys and GV.14 more for Heart. Both points regulate the spine, but GV.4 is more for spinal problems involving hips and legs and GV.14 for spinal problems involing neck, shoulders and arms.

With GV.11. Both points can be used to tonify Heart Yang or to calm the Spirit, but GV.14 has, in addition, the function of regulating the Yang of all the organs, since it is the meeting point of the six Yang channels.

With GV.12. Both points can be used to remove and prevent Exterior Wind Invasion and to strengthen the Dispersing function of the Lungs but GV.14 has additional specific and general functions listed earlier. For example, GV.14 is better to relieve fever or Summer Heat than GV.12.

With GV.15 and GV.16. All three points can be used to regulate speech, to calm and clear the mind and to treat local neck problems. However, GV.14 is more for shoulders and neck while GV.15 and GV.16 are more for neck and head. GV.14 is more for voice problems and GV.15 and GV.16 more for speech problems. Also, GV.14 is more to treat Lungs and throat, whilst GV.15 and GV.16 are more for tongue, nose, ear and eye problems.

With GV.20. Both points can regulate the movement of Yang into the head, but GV.14 is more related to Heart and GV.20 more to Liver. GV.20 is more to clear and calm the mind and to counteract Sinking of Qi, GV.14 is more to relieve Heat and remove Exterior Wind Invasion.

Combination of GV.14 with other GV points

Some important combinations are with GV.4, 11, 12, 15 or 16, 20.

With GV.4. Deficient Yang of Kidneys and Heart, Deficient Yang of all organ systems, spinal problems.

With GV.11. Deficient Yang and Fire of Heart, Disturbance of Spirit due to Hyperactive Yang or Heat.

With GV.12. Deficient Yang and Qi of Lungs with Stagnation of Lung Qi, Invasion of Lungs by Exterior Wind.

With GV.15 or GV.16. Upper spinal problems, speech and communication problems, mental and emotional problems due to Deficiency or to Disturbance of Spirit.

With GV.20. Disturbance of Spirit due to Hyperactive Yang, Heat or Interior Wind.

Syndromes

Spinal problems
External Wind Invasion
Heat
Internal Wind
Deficient Yang
Deficiency and Stagnation of Lung Qi

Spinal problems

Neck, shoulders and arms

Pulse. Various, maybe wiry, empty or thin.

Indications. Pain, stiffness or numbness in neck, shoulder and arms.

Example. Numbness and weakness from neck to right hand, aggravated by cold.

Combination. GV.14 Rf M; LI.5, LI.10, LI.14, LI.16 Rf M on right side; ST.40 Rf M on left side.

Neck, shoulder and head

Pulse. Wiry, maybe empty or thin, choppy or flooding.

Indications. Neck pain, headache, stiffness of shoulders, depression, agitation.

Example. Neck pain and headache with depression.

Combination. GV.4, GV.14, BL.10, BL.62, SI.3 E.

External Wind Invasion

Pulse. Superficial, tight.

Indications. Sneezing, runny nose, generalized muscle aches, ache in neck and occipital head, aversion to cold.

Example. Influenza with severe feeling of cold.

Combination. GV.13, GV.14, BL.10, BL.11, LI.4, ST.36 Rd M.

Heat

Wind Heat Invasion

Pulse. Superficial, rapid.

Indications. Sore throat, fever, cough, urticaria or eczema.

Example. Wind Heat urticaria, fever.

Combination. GV.14, LU.7, LI.4, BL.40 Rd.

Excess Heat — Acute Fever

Pulse. Full, rapid.

Indications. Acute fever, acute Excess Heat condition associated with Stomach, Heart, Lungs, Liver Fire.

Example. Acute fever.

Combination. GV.14, LI.4, LI.11 Rd; PC.9 B; HT.7 E.

Excess Heat — Heart Fire

Pulse. Rapid, full or flooding, maybe wiry or irregular.

Indications. Mania, hypertension, headache, menopausal flushes.

Example: Extreme stressful overenthusiasm and hyperactivity.

Combination. GV.14, GV.20, KI.1, HT.9 Rd; KI.3, HT.7 Rf.

Summer Heat

Pulse. Superficial, flooding.

Indications. Sunburn, sunstroke (Excess Heat phase).

Combination. GV.14, LI.4, SP.10 Rd; PC.3, PC.9, BL.40, shí xuān B.

Internal Wind

By regulating Heat and Yang this point can regulate Interior Wind in general. It is sometimes indicated for cerebrovascular accident, but GV.15, 16, 20 and 26 are more used for this.

Deficient Heart Yang

Pulse. Slow empty, maybe wiry or deep.

Indications. Sadness, depression.

Example. Melancholia with tiredness and cold extremities.

Combination. GV.4, GV.14, BL.15, BL.23, BL.60 Rf M; HT.7 Rf.

Alternation. CV.4, CV.17 Rf M; SP.4, PC.6 E.

Deficiency and Stagnation of Lung Qi

Pulse. Wiry, maybe empty or slippery, maybe slow or rapid.

Indications. Asthma, bronchitis.

Example. Asthma.

Points. GV.14, dìng chuǎn, BL.13, CV.17, ST.40, LU.6 Rd; KI.3 Rf.

GV.15 yǎ mén and GV.16 fēng fǔ

GV.15 is the Sea of Qi point; GV.16 is the Window of Heaven point, Sea of Marrow point, Crossing point of Yang Link and Governor. These two points are very similar, can be used together and indeed function almost as a unit. They constitute a regulatory gate to energy flow between neck and head and also represent the Throat energy centre concerned with speech and clear communication of ideas.

Clear Exterior Wind Invasion

Like GV.14, these points can be used to disperse Exterior Wind, but are more for symptoms of Exterior Wind in head and neck, whilst GV.14 is more for Exterior Wind in Lungs, shoulders and neck. Also GV.15 and GV.16 do not have the strong ability to tonify Yang possessed by GV.14.

Local neck and head problems

GV.15 and GV.16 are more for problems of upper neck and head, whilst GV.14 is more for problems of arms, shoulders and lower neck. GV.15 can also be used to treat deafness and GV.16 to treat problems of nose and eyes.

Internal Wind and Hyperactive Yang

GV.15 and GV.16 can act as a gate to control Interior Wind or Hyperactive Yang rising up the body to disturb consciousness and speech. They can thus be used for headache and dizziness, seizures such as apoplexy or epilepsy, or sequelae of apoplexy such as hemiplegia or speech problems.

Disturbance of Spirit

GV.15 and GV.16 can be used to regulate Disturbance of Spirit due to Interior Liver Wind or Hyperactive Liver Yang as described above, often associated with anger and irritability. In addition, they can be used for Heart disturbance with anxiety, mania, hysteria or delirium, and for Kidney disturbance with fear and fright.

Lack of mental clarity

This may be due to Deficient Kidney, Hyperactive Liver Yang, Deficient Qi and Blood or Phlegm disturbing the head. GV.15 and GV.16 are especially helpful if there is obstruction to the balanced flow of energy moving up the body in the Governor and Bladder channels to the head and brain. There may be stiffness of the neck with a congested or heavy feeling in the head accompanied by headache and depression.

Speech

The Throat energy centre, the focus of speech and communication, is represented on the back of the body by GV.15 and GV.16, and on the front of the body by GV.22 and GV.23. GV.14 and CV.22 govern the Lungs and the voice. GV.15 and GV.16 and CV.23 are more concerned with the upper throat, the tongue and speech. This is especially aided by the link, provided by GV.15 and GV.16, between speech and brain. Speech can be affected by disturbance of Spirit and by lack of mental clarity.

Syndromes (GV.15 and GV.16)

External Wind Invasion
Local and head problems
Internal Wind and Hyperactive Yang
Disturbance of Spirit
Lack of mental clarity
Speech problems

External Wind Invasion

Pulse. Superficial, tight.

Indications. Common cold or influenza.

Example. Common cold with rhinitis and neck ache.

Combination. GV.14 Rd M; GV.16, LI.4, LI.20, LU.7 Rd.

Local and head problems

Pulse. Wiry, maybe empty, slow or rapid.

Indications. Multiple sclerosis, cervical arthritis, sequela of neck injury, ankylosing spondylitis.

Example. Stiffness and pain in upper neck with occasional aches in head and lower neck.

Combination. GV.14, GV.15, GV.17, BL.9, BL.10, BL.62, SI.3 E.

Internal Wind and Hyperactive Yang

Pulse. Wiry, maybe empty or slippery, maybe rapid.

Indications. Dizziness, headache, epilepsy, CVA, hemiplegia, speech problems following CVA or head injury.

Example. Dizziness, neck ache, headache, mental confusion and lack of clarity.

Combination. GV.16, GV.20, LR.3, GB.20, GB.34 Rd; KI.3 Rf.

Disturbance of Spirit

Pulse. Various, for example, wiry, choppy, irregular, moving, scattered.

Indications. Emotional lability, whether of anger, fear or anxiety, mental irregularity, problems of speech.

Example. Neck ache and headache with anxiety and suppressed anger.

Combination. GV.15, BL.10, GB.21, GB.34, SI.3, SI.15 Rd; SP.6, HT.7 Rf.

Lack of mental clarity

Pulse. Maybe empty, wiry or slippery.

Indications. Neck ache, headache, heavy or congested feeling in the head, feeling of mental dullness, slowness or confusion.

Example. Damp and Phlegm invade the head with signs of heavy head and mental dullness.

Combination. GV.16, yìn táng, ST.40, ST.45, LI.1, LI.4 E.

Speech problems

Pulse. Various, for example, wiry or irregular, slow or rapid.

Indications. Stammering, confused speech, aphasia, slurred speech from cerebral damage, stage fright.

Example. Mild confusion of speech, worse with tiredness.

Combination. GV.16 yìn táng, HT.5 E; HT.7, SP.6 Rf.

Comparison of GV.15 and GV.16

These points are very similar and differences are partly due to location. GV.15 is lower on the neck and more for speech and deafness, while GV.16 is higher on the neck and slightly more for mental problems and for eye and nose problems.

GV.20 bǎi huì

Sea of Marrow point, Crossing point of all the Yang channels, Crossing point of Governor with internal Liver channel.

General

bǎi huì as an energy centre

GV.20 corresponds to the Crown chakra or energy centre, which is said to be especially concerned with spiritual development. In Qi Gong it is a main point through which the energies of Heaven enter the body and a main point through which energy circulates through and around the body.

bǎi huì and the CV–GV energy cycle

At GV.20, energy has come up the Governor channel as far as it can, and must now turn and go downward. This completes the vertical circulation of energy up the GV channel from GV.1 to GV.20, down the GV channel from GV.20 to GV.28 and down the CV channel from CV.24 to CV.1. The energy then flows from CV.1 to GV.1 and again ascends the spine.

bǎi huì as a point of polarity change

GV.20 has the usual properties of Governor channel points of regulation of Yang, but is especially important because like the Well points, it is a place where the energy flow in the channel changes direction. Such points have great effect upon the energy of the body, especially to calm severe disturbance of energy, when used with Reducing method, and also to stimulate severe collapse of energy, when used with Reinforcing method and moxa.

Syndromes

Disturbance of Energy
Hyperactive Liver Yang and Interior Wind
Disturbance of Heart Spirit from:
    Heat e.g. acute fever, Heart Fire, Liver Fire,
      Stomach Fire
    Fear
    Deficiency of Qi and Blood
Damp and Phlegm invade the head

Deficiency or Collapse of Yang
Loss of consciousnesss
Deficient Kidney Yang
Sinking of Spleen Qi
Deficient Heart Yang

Hyperactive Liver Yang and Interior Wind

Pulse. Wiry.

Indications. Hypertension, headache, dizziness, tinnitus, CVA and sequelae.

Example. Headache, stiff shoulders and neck, spinal stiffness and muscle cramps.

Combination. GV.1, GV.20, LR.3, LI.4 Rd.

Disturbance of Heart Spirit from Heart Fire

Pulse. Rapid, maybe wiry or irregular.

Indications. Restlessness, hyperactivity, mania, palpitations, insomnia, hypertension.

Example. Anxiety, hysteria, irrational behaviour.

Combination. GV.20, KI.1 Rd; SP.6, KI.3, HT.7 Rf.

Disturbance of Heart Spirit from Fear

Pulse. Maybe irregular or moving.

Indications. Shock, fright, fearful anxiety, suspicion and paranoia.

Example. Panic attacks in crowded places.

Combinations. GV.14, GV.20, PC.6 E; KI.7, SP.6, HT.7 Rf.

Disturbance of Heart Spirit from Deficiency of Qi and Blood

Pulse. Empty or thin, choppy, maybe irregular.

Indications. Dizziness, insomnia, palpitations, tiredness, emotional lability.

Example. Easily overexcited or tearful, feels vulnerable and easily hurt.

Combination. GV.20, SP.4, PC.6 E; SP.10, ST.36 Rf.

Damp and Phlegm invade the head

Pulse. Slippery, maybe wiry or empty.

Indications. Hypertension, headache, dizziness, heavy feeling in head and maybe chest and limbs.

Example. Oppressive full feeling in head, inability to

think clearly, restlessness, depression.

Combination. GV.20, GV.26, PC.5, PC.6, ST.40, ST.45, SP.9 Rd; HT.7 E.

Loss of consciousness

Pulse. Minute.

Indications. Loss of consciousness from exhaustion, heatstroke, food allergy, nervous tension, etc.

Example. Fainting from exhaustion and shock of first acupuncture treatment.

Combination. GV.20 E M; GV.26, PC.9 E.

Deficient Kidney Yang

Pulse. Empty to minute, choppy, deep, slow.

Indications. Exhaustion, depression, inability to concentrate, impotence, incontinence, tinnitus.

Example. Impotence, exhaustion and depression.

Combination. GV.4, GV.20, BL.23, BL.60 Rf M; BL.31, BL.33 E.

Alternation. CV.4, GV.20, KI.7, ST.36, Rf M; SP.6, HT.7 Rf.

Sinking of Spleen Qi

Pulse. Empty to minute, maybe deep, choppy or slow.

Indications. Gastroptosis, uterovaginal or rectal prolapse, abnormal vaginal bleeding, exhaustion, loss of appetite, desire to lie down and sleep.

Example. Forgetfulness, mental and physical exhaustion.

Combination. GV.1, GV.4, GV.6, GV.20, BL.20, ST.36, LI.4 Rf M.

Deficient Heart Yang

Pulse. Empty to minute, maybe deep, slow, irregular.

Indications. Depression, apathy, exhaustion, poor peripheral circulation.

Example. Tiredness and melancholy.

Combinations. GV.11, GV.20, BL.44, BL.62, HT.8 Rf M; HT.7 E.

Precautions in using GV.20

As with all GV points, it is essential to avoid moxa if there

are any Heat signs. Moxa on GV.20 should be avoided especially when treating depression, if there is a past history of alternation between depression and mania. Also, GV.20 should not have moxa if the patient has high blood pressure.

When using GV.20 to treat agitations, it should not be strongly reduced if the patient has underlying Deficiency. It is better to use GV.20 with Even method while simultaneously tonifying the Deficiency with points on the lower body, such as SP.6 or KI.3.

GV.23 shàng xīng and GV.24 shén tíng

GV.24 is the Crossing point of Governor and Stomach channels.

General

In Qi Gong, GV.20 represents the Crown energy centre and yìn táng represents the Brow centre. In acupuncture, GV.20 represents the stability of consciousness, with neither Excess nor Deficiency of Yang, whilst yìn táng represents calm and clear perception.

GV.23 and GV.24 are intermediate in function between GV.20 and yìn táng. GV.23 and especially GV.24, can be used for anxiety, palpitation, insomnia, fearfulness, schizophrenia and other mental disorders.

GV.23 and GV.24 for eye and nose problems

In common with the neighbouring points BL.3, 4, 5 and GB.13 and GB.15, GV.23 and GV.24 can be used to treat a variety of nose and eye problems.

Syndromes

Mental problems
Eye problems
Nose problems

Mental problems

Pulse. Various, maybe wiry or irregular.

Indications. Headache, vertigo, epilepsy, fearful anxiety, schizophrenia, insomnia.

Example. Worry, anxiety, obsessive thoughts (both day and night).

Combination. GV.24, GB.13, PC.7 E; SP.6, ST.36 Rf.

Eye problems

Pulse. Various, maybe tight and rapid.

Indications. Eye pain, redness and swelling, excessive lachrymation, myopia, sudden blindness.

Example. Acute conjunctivitis.

Combination. GV.24, GB.1, GB.14, GB.41, TE.3 E.

Nose problems

Pulse. Various, maybe tight or slippery.

Indications. Rhinitis, sinusitis, nasal polyps, epistaxis, frontal headache.

Example. Nasal obstruction with frontal headache.

Combination. GV.23, BL.2, BL.4, BL.67, LI.4, LI.20 E.

GV.26 rén zhōng

Meeting point of Governor, Stomach and Large Intestine channels.

General

GV.26, 27 and 28 are in the area where the Yang Governor channel meets the Yin Conception channel, so that these points can be used to regulate the balance of Yin–Yang in the body especially for mental disorders. GV.26 is the most used of these three points and like GV.20, CV.1 and the Well points, it can be used for loss of consciousness, since it is located where the energy changes polarity.

Syndromes

Disturbance of Spirit
Loss of consciousness
Acute lower back problems
Face problems
Nose problems

Disturbance of Spirit

Pulse. Maybe thin, choppy, rapid, irregular.

Indications. Severe anxiety, anxiety and depression, hysteria.

Example. Anxiety with incessant nervous talking.

Combination. GV.20, GV.26, CV.24, SP.4, PC.6, KI.3 E.

Loss of consciousness

Pulse. Minute.

Indication. Loss of consciousness from various causes.

Example. Fainting from shock due to allergic response to shellfish.

Combination. GV.26, HT.9 E.

Acute lower back problems

Pulse. Wiry.

Indication. Acute lower back sprain when pain is located in the spine. See p. 364 for details of use.

Combination. After GV.26 has been used, local points may be used also.

Face problems

Pulse. Various, maybe wiry or empty.

Indications. Trigeminal neuralgia, facial paralysis, toothache, facial swelling, skin problems,

Example. Severe acne, especially around mouth, chin and neck.

Combination. GV.26, CV.24, LI.4, LI.18, LI.20, ST.44 Rd.

Nose problems

Pulse. Maybe tight or slippery.

Indications. Rhinitis, sinusitis, epistaxis.

Example. Rhinitis.

Combination. GV.23, GV.25, GV.26, LI.4, LI.20, LU.7, Rd; ST.2 E.

Governor point comparisons and combinations

The functions of the main points of the GV channel are listed in Table 12.3.

Table 12.3 GV points comparisons

Point	Syndrome
GV.1	anal problems coccygeal problems
GV.2	sacral problems Internal Wind
GV.3	weakness of lower back and legs Deficient Kidney Yang
GV.4	spinal problems Deficient Kidney Yang and Jing Deficient Kidney Yang with Cold and Damp
GV.6	Deficient Spleen Yang Stagnant Qi of Spleen and Stomach
GV.8	Liver syndromes
GV.9	Liver syndromes spasm of diaphragm Stagnation of Qi in chest
GV.11	Heart syndromes
GV.12	Lung syndromes spinal problems
GV.13	Wind Heat, Interior Heat
GV.14	Wind Cold, Wind Heat Internal Heat Deficient Yang Deficient Lung Qi spinal problems Internal Wind
GV.15 and GV.16	External Wind Invasion neck and head problems Internal Wind and Hyperactive Yang disturbance of Spirit lack of mental clarity speech problems (GV.15 is better for speech and GV.16 is better for lack of mental clarity)
GV.20	Hyperactive Liver Yang and Interior Wind Disturbance of Spirit loss of consciousness Deficient Yang and Sinking of Qi
GV.23 and GV.24	mental problems eye problems nasal problems (GV.23 is more for nasal problems and GV.24 more for mental problems)
GV.26	Disturbance of Spirit loss of consciousness acute lower back sprain facial problems nasal problems

Some common combinations of GV channel points are summarized in Table 12.4.

Table 12.4 Combinations of GV points

Point	Combination	Syndromes	Example
GV.1	GV.2	Stagnation of Blood	coccygeal pain
GV.1	GV.8	Stagnation of Qi	spinal stiffness
GV.2	GV.3	Stagnation of Blood	sacral pain
GV.4	GV.3	Invasion of Cold and Damp	lumbar pain
GV.4	GV.6	Deficient Yang of Kidneys and Spleen	oedema
GV.4	GV.11	Deficient Yang of Kidneys and Heart	exhaustion and apathy
GV.4	GV.12	Deficient Yang of Kidneys and Lungs	bronchitis
GV.4	GV.14	Deficient Yang of all organs	exhaustion and coldness
GV.4	GV.20	Deficient Yang of Kidneys and Spleen	incontinence, impotence
GV.6	GV.20	Sinking of Spleen Qi	prolapses, diarrhoea
GV.8	GV.12	Stagnation of Liver Qi	spinal stiffness and pain
GV.11	GV.14	Deficient Heart Yang	poor circulation
GV.11	GV.15	Disturbance of Spirit	stammering
GV.11	GV.20	Deficient Heart Yin	hyperactivity
GV.12	GV.14	Deficient Lungs Qi	asthma
GV.13	GV.14	Stagnation of Blood	upper spinal problems
GV.14	GV.15	Wind Cold invasion	influenza and neck ache
GV.14	GV.16	Stagnation of Qi in GV channel	depression with feelings of heaviness in head
GV.15	GV.16	Stagnation of Blood	cervical trauma
GV.16	GV.20	Disturbance of Spirit by fear	fear and anxiety
GV.16	GV.23	Wind Cold invasion	rhinitis
GV.20	GV.8	Hyperactive Liver Yang	dizziness, muscle spasms
GV.20	GV.14	Disturbance of Spirit due to Internal Heat	acute fever
GV.20	GV.24	Disturbance of Spirit	anxiety, fear and suspicion
GV.20	GV.26	Collapse of Yang	fainting
GV.3	GV.4, 5	Invasion of Cold and Damp	lumbar pain
GV.4	GV.9, 12	Stagnation of Qi	spinal stiffness
GV.4	GV.11, 14	Deficient Yang of Heart and Kidneys	tiredness and depression
GV.4	GV.14, 20	Collapse of Yang	complete exhaustion
GV.11	GV.15, 20	Disturbance of Spirit	anxiety, mania, confused speech
GV.14	GV.15, 16	Invasion of Wind Cold and Stagnation of Blood	cervical arthritis
GV.14	GV.16, 20	Disturbance of Spirit and Stagnation of Qi	depression, anxiety, heavy feeling in head
GV.4	GV.6, 14, 20	Deficient Yang of Kidneys, Spleen and Heart	exhaustion, depression
GV.4	GV.9, 12, 15	Stagnation of Qi and Blood	ankylosing spondylitis

Kidney 13

Kidney channel

CHANNEL CONNECTIONS

MAIN CHANNEL PATHWAY

The external pathway starts under the fifth toe, runs to KI.1 on the sole of the foot, continues up the medial leg, through SP.6 to the groin and parallels the CV channel up the body from KI.11 to KI.27 below the clavicle.

The internal pathway runs from the groin to GV.1, ascends the lumbar spine and connects with the Kidney and the Bladder. From the Kidney, it passes through the Liver and the diaphragm, enters the Lungs, runs along the throat and ends at the root of the tongue.

A branch from the Lungs joins the Heart and flows into the chest to connect with the Pericardium channel.

CONNECTING CHANNEL PATHWAY

This channel starts at KI.4, crosses the heel and joins the Bladder channel. A branch follows the main Kidney channel upward to a point below the perineum, then spreads through the lumbar vertebrae.

CROSSING POINTS ON THE KIDNEY CHANNEL

The Thoroughfare channel borrows points KI.11–21 for part of its pathway and KI.8 and KT.9 are the Accumulating points for the Yin Heel and Yin Link channels respectively. Apart from these the Kidney channel does not have points where it meets with other channels. It is on the internal pathway of the main Kidney channel that the main connections are made: with Kidney, Bladder, Liver, Lung and Heart organs and with spine, diaphragm, throat and tongue.

THE KIDNEY CHANNEL AND THE ENERGY CENTRES

Through the links with the Governor and Conception channels, the Kidneys are connected with all the energy centres on the CV–GV energy circulation system. Indeed, between KI.11 and KI.21 on the abdomen, the Kidney channel is only 0.5 cm away from the Conception channel and the Kidney internal pathway flows through the spine.

The Kidneys are involved in the functions of each of the four lower centres in Table 13.1 and can be used to regulate the disharmonies of these centres, by the combination of appropriate Kidney and CV points.

Table 13.1 Kidneys and the lower energy centres

CV Point	Energy centre	Function	Example of problem
CV.14	Solar Plexus	survival of individual, growth and survival of ego	stress due to fear, anger and trying to control life
CV.4	Dan Tian	storage and distribution of energy	tiredness and depression from Deficiency and Stagnation
CV.3	Reproduction	regulation of sex, reproduction and development	infertility, dysmenorrhoea, impotence, etc.
CV.1	Perineal	regulation of lower orifices regulation of Yin–Yang	prostatitis, haemorrhoids loss of consciousness

THE KIDNEYS, THE HEART AND THE SOLAR PLEXUS CENTRE

The Kidneys represent the will, the ability to direct and focus energy and to maintain a determined effort to attain a goal. Expressing through the Solar Plexus centre, this becomes the will to achieve and the will to control situations to give maximum security to the individual and the ego. The fear of losing control can be very great, generating continual stress, fear, anger and the daily desperation of trying to maintain control over the situations of life. This stress can generate adrenalin and surges of adrenalin may be a main precipitating factor of heart attacks, the prime cause of death in the West.

In terms of Chinese medicine, we can say that Kidney fear invades the Heart, associated with the Liver anger, generated by the fear. Points can be selected from the Kidney, Conception and other channels to control this, but in these cases, acupuncture is most effective when combined with Qi Gong.

THE KIDNEYS AND THE ENERGY CENTRE ON THE SOLE OF THE FEET

Around KI.1, there is an energy centre on the sole of each foot which has a similar function to the acupuncture point. Just as KI.1 can be used to calm the mind by sinking Fire, Hyperactive Yang and Interior Wind, so by focusing attention on the soles of the feet, Qi Gong exercises can be used to treat hypertension, panic attacks, menopausal neurosis and many related problems.

FUNCTIONS OF KIDNEY POINTS

BALANCE THE WILL

The Kidneys give the ability to maintain a focused effort to achieve a goal. The combinations of CV.4 + KI.7 Rf can be used to strengthen the will, or the combination of GV.20 + KI.1 Rd can be used to relax the will. If because of underlying Deficiency, the effect of GV.20 + KI.1 Rd is likely to be too debilitating, the combination GV.20, KI.7 E; CV.4, KI.3, ST.36 Rf can be used as an intermediary measure.

BALANCE FEAR

Fear and will form a natural Yin–Yang balance. Will is expansive, fear is contractive. Fear sets limits upon the will, which in its turn controls fear by constantly striving to go beyond those limits.

The balance between will and fear is a natural and healthy situation, but excess of will or fear can create great damage within the body. Excess fear can lead to a desperate desire to control the material world and to create security, which can damage all body organs, including the Heart; as shown in Figure 13.2.

A common combination to control fear affecting the Heart is CV.14, HT.7 E; CV.4, KI.3 Rf.

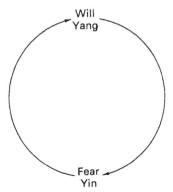

Fig. 13.1

AIR RECEPTION OF QI

One of the most basic exercises of Qi Gong is to bring the energy of the breath down the body to the Dan Tian on the inhalation, and to release this energy from the Dan Tian on the exhalation, so that it spreads through the body strengthening and vitalizing it. In Chinese medicine, the Lungs take in the pure Qi of air, and then have a descending action on the energy of the breath, directing it downwards to the Kidneys, which holds the Qi down. If they do not, it rebels upwards, causing cough, asthma and other breathing difficulties.

A useful combination for this is CV.17, LU.7 E; CV.4, ST.36, KI.3 Rf. This can be alternated with BL.13, BL.23 Rf.

REGULATE STORAGE AND RELEASE OF ENERGY

In Qi Gong, the Dan Tian is a centre for the reception, storage, release and distribution of energy. This function is related to the Kidneys and includes the concepts of Qi, Yuan Qi and Jing. The Kidneys, the Eight Extra channels and the main channels, together form a system for the storage and release of these energies. For this reason Kidney problems are largely of Deficiency and Kidney points are used to treat this. For example, CV.4, KI.3, KI.7, ST.36 Rf.

STABILIZE THE EMOTIONS

The Kidneys are a main store of Qi. A vital function of Qi is to hold things stable, homoeostasis, the ability to adapt to change yet keep internal fluctuations within acceptable limits. If there is not enough Kidney Qi, then energies which are very expansive and mobile, like Liver Yang or

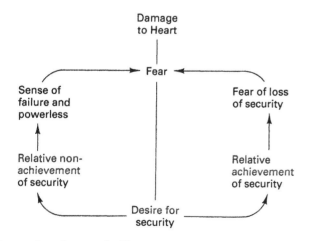

Fig. 13.2 Fear damages the Heart.

Heart Spirit, are likely to get out of proper control and cause emotional lability. Kidney points can regulate this. For example, GV.20, GB.20, GB.34 Rd; KI.3 Rf for irritability from Hyperactive Liver Yang with underlying Deficient Kidney Qi.

CONTROL OF THE LOWER ORIFICES

This same ability of Qi to hold things firm and in their proper place, controls the lower orifices and prevents leakage of sperm, discharge, bleeding and urinary and faecal incontinence. This holding aspect of Kidney Qi is closely associated with the ability of Spleen Qi to hold up flesh and organs and keep the blood in the vessels. For example, CV.4, KI.7, ST.36, SP.6 Rf for urinary incontinence.

REGULATE WATER METABOLISM

This is dependent upon a proper balance of Yin–Yang, sufficient Kidney energy to power water metabolism, and the ability of Kidney Qi to control the lower orifices. For example, BL.64, KI.3 Rf for frequent urination.

REGULATE THE BALANCE OF YIN–YANG

The Kidneys are said to be the foundation for all the Yin and Yang energies of the body. Often Deficiences of Yin or Yang within other organ systems are dependent on Deficiency of Kidney Yin or Kidney Yang and can be treated at least in part, by treating the associated Kidney Deficiency. For example, HT.6 + KI.6 Rf for Deficient Heart Yin.

REGULATE JING-RELATED FUNCTIONS

Owing to the association between Kidneys and Jing, Kidney points can be used to treat problems of reproduction, development, senescence, bones (especially the spine), brain and mental clarity. In this function they can often be combined with the Extra channel pairs, for example:

SI.3 + BL.62 with KI.6 for spinal problems
LU.7 + KI.6 with KI.13 for infertility
SP.4 + PC.6 with KI.1 for mental confusion.

KIDNEY SYNDROMES

Kidney syndromes are summarized in Table 13.2.

Table 13.2 Point combinations for Kidney and Bladder syndromes

Syndrome	Signs and symptoms	Pulse	Tongue	Point combination
Deficient Kidney Jing	declining vision, hearing, memory, concentration and sexual activity, hair loss, reduced mobility	thin, choppy, deep	various	CV.4, KI.3, KI.6, GB.39, ST.36 Rf alternate GV.4, BL.11, BL.23, BL.52 Rf
Deficient Kidney Qi	tiredness, no reserves of energy, lack of ambition, fear, weak knees and lower back, worse with tiredness or physical exertion	empty, maybe changing	pale, flabby	CV.4, KI.3, ST.36 Rf M
+ Excess will	+ strong will and unrealistic goals, resulting in exhaustion and depression	empty, maybe changing	pale, flabby	+ GV.20, KI.7 E
+ Deficient Heart Qi	+ depression or emotional lability, maybe palpitations	+ maybe irregular	+ maybe uneven at tip	+ GV.20, CV.17, HT.7 E
+ Fear invades Spleen and Stomach	+ indigestion or irritable bowel syndrome made worse by fear and insecurity	+ maybe moving	+ maybe trembling	+ CV.6, CV.14, PC.6, ST.21 or ST.25 E
+ Fear invades Lungs	+ asthma or dyspnoea made worse by fear	+ maybe moving and wiry	+ maybe white coat	+ CV.14, CV.17, LU.1, LU.7 E
+ Fear invades Heart	+ palpitations or discomfort in chest made worse by fear and anxiety, maybe panic attacks	+ maybe moving and irregular	+ trembling	+ GV.20, CV.14, CV.17, PC.6, HT.6 E
+ Hyperactive Liver Yang	+ emotional lability and irritation, dizziness, tinnitus or headache	+ wiry	+ maybe purplish	+ GV.20, GB.20, GB.40 Rd
+ Deficient Lung and Spleen Qi	+ easy to get infections, which linger in the body	+ deep	+ white coat	+ LU.7 E; KI.7 Rf M alternate BL.13, BL.20, BL.23 Rf M
Deficient Kidney Yang	exhaustion, cold extremities lower body, lack of interest, depression, impotence	empty, deep, slow	pale, swollen, moist, white coat	CV.4, CV.6, ST.36, KI.2, KI.7 Rf M
+ Kidney fails to receive Qi	+ shortness of breath on exertion, cough or asthma worse with exhaustion or cold	empty, deep, slow	pale, swollen, moist, white coat	+ CV.17, LU.7, KI.25 Rf
+ Kidney Qi not firm	+ incontinence of urine, faeces or sperm, frequent urination, or chronic white leucorrhoea	+ maybe choppy	+ maybe thin	as for Deficient Kidney Yang
+ Water Overflowing	+ oedema, abdominal distension, oliguria	+ maybe choppy	+ maybe thin	+ CV.9, ST.28, SP.6, SP.9 Rd M
+ Deficient Spleen Yang	+ desire to lie down, cold abdomen, watery phlegm in lungs, abdominal distension, loose watery stools	+ maybe choppy	+ maybe thin	+ CV.8 M; ST.25 M
+ Deficient Heart Yang	+ blue lips and nails, chest pain, shortness of breath, spontaneous sweating	+ maybe wiry	+ blue purple	+ GV.20, CV.17, KI.1 Rf M; PC.6 Rd
Deficient Kidney Yin	tired but restless, malar flush, sensation of heat in palms, soles or chest, chronic sore throat, thirst	thin, rapid	red, thin, dry, no coat	CV.4, KI.6, ST.36 Rf
+ Kidney Deficiency Fire	+ physically, emotionally and mentally restless and uncomfortable, insomnia, night sweats, feverish in afternoon, restless sexual overactivity	thin, rapid	red, thin, dry, no coat	+ KI.1, KI.2 Rd
+ Liver Fire and Hyperactive Yang	+ irritability, impatience, anger, dizziness and headache	+ wiry	+ dark red spots on edges	GV.20, LR.2, KI.1 Rd
+ Heart Fire	+ overenthusiasm, overexcitement, anxiety or mania, insomnia, palpitation or chest pain	+ hasty	+ trembling, dark red at tip	+ CV.14, PC.8, KI.1 Rd
Stagnation of Kidney Qi	fear of change, holding on to the past, maybe dysmenorrhoea, irregular menstruation or infertility	hindered, deep	pale, flabby	CV.3, CV.6, LU.7, KI.6, KI.13, ST.29 E M
Damp Heat in Bladder	burning, painful or difficult urination, cloudy urine or haematuria	rapid, slippery, maybe wiry, maybe thin or flooding	red, greasy, yellow coat	CV.3, CV.6, TE.6, ST.28, SP.6, SP.9 E

Rd, Reducing method; Rf, Reinforcing method; E, Even method; M, moxa.

Kidney points

KI.1 yǒng quán

Well point, Wood point, Sedation point.

General

The uses of KI.1 come from three main factors:

it is a well point
it is a Kidney point
it has a sinking action.

KI.1 as a Well point

Because they are located where the energy flow is changing direction, Well points can strongly affect the Yin–Yang balance. For example, they can all be used to clear Fire, to calm the Wind and to restore consciousness. They are especially useful in severe and acute conditions to produce a rapid improvement.

KI.1 as a Kidney point

Because KI.1 is a Well point on the Kidney channel, it can be used for rapid regulation of acute Kidney, Liver or Heart Fire, or for Hyperactive Liver Yang and Wind, with Disturbance of Heart Spirit.

Sinking action of KI.1

Fire, Yang and Wind are energies with expansive and irregular movement, which rise up the body causing disturbance to Heart and head. KI.1 at the opposite pole of the body, has a strong sinking action on these energies. Unlike the other Well points, the foot centres, around KI.1, can be used not only for acute situations, but in daily Qi Gong exercises for the long-term treatment and prevention of heart attacks and CVA for example due to the factors shown in Figure 13.2.

The centres on the soles of the feet represent contact with the earth, groundedness, and the ability to come out of the mental and emotional stress of the head and upper body, to bring awareness back into the physical body.

Syndromes

Liver Fire and Hyperactive Liver Yang
Heart Fire
Kidney Fire and Deficient Kidney Yin
Collapse of Yang

Liver Fire and Hyperactive Liver Yang

Pulse. Full, rapid, wiry.

Indications. Violent anger and aggression, severe headache, dizziness, restless irritability.

Example. Severe migraine.

Combination. KI.1, GV.20, LV.2 Rd; LV.1 B; KI.6 Rf.

Heart Fire

Pulse. Full, rapid, maybe irregular.

Indications. Hot flushes, hyperactivity, mania, raised blood pressure, insomnia.

Example. Extreme agitation and anxiety.

Combination. KI.1, GV.20, HT.8 Rd; HT.9 B; SP.6 E.

Kidney Fire and Deficient Kidney Yin

Pulse. Rapid, maybe full or thin.

Indications. Dry sore throat, dry mouth and tongue, cystitis, scrotal inflammation, hypertension.

Example. Sore throat, restlessness, insomnia.

Combination. KI.1, GV.20 Rd; HT.7 E; KI.6, KI.10, SP.6 Rf.

Collapse of Yang

Pulse. Minute.

Indications. Exhaustion, faintness, loss of consciousness.

Example. Feeling of great weakness, coldness and faintness.

Combination. KI.1, GV.20, CV.4, ST.36 Rf M; HT.7 Rf.

KI.2 rán gǔ

Fire point, Spring point, Starting point of Yin Heel.

General

KI.1 is used especially for acute Excess Fire conditions. Although KI.2 can also be used for these, it is not as powerful as KI.1 in acute situations and is more for Deficiency Fire with Deficient Kidney Yin. As with all Fire points, KI.2 can also be used, especially with moxa, to tonify Kidney Fire when it is Deficient. In certain cases, moxa can be used on KI.1, when there is Deficient Yin, to calm the wind by sinking the Deficiency Fire. KI.2 is not used in this way since it does not have the powerful sinking action of KI.1.

Syndromes

Deficiency Fire
  of Kidneys
  of Kidneys and Lungs
  of Kidneys and Heart

Deficient Kidney Yang

Deficiency Fire of Kidneys

Pulse. Thin, rapid, maybe wiry.

Indications. Feeling of heat in head or chest, thirst, dry throat, insomnia, night sweats, genital itching.

Example. Cystitis, restlessness, feverishness.

Combination. KI.2, CV.3 Rd; SP.6, KI.10, HT.7 Rf.

Deficiency Fire of Kidneys and Lungs

Pulse. Thin, rapid.

Indications. Dry cough with pain in chest, feelings of heat in head or chest, haemoptysis.

Example. Dry cough with aversion to dry, smoky environments, dry skin, thirst.

Combination. KI.2, LU.10 Rd; KI.10, LU.5 Rf.

Deficiency Fire of Kidneys and Heart

Pulse. Thin, rapid, maybe irregular.

Indications. Insomnia, hyperactivity, excessive sweating on physical exertion or with emotional stress.

Example. Excessively talkative, easily embarrassed.

Combination. KI.2, HT.8 Rd; SP.6, KI.10, HT.3 Rf.

Deficient Kidney Yang

Pulse. Empty, thin or minute, deep, slow, maybe choppy.

Indications. Impotence, frigidity, lack of drive.

Example. Apathy and tiredness.

Combination. KI.2, CV.2, CV.4, Rf M; KI.7, ST.36, HT.7 Rf; KI.1 M.

KI.3 tài xī

Source point, Earth point, Stream point.

General

As a Source point, KI.3 can call on Source Qi to tonify a Deficiency, and as a Source point of a Yin organ it is neutral and can tonify Yin or Yang. As an Earth point KI.3 not only supplies energy, but gives the Earth quality of stability. This combines with the ability of Kidney Qi to hold things stable and balanced, even under changing conditions. Thus, KI.3 can be used to strengthen and stabilize the emotions and help the person to adapt quickly and smoothly, like flowing water, to changes in the environment, without the fear of loss of control.

KI.3 can also be used to help the Kidneys hold down the energy of the breath, regulate water metabolism, control the lower orifices, and tonify Jing.

Regulating the Yin–Yang balance

Neutral points, e.g. Source points, Back Transporting points, CV.4 are very useful when there is a mixed condition of Deficient Yin and Deficient Yang together, or where there is a Deficiency of the one that, on treatment, might easily turn into the other. Also, Source points like KI.3, can be used to stabilize a rather polar treatment, e.g. KI.2 Rf M to tonify Kidney Fire or KI.2 Rd to drain Kidney Fire.

Strengthening and stabilizing mind and emotions

Will. The will must be kept in proper balance, if it is weak, then the person lacks drive and ambition and finds difficulty starting and completing tasks. If the will is too strong, then the person is ruthless with themselves and others and can deplete their energy, damage their health and damage their relationships.

Fear. Fear is necessary or a person behaves in a reckless and foolhardy manner, but too much fear can paralyse action, since the person sees danger and difficulties everywhere. Also, the continual stress of fear, and the anger it gives rise to, can damage the heart and cause death.

Emotional Lability. KI.3 can calm the mind by stabilizing the emotions. In the long term, this can save lives, because people who react to relatively minor stresses with great emotional and physiological response are at greater risk from heart attacks.

Syndromes

Deficient Kidney Jing
Deficient Kidney Yin
Deficient Kidney Yang
Deficient Kidney Yin and Deficient Kidney Yang
Deficient Kidney Qi
Unstable emotions

Deficient Kidney Jing

Pulse. Empty or thin, slow or rapid, choppy.

Indications. Premature ageing, infertility, arthritis in the elderly.

Example. Blurred vision in the elderly.

Combination. KI.3, SP.6, LR.3, GB.20, GB.37, CV.4 Rf.

Deficient Kidney Yin

Pulse. Thin, rapid, maybe choppy.

Indications. Tired but restless, insomnia, lower back problems, tinnitus, cystitis.

Example. Tiredness, finds life an effort, but is driven on by restlessness and willpower.

Combination. KI.3, KI.10, CV.4, SP.6 Rf; HT.6 E; KI.2 Rd.

Deficient Kidney Yang

Pulse. Empty to minute, slow, deep, maybe choppy.

Indications. Tiredness, coldness, oedema, urinary frequency, urinary incontinence, impotence.

Example. Depression with lower back pain and abdominal distension.

Combination. KI.3, BL.20, BL.23, BL.60, Rf M; SP.6, BL.15, HT.7 Rf.

Deficient Kidney Yin and Deficient Kidney Yang

Pulse. Empty or thin, maybe changing between rapid and slow or normal.

Indications. Coldness in extremities or lower body aggravated by tiredness, occasional feelings of heat in upper body or head aggravated by stress.

Example. Depression and inactivity, alternating with hyperactivity and anxiety.

Combination. KI.3, CV.4, SP.4, Rf; PC.6, HT.7, CV.17 E.

Deficient Kidney Qi

Pulse. Empty, maybe choppy, changing (see Appendix, p. 459), flooding with underlying emptiness, scattered.

Indications. Tiredness aggravated by physical exertion, lower back problems, recurring urinary infections.

Example. Asthma and shortness of breath aggravated by physical exertion.

Combination. KI.3, LU.9, BL.13, BL.23, ST.36 Rf; dìng chuǎn Rd.

Unstable emotions

Pulse. Empty, maybe choppy, deep or changing.

Indications. Weak will, emotional lability, fearfulness, insomnia with frightening dreams.

Example. Difficulty in starting or finishing tasks, seeing danger or difficulty everywhere.

Combination. KI.3, KI.7, CV.4, BL.62, SI.3, HT.7 Rf.

KI.4 dà zhōng

Connecting point. KI.4 can be used for chronic lower back problems since it connects the Kidney and Bladder channels. It has similar function to KI.3 in tonifying Kidney Qi and can be used to stabilize the emotions or to raise the spirits in depression due to Deficient Kidney Qi.

KI.5 shuǐ quán

As the Accumulation point, KI.5 can be used for acute painful conditions related to the Kidney channels, e.g. acute cystitis, dysmenorrhoea, periumbilical pain.

KI.6 zhào hǎi

Opening point of Yin Heel channel.

General

The properties of KI.6 depend on the internal connections of the Kidney channel, e.g. to the throat and to the uterus, the ability of KI.6 to tonify Yin and the fact that KI.6 is the Opening point of the Yin Heel channel.

KI.6 tonifies Yin

This is the main point of the Kidney channel for treating Deficient Yin. KI.1 can tonify Yin, but this is mainly in the context of Excess Fire. KI.2 can remove the Deficiency Heat that may accompany Deficient Yin. KI.3 is a neutral point which can tonify Deficient Yin or Deficient Yang. KI.9 has a similar action to KI.6 in tonifying Yin but perhaps not as strongly. KI.10 can tonify Kidney Water and Kidney Yin and, as a water point, also cool Excess or Deficiency Fire.

Because it tonifies Yin, KI.6 can calm the mind, treat dryness and soreness of the throat, and help skin conditions associated with Deficient Kidney Yin and Heat in the Blood.

Regulation of Yin Heel channel

KI.6 as the Opening point of the Yin Heel channel, can be used to treat amenorrhoea or infertility due to Kidney Deficiency, especially if it is combined with LU.7, the Opening point for the Conception channel, which is paired with the Yin Heel. Since the Yin Heel and Kidney channels pass through the chest, KI.6 can be used, especially in combination with LU.7 or PC.6 for chest pain or discomfort.

The Yin Heel can also be paired with the Yang Heel to regulate sleep, since both these channels flow up to the eyes.

Syndromes

Deficient Yin
Disharmony of Yin Heel channel

Deficient Yin

Pulse. Thin, maybe rapid, maybe choppy.

Indications. Insomnia, restlessness, sore throat, fear and anxiety.

Example. Menopausal anxiety and hot flushes.

Combination. KI.6, KI.10, SP.6, HT.6, HT.3 Rf; KI.2 Rd.

Disharmony of Yin Heel channel

Pulse. Maybe empty or thin or choppy.

Indications. Amenorrhoea, infertility, eye diseases in the elderly.

Example. Somnolence.

Combinations. KI.6, Rd; BL.62 Rf; BL.1 E.

KI.7 fù liū

Metal point, Tonification point, River point.

General

As the Metal point, KI.7 can tonify the Kidneys according to the Five Phase theory. However, it is not as effective as KI.3 to tonify Kidney Qi and is mainly used to tonify Kidney Yang. Its contribution as a Metal point is mainly that it gives structure and firmness to the Kidneys, which can strengthen the will, reduce fear, stop sweating and reduce discharges or leakages of urine or semen.

Regulates sweating

KI.7 can be used with LI.4, both with Reducing method to cause sweating in the excess condition of Exterior Wind Cold. KI.7 and HT.6 with Reinforcing method, can be used to reduce sweating due to Deficiency of Kidney Yin, as in hyperthyroidism or menopausal flushes.

KI.7 can be combined with LI.4 and ST.36 with Reinforcing method when there is spontaneous sweating or when there is excessive sweating during physical exercise, due to Deficient Qi and Yang.

Regulates water metabolism

KI.7 is important in regulating Damp Cold, Damp Heat and urinary retention or incontinence due to Deficient Kidneys. It is perhaps more used for Cold and Damp associated with Deficient Qi and Yang, than for Damp Heat.

Syndromes

Kidney Qi not firm
Deficient Kidney Yang
Damp Heat

Kidney Qi not firm

Pulse. Empty, maybe changing.

Indications. Lack of drive, lack of ambition, incontinence, leucorrhoea, excessive perspiration.

Example. Weak and spineless character with no perseverance or determination.

Combination. KI.7, GV.4, GV.20, BL.52, BL.67, SI.7 Rf M.

Deficient Kidney Yang

Pulse. Empty to minute, slow, deep, maybe scattered.

Indications. Coldness, exhaustion, oedema, urinary retention or incontinence, depression.

Example. Mental and physical exhaustion with inability to concentrate.

Combination. KI.3, KI.7, BL.64, BL.67, CV.4, ST.36 Rf M; KI.2 Rf.

Damp Heat

Pulse. Rapid, maybe slippery, empty or thin.

Indications. Recurring urinary infections, leucorrhoea.

Example. Urinary tract infection.

Combination. KI.7, KI.9, BL.58, ST.29 E.

KI.8 jiāo xìn

Accumulation point of Yin Heel. As an Accumulation point, KI.8 is used for Stagnation of Qi, with pain, stiffness, swelling or lumps, in the pathways of the Yin Heel and Kidney channels. It can therefore treat irregular menstruation, dysmenorrhoea, pain in kidneys, back or abdomen and orchitis.

Syndrome: Stagnation of Qi and Blood

Pulse. Wiry.

Indications. Abdominal masses, fibroids, retention of placenta.

Example. Irregular, painful menstruation with excess bleeding.

Combination. KI.8, KI.13, CV.3, ST.29, SP.6 Rd.

KI.9 zhù bīn

Accumulation point of Yin Link.

General

KI.9 is the starting point and Accumulation point of the Yin Link channel, which links and stabilizes Heart and Kidneys. In addition to the ability of KI.9 to tonify Yin, this means that it can be used to calm the mind and reduce the palpitations and feelings of oppression, tightness or pain in the chest that often accompany anxiety or apprehension.

Syndrome: Deficient Kidney Yin and Disturbance of Spirit

Pulse. Thin, rapid, maybe irregular.

Indications. Tiredness, restlessness, depression, anxiety, insomnia.

Example. Palpitations, fear, apprehension, feeling of heat and agitation in the chest.

Combination. KI.9, SP.4, PC.6, HT.6, CV.14 E; CV.4 Rf.

KI.10 yīn gǔ

Water point, Sea point.

General

KI.10 and KI.7 may be combined, since they both regulate Damp in the Lower Energizer and can treat oedema and urinary problems. KI.10 and KI.2 may be combined, as Water and Fire points, for example reinforcing KI.10 and reducing KI.2 to control Excess or Deficiency Kidney Fire. KI.10, KI.9 and KI.6 all tonify Yin of the Kidneys and all also help to stabilize the Kidney–Heart relationship. However, KI.10 is best for cooling Fire; KI.9 on the Yin Link is best for calming the mind and opening the chest; KI.6 on the Yin Heel, has similar functions to KI.9, but in addition, treats dry eyes, dry throat and asthma.

Syndromes

Deficient Kidney Yin
Deficiency Fire of Kidneys and Heart
Accumulation of Damp

Deficient Kidney Yin

Pulse. Thin, maybe rapid, maybe choppy.

Indications. Dry mouth and throat, dry skin, thirst, vaginal dryness, restlessness.

Example. Vaginitis and vaginal dryness.

Combination. KI.3, KI.10, SP.6, TE.2, TE.6 Rf, CV.3.

Deficiency Fire of Kidneys and Heart

Pulse. Rapid, thin, maybe irregular.

Indications. Restlessness, insomnia, feelings of heat in chest and head, hyperactivity.

Example. Overenthusiasm followed by tiredness.

Combination. KI.2, HT.8 Rd; KI.10, HT.3, CV.4, SP.6 Rf; GV.20 E.

Accumulation of Damp

Pulse. Maybe empty or thin, slow or rapid, slippery or wiry.

Indications. Oedema, difficulty, pain or frequency or urination, leucorrhoea, genital pain and itching.

Example. Painful urination with feelings of cold in lower abdomen.

Combination. KI.8, KI.10, CV.3 Rd; CV.6 Rf M.

KI.11, KI.12 and KI.13 héng gǔ, dà hè, and qì xué

Segmental action

CV.4   KI.13   ST.28: energy and fluid metabolism
CV.3   KI.12   ST.29: menstruation, sexuality
CV.2   KI.11   ST.30: groin, external genitals

The points KI.11–13 have a segmental action according to their anatomical level on the abdomen, shared by the CV and Stomach points at the same level as shown above (allowing for considerable overlap in function).

Energy centres

KI.12 and KI.13 are also related to the Reproduction and Dan Tian energy centres respectively. However, the CV points are far more effective in regulating these centres, and the Kidney points have a secondary function. For example, KI.13 can be used to tonify Kidney Jing and Qi.

Points on Thoroughfare channel

KI.11–KI.21 are points borrowed by the Thoroughfare channel on its path up the abdomen. The Thoroughfare channel is linked both to the Kidneys and the uterus so that points like KI.12–14 can be used for Stagnation of Qi and Blood in the abdomen and in the uterus in particular. For example, KI.13 can be used for infertility due to a combination of Deficiency and Stagnation of Kidney Qi.

KI.24, KI.25 and KI.26 líng xū, shén cáng and yù zhōng

These three points derive their functions from their location on the chest. KI.24 and KI.25 are nearer to the heart and can be used to calm the mind, especially when Deficiency of Kidney and Heart cause restlessness, anxiety and nervous tension. For example, these points could be combined with a Thoroughfare and Yin Link treatment involving SP.4 and PC.6.

KI.25 and KI.26 have more effect on the Lungs and the balance between the Lungs and Kidneys in sending down and holding down the energy of the breath. KI.25 and KI.26 could therefore be combined with a CV and Yin Heel treatment for asthma or cough, involving LU.7 and KI.6.

KI.27 shū fǔ

KI.27 is an important local point for asthma, bronchitis and pain or discomfort of the chest. It can be combined with KI.6 + LU.7 to open up the chest in asthma, or with KI.6 and PC.6 for chest pain.

KI.27 can be used to tonify the Kidneys, especially Kidney Yang, often in combination with KI.3 or KI.7, for example for physical or mental tiredness with disorientation and depression.

Kidney point comparisons and combinations

The functions of the main points of the Kidney channel are listed in Table 13.3.

Table 13.3 Kidney point comparison

Point	Point type	Syndrome
KI.1	Well point Wood point	Liver Fire and Hyperactive Yang Heart Fire Kidney Fire and Deficient Kidney Yin Collapse of Yang
KI.2	Spring point Fire point	Kidney Deficiency Fire Deficient Kidney Yang
KI.3	Source point Earth point	Deficient Kidney Jing Deficient Kidney Yin Deficient Kidney Yang Deficient Kidney Yin and Deficient Kidney Yang Deficient Kidney Qi Unstable emotions
KI.6	Opening point of Yin Heel	Deficient Kidney Yin Disharmony of Yin Heel channel
KI.7	Metal point	Kidney Qi not firm Deficient Kidney Yang Damp Heat
KI.8	Accumulation point of Yin Heel	Stagnation of Qi in Kidney and Yin Heel channels
KI.9	Accumulation point of Yin Link	Deficient Kidney Yin and Disturbance of Spirit
KI.10	Water point	Deficient Kidney Yin Deficiency Fire of Kidneys and Heart Accumulation of Damp
KI.13		Deficient Kidney Qi and Jing Stagnation of Qi in uterus
KI.27		Stagnation of Qi in chest Deficient Kidney Yang

Some combinations of the Kidney channel points are summarized in Table 13.4.

Table 13.4 Combinations of Kidney points

Point	Combination	Syndrome	Example
KI.1	KI.2	Excess Kidney Fire	hypertension
KI.1	KI.6	Kidney Fire + Deficient Kidney Yin	severe restlessness and insomnia
KI.2	KI.3	Deficient Kidney Qi and Yang	coldness and exhaustion
KI.2	KI.10	Deficiency Fire of Kidney	menopausal hyperactivity
KI.2	KI.13	Deficient Kidney Qi and Yang	impotence
KI.2	KI.27	Deficient Kidney Yang	depression and disorientation
KI.3	KI.6	Deficient Kidney Qi and Yin	dry, weak cough
KI.3	KI.7	Kidney Qi not firm	urinary incontinence
KI.3	KI.10	Deficient Kidney Qi	weak legs and knees
KI.3	KI.24	Deficient Kidney and Heart Qi	palpitations and anxiety
KI.3	KI.26	Deficient Kidney Qi	asthma and cough
KI.3	KI.27	Deficient Kidney Qi and Yang	tiredness and cold
KI.6	KI.10	Deficient Kidney Yin	chronic sore throat
KI.6	KI.12	Stagnation of Qi	amenorrhoea
KI.6	KI.25	Deficiency and Stagnation of Kidney Qi	shortness of breath and asthma
KI.7	KI.10	Damp Cold in Lower Jiao	oedema
KI.7	KI.12	Kidney Qi not firm	leucorrhoea
KI.7	KI.27	Deficient Kidney Yang	lack of drive
KI.8	KI.13	Stagnation of Qi	dysmenorrhoea
KI.9	KI.6	Deficient Kidney Yin and Disturbance of Spirit	anxiety with palpitation
KI.9	KI.24	Deficiency Kidney Yin and Stagnation of chest Qi	chest pain and palpitations
KI.10	KI.13	Deficient Kidney Qi and Accumulation of Damp	retention of urine
KI.27	KI.6	Deficient Kidney Qi	cough and chest pain
KI.2	KI.3, 27	Deficient Kidney Qi and Yang	apathy and depression
KI.2	KI.7, 27	Kidney Qi not firm	weak will, no determination
KI.2	KI.3, 10	Deficient Kidney Qi and Kidney Deficiency Fire	restless with sudden mood changes
KI.3	KI.6, 10	Deficient Kidney Jing and Yin	dry eyes and blurred vision
KI.3	KI.6, 13	Deficient Kidney Qi Jing and Yin	infertility

Bladder 14

Bladder channel

CHANNEL CONNECTIONS

MAIN CHANNEL PATHWAY

Starting at BL.1 at the inner canthus, it ascends the forehead, crossing the Governor channel at GV.24 and the Gallbladder Channel at GB.15. It ascends to the vertex crossing the Governor channel at GV.20, from where a branch runs to meet the Gallbladder channel above the ear. A branch enters the brain from the vertex, crosses with the Governor channel at GV.17 and then descends either side of the neck from BL.10 and runs down the back, entering the Kidney and the Bladder from the lumbar region. Another branch from the occiput flows down the back medial to the scapula, through GB.30, down to the popliteal fossa. Here it meets the previous branch and descends the posterior leg to end at BL.67 on the lateral side of the tip of the little toe, where it links with the Kidney channel.

CONNECTING CHANNEL PATHWAY

This channel starts from BL.58 on the leg and then runs down to the medial aspect of the leg to connect with the Kidney channel.

The Bladder Divergent channel connects with the Heart area.

Table 14.1 Crossing points on the Bladder channel

Point	Crossing	Other function
BL.1	BL, SI, ST, Yin Heel, Yang Heel	
BL.11	BL, SI	Sea of Blood point, Gathering point for bones
BL.61	BL, Yang Heel	
BL.63	BL, Yang Link	

THE BLADDER CHANNEL AND THE ENERGY CENTRES

SEGMENTAL ARRANGEMENT OF THE BACK TRANSPORTING POINTS

The Bladder points on the back, like the GV points, are arranged upon a segmental basis. In terms of Western medicine, this means they can be associated with the spinal nerves, dermatome and myotome of the spinal segment in which they are found. In terms of Chinese medicine, it means they can be associated with the vertebrae, flesh and organ systems linked with their level on the spine. In terms of energy theory, it means that, along with the GV points, they can be related to specific energy centres, as shown in Table 14.2.

Table 14.2 Back Transporting points and energy centres

Centre	Below vertebra (or other)	GV	Inner BL (or other)	Outer BL
Throat	C.1	GV.15	BL.10	–
Heart	T.5	GV.11	BL.15	BL.44
Solar Plexus	T.7	GV.9	BL.17	BL.46
Spleen	T.11	GV.6	BL.20	BL.49
Dan Tian	L.2	GV.4	BL.23	BL.52
Reproduction	c.mid-sacrum	GV.2–3	BL.32–33	–
Perineal	tip of coccyx	GV.1	–	–

SPINAL SEGMENTS AND THE FIVE YIN ORGAN SYSTEMS

Specific to Chinese medicine is the concept that points in a specific spinal segment not only relate to the physical patterns associated with the organ system of that segment (or segments), but also with the mental and emotional patterns associated with the organ systems. So in the sense of selecting Governor and Bladder points to use in treatment, we can say that the emotions and the mental faculties have a segmental representation on the back.

COMPARISON OF THE GV–BL AND CV–KI SYSTEMS

The Bladder points on the back have a similar relationship to the energy centres and the Governor points to that of the Kidney points with centres and Conception points on the front. However, on the front the conception points are more used than the Kidney points to activate organs and energy centres, whereas on the back the Bladder points are more often used than the Governor points for these effects. Whereas on the front the Kidney points are not often combined with the Conception points at the same level, perhaps because the Kidney and Conception channels are so close, on the back the Governor points are commonly combined with the inner or outer Bladder channel points.

To affect the energy centres on the back, it may be more effective to use the inner Bladder line points in combination with Governor points, but to regulate the mental and emotional aspects of the organ systems, it may be better to combine outer and inner Bladder line points, or outer Bladder line points with those on the Governor channel.

FUNCTIONS OF BLADDER POINTS

TREAT CHANNEL PROBLEMS

The Bladder channel is the longest on the body and can be used to treat the areas through which it passes, including foot, posterior leg, hip, back, neck, occiput, vertex, frontal head, eyes and nose. For example, BL.1 and BL.4 can be combined as local points for rhinitis, and BL.67 can be added as a distal point.

TREAT SEGMENTAL CONNECTIONS

The Bladder channel, on the back, is unique amongst the main meridians in the power of its segmental connections to organ systems. Its segmental effects are much greater than those of the Kidney and Stomach channels on the front of the body. The Back Transporting points are discussed in detail in Chapter 8.

For example, BL.23 and BL.52 can be combined to treat back pain at the level of the second lumbar vertebra.

TREAT KIDNEY PROBLEMS

The Bladder and Kidneys form a Yang–Yin pair and Bladder points can be used for some of the systems and attributes governed by the Kidneys, for example for problems of will, fear, ears, uterus and lower orifices. For example, CV.4, BL.22, SI.3 Rf can treat fear.

However, Bladder points do not have the power to tonify Qi possessed by Kidney points, nor can Bladder points on the legs tonify Yin.

TREAT THE BRAIN

The Kidneys govern the brain through the Jing from which the brain is formed. The Bladder channel links with the Governor and Kidney channels and with the brain itself. Bladder points, such as BL.67, BL.62 and

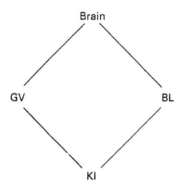

Fig. 14.1

BL.1–10 can be used to clear the brain and improve the ability to focus the mind and to concentrate and think clearly.

TREAT SIX DIVISION PAIRS

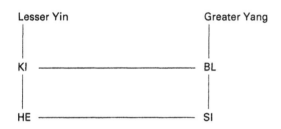

Fig. 14.2

The Six Division classification links Kidneys to Heart and Bladder to Small Intestine, which is paired with Heart according to the Yin–Yang channel couples. Bladder points such as BL.62 and BL.64 can regulate the balance between Heart and Kidneys, and treat fear and mania.

TREAT EXTRA VESSELS

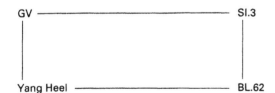

Fig. 14.3

BL.62, the Opening point for the Yang Heel channel may be paired with SI.3 to use the Governor and Yang Heel as a pair, for example, for spinal problems with depression.

Since Governor is linked to Conception and Yang Heel to Yin Heel in the Yin–Yang pairs of the Extra channels

(see Fig. 14.4) SI.3 + BL.62 can be combined with LU.7 + KI.6 to treat panic attacks with fear of loss of control, palpitations and dyspnoea.

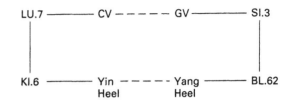

Fig. 14.4

TREAT THE HEART

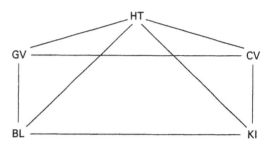

Fig. 14.5

Bladder, Governor and Kidney channels all connect with the Heart on their deep pathways. While the Conception channel is not listed as connecting with the Heart, CV.17 controls Heart function. Through these relationships Bladder points, such as BL.60, 62 or 64, can be used to calm the Spirit when it is disturbed by anxiety or fear.

TREAT INTERIOR WIND

Bladder points, at the extremities of the body, for example BL.7 on the head or BL.60 on the ankle, may be used to control Interior Wind disturbing the Spirit and the brain and causing vertigo, dizziness, headache, epilepsy, hemiplegia or convulsions in children.

TREAT WATER METABOLISM

Surprisingly, Bladder points are not so much used to control water metabolism as are the points of Spleen, Conception and Kidneys. The Bladder points that are involved in this, e.g. BL.22, 23 and 39, do so because they are the Back Transporting points for the Triple Energizer and Kidneys, and the Lower Sea point of Triple Energizer, respectively.

BLADDER SYNDROMES

Bladder syndromes are included in Table 13.3 with the Kidney syndromes.

Bladder points

BL.1 and BL.2 jīng míng and zǎn zhú

BL.1 is the Crossing point of BL, ST, Yang Heel and Yin Heel channels.

General

BL.1 is the more powerful of the two points for eye problems, endocrine problems and insomnia. BL.2 is better for nasal and facial problems. Since it is relatively easy to cause black eyes if BL.1 is used regularly, the author prefers, in nearly all cases, to use BL.2 with the needle running under the skin almost to BL.1. This method avoids black eyes and is almost as powerful as BL.1 for most purposes. *BL.2 is needled in this way in all combinations in this book, unless otherwise stated.*

Eye problems

BL.1 and BL.2 are perhaps the best two points for eye problems of all kinds from early-stage cataract or glaucoma to hysteria with vision loss. They are also used for problems from conjunctivitis due to Wind Heat and Liver Heat, to blurred vision in the elderly due to Deficient Jing and Blood.

Cerebral and endocrine problems

BL.2 can be used in combination with either or both of the Extra channels Yang Heel and Yin Heel to treat cerebral problems such as postconcussion syndrome, hypersomnia or hyposomnia and epilepsy.

Opening point of Yang Heel + BL.62	± BL.61 Meeting point of BL and Yang Heel
or	
+ KI.6 Opening point of Yin Heel	± KI.8 Accumulation point of Yin Heel

These point combinations have been listed to treat disorders of pineal and pituitary glands and hypothalamus.

Syndromes

Eye problems
Nasal problems
Facial problems
Problems of the nervous system

Eye problems

Pulse. Various

Indications. Conjunctivitis, spasms of the eyelid, headaches from eyestrain, early-stage cataract.

Example. Early-stage glaucoma.

Combination. BL.2, GB.1, GB.20, LR.3, KI.6, LI.4 E.

Nasal problems

Pulse. Various, maybe slippery.

Indications. Allergic rhinitis, nasal polyps, sinusitis, sinus, headaches.

Example. Sinusitis from Heat in Bright Yang.

Combination. BL.2, ST.2 E; ST.40, ST.44, LI.5, LI.20 Rd.

Facial problems

Pulse. Maybe tight or wiry, empty or thin.

Indications. Facial paralysis, eczema around eyes, trigeminal neuralgia.

Example. Supraorbital pain.

Combination. BL.2, BL.67 E; KI.3, GB.43. LI.4 Rd.

Problems of the nervous system

Pulse. Various

Indication. Hypersomnia or hyposomnia, postconcussion syndromes, dizziness.

Example. Mental exhaustion with inability to concentrate.

Combination. BL.2, BL.67 E; KI.3, ST.36, CV.4, LI.4 Rf.

BL.7 tōng tiān

General

BL.7 has two main functions – for Exterior Wind and for Interior Wind. The Exterior Wind can be Wind Cold or Wind Heat and the Interior Wind may be associated with either Hyperactive Liver Yang or Deficient Liver Blood.

It should be remembered that the Bladder channel ascends to the vertex, crossing the GV channel at GV.20 (where the internal pathway of the Liver meets the Governor channel). From GV.20, one branch of the Bladder channel enters the brain and another branch runs to meet the Gallbladder channel above the ear. BL.7 can therefore be used for dizziness or vertex headache from rising Liver Yang, in preference to GV.20, when the tension from the Liver Yang is also affecting neck, shoulder or eyes.

Syndromes

Exterior Wind
Hyperactive Liver Yang

Exterior Wind

Pulse. Superficial and tight or empty and tight.

Indications. Excessive lachrymation, rhinitis, headache, facial paralysis, epistaxis, sinusitis.

Example. Rhinitis and headaches from Wind Cold.

Combination. BL.2 E; BL.7, BL.67, SI.3 Rd.

Hyperactive Yang

Pulse. Wiry, maybe empty, thin or choppy.

Indications. Convulsions, vertigo, vertex headache.

Example. Vertex headache with dizziness and disorientation.

Combination. BL.7, BL.62. SI.3, KI.6 E; LR.3 Rd.

BL.10 tiān zhù

Window of Heaven point.

Cerebral problems

BL.10 is where the Bladder channel emerges from the brain and so can be used to treat memory and concentration problems, especially where these are due to Deficient Kidney.

Psychological problems

BL.10 is a Window of Heaven point, and a gate to energy flow between the body and the head. It can therefore be used for depression, disorientation and heavy feelings in the head linked with fear. It can also be used for hysteria.

Eye problems

It can treat eye disorders due to both Exterior Wind and to Deficiency of Kidney Qi.

External Wind Invasion

The neck is one of the main points of Wind Invasion and BL.10 can be used for effects such as ache in the neck and head, nasal congestion and loss of smell, cough and asthma, and throat pain and swelling.

Neck and head problems.

BL.10 can be used for a variety of neck and head pains, including Wind Cold Invasion, acute trauma, chronic Stagnation and Deficiency of Qi associated with old injury or arthritis, tension in neck and head from Hyperactive Liver Yang.

Since it can regulate the lower back as well as the neck it is very often included in treatments to regulate the whole of the spine, as in the chronic diseases multiple sclerosis and ankylosing spondylitis.

Syndromes

Cerebral problems
Psychological problems
Eye problems
Exterior Wind Invasion
Neck and head problems

Cerebral problems

Pulse. Empty or thin, maybe choppy or deep.

Indications. Mental exhaustion, mental overstrain, inability to think clearly or for long periods.

Example. Desperation from inability to concentrate.

Combination. BL.10, BL.23, BL.64, BL.67, GV.20, KI.6, HT.6 Rf.

Psychological problems

Pulse. Maybe wiry and empty or choppy.

Indications. Depression, tiredness, fear, feeling of loss of contact with the body or the environment.

Example. Feeling of being shut inside the head.

Combination. BL.10, BL.62, SI.3 E; KI.6 Rf; KI.1 M.

Eye problems

Pulse. Various.

Indications. Conjunctivitis, blurred vision.

Example. Decline in vision with age or tiredness, the room seeming to get darker with a reduced visual field.

Combination. BL.2, BL.10, BL.62, KI.6, ST.36 Rf.

Exterior Wind Invasion

Pulse. Superficial, tight, maybe empty or choppy.

Indications. Sneezing, cough, asthma, sore throat, aches in shoulders, neck and back.

Example. Common cold with nasal congestion and inability to smell.

Combination. BL.2 Rf; BL.10 Rd M; GV.23, LU.7, LI.4, LI.20 Rd.

Neck and head problems

Pulse. Tight or wiry, empty, thin or choppy, maybe flooding.

Indications. Acute injury, chronic injury, sequelae, multiple sclerosis, arthritis, ankylosing spondylitis.

Example. Neck and shoulder ache from Deficient Kidney and Hyperactive Liver Yang.

Combination. BL.10, BL.66, SI.3, SI.15, GB.20, GB.21, GB.41 E; KI.6 Rf.

BL.11 dà zhù

Crossing point of Bladder and Small Intestine, Gathering point for bones, point of Sea of Blood.

Connections of BL.11

There is a link at GV.13 between the Governor and Bladder channels. Since dà zhù is also the Crossing point of Bladder and Small Intestine, it acts as a junction between Bladder, Governor and Small Intestine channels (see Fig. 14.6). Not only does this make it an important

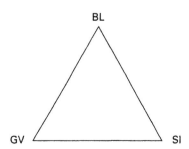

Fig. 14.6

point for local neck and shoulder problems, especially those with Wind Invasion, but also links it to the Extra channel system.

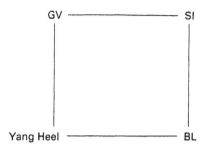

Fig. 14.7

The Bladder channel links with Kidneys, which rules the bones, and BL.11, as the Gathering point of the bones, can treat skeletal problems in general and not just locally in the neck region.

BL.11 can be combined with Extra channel treatments for bone and joint problems (see Fig. 14.8).

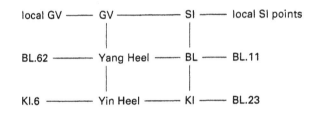

Fig. 14.8

In many spinal problems, BL.62 and KI.6 are used together to combine the Yang effect of strengthening the joints with the Yin effect of providing fluid to lubricate them.

BL.11 tonifies the Blood

BL.11, 12, 13 and GV.14 may help to prevent Exterior Invasion by tonifying Defensive and Nutritive Qi. In addition, BL.11 may also help to make invasion less easy by tonifying Blood. BL.11 can be incorporated into treatment to tonify the Blood, for example: BL.11, 20, 23, 43 Rf M.

Syndromes

Exterior Wind Invasion ⎫
Neck and head problems ⎬ see BL.10
Bone and joint problems ⎭

Bone and joint problems

Pulse. Maybe empty, thin, choppy or deep.

Indications. Painful arthritis with joint deformation, neck and spinal stiffness, pain and stiffness in knees.

Example. Bone degeneration in the elderly.

Combination. BL.11, BL.23, BL.62, KI.6, GB.39 Rf; local points E.

BL.12 fēng mén

Crossing point of GV and BL channels.

General

This point is similar in function to BL.13, since it clears Exterior invasion and regulates Lungs. However, BL.13 is more used to treat Lungs and the main function of BL.12 is to release Exterior Wind, especially by cupping. Also, BL.12 is better for nasal problems and BL.13 for throat problems.

BL.13 fèi shū

As the Back Transporting point of the Lungs, BL.13 can treat all Lung problems. However, the outer Bladder channel point BL.42, is considered better for emotional and behavioural problems of the Lungs, or BL.13 and BL.42 can be combined.

Syndromes

Wind Cold
Wind Heat
Wind Dryness
Deficient Lung Qi
Deficient Lung Yin
Accumulation of Phlegm Cold in Lungs
Accumulation of Phlegm Heat in Lungs
Stagnation of Lung Qi

Wind Cold invades Lungs

Pulse. Tight at superficial level, maybe empty at middle or deep level.

Indications. Common cold, influenza.

Example. Sneezing, itchy throat, aching upper back.

Combination. BL.12, BL.13 Rd M; LU.7, LI.14, CV.22 Rd.

Wind Heat

Pulse. Superficial, rapid.

Indications. Common cold, influenza.

Example. Sore throat with dry cough.

Combination. BL.13, LU.10, LI.4, SI.17 Rd.

Wind Dryness

Pulse. Superficial.

Indications. Dry cough, dry nose, throat and mouth.

Example. Over-reaction to dry atmospheres.

Combination. BL.13, LU.7, LI.14 Rd; LU.5, LU.9, KI.6 Rf.

Deficient Lung Qi

Pulse. Empty or big

Indications. Asthma, bronchitis or cough.

Example. Chronic dry sore throat.

Combination. BL.13, BL.23, LU.7, KI.6, CV.22 Rf.

Deficient Lung Yin

Pulse. Thin, rapid

Indications. Chronic dry cough, pulmonary tuberculosis.

Example. Chronic sore throat with restlessness.

Combination. BL.13, LU.9, LU.5, ST.36, SP.6 Rf.

Accumulation of Phlegm Cold in Lungs

Pulse. Slippery, full or flooding, maybe wiry.

Indications. Bronchitis, asthma.

Example. Reaction of profuse nasopharyngeal catarrh to excessive consumption of dairy products.

Combination. BL.13, BL.20, LU.9, SP.3 Rd; LU.6, ST.40, LI.20 Rd.

Accumulation of Phlegm Heat in Lungs

Pulse. Slippery, rapid, full or flooding, maybe wiry.

Indications. Acute bronchitis, bronchiectasis.

Example. Acute aggravation of chronic bronchitis, resistant to antibiotics.

Combination. BL.13, GV.14, LU.1, LU.10, LI.4, ST.40 Rd.

Stagnation of Lung Qi

Pulse. Hindered or wiry.

Indications. Dyspnoea, cough, grief, withdrawal, living in the past.

Example. Unresolved grief and depression.

Combination. BL.13, CV.17, CV.22, LU.1, LU.6, LU.7 Rd; ST.36 Rf.

BL.14 jué yīn shū

BL.14 can be used as a supplementary point to BL.15 for Heart conditions. Also BL.14 can be used to treat pain and discomfort in chest, hypogastrium and epigastrium, due to Stagnation of Liver Qi, and also dyspnoea, hiccups and vomiting.

BL.15 xīn shū

Back Transporting point of the Heart.

Syndromes

Deficient Heart Qi
Deficient Heart Yang
Deficient Heart Blood
Deficient Heart Yin
Heart Fire
Heart Phlegm
Stagnant Heart Qi
Stagnant Heart Blood

Deficient Heart Qi

Pulse. Empty, maybe changing, choppy or irregular.

Indications. Tiredness, emotional lability, palpitations.

Example. Enthusiasm alternating with tiredness and lack of interest.

Combination. BL.15, HT.7, SI.3, BL.64, KI.3.

Deficient Heart Yang

Pulse. Empty to minute, deep, slow.

Indications. Exhaustion, cold extremities, depression, lack of interest.

Example. Apathy and exhaustion.

Combination. BL.15, BL.23, GV.4, GV.20, BL.62 Rf; HT.7 Rf.

Deficient Heart Blood

Pulse. Thin, choppy.

Indications. Poor memory, lack of concentration, tiredness, palpitations, dizziness.

Example. Insomnia and feelings of vulnerability.

Combination. BL.15, BL.20, ST.36, SP.4, SP.10, HT.7 Rf; PC.6, ān mián Rd.

Deficient Heart Yin

Pulse. Thin, rapid, maybe hasty.

Indications. Menopausal syndromes, night sweats and insomnia, anxiety.

Example. Inability to relax and find peace.

Combination. BL.15, BL.23, KI.1, HT.6, KI.6 E.

Heart Fire

Pulse. Rapid, full or flooding.

Indications. Mania, manic depression, hypertension, headache.

Example. Menopausal syndrome with extreme hyperactivity and agitation.

Combination. BL.15, BL.44, KI.1, GV.20, HT.8 Rd; HT.3, KI.10 Rf.

Heart Phlegm

Pulse. Slippery, maybe slow or rapid, maybe irregular.

Indications. Disorientation, forgetfulness, mental confusion, disturbed speech, depression.

Example. Mental confusion, oppressive feeling in chest.

Combination. BL.15, BL.44, GV.15, ST.40, PC.6 Rd.

Stagnant Heart Qi

Pulse. Hindered, wiry or jerky.

Indications. Depression, sadness, pain or discomfort in chest.

Example. Frustration and difficulty in relationships.

Combination. BL.13, BL.15, PC.4, HT.6 Rd; KI.4 E.

Stagnant Heart Blood

Pulse. Wiry, maybe choppy.

Indications. Chest pain, especially if radiating to the back.

Combination. BL.15, BL.16, SP.4, PC.6 Rd.

BL.17 gé shū

Influential point of the Blood, Back Transporting point of the diaphragm.

BL.17 governs the Blood

Depending on the situation, BL.17 can tonify, move, cool and contain the Blood. For example, BL.17 + BL.43 Rf M can be used to tonify a general condition of Deficient Blood and Qi. Alternatively, BL.17 can be combined with BL.15 or BL.18 or BL.20 as in Table 14.3, to tonify the Blood of specific organs, or, BL.15, 17, 18 and 20 can all be used together to treat generalized Deficient Blood.

Table 14.3 Combinations of BL.17 to govern the Blood

Syndrome	Example	Back point	Other point
Deficient Blood			
Deficient Heart Blood	insomnia and palpitations	BL.15	HT.7
Deficient Liver Blood	blurred vision	BL.17	LR.3
Deficient Spleen Blood	weak muscles	BL.20	SP.3
Stagnation Blood and Qi			
Heart Stagnation	chest pain	BL.15	PC.6
Liver Stagnation	dysmenorrhoea	BL.17	LR.3
Spleen Stagnation	varicose veins	BL.20	SP.4
Bleeding and Heat in the Blood			
Heart Fire	eczema	BL.15	HT.8
Liver Fire	menorrhagia	BL.18	LR.1
Heat in Bright Yang	allergic skin reaction to food	BL.21	SP.10
Fire Poison	acne	BL.25	GV.7

BL.17 regulates diaphragm

BL.17, BL.46 and GV.9 below the seventh thoracic vertebra, relate to the Solar Plexus centre and share some functions with CV.14 and CV.15. The diaphragm separates the Upper from the Middle and Lower Energizer, and the Solar Plexus centre can act as a focal point for emotional impressions. Fear and anger especially can disturb digestion, tighten the diaphragm, restrict breathing and change the heart beat rate.

BL.17 treats skin disorders

Since BL.17 can be used to tonify, move and cool the Blood it can be used for skin disorders including urticaria, boils and psoriasis. By calming the Solar Plexus centre, this point can relieve some of the emotional tensions that contribute to dermatological ailments. BL.17 can be combined with BL.20 for worry, BL.18 for frustration and suppressed anger, or with BL.15 for overexcitement or the pressure of personal relationships, as these factors affect the skin.

Syndromes

Deficient Blood
Stagnant Blood
Heat in the Blood
Problems of diaphragm and chest
Skin disorders

Deficient Blood

Pulse. Thin and choppy, maybe wiry, irregular or empty.

Indications. Insomnia, palpitations, anaemia, weak muscles.

Examples. Excessive study and worry with blurred vision and poor memory.

Combinations. BL.17, BL.18, BL.20, GV.20, ST.36, LI.4 E.

Stagnant Blood

Pulse. Wiry, choppy.

Indications. Chest pain, epigastric pain, abdominal pain and lumps, dysmenorrhoea.

Example. Varicose veins and poor peripheral circulation.

Combinations. BL.17, BL.18, BL.20, SP.4, PC.6 E.

Alternation. SP.1, SP.4, SP.8, SP.10, ST.40, PC.6 E.

Heat in the Blood

Pulse. Rapid, maybe full or flooding, thin or wiry.

Indications. Menorrhagia, epistaxis, haemoptysis.

Example. Acute psoriasis with hot, red skin lesions.

Combinations. BL.15, BL.17, BL.18, LI.4, LI.11, SP.6, ST.40 Rd.

Problems of diaphragm and chest

Pulse. Hindered or wiry.

Indications. Chest pain, diaphragmatic spasm, hiccups, vomiting, dyspnoea.

Example. Belching with nausea and epigastric discomfort.

Combinations. BL.17, BL.21, SP.4, PC.6 Rd.

Alternation. CV.12, CV.14, SP.4, PC.6 Rd.

Skin disorders

Pulse. Various.

Indications. Boils, acne, eczema, urticaria.

Example. Psoriasis, resistant to treatment, with purple lesions with much squamation.

Combinations. BL.17, BL.18, BL.20, TE.6, GV.9, SP.6 Rd.

BL.18 gān shū

Back Transporting point for the Liver.

General

GV.8, BL.18 and BL.47, below the ninth thoracic vertebra, relate to the Wood element and to the functions of the Liver. BL.18 is not so much used to calm Liver Fire and Hyperactive Yang, but to strengthen Liver Qi, move Liver Qi, tonify Liver Blood and clear Damp Heat in Liver and Gallbladder.

GV.8, BL.18 and BL.47 are effective in balancing the Wood element. For the Yin Wood type, these points can be used to treat lack of self-confidence, lack of assertiveness, indecision and self-doubt. For the Yang Wood type these points can be used to treat the impatience, intolerance, abrasive and abrupt behaviour associated with the person not acting in harmony with their own inner-self and the needs of other people around them. Both Yin and Yang Wood types will tend to feel easily blocked and obstructed in their outer lives and inner feelings.

Syndromes

Deficient Liver Qi
Stagnant Liver Qi
Deficient Liver Blood
Damp Heat in Liver and Gallbladder

Deficient Liver Qi

Pulse. Empty, maybe choppy or wiry.

Indications. Indecision, lack of self-confidence, depression, headache.

Example. Lack of assertion, associated with lack of energy and lack of contact with inner strength and certainty.

Combinations. BL.18, BL.23, BL.47, BL.52, LR.3, GB.40, KI.7 Rf.

Stagnant Liver Qi

Pulse. Wiry or hindered.

Indications. Nausea, chest pain, headache, muscle spasm, dysmenorrhoea, depression.

Example. Tendency to feel easily blocked.

Combinations. BL.18, BL.47, LR.3, PC.6 Rd or E.

Deficient Liver Blood

Pulse. Thin, choppy, maybe wiry.

Indications. Blurred vision, muscle spasm and weakness, brittle nails, dizziness.

Example. Feelings of tiredness and vulnerability, feelings of not having solidity and strength of character.

Combinations. BL.18, BL.20, LR.3, SP.3, GB.40, ST.36 Rf.

Damp Heat in Liver and Gallbladder

Pulse. Rapid, slippery, wiry, maybe thin or flooding.

Indications. Otitis media, cholecystitis, irritability, eczema.

Example. Lingering feelings of bitterness, resentment and hatred, tendency to blame self and other people.

Combinations. BL.18, BL.20, LR.3, SP.3, GB.40, TE.6 Rd.

BL.19 dǎn shū

Back Transporting point for the Gallbladder.

General

GV.7, BL.19 and BL.48, below the tenth thoracic vertebra, relate to the Wood element and the functions of the Gallbladder. These points can be used in combination with GV.8, BL.18 and BL.48 for problems of both Liver and Gallbladder. The points for the Liver have wider application, including problems of the Gallbladder. The points of the Gallbladder tend to be of a more limited application, relating mainly to problems of the Gallbladder itself.

Liver and Gallbladder

Yin	Yang
Liver	Gallbladder
inner	outer

BL.18 and BL.47 can be used to treat the more Yin, internal problems of poor planning ability, and BL.19 and BL.46 can be used to treat the more Yang, outer problems of the decisions and judgements which translate these internal plans into external action. However, BL.18 and BL.47 are often used to treat both planning and decision-making abilities, especially where there is lack of connection between Liver and Gallbladder in that, for example, snap decisions are being made without relation to proper plans.

Liver, Gallbladder and Kidneys

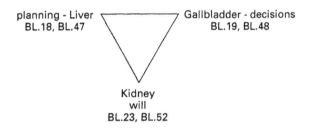

Fig. 14.9

Kidneys, Liver and Gallbladder are interdependent. For planning and decision-making to be effective, there must be a clearly defined goal, activated by a sustained effort of will. Yet, even if the will is strong it cannot create anything in the outer world, unless there is a clear plan for it to flow through.

Syndromes

Damp Heat in Liver and Gallbladder — see BL.18
Deficient Gallbladder Qi

Deficient Gallbladder Qi

Pulse. Empty, thin, maybe choppy or wiry.

Indications. Timidity, indecision, muscular tension, eye strain, headache.

Example. Person does not feel strong or certain enough to act with resolution or decision.

Combinations. BL.19, BL.23, KI.3, GB.40, TE.4 RF.

BL.20 pí shū

Back Transporting point of the Spleen.

General

GV.6, BL.20 and BL.49, below the eleventh thoracic vertebra, relate to the Earth element and to the functions of the Spleen. They correspond to the Spleen energy centre and to CV.12 on the front of the body.

BL.20 and Spleen Deficiency

By tonifying a Deficient Spleen, BL.20 can tonify Qi and Blood for the whole body, and also resolve Damp and Phlegm. The use of the Reinforcing method and moxa on BL.20 can tonify Spleen Qi and Yang, remove Cold and Damp, and help the Spleen functions of holding in the Blood and holding up the organs. Use of BL.20 can move Stagnation of Qi of the Middle Energizer, although more for chronic conditions than for acute pain. It can also resolve Damp Heat, although it is more used for Damp Cold.

BL.20 and the emotions

GV.6, BL.20 and BL.48 can be used singly or in combination to balance the behaviour of Earth element types. The Yin Earth type can create an internal world of worry and preoccupation, where excessive thinking cripples action. The Yang Earth people are more outgoing and intrude into the lives of others by projecting their worries on to them. Their possessiveness and overconcern can dominate and stifle the free expression and development in the lives of other people, causing problems in relationships.

Syndromes

Deficient Spleen Qi
Deficient Spleen Blood
Deficient Spleen Yang
Damp and Phlegm
Stagnation in the Middle Energizer

Deficient Spleen Qi

Pulse. Empty.

Indications. Tiredness, lethargy, abdominal distension, worry, loose stool.

Example. Tiredness and weak, flaccid muscles and overweight.

Combinations. BL.20, GV.6, SP.3, ST.36, LI.4 Rf.

Deficient Spleen Blood

Pulse. Thin, choppy.

Indications. Muscle weakness and atrophy, dry skin, dizziness, chronic tiredness.

Example. Exhaustion following heavy blood loss in childbirth.

Combinations. BL.17, BL.20, BL.43, ST.36, LI.4 Rf M.

Deficient Spleen Yang

Pulse. Empty, maybe slow deep.

Indications. Exhaustion, cold extremities, prolapses, haemorrhages, abdominal distension, oedema.

Example. Extreme tiredness and flaccidity of personality, person needs something to 'pick them up off the ground', to lift them up.

Combinations. BL.20, BL.23, GV.20, ST.36, KI.7 Rf M.

Alternation. CV.4, CV.12, GV.20, ST.36, KI.7.

Damp and Phlegm

Pulse. Slippery, maybe empty or flooding, maybe slow or rapid.

Indications. Oedema, obesity, lethargy, mental dullness or confusion, heavy feeling in limbs, body or head.

Example. Pleasant but sluggish lazy person, overweight from great pleasure in eating.

Combinations. BL.20, BL.21, BL.49, BL.50, SP.3, ST.40 Rf M.

Stagnation in the Middle Energizer

Pulse. Wiry, maybe flooding or full, maybe slippery.

Indications. Epigastric discomfort, abdominal distension, nausea.

Example. Intrusive overconcern in the lives of others with indigestion.

Combinations. BL.20, BL.21, SP.1, SP.4, ST.40, ST.45 Rd.

BL.21 wèi shū

Back Transporting point of Stomach.

General

BL.20 and BL.21 have overlapping uses, but BL.20 has far more general application, while BL.21 is more limited to Stomach function. BL.21 is more used for Excess syndromes such as Stagnation or Rebellion of Stomach Qi, with nausea, belching, hiccup or vomiting, or for retention of food in the stomach with epigastric distension and sour belching. BL.20 is more used to tonify Deficiency.

BL.22 sān jiāo shū

Back Transporting point for the Triple Energizer.

General

Because of its location, this point tonifies the Kidneys and resolves Damp in the Lower Energizer, e.g. it treats oedema, dysuria and urinary retention. It is interesting that it does not have indications relating to the Triple Energizer as the heating system of the body or as 'the thermostat of the body', perhaps because these concepts are more Western than Chinese.

Combinations

BL.22 can be combined with BL.20 and/or BL.23 to treat Damp. If combined with BL.20 it would treat Damp relating to oedema with abdominal distension, borborygmus and diarrhoea; if combined with BL.23 it would treat Damp associated with urinary problems, Kidney stones or lower back pain. It can be combined with BL.39, the Lower Sea point of the Triple Energizer, and with TE.6 to move Stagnation of Qi and Fluids in the Lower Energizer.

BL.23 shèn shū

Back Transporting point of the Kidneys.

General

GV.4, BL.23 and BL.52, below the second lumbar vertebra, correspond to the Water element and to the functions of the Kidneys. These points are associated with the Dan Tian energy centre, which is represented on the front of the body by the points CV.4, 5 and 6. The Dan Tian

Table 14.4 Comparison of GV.4, BL.23, KI.3 and CV.4

| Indication | Yang ← | | | → Yin |
	GV.4	BL.23	KI.3	CV.4
Deficient Jing	X	X	X	X
Deficient Qi	x	X	X	X
KI Qi not firm	X	X	X	X
Deficient Yang	X	X	X	X
Internal Cold	X	X	X	X
Internal Damp	X	X	X	X
Deficient Yin	–	X	X	X
Deficient Blood	–	x	–	X
Damp Heat in Bladder	–	X	–	–

X, primary use; x, secondary use.

energy centre can be used for tonification via points BL.23, BL.52, GV.4 and CV.4 for example, but each point has slightly different functions, as shown in Table 14.4. From the table it can be seen that whereas GV.4 has a strong action to tonify Yang, but does not tonify Yin, the other three points have the ability to tonify both Yin and Yang. CV.4 has the strongest action to tonify Blood, since it is the most Yin of the four points, but BL.23 can be combined with BL.20 to tonify the Blood, since the Kidneys have a role in Blood formation. BL.23 is the best of these points to treat Damp Heat in the Bladder for cystitis and dysuria, and to move Stagnation of Qi in the Kidneys and lower back. In these two functions BL.23 is similar to CV.6, and indeed both points can be used to expel stones in the Kidneys and upper urinary tract.

BL.23 and psychological problems

BL.23, BL.52, KI.3 and CV.4 can be said to treat four main types of emotional problem associated with the Kidneys:

disharmonies of will
fear
depression
emotional lability.

Each of these problems can affect not only the Kidneys, but the other four systems, Lungs, Heart, Liver and Spleen. BL.23 can then be combined with BL.13, 15, 18 or 20. For example, if Kidney fear is affecting the Heart and there is fearful anxiety, BL.23 can be combined with BL.15. Or if lack of will combined with pensiveness is allowing excessive thought to paralyse action, BL.23 can be combined with BL.20.

Table 14.5 shows how each of the four emotional problems of the Kidneys can affect each of the other four organ systems, indicating which back point to combine with BL.23. The outer Bladder line points, BL.42, 44, 47, 49 and 52, can be used instead of, or in combination with the inner Bladder line points for these psychological problems. For example, if the focusing and concentrating abilities of Kidney will are not balancing the expansive energies of the Liver creativity, so that the person is frittering their energy away in too many directions, BL.18 and BL.23 can be combined with BL.47 and BL.52 to harmonize the energies.

BL.23 and the ageing process

Since BL.23 can tonify Kidney Jing, it can be used to treat symptoms associated with ageing including degeneration of bones, teeth, joints, eyes, hair and sexuality. However, since Jing is closely associated with Blood in its functions, it is often advisable to combine BL.23 with BL.18 and BL.20 to treat symptoms associated with senescence.

Table 14.5 Combinations with BL.23 for Kidney psychological problems

	Combine BL.23 with	Psychological problems
Disharmonies of will	BL.13	lack of coordination of rhythmic order in breathing, in Qi circulation and in the life
	BL.15	unfocused and exhausting overenthusiasm when expansion of Spirit is not balanced by concentration of will
	BL.18	scattering of the energies in too many areas when energies are not focused by the will into an integrated life-plan
	BL.20	aimless thinking due to lack of focusing and direction of the will on to some specific task
Fear	BL.13	fear of loss, fear of the pain of letting go, avoidance of grief by avoidance of relationships in depth
	BL.15	fearful restless anxiety, fear scatters the Spirit, reducing coordination of thought, speech and behaviour
	BL.18	anger borne from fear and insecurity
	BL.20	fearfulness and worry arising from insecurity, lack of solidity and stability
Depression	BL.13	depression and inaction with lack of interest in the present and withdrawal into memories of the past
	BL.15	apathy and depression associated with lack of active interest and enjoyment in life
	BL.18	depression with timidity, lack of confidence, and lack of feeling of strength and certainty in self
	BL.20	depression with lethargy, dull mind, aimless thoughts and vague worries
Emotional	BL.13	person alternates between moods of withdrawal and liability to tearfulness
	BL.15	person is jumpy, nervous and overexcitable with up and down swings of mood
	BL.18	person is hypersensitive, easily irritated and greatly disturbed by anger
	BL.20	relatively small insecurities can produce great worry or clinging, whining possessive behaviour

For example, Deficient Jing and Blood can lead to restricted movement and restricted lives in the elderly, due to brittle bones, stiff joints, weak muscles and declining coordination, concentration, balance and memory.

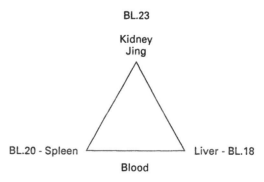

Fig 14.10

The importance of combining BL.23 and BL.20

Apart from tonifying Blood Jing and Qi, and stabilizing the emotions, this combination of points can be used with Reinforcing method and moxa, to firm Spleen and Kidney Qi and tonify Spleen and Kidney Yang. This has the function of resolving Damp and Phlegm and treating urinary problems and oedema and of assisting the Qi to hold things up and in, to treat prolapses, flaccid skin, and muscles, haemorrhages and incontinences.

If BL.23 and BL.20 are combined with BL.13, then this can tonify the Qi of the whole body, improving the production storage and circulation of Qi by Lungs, Spleen and Kidneys, and so increasing the strength of the body to resist infection. This combination can also treat chronic respiratory disorders like asthma and bronchitis, associated with Deficiency of Lungs and Spleen and the failure of the Kidneys to hold down the Qi.

BL.23 and the balance of Yin–Yang

To treat Deficient Yin or Deficient Yang successfully, it is necessary to tonify Qi in general and to tonify *both* Yin and Yang. Points such as BL.23 and KI.3, which do this, can be used to tonify Kidney Yin or Kidney Yang, and can stabilize a fluctuating Yin–Yang balance, where the patient either alternatively or simultaneously shows signs of both Deficient Yang and Deficient Yin.

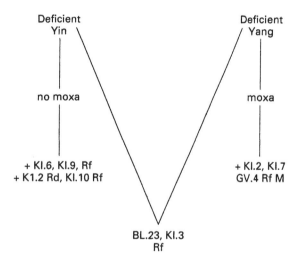

Fig. 14.11

While moxa is often used to emphasize the tonification of Yang, it should be avoided in cases of Deficient Yin and used with great caution where there is fluctuating Yin–Yang balance. In addition, BL.23 and KI.3 can be used in combination with other back points to stabilize Deficient Yang or Deficient Yin in other organs, as shown in Table 14.6.

Table 14.6 Combinations with BL.23 and KI.3 to stabilize Yang and Yin

Syndromes	Back Transporting point	Other points
Deficient Yang of Lungs	BL.13 Rf M	LU.9 Rf; LU.10 Rf M
Deficient Yin of Lungs	BL.13 Rf	L.U9 Rf; LU.5 Rf
Deficient Yang of Liver	BL.18 Rf M	LR.3 Rf; LR.2 Rf M
Deficient Yin of Liver	BL.18 Rf	LR.3 Rf; LR.8 Rf
Deficient Yang of Heart	BL.15 Rf M	HT.7 Rf; HT.8 Rf M
Deficient Yang of Spleen and Stomach	BL.20 Rf M	SP.3, ST.36 Rf M
Deficient Yin of Stomach	BL.21 Rf	ST.36, SP.6 Rf

Rf, Reinforcing method; M, moxa.

In all cases, caution should be used when moxa is used on the Fire point of the organ, and tongue and pulse checked for signs of excessive heat.

Syndromes

Deficient Kidney Jing
Deficient Kidney Yin
Deficient Kidney Yang
Deficient Kidney Yin and Deficient Kidney Yang
Deficient Kidney Qi
Disharmonies of will
Fear
Depression
Emotional lability
Problems of bones, spine and joints
Problems of ageing.

Since most of these syndromes have been dealt with under KI.3 in Chapter 13, the syndromes of BL.23 are here summarized in Table 14.7.

BL.24 qì hǎi shū

This point is mainly used for acute or chronic lower back pain, either as a primary point, or as a secondary local point following the use of a distal point such as yāo tòng diǎn. See Back pain in Chapter 27.

BL.25 dà cháng shū

Back Transporting point of the Large Intestine.

General

This point regulates the Large Intestine and anus and can also be used as a local point for back pain.

Syndromes

Deficiency and Stagnation of Qi of Spleen and Large

Table 14.7 Summary of the syndromes of BL.23

Syndrome	Example of ailment	Example of combination
Deficient Kidney Jing	declining eyesight	BL.10, BL.18, BL.20, BL.23, KI.6, TE.3 Rf
Deficient Kidney Yin	cystitis	BL.23, BL.28, BL.31, SP.6, HT.8 E
Deficient Kidney Yang	oedema	BL.20, BL.22, BL.23, SP.6, ST.40, TE.6 E
Deficient Kidney Yin and Deficient Kidney Yang	menopausal anxiety and depression	BL.23, BL.52, KI.3, KI.6 Rf; BL.15, BL.44, HT.6 E
Deficient Kidney Qi	asthma and tiredness	BL.13, BL.23, KI.3, KI.6, LU.9 Rf dìng chuǎn, LU.7 Rd
Disharmonies of will	difficulties completing tasks	BL.23, BL.52, GV.4, KI.7, BL.60 Rf M
Fear	fear of the dark	BL.23, BL.52, KI.3, BL.64, SI.3, HT.7 E
Depression	fear of failure discouragement at setbacks	BL.23, BL.52, BL.64, BL.67, KI.1, KI.3, GV.20 Rf
Emotional lability	jumpy and fearful	BL.15, BL.20, BL.23, ST.36, KI.3, HT.7 E
Skeletal problems	stiffness and weakness of spine	BL.1, BL.23, BL.62, GV.4, GV.14, SI.3 E
Problems of ageing	deafness and tinnitus	BL.18, BL.23, KI.3, GB.20, GB.34, TE.3, TE.17 E

Intestine
Deficiency of Qi and Yang of Spleen and Large
Intestine
Damp Heat in Intestines

Deficiency and Stagnation of Qi of Spleen and Large Intestine

Pulse. Empty, maybe wiry or flooding.

Indications. Abdominal pain and distension, borborygmus, flatulence, constipation especially with lower back pain.

Example. Constipation alternating with diarrhoea.

Combinations. BL.18, BL.20, BL.25, LR.3, GB.34, LI.10, TE.6 E.

Deficiency of Qi and Yang of Spleen and Large Intestine

Pulse. Empty, maybe deep, slow and slippery.

Indications. Rectal haemorrhage, prolapse of anus, haemorrhoids.

Example. Faecal incontinence and diarrhoea.

Combinations. BL.20, BL.23, BL.25, ST.36, GV.20 Rf M.

Damp Heat in Intestines

Pulse. Rapid, slippery, maybe full or flooding.

Indications. Dysentery, diarrhoea, bleeding, haemorrhoids.

Example. Diarrhoea with pain and burning sensation.

Combinations. BL.20, BL.25, BL.27, LI.11, ST.37 Rd.

Alternation. CV.3, CV.12, SP.6, SP.9, LI.11, ST.37 Rd.

BL.26 guān yuàn shū

Owing to its specific segmental location, this point can be combined with other back points to treat lower back pain and the following disorders:

+ BL.23 urinary problems
+ BL.24 leg weakness
+ BL.25 constipation and diarrhoea
+ BL.27 enteritis
+ BL.28 cystitis.

BL.27 xiǎo cháng shū

Back Transporting point for Small Intestine.

General

The functions of this point relate to the syndromes of the Small Intestine discussed on page 284.

Syndromes

Deficiency and Cold in Small Intestine
Stagnation of Qi in Small Intestine
Damp Heat in Intestines
Heat in Small Intestine

Deficiency and Cold in Small Intestine

Pulse. Empty, deep, slow, maybe wiry.

Indications. Abdominal pain, diarrhoea, urinary frequency.

Example. Diarrhoea, desire for warmth and hot drinks.

Combinations. BL.20, BL.23, BL.27, ST.36, ST.39 Rf M.

Alternation. CV.6, CV.12, ST.25, ST.36, ST.39 Rf M.

Stagnation of Qi in Small Intestine

Pulse. Wiry, maybe deep.

Indications. Appendicitis, lower abdominal pain which

is mild to violent, abdominal distension, flatulence, constipation.

Example.   Irritable bowel syndrome.

Combinations.   BL.18, BL.20, BL.27, LR.3, ST.39, LI.4 E.

Alternation.   CV.6, LR.3, LR.13, SP.15, GV.28, ST.39 E.

Damp Heat in Intestines

Pulse.   Slippery, rapid, maybe full, flooding or wiry.

Indications.   Dysentery, diarrhoea, enteritis.

Example.   Diarrhoea with pus and blood.

Combinations.   BL.20, BL.25, BL.27, SP.1, SP.2 Rd.

Alternation.   CV.6 E; SP.1, SP.2, SP.15, CV.3, ST.39 Rd.

Heat in Small Intestine

Pulse.   Rapid, full or flooding, maybe wiry.

Indications.   Dysuria, menorrhagia, tongue ulcers.

Example.   Abdominal pain with heat sensation in the chest.

Combinations.   BL.15, BL.27, ST.39, SI.5, HT.5, HT.8 Rd.

BL.28 páng guāng shū

Back Transporting point of the Bladder.

General

The functions of this point relate to the syndromes of the Bladder discussed on page 168.

Syndromes

  Deficiency of Qi of Spleen, Kidneys and Bladder
  Damp Heat in Bladder
  Lower back pain

Deficiency of Qi of Spleen, Kidneys and Bladder

Pulse.   Empty, maybe slippery.

Indications.   Prostatitis, urinary frequency or retention, oedema.

Example.   Incomplete urination with discomfort.

Combinations.   BL.20, BL.23, BL.28, BL.39, ST.36, SP.6 Rf.

Damp Heat in Bladder

Pulse.   Slippery, rapid, maybe wiry, thin or flooding.

Indications.   Cystitis, urinary tract infection.

Example.   Dysuria with blood in urine.

Combinations.   BL.17, BL.28, KI.2, HT.8 Rd; SP.6 E.

Alternation.   CV.3, SP.9, KI.2, HT.8 Rd; SP.6 E.

Lower back pain

Pulse.   Empty or thin, maybe wiry.

Indications.   Lower back pain, sciatica, leg pain.

Example.   Cold, painful sacral and lumbar region.

Combinations.   BL.23, BL.28, BL.32, BL.60, GV.3 Rf M.

BL.30 bái huán shū

This point is similar in function to BL.31–34, in that it treats anal, urogenital and local sacral problems. It is mainly used for anal problems such as constipation with painful defecation, haemorrhoids, anal prolapse and incontinence.

BL.31–34 shàng liáo, cì liáo, zhōng liáo, xià liáo

General

The sacral segments in which BL.31–34 are located are associated in Western medicine with the pelvic plexuses of the autonomic nervous system with control of rectum, bladder and genitals. The sacral area also corresponds to the Reproduction energy centre, which is represented on the front of the body by CV.2 and CV.3.

Since they represent the Reproduction centre, the bā liáo points and CV.3 are very similar in function and can both be used with moxa to tonify Jing for the treatment of infertility and impotence. Both BL.31–34 and CV.4 can be used to treat Damp Heat in the Lower Energizer, whether in Bladder, Intestines or genitals. Both BL.31–34 and CV.3 can be used to move Stagnant Qi and Blood in the uterus for dysmenorrhoea, but BL.31–34 is safer for difficult or delayed labour.

Syndromes

  Damp Heat in the Lower Energizer
    Damp Heat in Large Intestine
    Damp Heat in Bladder
    Damp Heat in genitals
  Stagnation of Qi and Blood in uterus
  Deficient Kidney Jing

Kidney Qi not Firm
Lower back problems

Damp Heat in the Lower Energizer

Pulse. Slippery, rapid, maybe thin, flooding or wiry.

Damp Heat in Large Intestine.

Examples. Diarrhoea, tenesmus.

Combination. BL.32 + BL.25, ST.37, SP.6, SP.9 Rd.

Damp Heat in Bladder

Examples. Urinary tract infection.

Combination. BL.32 + BL.28, BL.39, SP.6, SP.9 Rd.

Damp Heat in genitals

Examples. Pruritus, leucorrhoea.

Combination. BL.32 + BL.26, GB.34, SP.6, SP.9 Rd.

Stagnation of Qi and Blood in uterus

Pulse. Wiry, choppy.

Indications. Delayed or difficult childbirth, dysmenorrhoea.

Example. Uterine and ovarian pain.

Combinations. BL.24, BL.32, BL.60, BL.67, LI.4 Rd.

Deficient Kidney Jing

Pulse. Thin or empty, choppy, maybe deep and slow.

Indications. Prostatitis, impotence, infertility.

Example. Impotence, prostatitis and depression.

Combinations. BL.23, BL.32, BL.52, BL.60, KI.7, GV.4, GV.20 Rf M.

Alternation. CV.4, CV.17, GV.20, KI.7 Rf M; SP.6, PC.6 E.

Kidney Qi not firm

Pulse. Empty, scattered, choppy or changing.

Indications. Leucorrhoea, prolapse of uterus, vagina or anus.

Example. Urinary frequency, haemorrhoids, weak lower back.

Combinations. BL.23, BL.32, BL.54, BL.57.

Lower back problems

Pulse. Empty, maybe slow and deep or wiry.

Indications. Pain, stiffness and weakness of lower back and sacrum, sciatica, leg problems.

Example. Sacrum and leg pain, worse with cold.

Combinations. BL.28, BL.32, BL.60, GV.2, GV.3.

BL.35 huì yáng

Although this point can be used for the various Damp Heat syndromes of the Lower Energizer, BL.31–34 are more effective. The author mainly uses BL.35 for coccygeal problems, with the needles angled towards GV.1, which can be used in combination with BL.35.

BL.36 and BL.37 chéng fú and yǐn mén

These points are mainly used for pain in lower back, sacrum, coccyx or hip, with radiation of pain through the buttock or down the leg. They are usually used as part of the chain of points on the Bladder and/or Gallbladder channels, for example:

BL.23, BL.26, BL.36, BL.37, BL.40, BL.60 E M for pain along Bladder channel
BL.36, BL.37, BL.54, BL.60, GB.30, GB.34 Rd for pain along Bladder and Gallbladder channels

BL.39 wěi yáng

Lower Sea point of Triple Energizer channel. BL.39 can be used with Reducing method for Damp syndromes of Excess and Stagnation, such as oedema and urinary retention or Damp Heat cystitis. It can also be used with Reinforcing method for Damp syndromes due to Deficiency, such as urinary frequency or incontinence. For example:

| Damp + Stagnation of Qi | e.g. cystitis | BL.39 + BL.28, BL.32, SP.6, SP.9 Rd |
| Damp + Deficient Qi | e.g. frequency | BL.39 + BL.20, BL.22, KI.7, SP.9 Rf |

BL.40 wěi zhōng

Earth point of Bladder channel.

General

BL.40 has three main areas of use: Bladder channel problems, Bladder organ problems and skin diseases. It is mainly used with Reducing method or bleeding for acute or chronic Excess conditions. These may be Stagnation of Qi and Blood affecting the Bladder organ, or Summer Heat, Heat in the Blood, Damp Heat or Fire poison affecting the skin.

BL.40 is generally used for Excess types of lower back pain with bleeding or Reducing method. For Deficiency type lower back pain it is often replaced by BL.60 with Reinforcing method and moxa, since BL.40 is not generally used with moxa. However, BL.40 can be used for numbness, weakness and atrophy of the legs providing it is combined with other points which are used with moxa, e.g. BL.54 and BL.60.

Syndromes

  Lower back problems
  Damp Heat in the Bladder
  Skin diseases
    Summer Heat
    Heat in the Blood
    Damp Heat
    Fire poison

Lower back problems

Pulse. Wiry,

Indications. Pain or stiffness along Bladder channel in lower back, hip, knee or gastrocnemius muscle.

Example. Acute lower back sprain.

Combinations. Bleed BL.40, then use local points such as BL.24 and 26, with distal points, e.g. BL.60 Rd.

Damp Heat in the Bladder

Pulse. Rapid, slippery, wiry.

Indications. Cystitis, urinary tract infections.

Example. Dysuria and lower back pain.

Combinations. BL.23, BL.28, BL.40, BL.60, TE.6 Rd.

Skin diseases

Summer Heat

Pulse. Superficial, scattered or flooding.

Indications. Sunstroke, fever, delirium, fainting, sunburn.

Example. Sunburn with faintness and nausea.

Combinations. BL.40, PC.9 B; PC.6, GV.14 Rd.

Heat in the Blood

Pulse. Rapid, full or thin.

Indications. Eczema, psoriasis, urticaria, restless fetus.

Example. Eczema with red, hot, itching, painful skin.

Combinations. BL.40, PC.3, PC.9, SP.1 B; LI.4, LI.11, SP.6 Rd.

Damp Heat

Pulse. Slippery, rapid, maybe wiry.

Indications. Herpes zoster, eczema, seborrhoeic dermatitis.

Example. Eczema with fluid-filled blisters and exudation.

Combinations. BL.40, SP.6, SP.9, GB.34, TE.6 Rd.

Fire Poison

Pulse. Maybe rapid, slippery, wiry and flooding.

Indications. Acne, boils, swollen lymph or salivary glands.

Example. Acne with hard, red, painful boil-like swellings which cannot be discharged.

Combinations. BL.40 B; LI.5, LI.11, LI.17, LI.18, SI.5, SI.16 Rd.

Outer Bladder line points BL.42, 43, 44, 47, 49 and 52

General

BL.42, 44, 47, 49 and 52 are the outer Bladder line points for the Lungs, Heart, Liver, Spleen and Kidneys respectively. BL.43 is the outer Bladder line point for the Pericardium, level with BL.14, below the level of the spinous process of the fourth thoracic vertebra.

BL.43 gāo huāng shū

This point has some overlapping functions with BL.13, in that it tonifies the Lungs and transforms Phlegm, but its main function is to tonify Qi and Blood in chronic exhaustion and debility, for example after long illness, especially when used with moxa cones. For example, BL.43 can be combined with BL.17 and BL.20 with Reinforcing method and moxa to tonify Blood.

BL.43 can strengthen the Lung Yin, to relieve pulmonary tuberculosis; Reinforcing method is used without moxa. By tonifying Kidney Jing, BL.43 can improve reduced sexual drive and by tonifying the Yang of Kidney and Heart, it can invigorate the brain and the Spirit to improve memory and to disperse depression after chronic illness. In common with BL.15 and BL.44 it can also calm the Spirit.

BL.42, 44, 47, 49 and 52 pò hù, shén táng, hún mén, yì shè and zhì shì

The outer and inner Bladder line points on the back can be used for both physiological and psychological conditions. Traditionally, the outer line points are used more for psychological disorders. Table 14.8 gives the psychological problems associated with each of the five main outer line points, and also gives points which can be combined with them; the inner Bladder line and GV points at the same spinal level; the CV points that can be used as an alternative treatment; the Source points corresponding to the organ system and the related Window of Heaven points.

BL.54 zhì biān

This is a useful local point for lower back pain radiating through buttocks and legs. It is used with a needle depth of 1.5–2 units, aiming to obtain a needle sensation radiating down the leg, with the use of moxa where appropriate. It can be combined with such points as BL.23, 32, 36, 37, 40 and 60, for back, buttock and leg problems.

BL.57 chéng shān

The main uses of this point are cramps for the gastrocnemius muscle, lower back pain and haemorrhoids.

Syndromes

Stagnant Qi and Blood in the Bladder channel
  Lower back pain and sciatica
  Gastrocnemius spasm
Damp Heat in the Lower Energizer
  Damp Heat in the Large Intestine
  Damp Heat in the Bladder

Stagnant Qi and Blood in the Bladder channel

Lower back pain and sciatica

Pulse. Wiry.

Indications. Pain and stiffness in lower back, hip and leg.

Example. Sciatica with pain down both Bladder and Gallbladder channels.

Combinations. BL.26, BL.31, BL.54, BL.57, GB.30, GB.34, GB.40 Rd.

Gastrocnemius spasm

Pulse. Wiry.

Indications. Localized gastrocnemius spasm, general tension of muscles, night cramps.

Example. Gastrocnemius spasm with generalized nervous and muscle tension.

Combinations. BL.56, BL.57, BL.59, GB.20, GB.34, LR.3 Rd.

Table 14.8 Using outer Bladder line points for psychological problems

Outer BL	Inner BL	GV	CV	Source	WoH	Psychological problems
BL.42 (LU)	BL.13	GV.12	CV.17	LU.9	LU.3 LI.18	rejection of the rhythmic aspect of gain and loss, failure to gain wisdom by assimilating the experience of loss, unwillingness to participate deeply in life from fear of loss
BL.44 (HT)	BL.15	GV.11	CV.17 CV.14	HT.7	PC.1 SI.16 SI.17	disharmony in the expression of the two aspects of Spirit, life and love; not only under- or over-animation, but also difficulties in the expression and communication of love and affection
BL.47 (LR)	BL.18	GV.8	CV.14 CV.12	LR.3	–	lack of contact with intuition, the inner sense of direction in life, uncertainty or frustration from using plans or decisions not related to the person's own inner needs or to the needs of other people
BL.49 (SP)	BL.20	GV.6	CV.12	SP.3	ST.9	insecurity, not feeling strong, rooted and stable in the physical body and in the physical world, living in a world of repetitive thought untranslated into action, lack of coordination between Spirit, intelligence and physical body
BL.52 (KI)	BL.23	GV.4	CV.6 CV.4	KI.3	BL.10	feelings of powerlessness and inadequacy, fear of the unknown, fear of failure, fear of death, lack of endurance, lack of perseverance

Damp Heat in the Lower Energizer

Damp Heat in the Large Intestine

Pulse. Slippery, rapid, maybe full, flooding or wiry.

Indications. Constipation, diarrhoea, haemorrhoids.

Example. Bleeding haemorrhoids.

Combinations. BL.35, BL.57, BL.59, GV.1, SP.1, SP.6 Rd.

Damp Heat in the Bladder

Pulse. Slippery, rapid, maybe wiry, maybe thin or flooding.

Indications. Cystitis, urethritis.

Example. Urinary tract infection with haematuria.

Combinations. BL.28, BL.32, BL.57, SP.1, TE.6 Rd.

BL.58 fēi yáng

Connection point of Bladder channel.

General

This point can treat back pain and sciatica, like BL.57, especially if the pain goes down the leg either on both Bladder and Gallbladder channels, or between the two channels. Again, like BL.57, it can be used to treat haemorrhoids. What is important about this point relates to its function as Connecting point on the Bladder channel. It tonifies the Kidneys and thus controls upper and moving Yang, to treat seizures, headaches and dizziness. It can dispel both Interior and Exterior Wind to treat nasal obstruction and Wind-type arthritis of the legs.

Syndromes

Lower back pain and sciatica ⎫
Damp Heat in the Bladder ⎬ see BL.57
Deficient Kidney Qi and Hyperactive Yang
Exterior Wind invasion ⎭

Deficient Kidney Qi and Hyperactive Yang

Pulse. Empty, wiry.

Indications. Seizures, headache, dizziness.

Example. Headache with blurred vision.

Combinations. BL.2, BL.10, BL.58, SI.3 E; KI.3 Rf.

Exterior Wind invasion

Pulse. Superficial, tight.

Indications. Nasal obstruction, headache, arthritis of the legs.

Example. Nasal obstruction and aching limbs.

Combinations. BL.2, BL.10, BL.12, BL.58, BL.62, SI.3, LI.20 Rd.

BL.59 fū yáng

Accumulating point of Yang Heel channel.

General

From BL.36 through to BL.57 on the leg, the points have local effects, or effects mainly on the lower body. However, from BL.58 to BL.67, the points have an increasingly powerful effect on the upper body. This is because the nearer to the point of change of polarity and direction of energy at BL.67, the greater the effect the points have at the opposite end of the meridian, the head and face.

BL.59 is similar in function to BL.58, but its main function is to assist freedom and agility of movement by treating pain or stiffness in the calf, ankle and foot, since it is the Accumulation point for the Yang Heel channel.

Back, leg and ankle problems

Pulse. Wiry, maybe empty.

Indications. Pain or stiffness in back, hip, leg and lateral ankle or foot.

Example. Pain in external malleolus.

Combinations. BL.57, BL.59, BL.62 Rd on affected side; SI.4, SI.5, SI.6 Rd on opposite side.

BL.60 kūn lún

Fire point of Bladder channel.

General

BL.60, like BL.62, 64 and 65, can treat problems along the whole pathway of the Bladder channel, from head to foot.

Back pain

While BL.40 is for acute or chronic back pain mainly of the Excess type, BL.60 is more used for chronic back pain of the Deficiency type, especially with invasion by Cold. This is because BL.60, as the Fire point of the Bladder, can have a warming effect and because BL.60 tonifies the Kidneys.

Shoulder, neck and occipital problems

A further difference between BL.40 and BL.60 is that while BL.40 is mainly for lower back and leg problems, BL.60 can also treat pain in the upper back, shoulders, neck and head, both by tonifying and warming the Kidneys and the Bladder channel, and by dispersing Exterior Wind Cold.

BL.60 as a Fire point

Because it is a Fire point and because it tonifies the Kidneys, BL.60 can be used to tonify Kidney Yang and Kidney Fire, to treat depression and exhaustion, especially when the patient also has aching neck, shoulder and head. BL.60 can be combined with KI.2, the Fire point of the Kidneys, and the effect can be stabilized and strengthened by adding the Source points, BL.64 and KI.3. To further enhance the combination, GV.4 or CV.4 can be added, or treatment on the back can be alternated with treatment on the front of the body. Alternatively, like KI.2, BL.60 can be used with Reducing method to clear Heat or Damp Heat in the Bladder, as in cystitis, perhaps in combination with BL.66 and KI.10.

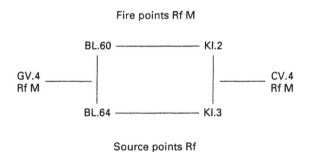

Fig. 14.12

Stagnant Qi and Blood in the uterus

Both BL.60 and BL.67 can move Stagnant Qi and Blood to regulate uterine spasms. BL.60 can treat dysmenorrhoea or be used for difficult labour and retained placenta.

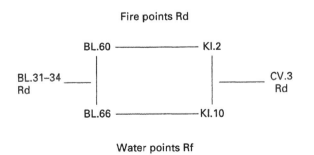

Fig. 14.13

Syndromes

Back, shoulder, neck and occipital problems
Deficient Kidney Yang
Heat in the Bladder
Stagnant Blood in the uterus

Back, shoulder, neck and occipital problems

Pulse. Wiry, empty, maybe deep and slow, maybe superficial and tight.

Indications. Pain, stiffness or weakness in occiput, neck, shoulders, back, hip, leg or foot, worse with tiredness or cold.

Example. Back pain with occipital headache.

Combinations. BL.10, BL.11, SI.3, SI.11, SI.15 Rd; BL.60, KI.3 Rf M.

Deficient Kidney Yang

Pulse. Empty, slow, deep.

Indications. Depression, back pain, neck pain, occipital headache.

Example. Cold extremities and lower back, apathy and depression.

Combinations. BL.23, BL.60, KI.2, GV.4, GV.14, GV.20 Rf M.

Heat in the Bladder

Pulse. Rapid, maybe thin and wiry.

Indications. Dysuria, haematuria, restlessness, feeling of heat in the chest, tongue ulcers.

Example. Cystitis, pruritus and insomnia.

Combinations. BL.32, BL.60, KI.2, HT.8 Rd; BL.66, KI.10, HT.3 Rf.

Stagnant Blood in the uterus

Pulse. Wiry, choppy.

Indications. Dysmenorrhoea, difficult labour, retention of placenta.

Example. Dysmenorrhoea with lower back pain.

Combinations. BL.24, BL.32, BL.60, SP.6, LI.4 Rd. **Contraindicated during pregnancy.**

BL.62 shēn mài

Opening point of the Yang Heel channel.

General

As a Bladder point on the lower leg, BL.62, like BL.60 and BL.64, can treat problems along the whole course of the Bladder channel, from ankle stiffness to nasal congestion. However, the special emphasis of BL.62 derives from its function as the Opening point of the Yang Heel channel. This channel can be seen as an extension of the Bladder channel and the Kidney organ. As an Extra channel pathway, the Yang Heel can absorb Excess energy in the Bladder channel, whether this originates from Stagnation of Qi and Blood, Wind invasions, or rising Yang. Alternatively, use of BL.62 with Reinforcing method, can tonify Deficiency of Qi in the Bladder channel deriving from Deficient Qi of the Kidneys.

Because of its connections with BL.1, the Yang Heel channel can be used to treat ear and nose problems, and because it enters the brain at GV.16 the Yang Heel pathway can be used to calm Interior Wind, and treat insomnia, dizziness and postconcussion syndromes.

Using BL.62 in combination with SI.3

These two points operate the Yang Heel and Governor channels as a pair, to increase flexibility of the whole skeletal system. In certain patients, stiffness and lack of flexibility of the spine seems to be associated with rigidity and inflexibility of the personality and BL.62 and SI.3 in combination can treat this. In this case, the Window of Heaven points BL.10, SI.16 and SI.17 can be added to expand the feeling of limitation.

Syndromes

Table 14.9 shows additional points that can be added to the BL.62 + SI.3 combination to treat a variety of ailments.

BL.63 jī mén

Accumulation point of Bladder channel, Beginning point of the Yang Link channel. BL.63 has some interesting indications which it shares with BL.64, such as childhood convulsions and fear and agitation in children. However, its main use is as an Accumulation point to treat acute pain on the Bladder channel, acute cystitis, and also acute abdominal pain.

BL.64 jīng gǔ

Source point of the Bladder channel.

BL.64 as a Source point

Like all Source points, BL.64 can tonify Qi and tonify both Yin and Yang, to treat back pain, headache, dizziness or eye problems associated with Deficient Kidney Qi. To tonify the Qi of Kidneys and Bladder together the two Source points BL.64 and KI.3 can be combined. The action of these two points to tonify the Source Qi can be strengthened by adding CV.4 or GV.4 to the combination.

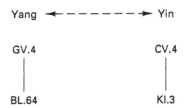

Combining Greater Yang with Lesser Yin to calm the Spirit

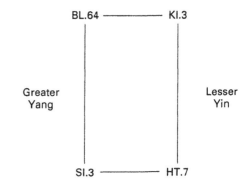

Fig. 14.14

Table 14.9 BL.62 syndromes: combining BL.62 + SI.3 with other points

Syndromes	Example	Other points
Excess		
Stagnation of Qi and Blood in Bladder channel	chronic stiffness and pain in shoulder	+ BL.40, SI.10
	mental and spinal rigidity and inflexibility	+ BL.10, SI.16
Invasion of Wind Cold	stiffness in neck, shoulders and back	+ BL.10, SI.12
	frontal headache and nasal discharge	+ BL.2, BL.10
Yang rising to head	occipital headache, stiff neck and disorientation	+ BL.58, GV.15
Interior Wind	hemiplegia and voice loss	+ BL.7, GV.15
Deficiency		
Deficient Yin of Kidney and of Bladder channel	arthritis in neck	+ BL.11, KI.6
Deficient Qi of Kidney and of Bladder channel	bone degeneration in spine	+ BL.11, KI.3
	fatigue, disorientation and depression	+ BL.23, SI.5
	declining vision	+ BL.2, BL.23

In addition to the relationship between the Yin–Yang pair, Bladder and Kidney, the pair Bladder and Small Intestine comprise the Greater Yang division and the pair Kidney and Heart the Lesser Yin division of the Six Divisions classification.

The four Source points, BL.64, KI.3, SI.3 and HT.7 can be used together to stabilize and calm the Spirit, since both BL.64 and SI.3 can treat Heart psychological problems. Figure 14.15 shows further possible point combinations with BL.64 and KI.3 to strengthen the Spirit (GV.4, GV.11, CV.17), or to calm the Spirit (GV.14, CV.14). BL.15, 23, 44 and 52 can be used either to strengthen or to calm.

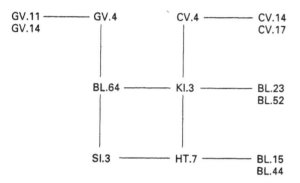

Fig. 14.15

Syndromes

Deficient Qi of Kidneys and of Bladder channel
Fear disturbing the Spirit

Deficient Qi of Kidneys and of Bladder channel

Pulse. Empty, maybe choppy or changing.

Indications. Ache in back or legs, headache, dizziness, blurred vision.

Example. Mental exhaustion and lack of mental clarity.

Combinations. BL.10, BL.23, BL.64, BL.67 E; KI.3 Rf.

Fear disturbing the Spirit

Pulse. Empty or thin, maybe choppy, changing or even moving, scattered or irregular.

Indications. Fear and agitation in children, enuresis, dream-disturbed sleep, fearful anxiety, palpitations.

Example. Fearful dreams and fear of the dark.

Combinations. BL.44, BL.52, BL.64, GV.20, KI.3, HT.7 Rf.

BL.66 zú tōng gǔ

Water point of Bladder channel, Spring point.

General

As both a Water point and a Spring point BL.66 can be used to clear Heat, and as discussed under BL.60, can be combined with BL.60, KI.2 and KI.10 to clear Heat from the Bladder as in cystitis. BL.66 can be combined with the Water point and Spring point of the Small Intestine channel, SI.2, to treat dizziness, headache, neck stiffness, feverishness and disturbance of the Spirit.

Combination of BL.66 to calm the Spirit

BL.66 + SI.2, the Water points, used with Reinforcing method, can be further combined with the Fire points, BL.60 and SI.5, with Reducing method for fear, mania and incoherent speech. Both Bladder Divergent channel and the Small Intestine main channel connect with the Heart.

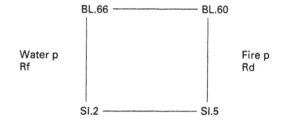

Fig. 14.16

Syndromes

Heat in the Bladder – see BL.60
Exterior and Interior Wind and Heat
Fear disturbing the Spirit

Exterior and Interior Wind and Heat

Pulse. Superficial or wiry, rapid.

Indications. Fever, neck stiffness, headache, dizziness, epistaxis.

Example. Occipital headache and fever.

Combinations. BL.66, LI.4, GV.14, GV.16 Rd.

Fear disturbing the Spirit

Pulse. Rapid, thin, maybe hasty.

Indications. Restlessness, hot feeling in chest or head, fear, anxiety.

Example. Mental restlessness and agitation.

Combinations. BL.7, BL.60, SI.5 Rd; BL.66, SI.2 Rf.

BL.67 zhì yīn

Metal point, Well point and Tonification point of Bladder channel.

General

BL.67 can be used as a local point for foot problems, for example, since the Kidney and Bladder channels link in the fifth toe, BL.67 can be used for sensation of heat in the soles. However, it is at the other end of the channel that BL.67 has its greatest effect.

BL.67 as a Well point

A Well point has such a powerful effect on the channel in general, and the far end of the channel in particular, because at a Well point the energy is changing polarity and direction, and is therefore especially amenable to change by acupuncture treatment. BL.67 can invigorate the whole channel and especially improve eyesight, nasal obstruction and mental dullness because it has a Well point's rapid awakening effect on the channel, removing Stagnation and stimulating the circulation of Qi.

Combination of points at the two ends of the channel

As with other Well points the effect of BL.67 is enhanced by combining with BL.1 or BL.2. This can awaken the mind and improve mental clarity, especially when BL.67 and BL.1 are combined with ST.45 and LI.1.

Invigoration and tonification

However, BL.67 like all Well points, and despite the fact it is the Tonification point on the Bladder channel, does not so much tonify as invigorate.

Invigoration is more a quick stimulation of an acute Stagnation, while tonification is a slower but steady supply of energy to a chronically Deficient condition. The two effects can be combined, for example if BL.64 and/or BL.60 are added to BL.67 and BL.1.

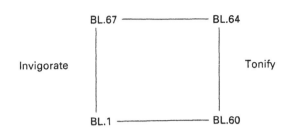

Fig. 14.17

Regulates the uterus

Like BL.60, BL.67 can be used for difficult labour and retention of placenta. BL.67 can also be used for malposition of fetus, with the practitioner using moxa cones or the patient using moxa stick on BL.67. There should be regular checks on fetal position, and as soon as the fetus is turned the treatment should stop.

Syndromes

Stagnation of Qi in the Bladder channel
Nose and eye problems
Obstetric problems

Stagnation of Qi in the Bladder channel

Pulse. Maybe empty, hindered or wiry.

Indications. Melancholy, head and neck ache, mental dullness.

Example. Occipital headache.

Combinations. BL.67, GB.20.

Nose and eye problems

Pulse. Various.

Indications. Nasal obstruction, nasal discharge, epistaxis, conjunctivitis, blurred vision.

Example. Blurred vision and eye strain.

Combinations. BL.2, BL.10, BL.67, SI.3, GB.1 E.

Obstetric problems

Pulse. Various.

Indications. Malposition of fetus, difficult labour, retention of placenta.

Example. Retention of placenta.

Combinations. BL.60, BL.67, CV.2 Rd; CV.4 Rf.

Bladder point comparisons and combinations

The functions of the main Bladder points are listed in Table 14.10.

Table 14.10 Bladder points comparisons

Point	Point type	Syndrome
BL.1	Point of Yang and Yin Heel Crossing point of Bladder, Small Intestine, Stomach	eye problems
BL.2		nasal problems, facial problems problems of the nervous system
BL.7		External Wind Hyperactive Yang
BL.10		cerebral problems, psychological problems eye problems External Wind neck and head problems
BL.11	Gathering point of bones Sea of Blood point	External Wind neck and head problems bone and joint problems
BL.13 BL.42	Back Transporting point for Lungs	Wind Cold Wind Heat, Wind Dryness Deficient Lung Qi, Deficient Lung Yin Accumulation of Phlegm Cold in Lungs Accumulation of Phlegm Heat in Lungs Stagnation of Lung Qi
BL.15 BL.44	Back Transporting point of Heart	Deficient Heart Qi Deficient Heart Yang Deficient Heart Blood Deficient Heart Yin Heart Fire Heart Phlegm Stagnant Heart Qi Stagnant Heart Blood
BL.17 BL.46	Gathering point of Blood Back Transporting point for diaphragm	Deficient Blood Stagnant Blood Heat in the Blood problems of diaphragm and chest skin disorders
BL.18 BL.47	Back Transporting point for Liver	Deficient Liver Qi Stagnant Liver Qi Deficient Liver Blood Damp Heat in Liver and Gallbladder
BL.19 BL.48	Back Transporting point for Gallbladder	Damp Heat in Liver and Gallbladder Deficient Gallbladder Qi
BL.20 BL.49	Back Transporting point for Spleen	Deficient Spleen Qi Deficient Spleen Blood Deficient Spleen Yang Stagnation in Middle Energizer Damp and Phlegm
BL.21 BL.50	Back Transporting point for Stomach	Retention of food in stomach Rebellion of Stomach Qi
BL.22	Back Transporting point for Triple Energizer	Damp in the Lower Energizer
BL.23 BL.52	Back Transporting point for Kidneys	Deficient Kidney Jing Deficient Kidney Yin Deficient Kidney Yang Deficient Kidney Yin and Deficient Kidney Yang Deficient Kidney Qi Disharmonies of will fear depression emotional lability problems of bones, spine and joints problems of ageing
BL.24		lower back problems

Table 14.10 (cont'd)

Point	Point type	Syndrome
BL.25	Back Transporting point of Large Intestine	Deficiency and Stagnation of Qi in Spleen and Liver
		Deficiency of Qi and Yang in Spleen and Liver
		Damp Heat in Intestines
BL.26		lower back pain
BL.27	Back Transporting point of Small Intestine	Deficiency and Cold in Small Intestine
		Stagnation of Qi in Small Intestine
		Damp Heat in Intestines
		Heat in Small Intestine
BL.28	Back Transporting point of Bladder	Deficiency of Kidneys, Spleen and Bladder
		Damp Heat in Bladder
		lower back pain
BL.31–34	bā liáo	Damp Heat in Lower Energizer
		Stagnation of Qi and Blood in uterus
		Deficient Kidney Jing
		Kidney Qi not firm
		lower back pain
BL.35		coccygeal problems
BL.36 ⎤ BL.37 ⎦		lower back, buttock and leg pain
BL.39	Lower Sea point of TE	Stagnation of Qi and Damp in Lower Energizer
		Deficient Qi and Damp in Lower Energizer
BL.40	Earth point	lower back problems
		Damp Heat in Bladder
		skin diseases
BL.43		Deficient Blood
BL.54		lower back and leg pain
BL.57		Lower back and leg pain
		gastrocnemius spasm
		Damp Heat in Bladder
		Damp Heat in Large Intestine
BL.58	Connecting point	lower back and leg pain
		Damp Heat in Bladder
		Deficient Kidney Qi and Hyperative Liver Yang
		Exterior Wind invasion
BL.59	Accumulation point of Yang Heel	back, leg and ankle problems
BL.60	Fire point	Back, shoulder, neck and occipital problems
		Deficient Kidney Yang
		Heat in Bladder
		Stagnant Blood in uterus
BL.62	Opening point of Yang Heel	Stagnation of Qi and Blood in Bladder channel
		Invasion of Bladder channel by Wind Cold
		Yang and Interior Wind to the head
		Deficient Yin of Kidney and of Bladder channel
		Deficient Qi of Kidney and of Bladder channel
BL.64	Source point	Deficient Qi of Kidney and of Bladder channel
		Fear disturbing Spirit
BL.66	Spring point	Heat in Bladder
	Water point	Exterior and Interior Wind and Heat
		Fear disturbing Spirit
BL.67	Well point	Stagnation of Qi in Bladder channel
	Metal point	nose and eye problems
		obstetric problems

Some common combinations of Bladder points are summarized in Table 14.11.

Table 14.11 Combinations of Bladder points. It is possible to make horizontal chains of points, in one spinal segment, across the back, e.g.GV.4 + BL.23 + BL.52; or to make vertical chains of points, e.g. BL.10 + BL.14 + BL.23 + BL.62.

Point	Combination	Syndromes	Example
BL.2	BL.10	Various	eye, nose and head problems
BL.2	BL.12	Wind Cold	nasal congestion
BL.2	BL.18	Wind Heat and Liver Fire	conjunctivitis
BL.2	BL.62	Deficient Kidney Jing	blurred vision in the old
BL.2	BL.64	Deficient Kidney Qi	difficulty in concentration
BL.2	BL.67	Wind Cold or Wind Heat	allergic rhinitis
BL.7	BL.67	Wind Cold or Wind Heat	sinusitis
BL.10	BL.11	Stagnation of Blood in Bladder channel	traumatic neck injury
BL.10	BL.23	Deficient Kidney Jing	poor memory
BL.10	BL.52	Deficient Kidney Qi	depression, lack of drive
BL.10	BL.60	Wind Cold	aches in neck and back
BL.10	BL.67	Stagnation of Blood in Bladder channel	cervical spondylitis
BL.11	BL.12	Wind Cold	influenza
BL.11	BL.13	Wind Heat and Lung Heat	pneumonia
BL.11	BL.23	Deficient Kidney Jing	osteoporosis
BL.11	BL.62	Deficient Kidney Jing	weak bones and joints in the old
BL.12	BL.13	Deficient Lung Qi and Wind Cold	common cold
BL.13	BL.15	Stagnation of Qi of Lung and Heart	sadness and depression
BL.13	BL.17	Stagnation of Lung Qi	dyspnoea
BL.13	BL.18	Liver invades Lungs	cough with chest pain
BL.13	BL.20	Deficient Qi of Lungs and Spleen	bronchitis
BL.13	BL.23	Deficient Qi of Lungs and Kidney	asthma
BL.15	BL.17	Stagnant Blood of Heart	angina pectoris
BL.15	BL.18	Liver invades Heart	frustration in relationships
BL.15	BL.20	Deficient Blood of Heart and Spleen	insomnia and dizziness
BL.15	BL.21	Stomach Fire invades Heart	restless insomnia
BL.15	BL.23	Deficient Yang of Heart and Kidneys	cold limbs
BL.17	BL.18	Stagnation of Liver Blood	dysmenorrhoea
BL.17	BL.20	Deficient Spleen Blood	dry, rough skin
BL.17	BL.40	Heat in the Blood	psoriasis
BL.19	BL.23	Deficient Qi of Kidney and Gallbladder	timidity and lack of confidence
BL.20	BL.21	Stagnation in Middle Energizer	indigestion and flatulence
BL.20	BL.23	Deficient Yang of Spleen and Kidney	oedema
BL.20	BL.27	Damp Heat in Spleen and Intestine	diarrhoea
BL.21	BL.25	Stagnation of Qi in Bright Yang	epigastric distension and constipation
BL.23	BL.24	Internal cold	lower back pain
BL.23	BL.28	Deficient Bladder Qi	urinary frequency
BL.23	BL 31–34	Damp Heat in Lower Energizer	urinary tract infection
BL.23	BL.35–37	Stagnation in Bladder channel	lumbar, sacral, buttock, and upper leg pain
BL.23	BL.39	Deficient Bladder Qi	urinary retention
BL.23	BL.40	Stagnation in Bladder channel	acute or chronic lumbar pain
BL.23	BL.57–58	Stagnation in Bladder channel	back pain, lower leg pain
BL.23	BL.60	Deficient Kidney Yang	mental and physical exhaustion
BL.23	BL.62	Deficient Kidney Jing	infertility, impotence
BL.23	BL.64	Deficient Kidney Qi	fear and depression
BL.24	BL.26	Internal Cold and Damp	local back pain
BL.25	BL.27	Damp Heat in Intestines	diarrhoea and tenesmus
BL.25	BL.35, or 36, or 39, or 40 or 57, or 58, or 59	Damp Heat in Large Intestine	haemorrhoids and rectal pain
BL.28	BL.31, or 32, or 33, or 34	Deficiency and Stagnation of Bladder Qi	prostatitis
BL.30	BL.35	Stagnation in Bladder channel	coccygeal pain
BL.30	BL.57	Damp Heat in Bladder	haemorrhoids
BL.31–34	BL.35	Stagnation in Bladder channel	sacral and coccygeal pain
BL.31–34	BL.40	Damp Heat in Bladder	cystitis
BL.31–34	BL.57	Stagnation of Qi in Lower Energizer	constipation
BL.31–34	BL.60	Internal Cold	sacral pain and sciatica
BL.31–34	BL.62	Deficient Kidney Jing and Qi	amenorrhoea
BL.36	BL.37	Stagnation in Bladder Channel	back, buttock and thigh pain
BL.36	BL.40	Stagnation in Bladder channel	back and knee pain
BL.39	BL.51	Deficient Qi of Triple Energizer	oedema
BL.39	BL.40	Deficient Kidney Qi	weak knees
BL.40	BL.54	Stagnation in Bladder channel	back, buttock and knee pain
BL.40	BL.57	Stagnation in Bladder channel	gastrocnemius spasm

Table 14.11 (cont'd)

Point	Combination	Syndromes	Example
BL.40	BL.60	Stagnation and Cold in Bladder channel	chronic lumbar pain
BL.58	BL.62	Deficient Kidney Qi and Hyperactive Yang	headache and dizziness
BL.60	BL.52	Deficient Kidney Yang	lack of clear goals
BL.60	BL.64	Deficient Kidney Qi and Yang	chronic weak cold back
BL.60	BL.66	Heat in the Bladder	dysuria and haematuria
BL.62	BL.67	Deficiency in Bladder channel	blurred vision and poor memory
BL.64	BL.67	Deficiency and Stagnation in Bladder channel	mental exhaustion and lack of interest in work
BL.2	BL.7, 10	Disturbance of Spirit and Deficient Kidney Qi	mental disorientation
BL.2	BL.10, 12	Wind Cold	nasal congestion
BL.2	BL.10, 23	Deficient Kidney Jing and Qi	degeneration of vision
BL.2	BL.10, 67	Wind Cold and Deficient Kidney Qi	conjunctivitis
BL.2	BL.62, 67	Deficient Kidney Jing and Qi	lack of concentration
BL.7	BL.58, 62	Deficient Kidney Qi and Hyperactive Yang	headache, dizziness
BL.10	BL.11, 13	Deficient Lung Qi and Wind Cold	influenza and neck ache
BL.10	BL.11, 23	Deficient Kidney Qi and Stagnation in Bladder channel	pain and stiffness of neck and back
BL.10	BL.18, 23	Deficient Kidney Qi and Hyperactive Liver Yang	spasm and stiffness in neck and back
BL.10	BL.23, 60	Deficient Kidney Yang	coldness and pain in neck, back and legs
BL.11	BL.23, 62	Deficient Kidney Qi	brittle bones in the elderly
BL.11	BL.12, 13	Wind Cold	influenza and muscle aches in upper back
BL.13	BL.20, 23	Deficient Qi of Lungs, Spleen and Kidneys	asthma
BL.13	BL.23, 43	Deficient Qi and Yin of Lungs and Kidneys	recovery from chronic illness
BL.15	BL.17, 23	Disturbance of Spirit by fear	anxiety, paranoia, suspicion
BL.15	BL.18, 20	Deficient Blood of Heart, Liver and Spleen	insomnia and exhaustion
BL.15	BL.18, 23	Deficient Qi of Heart, Liver and Kidneys	emotional instability
BL.15	BL.20, 23	Deficient Qi of Heart, Spleen and Kidneys	nervous anxiety and no reserves of energy
BL.17	BL.18, 20	Deficient Blood of Spleen and Liver	weak muscles and lethargy
BL.17	BL.21, 25	Heat in the Blood and Heat in Bright Yang	acute allergic skin reaction to food
BL.17	BL.40, 67	Wind Heat and Heat in the Blood	urticaria with generalized itching
BL.17	BL.26, 32	Stagnant Blood in the uterus	dysmenorrhoea
BL.18	BL.20, 21	Liver invades Spleen and Stomach	belching and abdominal distension
BL.18	BL.23, 62	Deficient Kidney Jing and Deficient Liver Blood	stiffness and weakness of joints and muscles
BL.18	BL.25, 27	Liver invades Intestines	irritable bowel syndrome
BL.20	BL.21, 27	Deficient Qi of Spleen, Stomach and Intestines	malabsorption syndrome
BL.20	BL.22, 23	Deficient Qi and Yang of Spleen and Kidneys	oedema of lower body
BL.23	BL.28, 32	Damp Heat in Bladder and Deficient Kidney Yin	cystitis and nervous restlessness
BL.23	BL.32, 54	Stagnation in Bladder channel	lumbar and sacral pain
BL.23	BL.32, 57	Stagnation in Bladder channel and Deficient Kidney Yin	lumbar pain and cystitis
BL.23	BL.36, 58	Stagnation in Bladder channel and Deficient Kidney Qi	sciatica, worse with tiredness
BL.23	BL.60, 64	Deficient Kidney Qi and Yang	cold, weak lower back
BL.24	BL.26, 32	Stagnation in Bladder channel and uterus	dysmenorrhoea and back pain
BL.31–34	BL.40, 60	Damp Heat in Lower Energizer	cystitis and vaginitis
BL.31–34	BL.60, 66	Heat in Bladder	cystitis with restlessness and insomnia
BL.10	BL.11, 23, 62	Deficient Kidney Qi and Jing	ankylosing spondylitis
BL.10	BL.18, 23, 62	Deficient Jing and Blood	degenerating vision in the elderly
BL.10	BL.11, 23, 60	Deficient Kidney Yang and Internal Cold	coldness and stiffness of neck, back and legs
BL.10	BL.11, 13, 23	Wind Cold and Deficient Qi of Lungs and Kidneys	repeated colds with slow recovery
BL.17	BL.20, 23, 43	Deficient Blood	exhaustion after childbirth
BL.23	BL.32, 54, 57	Stagnation in Bladder channel	back and sacral pain
BL.26	BL.32, 40, 58	Stagnation in Bladder channel	sciatica

Spleen 15

Spleen channel

CHANNEL CONNECTIONS

MAIN CHANNEL PATHWAY

Starting from SP.1 on the big toe, the main pathway runs up the medial aspect of the leg to SP.12 and SP.13; and then ascends the abdomen, crossing the Conception channel at CV.3 and CV.4. From CV.4 it runs up to SP.14 and SP.15, and then to meet again with the Conception channel at CV.10, before running up the lateral abdomen and chest through SP.16, GB.24, LR.14 and SP.20 to end at SP.21. From CV.10, one internal pathway enters the abdomen and connects with the spleen and stomach. Another internal pathway from CV.10 connects with the heart, and a third branch from SP.20 runs through LU.1 up the oesophagus, to disperse in the lower surface of the tongue.

CONNECTING CHANNEL PATHWAY

One branch from SP.4 joins the Stomach channel and another branch runs up to the abdomen to connect with the stomach and intestines. The Great Connecting channel of the Spleen starts from SP.21 and spreads through the chest and hypochondrium. The Muscle Region of the Spleen runs up the leg to the external genitals, and then up inside the abdomen to supply the ribs, before ending in the spine.

Table 15.1 Crossing points on the Spleen channel

Point	Crossing
SP.6	Liver, Kidneys
SP.12	Liver
SP.13	Liver, Yin Link
SP.15	Yin Link
SP.16	Yin Link

THE SPLEEN ENERGY CENTRE

THE FUNCTION OF THE SPLEEN ENERGY CENTRE

The function of the Spleen energy centre is nourishment, to receive energy coming into the body from the sun, the Yang energy of Heaven, or from the planet, the more Yin energy of Earth, and to distribute these incoming energies to all parts of the energy body. The spleen organ is the physical counterpart of the Spleen energy centre.

THE FUNCTION OF THE SPLEEN ORGAN SYSTEM

In Chinese medicine, the function of the Spleen organ system is nourishment; not only physical nourishment, but emotional and mental nourishment also.

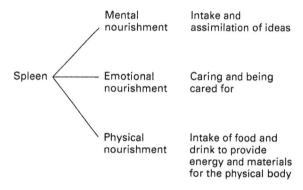

Fig. 15.1

SPLEEN ORGAN SYSTEM DISHARMONIES

If this nutrition function is imbalanced, it may express as Yin or Yang type disharmonies as shown in Table 15.2.

Table 15.2 Yin and Yang disharmonies of the Spleen

	Yin or Deficient disharmony	Yang or Excess disharmony
Mental	intellectual malnutrition	overstudy, mental congestion
Emotional	insecurity, internalized worries	overconcern for others, tending to dominate or intrude
Physical	malnutrition, weakness	overeating, obesity

THE DIFFERENCE BETWEEN THE SPLEEN ENERGY CENTRE AND THE SPLEEN ORGAN SYSTEM

The intake of the Spleen energy centre is considered more as energy radiations from the sun or the planet, while the intake of the Spleen organ system is from the more immediate environment, and, although it includes nour-ishment on the emotional and mental levels, also includes intake of physical material in the form of food and drink.

Relative to the Lungs, the Spleen organ system can be seen as Yin, since the Lungs take in the lighter material of air (Heaven), whilst the Spleen takes in the more solid material of food (Earth). However, compared with the Spleen energy centre, both Lung and Spleen organ systems are Yin, since both air and food are energy as molecules rather than energy as radiation.

RELATIONSHIPS OF THE SPLEEN TO OTHER ORGANS

THE DIGESTIVE SYSTEM

The Spleen rules the digestive system, consisting of the Spleen, Stomach and Intestines. Points such as SP.3, SP.6 and SP.15, can tonify not only the Spleen and Stomach, but also the Small and Large Intestines.

THE SPLEEN AND THE LIVER

The Liver may invade any of the digestive organs with Stagnant Qi, Hyperactive Yang, or Fire as shown in Figure 15.2. SP.1, SP.4, SP.6 and SP.15 can treat Stagnant Liver Qi invading the digestive organs, SP.6 can treat invasion by Hyperactive Liver Yang, and SP.1, SP.2, SP.6 and SP.15 can treat invasion by Liver Fire.

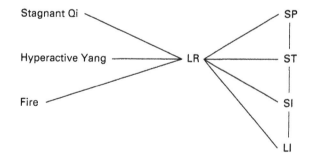

Fig. 15.2

THE SPLEEN AND THE HEART

The Spleen and Stomach provide the Qi and Blood that nourishes the Heart, promote circulation of the Blood, and hold the Spirit stable. Also, a healthy Spleen prevents the accumulation of Damp and Phlegm which could lead to disturbance of mind, emotions, speech and behaviour.

Spleen points such as SP.1, 2, 3, 4 and 6 are therefore main points for mental and emotional problems.

THE SPLEEN AND THE LUNGS

The Spleen and Stomach provide the Qi that enables the Lungs to perform their functions of breathing and control of Qi. Also, the Spleen and Stomach prevent Damp and Phlegm forming, which might then accumulate in chest, throat, nose, sinuses or Eustachian tubes.

SP.3 is often combined with ST.36 to help the Spleen to strengthen the Lungs, and SP.1 and SP.21 can be used for chest pain from Stagnation of Qi and Phlegm in the Lungs.

THE SPLEEN AND THE KIDNEYS

The Spleen and Stomach provide the postnatal energy that is stored and distributed by the Kidneys. If the two organs are deficient, the person is exhausted and points like SP.4 and SP.6 can be used since they tonify both Spleen and Kidneys. Spleen and Kidneys together dominate Fluid metabolism, so that points like SP.3, SP.6 and SP.9 can be used for oedema due to Deficient Spleen and Kidney Qi. When there is joint Deficiency of Spleen and Kidney Yang, moxa on SP.1, SP.2 or SP.3, can strengthen the ability of Spleen and Kidneys to warm and energize the body, hold up the organs and hold in the blood, to treat exhaustion, depression, poor circulation, prolapse and bleeding.

These organ relationships of the Spleen are summarized in Figure 15.3.

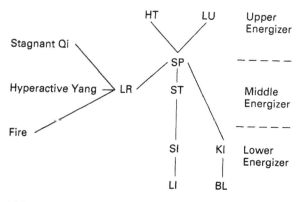

Fig. 15.3

THE RELATIONSHIP BETWEEN SPLEEN, LUNGS AND KIDNEYS

There is a close relationship between these three systems. The Lungs receive the pure Qi of air, and in breathing, the Kidneys hold down the breath. The Spleen is responsible for providing energy from food and drink, which then combines with the energy of air to provide the energy of the body, which can be stored by the Kidneys. The Kidneys provide the mix of prenatal and postnatal energies which activate and catalyse the process of breathing and digestion.

If these three systems are Deficient, the patient is tired, weak and often insecure and depressed. One combination to treat simultaneous Deficiency of Spleen, Lungs and Kidneys, is the three Earth points plus the Conception point corresponding to each system:

KI.3, SP.3, LU.9, CV.4, CV.12, CV.17.

FUNCTIONS OF SPLEEN POINTS

TONIFY QI AND BLOOD

The Earth element, the Spleen and Stomach, not only supply Qi and Blood as sources of energy for the physical, emotional and mental activities of the body, but also as the materials for its solid physical structure. The Spirit can only manifest when clothed in matter, and this supply of physical matter is one of the functions of the Spleen.

SP.3 or SP.6 are usually combined with ST.36 to tonify Qi and Blood.

TREAT INSECURITY

People need to feel the solidity and stability of the Earth element within themselves, or they may be worried and insecure. For example, lack of sufficient physical nourishment or emotional caring in early childhood can lead to the constant feeling or fear in later life of never having enough, the need to be surrounded with material possessions, the fear of loss of material security, or the need to cling in a relationship. When people feel insecure in their environment, or feel this emptiness within, they may compensate by overeating and obesity, which gives them the reassuring feeling of being physically solid, protected by a heavy fleshy envelope.

The Earth element is necessary to give a feeling of being rooted or grounded in oneself, or in the environment. Points such as SP.3, SP.6, ST.36, BL.20 and BL.49 can be used to increase emotional security.

STABILIZE THE EMOTIONS

The lighter, active, expansive energies of the Heart and Liver need to be balanced and held down by the heavier material component of the energies of Earth. The Qi and Blood produced by the Spleen, and stored by the Kidneys and Liver respectively, are necessary to stabilize Heart

Spirit and Liver Yang, and prevent them from rising up the body in an imbalanced way to disturb the mind and emotions.

For example, when Deficient Kidney Qi leads to over-excitability, since there is not enough Qi to hold the Heart Spirit stable, SP.3 can be combined with KI.3 and HT.7. Or, when Deficient Liver Blood leads to emotional hyper-sensitivity, since there is not enough Blood to stabilize Liver Yang, SP.6 can be combined with LR.3 and LR.8.

TRANSFORM DAMP

The transforming and transporting functions of the Spleen prevent the accumulation and stagnation of the body fluids as Damp and Phlegm. Damp can result in dullness, heaviness and lethargy of body, emotions and mind, and Phlegm can result in disturbance and confusion of speech and behaviour, as well as catarrh or fat.

Points such as SP.1, SP.2, SP.3, SP.6 and SP.9 can all assist the function of Transforming Damp, especially when combined with ST.36, ST.40, CV.12 or BL.20. SP.6 and SP.9 are the most effective for Damp Heat, while CV.12, ST.36, SP.1, SP.2 and SP.3, with needle and moxa, are the most effective for Damp Cold. ST.40 is the premier point for Phlegm, while BL.20 can be used for Phlegm, Damp Heat or Damp Cold.

REGULATE DIGESTION

Spleen points, like SP.3 can be used to strengthen a weak digestion, or, like SP.1, SP.2, SP.4 or SP.6 move Stagnant Qi in the Middle Energizer, to ease indigestion and epigastric pain. SP.4, SP.15 can regulate the Qi of the Intestines to treat lower abdominal pain and distension.

MOVE QI AND BLOOD

Many Spleen points, especially SP.1, SP.4, SP.6, SP.8 and SP.21 are powerful in moving Stagnant Qi and Blood. SP.8 is more for the Lower Energizer and legs and SP.21 for the chest, but SP.4 especially, can move Stagnation in the Lower, Middle and Upper Energizer, to treat pain, distension and depression.

REGULATE THE MIND

The Spleen regulates the ability to assimilate and analyse information. It regulates the intellectual faculties of mem-ory and logic. Mental drive and clarity is provided by the Kidneys; vivacity of the mind and conscious awareness are provided by the Heart; imagination and intuition by the Liver; wisdom, and ability to let go of unnecessary structures to experience the clear truth, is provided by the Lungs; but the Spleen provides the ability to ponder and reflect.

If the Spleen Qi is Deficient or Stagnant, memory may become weak and the mind may become congested or slow to take in and digest information. Alternatively, there may be worry, preoccupation or obsessive thoughts and behaviour.

SP.3, SP.6 and SP.10 can strengthen the mind by tonifying Qi and Blood; SP.6 can calm the mind by tonifying the Yin or Stomach, Lungs, Heart, Liver and Kidneys; and SP.1 can invigorate the mind by moving Stagnation.

HOLD UP THE ORGANS AND STOP BLEEDING

Points like SP.3 and SP.6 can be tonified to reduce organ prolapse, or to improve skin and muscle tone, and SP.1 and SP.10 can be used to stop bleeding, either due to Deficient Spleen Qi or to Heat in the Blood.

REMOVE HEAT IN THE BLOOD

SP.1, SP.2, SP.6, and SP.10 can be used to remove Heat in the Blood to treat bleeding in the digestive, urinary, or reproductive systems.

REGULATE THE SKIN

Spleen points are especially important for the treatment of skin disorders as shown in Table 15.3.

Table 15.3 Spleen points for skin disorders

Aetiology	Spleen points
Deficient Blood	SP.6, SP.10 Rf
Deficient Yin	SP.6 Rf
Dryness	SP.6, SP.10 Rf
Heat in the Blood	SP.1, SP.2, SP.6, SP.10 Rd
Damp Heat	SP.6, SP.9 Rd
Stagnant Blood	SP.1, SP.6, SP.8, SP.10 Rd

SPLEEN SYNDROMES

Spleen syndromes are summarized in Table 15.4.

Table 15.4 Point combinations for Spleen syndromes

Syndrome	Signs and symptoms	Pulse	Tongue	Point combination
Deficient Spleen Qi	tiredness, lethargy, weakness, appetite problems, abdominal distension, loose stools, worry and insecurity	empty	pale and flabby, toothmarks	CV.12, ST.36, SP.3 Rf M
+ Deficient Lung Qi	+ bright white face, weak voice, shortness of breath	empty	pale and flabby, toothmarks	+ CV.17 Rf M; LU.9 Rf
+ Deficient Kidney Qi	+ oedema, urinary retention or frequency, back pain, fearfulness	+ deep, maybe choppy	pale and flabby, toothmarks	+ CV.4, KI.3 Rf
+ Deficient Heart Qi	+ cold hands and feet, palpitations, emotional lability, anxiety	+ maybe irregular	+ uneven at tip	+ CV.14, CV.17 Rf M; HT.7 Rf
+ Spleen not holding Blood	+ bleeding in urine or stools, menorrhagia, dull pale face, maybe dizziness	+ choppy	+ maybe very pale	+ SP.1 M; SP.10 Rf M
+ Sinking of Spleen Qi	+ prolapses, poor skin and muscle tone, desire to lie down and rest	+ deep	pale and flabby, toothmarks	+ GV.20, CV.6 Rf M
+ Damp	+ feeling of heaviness in head, limbs, or body, maybe nausea, white discharges or fluid-filled skin eruptions	+ slippery	+ moist greasy white coat	+ CV.6, CV.9 M; SP.9 Rd
+ Phlegm in Lungs	+ catarrh in nose, throat or chest	+ slippery, full in Lung position	+ thick greasy white coat	+ CV.17, BL.13, LU.6, LU.7 E or Rd
+ Phlegm – Damp invades the head	+ dizziness or headache, feeling of heaviness or dullness in the head, mental confusion	+ slippery, maybe flooding	+ greasy white coat	+ GV.20 yìn táng, ST.8, ST.40 Rd
+ Stagnant Liver Qi	+ frustration, depression, nausea, epigastric or abdominal distension or discomfort	+ wiry	+ maybe purplish	+ PC.6, LR.3, LR.13 E or Rd
+ Hyperactive Liver Yang	+ feelings of tiredness, faintness, irritability and headache unless eat at frequent intervals	+ wiry, maybe choppy	+ maybe trembling	+ GV.20, GB.20, GB.40 E
Deficient Spleen Yang	feeling of cold, cold limbs and abdomen, desire for warmth, exhaustion, oedema, undigested food in stools	empty, deep, slow, maybe slippery	pale, moist, maybe swollen, white coat	CV.6, CV.12, ST.28, ST.36, KI.7 Rf M
+ Cold Damp in Spleen	+ acute feeling of coldness, heaviness, lethargy and loss of appetite following exposure to Exterior Cold and Damp	+ flooding or tight	pale, moist, maybe swollen, white coat	+ CV.9, SP.9 Rd M; SP.2 Rf M
Stagnant Spleen and Stomach Qi	feeling of fullness in epigastrium or abdomen, mental congestion, overconcern or clinging possessiveness	flooding, maybe slippery	maybe greasy coat	CV.6, CV.12, LI.10, ST.40, SP.4 E or Rd
+ Stagnant Liver Qi	+ frustration, depression, suppressed anger, nausea or abdominal pain	+ wiry	+ maybe purplish	+ PC.6, LR.1, LR.3, LR.13 Rd

Rf, Reinforcing method; Rd, Reducing method; E, Even method; M, moxa.

Spleen points

SP.1 yĭn bái

Well point, Wood point.

General

SP.1 has three main functions:

invigorates the Spleen
stops bleeding
regulates the mind.

Invigorates the Spleen

As a Well point, SP.1 can invigorate the Spleen and the Spleen channel, to move Stagnation in each of the three Energizers:

Upper Energizer   e.g. chest fullness and pain

Middle Energizer   e.g. epigastric fullness and pain, nausea

Lower Energizer   e.g. abdominal distension, menstrual irregularities.

SP.1 is especially used in acute situations of Stagnation and local Excess.

Stops bleeding

SP.1 strengthens the Spleen's function of holding in the blood and can be used with either needle or moxa cones to stop bleeding from nose, stomach, intestines, bladder or uterus, whether the bleeding is due to Deficiency or to Heat in the Blood.

Regulates the mind

SP.1 can treat psychological problems associated with the effects of Heat or Stagnation on the Heart and Spleen:

Excess Heat

Heart Stagnation
Spleen Stagnation
Appetite problems.

Excess Heat. As a Well point, SP.1 can clear Heat and Interior Wind to treat severe acute conditions such as convulsions and mania.

Heart Stagnation. SP.1 can not only treat chest pain or feelings of oppression in the chest, but also depression, melancholy, insomnia and excessive dreaming.

Spleen Stagnation. SP.1 can be used for feelings of mental congestion, or for when the mind seems blocked and overheated from excessive worry or study.

Appetite problems. SP.1 can help to regulate overweight and overeating, especially when these are associated with worry and depression. It can be used with Reducing method to decrease craving for sweet foods, or it can be used with Reinforcing method and moxa to stimulate appetite and weight gain in cases of Deficient Spleen Yang with Stagnant Spleen Qi.

Syndromes

Stagnant Qi in the Spleen channel
Bleeding
Psychological problems

Stagnant Qi in the Spleen channel

Pulse. Wiry, maybe full, flooding or slippery.

Indications. Chest pain, epigastric pain, lower abdominal distension, menstrual irregularities.

Example. Sensations of cold in the legs.

Combination. SP.1, SP.4, SP.8, ST.41, CV.4 E M; PC.6 E.

Bleeding

Pulse. Maybe empty, thin, choppy and slow; or wiry, full and rapid.

Indications. Epistaxis, bleeding haemorrhoids, haematuria.

Example. Rectal bleeding.

Combination. SP.1 M; SP.6 E; ST.36, CV.4, GV.20 Rf M.

Psychological problems

Heart Stagnation

Pulse. Hindered or wiry, maybe choppy or irregular.

Indications. Depression, dream-disturbed sleep.

Example. Oppressive feeling round the heart with melancholia and mental restlessness.

Combination. SP.1, SP.21, CV.17, PC.1, PC.5 Rd.

Spleen Stagnation

Pulse. Hindered or wiry, maybe slippery or rapid.

Indications. Feelings, mental dullness, congestion or blockage.

Example. Worry, repeating thoughts, repeating dreams and restless sleep.

Combination. SP.1, SP.6, SP.21, CV.17, yìn táng, ān mián, HT.5 Rd.

Appetite problems

Pulse. Wiry, slippery and flooding; or empty and hindered.

Indications. Bulimia, obesity.

Example. Overeating with craving for sweets.

Combination. SP.1, SP.4, ST.36, LR.1, LR.3, LR.13, CV.12, LI.4 Rd.

SP.2 dà dū

Spring point, Fire point, Tonification point.

General

SP.2 can be used like SP.1 to move Stagnation in the Spleen channel affecting the Lower, Middle or Upper Energizer. However, its specific indications are as the Fire point, either to clear Heat, or to tonify Spleen Yang and Fire.

SP.2 to clear fire

SP.2 is the Fire point of the Spleen channel and also a Spring point. It can be used in fevers to remove Exterior Heat and to cause sweating, but its main function is to clear Heart or Damp Heat in the Spleen or Stomach, with such signs as epigastric pain, vomiting or diarrhoea.

SP.2 to tonify Spleen Yang

While SP.2 is seldom used to tonify Spleen Qi, since SP.3, SP.4, SP.6 and ST.36 are more effective, it can be used to tonify Spleen Yang and Fire, with signs of Deficiency, Cold and Damp. For this purpose it is used with Reinforcing method and moxa, and often combined with ST.36 and CV.4.

Syndromes

Heat in Spleen or Stomach
Deficient Spleen Yang

Heat in Spleen or Stomach

Pulse. Rapid, maybe wiry, slippery or flooding.

Indications. Epigastric pain, vomiting, diarrhoea.

Example. Gastritis with nausea, restlessness and insomnia.

Combination. SP.2, ST.21, ST.36, ST.44, PC.3, PC.8 Rd.

Deficient Spleen Yang

Pulse. Empty, maybe deep and slow.

Indications. Loss of appetite, abdominal distension, lethargy, cold hands and feet.

Example. Mental tiredness and dullness.

Combination. SP.1, SP.2, ST.36, ST.45, CV.12, GV.20, LI.1 Rf M; LI.4 E.

SP.3 tài bái

Source point, Stream point, Earth point.

General

SP.3 can be used with Reducing method to move Stagnant Spleen Qi, e.g. for epigastric pain, or to drain Damp Heat, e.g. acute gastroenteritis. However, its main use is to tonify Deficiency, and indeed SP.3 and ST.36 are the two most important points to strengthen the Spleen.

The main tonic effects of SP.3 are summarized in Table 15.5.

Table 15.5 Tonic actions of SP.3

Disorder	Example	Combination
Deficient Qi	tiredness	SP.3, ST.36, LU.9 LI.4 Rf
Deficient Yang	coldness	SP.3, KI.3, ST.36, CV.4 Rf M
Spleen Qi sinking	prolapses	SP.3, KI.7, ST.36, GV.20 Rf M
Damp and Deficiency	oedema	SP.3, SP.9, CV.4, CV.9, Rf M
Phlegm and Deficiency	bronchitis	SP.3, Rf M; ST.40, CV.17, LU.7 E
Deficient Blood	dizziness	SP.3, SP.10, ST.36, LR.3, GV.20, LI.4 Rf
Psychological problems	worry and mental exhaustion	SP.1, SP.3, ST.36, LI.4 yìn táng Rf
Chronic back problems	lumbar ache and weakness	SP.3, BL.23, BL.60 Rf M

The psychological problems treated by SP.3 include mental exhaustion from Deficient Spleen Qi and Yang, mental cloudiness from Damp and Phlegm, and mental restlessness and poor memory from Deficient Blood.

SP.3 can treat chronic back problems of the Deficiency type because it is the Source point and because the Spleen Muscle Region ends in the spine.

Syndromes

Deficient Spleen Qi and Yang
Damp and Phlegm
Deficient Blood
Psychological problems

Deficient Spleen Qi and Yang

Pulse. Empty, maybe deep, slow or slippery.

Indications. Loss of appetite or comfort eating, weight loss or weight gain, tiredness, coldness.

Example. Abdominal distension with empty, cold feeling and borborygmus.

Combination. SP.3, SP.15, ST.36, CV.4, CV.12 Rf M; LI.4 E.

Damp and Phlegm

Pulse. Slippery, maybe empty or flooding.

Indications. Sinus catarrh, bronchitis, oedema, lethargy and heavy sensation in head and limbs.

Example. Arthritis of the knees, worse with tiredness, cold and damp.

Combination. SP.3, SP.9, SP.10, ST.35, ST.36, TE.6 Rf M.

Deficient Blood

Pulse. Thin, choppy.

Indications. Tiredness, blurred vision, insomnia.

Example. Weak muscles and dry skin.

Combination. SP.3, ST.36, BL.18, BL.20 Rf M; LI.4 Rf.

Psychological problems

Pulse. Empty, choppy or slippery.

Indications. Mental exhaustion, poor memory, worry.

Example. Mind seems tired, heavy, vague and dull.

Combination. SP.1, SP.3, SP.9, ST.8, ST.40, ST.45, GV.20, LI.4 Rf.

SP.4 gōng sūn

Connecting point, Opening point of Thoroughfare channel.

General

SP.4 is the Connecting point between the Spleen and Stomach channels and can be used for patterns involving Stomach and Spleen together, e.g. indigestion with chronic loose stools.

SP.4 is the Opening point of the Thoroughfare channel, and most of the indications of SP.4 relate to the functions of this Extra channel. The most important connections of the Thoroughfare channel are to the Kidneys and uterus in the Lower Energizer, the Stomach in the Lower Energizer and the Heart and chest in the Upper Energizer.

The main function of SP.4 and the Thoroughfare channel is to move Stagnation and because the Thoroughfare channel passes through the three Energizers before dispersing in the chest, SP.4 can be used for Stagnant Qi and Blood in the Lower, Middle or Upper Energizer.

Functions of SP.4

The functions of SP.4 are:

  moves Qi and Blood in the legs
  moves Qi and Blood in the uterus
  moves Qi and Blood in the Lower Energizer
  moves Qi and Blood in the Stomach and calms Rebellious Stomach Qi
  moves Qi and Blood in the Heart and chest
  tonifies Qi of Kidneys, Stomach and Spleen.

Moves Qi and Blood in the legs

The Thoroughfare channel represented by SP.4 is important in circulatory disorders because:

- it can move Stagnant Qi and Blood in the legs, especially when combined with ST.30 and ST.31

- it can move Stagnant Blood due to Stagnation in the Heart itself, especially when combined with CV.17 and PC.6

- it can move Stagnant Blood associated with Deficient Blood especially when combined with ST.36 and SP.10

- it can move Stagnant Blood associated with Deficient Kidney Qi or Deficient Kidney Yang, especially when combined with CV.4.

Moves Qi and Blood in the uterus

The Conception channel and the Thoroughfare channel both regulate the uterus. The Conception channel is more concerned with Deficiency of Kidney Qi and with Stagnation of Qi flow, whereas the Thoroughfare channel is more concerned with Deficiency of Blood and Stagnation of Blood. However, by combining SP.4 and PC.6 with Conception channel points, the Conception and Thoroughfare channels can be treated simultaneously. For example, for amenorrhoea due to Deficient Kidney Qi and Deficient Blood, SP.4 and PC.6 can be combined with CV.4; or for dysmenorrhoea due to Stagnant Qi and Stagnant Blood, SP.4 and PC.6 can be combined with CV.3 or CV.6.

Moves Qi and Blood in the Lower Energizer

SP.4 can regulate Stagnant Qi in the Intestines, including problems where Damp or Damp Heat are associated with the Stagnation of Qi, for example borborgymus, abdominal distension or diarrhoea. SP.4 can be used for conditions involving both the Middle and Lower Energizers, for example gastroenteritis involving both Stomach and Intestines. Also, SP.4 can treat abdominal masses or painful conditions of Stagnant Blood in the Lower Energizer, e.g. following trauma or surgery.

Moves Qi and Blood in the Stomach and calms Rebellious Stomach Qi

SP.4 can be used with PC.6 both to move Stagnation in the Stomach, for example epigastric pain and bleeding often in combination with CV.12; and also to calm Rebellious Stomach Qi, e.g. nausea and vomiting, often in combination with CV.14.

Moves Qi and Blood in the Heart and chest

SP.4 is usually combined with PC.6 and CV.17 for this syndrome, and if there is general Stagnation of Qi, CV.6 may be added. In addition, SP.4 may be combined with SP.21, the point of the Great Connecting channel of the Spleen, which radiates through the chest.

SP.4 is not as powerful as SP.6 in calming the mind, and if it is used for this purpose is generally combined with PC.6 which has a powerful effect on the Heart. SP.4 can combine with SP.1 to move Stagnation of Qi in the chest, associated with depression, melancholy and emotional stagnation, but again would generally be combined with CV.17 and PC.6 for this purpose.

Tonifies Qi of Kidneys, Stomach and Spleen

The Thoroughfare channel links the prenatal energies of the Kidney with the postnatal energies of Stomach and Spleen. SP.4 can be used with Reinforcing method to tonify the capacity of the Spleen to form energy and the capacity of the Kidneys to store both the prenatal and postnatal energies and to release these when required for the needs of the body. SP.4 can therefore be used when there is chronic tiredness and weakness associated with both inherited weakness of constitution and weak digestion. SP.4, PC.6 and CV.4 are usually combined for this problem, which is often accompanied by poor peripheral circulation, especially in the lower legs. This pattern may be accompanied by anxiety, depression or both and variations of the basic SP.4, PC.6, CV.4 combination are discussed on page 114 in the section on Eight Extra channels.

Syndromes

Stagnant Qi and Blood in the legs
Stagnant Qi and Blood in the uterus
Stagnant Qi and Blood in the Lower Energizer
Stagnant Qi and Blood in the Stomach and Rebellious Stomach Qi
Stagnant Qi and Blood in the Heart and chest
Deficient Qi of Kidneys, Stomach and Spleen

Stagnant Qi and Blood in the legs

Pulse. Wiry, slippery.

Indications. Varicose veins, Raynaud's disease, Buerger's disease.

Example. Poor circulation in the legs.

Combination. SP.1, SP.4, SP.8, ST.30, ST.31, ST.41, PC.6 Rd; CV.6 Rf M.

Stagnant Qi and Blood in the uterus

Pulse. Wiry, choppy, maybe empty or full.

Indications. Irregular menstruation, dysmenorrhoea, endometriosis.

Example. Dysmenorrhoea with heavy bleeding.

Combination. SP.1, SP.4, ST.29, PC.6 Rd; CV.3 E.

Stagnant Qi and Blood in the Lower Energizer

Pulse. Wiry, maybe slippery.

Indications. Abdominal masses, abdominal pain and distension, abdominal trauma, diarrhoea.

Example. Pain and distension from uterine fibroid.

Combination. SP.4, PC.6, ST.30, CV.3 Rd.

Stagnant Qi and Blood in the Stomach and Rebellious Stomach Qi

Pulse. Wiry, maybe slippery, maybe flooding.

Indications. Epigastric pain, gastric bleeding, nausea, vomiting.

Example. Gastroenteritis.

Combination. SP.4, PC.6, CV.12, CV.6, ST.39 Rd.

Stagnant Qi and Blood in the Heart and chest

Pulse. Wiry, choppy, maybe jerky or irregular.

Indications. Chest or heart pain and discomfort in the chest with depression and loneliness.

Combination. SP.1, SP.4, SP.21, PC.6 Rd; CV.6, CV.17 E.

Deficient Qi of Kidneys, Stomach and Spleen

Pulse. Empty, maybe deep and choppy.

Indications. Weak constitution, exhaustion, weak digestion, poor circulation.

Example. Exhaustion with anxiety and depression.

Combination. SP.4, PC.6, CV.4, CV.14, CV.17 Rf.

SP.6 sān yīn jiāo

Crossing point of Spleen, Liver and Kidney channels.

General

SP.6 is one of the major points of acupuncture and the range of its functions is listed here:

tonifies the Spleen
tonifies Qi and Blood
raises Qi
holds in the Blood
regulates Liver Qi
softens masses
moves the Blood and stops pain
resolves Damp
tonifies Yin
cools the Blood
calms the mind
regulates the skin
regulates the joints

regulates the circulatory system
regulates digestive problems
regulates the urinary system
regulates the reproductive system.

Tonifies the Spleen

Any point that tonifies the Spleen, e.g. SP.3, SP.6, ST.36, BL.20 or CV.12, will have five related functions:

tonifies the digestive system	SP.6 + CV.12
tonifies Qi and Blood of the whole body	SP.6 + ST.36
resolves Damp	SP.6 + SP.9
raises Qi	SP.6 + GV.20
holds in the Blood	SP.6 + SP.1.

Illustrative combinations with SP.6 are given for each of the five functions.

SP.6 differs from SP.3, in that SP.6 is better for Deficient Spleen Qi with Stagnant Qi in the digestive system, with Even method, while SP.3 is better for Deficient Spleen Qi and Yang, with Reinforcing method and moxa. SP.6 is often combined with CV.12, since these two points have both tonifying and moving action, and SP.3 is often combined with CV.4, since these two points together tonify Spleen and Kidneys, via the Source Qi.

Tonifies Qi and Blood

The combination of SP.6 and ST.36 treats chronic tiredness due to Deficient Qi and Blood, and other points may be added depending on the overall pattern. For example, for chronic tiredness with inability to concentrate, yìn táng can be added, or for chronic tiredness with a desire to lie down, GV.20 can be included.

Raises Qi

Since it tonifies Spleen Qi, SP.6 can be included in combinations to raise the Qi of the Middle and Lower Energizers, to treat a variety of organ prolapses and also to improve skin and muscle tone.

Stops bleeding

SP.6 can be combined with other points such as SP.1, LR.1 and GV.20 to increase the capacity to hold the blood in the vessels. This is partly because SP.6 cools Heat in the Blood and drains Damp Heat, and partly because it raises Spleen Qi.

Regulates Liver Qi

SP.6 affects the Liver in various ways:

moves Stagnant Liver Qi
calms Hyperactive Liver Yang
tonifies Liver Yin
tonifies Liver Blood.

It can be used when Stagnant Liver Qi is affecting the Lower Energizer, such as abdominal pain and distension or dysmenorrhoea. It can also be used in hypertension associated with Deficient Liver Yin and Hyperactive Liver Yang or Liver Fire, with symptoms such as headache, migraine, dizziness.

Softens masses

SP.6 can be used to treat enlargement of lymph glands, spleen or liver, and to treat abdominal masses such as fibroids or cysts. This is due to its ability to move Liver Qi and to move Blood.

Moves the Blood and stops pain

SP.6 is one of the main points to move Stagnant Blood and relieve pain, especially in the lower abdomen and legs. It is often combined with LI.4, and electroacupuncture may be used if the pain is severe or does not respond to normal Reducing method, for example dysmenorrhoea or pain in childbirth.

Resolves Damp

SP.6, often in combination with SP.9, can help to resolve Damp, especially in the Lower Energizer, e.g. diarrhoea, cystitis, oedema, leucorrhoea. It can resolve Damp Cold or Damp Heat, and can be used to remove Damp in skin conditions and arthritis.

Tonifies Yin

Table 15.6 shows the points that can be combined with SP.6 to treat the Yin Deficiency syndrome, and the points that can be added to these combinations, when there is also Deficiency Fire.

Table 15.6 SP.6 combinations for deficient Yin

Syndrome	Point for Deficient Yin	Point for Deficiency Fire	Example
Deficient Kidney Yin	KI.6	KI.2	dry skin
Deficient Liver Yin	LR.8	LR.2	dry eyes
Deficient Stomach Yin	ST.36	ST.44	gastritis
Deficient Heart Yin	HT.6	HT.8	insomnia
Deficient Lung Yin	LU.3	LU.10	dry cough

SP.6 can be used as the basis of a combination to treat Deficient Yin or Deficiency Fire of two or more organs together, for example:

Deficient Heart and + Deficiency Heart   e.g. restless-
Kidney Yin   and Kidney Fire   ness and
SP.6, HT.6, KI.6 Rf + HT.8, KI.2 Rd   insomnia

Deficient Lung and   + Deficiency Lung   e.g. dry
Kidney Yin   and Kidney Fire   cough and
SP.6, LU.3, KI.6   + LU.10, KI.2 Rd   sore throat

Cools the Blood

SP.5 is a major point to cool the Blood, for example, to stop bleeding or to treat skin disorders. This is partly due to the ability of SP.6 to tonify Yin.

Calms the mind

SP.6 can regulate the mind and emotions for a variety of reasons.

- by moving Stagnant Liver Qi it can relieve depression, frustration and blocked anger

- by moving Stagnant Blood it can relieve pain

- it can tonify the Blood so that the Heart and Liver Spirits are properly balanced

- it can tonify Yin of Kidneys, Heart, Liver and Stomach, and relieve Deficiency Fire syndromes of these organs

- it can calm Hyperactive Liver Yang to treat hypersensitivity, irritability and emotional lability

- by cooling the Blood, it can relieve the distress associated with severe skin irritation.

Table 15.7 SP.6 combinations to calm the mind

Syndrome	Example	Combination
Stagnant Liver Qi	frustration and depression	SP.6, SP.21, LR.3, LR.14, CV.17 Rd
Stagnant Blood	anxiety from chest pain	SP.6, SP.21, PC.1, PC.6, CV.14, CV.17 Rd
Deficient Spleen and Heart Blood	insomnia and feeling of vulnerability	SP.6, ST.36, GV.20, CV.4 Rf; HT.7 Rd
Deficient Heart Yin and Heart Fire	menopausal neurosis	SP.6, HT.3, KI.6 Rf; HT.8, CV.14 Rd
Hyperactive Liver Yang and Deficient Kidney Qi	irritability and emotional lability	SP.6, KI.3 Rf; LR.3, GB.34, GV.20 Rd
Heat in the Blood	extreme distress from skin irritation	SP.6, SP.10, PC.3, PC.8, HT.7 Rd

Rd, Reducing method; Rf, Reinforcing method

Regulates the skin

SP.6 is a basic point for skin problems, discussed in Chapter 33, since it can be used, according to the situation for skin patterns associated with:

Damp
Damp Heat
Dryness
Deficient Blood
Deficient Yin
Deficiency Fire
Heat in the Blood
Stagnant Qi and Blood.

Regulates the joints

SP.6 can be used to resolve Damp in arthritis, whether Damp Cold or Damp Heat, often in combination with SP.9 and suitable local points.

Regulates the circulatory system

Hypertension. SP.6 can be used to treat hypertension, since it moves Liver Qi, calms Hyperactive Liver Yang, tonifies Kidney, Liver and Heart Yin, and relieves Deficiency Fire of these organs. SP.6 can also resolve Damp to treat hypertension due to Damp affecting the head.

Heart disease. While SP.4 is better for heart and chest pain, especially when combined with SP.21 and SP.1, SP.6 is better to control Heart patterns associated with Deficient Heart Yin and Deficiency Heart Fire. SP.6 is therefore preferable for palpitations accompanied by restlessness, insomnia and feverish agitation. SP.6 has been used successfully for rheumatic heart disease in combination with HT.7, PC.6, PC.7 and CV.17.

Peripheral circulation. SP.4 and PC.6 are commonly combined for cold hands and feet or for more serious circulatory disorders, such as Buerger's disease. However, SP.6 and PC.6 is an alternative combination, and may be preferable especially when the restriction is intermittent and related to stress, as in Raynaud's disease.

Varicose veins. All the Spleen points on the lower leg, especially SP.1, 4, 6 and 8, are effective for varicose veins. However, there is often varicose ulceration or thinning and hardening of the skin around SP.6 and this point cannot be used and other Spleen points may have to be substituted.

Regulates the digestive system

Some of the uses of SP.6 for digestive problems are given in Table 15.8.

Table 15.8 SP.6 combinations for digestive problems

Syndrome	Example	Combination
Deficient Spleen and Stomach Qi	epigastric distension and discomfort	SP.6, ST.36, CV.12 Rf M
Deficient Qi and Yin of Intestines	constipation	SP.6, SP.15, CV.6, TE.6 E
Spleen not holding the Blood	gastrointestinal bleeding	SP.1, SP.6, SP.10, CV.4 Rf M
Stagnation of Qi in Intestines	abdominal distension and pain	SP.6, ST.39, LI.10, CV.6 Rd
Damp Heat in Intestines	diarrhoea	SP.6, SP.9, ST.25, CV.6 Rd
Deficient Stomach Yin and Stomach Fire	gastritis	SP.6, ST.21, ST.36, ST.44, PC.6 E

Regulates the urinary system

Since SP.6 moves Stagnant Qi in the Lower Energizer and resolves Damp, whether Damp Cold or Damp Heat, it is a most important point to treat oedema and urinary problems, such as cystitis, nephritis and urinary incontinence or retention. Prostatitis is included in this section, and SP.6 is a main point for this disorder.

Regulates the reproductive system

The multiple function of SP.6 enables it to treat a very wide range of reproductive disorders, some examples being shown in Table 15.9.

Table 15.9 SP.6 combinations for reproductive disroders

Syndrome	Example	Combination
Deficient Kidney Yang and Stagnation of Qi	impotence with depression	SP.6, HT.7, LR.5 E; CV.4 Rf M
Stagnation of Qi and Blood in the uterus	dysmenorrhoea	SP.6, ST.29, CV.3 Rd
Heat in the Blood	menorrhagia	SP.1, SP.6, LR.1, CV.7 Rd
Sinking of Spleen Qi	uterine prolapse	SP.6, GB.28, ST.30, CV.6, GV.20 Rf
Damp Heat in Lower Energizer	leucorrhoea	SP.6, GB.26, CV.3 Rd
Deficient Yin of Heart and Liver	menopausal syndrome	SP.6, HT.6, KI.6 Rf; LR.2, TE.6 Rd

Syndromes

Deficient Qi and Blood
Sinking of Spleen Qi
Skin disorders
Arthritis disorders
Circulatory disorders
Digestive disorders
Urinary disorders

Reproductive disorders
Psychological disorders

Deficient Qi and Blood

Pulse. Empty, choppy, maybe changing or deep.

Indications. Exhaustion, poor skin and muscle tone, lack of interest or emotional lability.

Example. Tiredness, blurred vision and lack of concentration.

Combination. SP.6, ST.36, BL.20, BL.43, GV.20 Rf.

Sinking of Spleen Qi

Pulse. Empty, deep, maybe slow.

Indications. Prolapses, desire to lie down, muscular weakness.

Example. Haemorrhoids, worse with tiredness.

Combination. SP.6, GV.1, GV.20, ST.36 Rf M.

Skin disorders

Pulse. Various.

Indications. Eczema, psoriasis, dry skin.

Example. Vaginal irritation and discharge.

Combination. SP.6, SP.9, GB.26, GB.34, CV.3 Rd.

Arthritis disorders

Pulse. Slippery, thin or flooding, maybe choppy or rapid and wiry.

Indications. All arthritic disorders associated with Damp.

Example. Rheumatoid arthritis of thumb and first two fingers.

Combination. SP.6, SP.9, LU.10, special point in line with LU.10 at the base of the metacarpal, bāxié Rd; sìfèng B.

Circulatory disorders

Pulse. Often wiry, maybe slippery, choppy, thin or flooding.

Indications. Hypertension, heart pain, palpitations, poor peripheral circulation, varicose veins.

Example. Hypertension due to Deficient Liver Yin and Hyperactive Liver Yang.

Combination. SP.6 Rf; LR.3, GB.20, GB.34, LI.4 Rd.

Digestive disorders

Pulse. Maybe wiry, slippery, empty or flooding.

Indications. Epigastric or abdominal pain or distension, constipation or diarrhoea, stomach prolapse.

Example. Gastritis and restlessness from excessive tea consumption.

Combination. SP.6, ST.21, ST.36, ST.44, GV.20, HT.6 E.

Urinary disorders

Pulse. Often slippery and wiry, maybe empty deep and slow, or flooding and fast.

Indications. Oedema, nephritis, renal pain, cystitis, incontinence.

Example. Prostatitis and exhaustion.

Combination. SP.6, ST.29, CV.2, LI.4 E; ST.36, CV.4 Rf M.

Reproductive disorders

Pulse. Various.

Indications. Impotence, infertility, irregular menstruation, difficult labour, menopausal syndrome.

Example. Infertility.

Combination. SP.6, KI.6, ST.29, CV.3, LI.4 E.

Psychological disorders

Pulse. Various.

Indications. Insomnia, restlessness, hypersensitivity, emotional lability.

Example. Difficulty in concentration, feelings of unreality and restlessness.

Combination. SP.6, ST.36, LI.4, GV.20 E.

SP.8 dì jī

Accumulation point.

General

The main function of SP.8 is to move Stagnant Blood and relieve pain, especially in the lower abdomen and the legs. SP.8 is also used to treat Stagnant Qi in the Lower Energizer with abdominal distension, discomfort and oedema. Although SP.8 is specific for severe acute painful conditions, e.g. dysmenorrhoea, it can also be used for chronic conditions of Stagnant Qi and Blood, such as oedema or varicose veins.

Syndromes

Stagnant Blood in the uterus
Stagnant Qi and Blood in the legs
Stagnant Qi in the abdomen

Stagnant Blood in the uterus

Pulse. Wiry, maybe full or choppy.

Indications. Irregular menstruation, amenorrhoea, menorrhagia, dysmenorrhoea.

Example. Dysmenorrhoea due to Stagnant Blood.

Combination. SP.8, LI.4, ST.30, CV.3 Rd.

Stagnant Qi and Blood in the legs

Pulse. Wiry, choppy.

Indications. Peripheral circulation problems, varicose veins, leg oedema.

Example. Varicose veins and cold feet.

Combination. SP.4, SP.8, PC.6 Rd; CV.4 Rf M.

Stagnant Qi in the abdomen

Pulse. Wiry, slippery.

Indications. Abdominal pain and distension, oedema, dysuria.

Example. Oedema of abdomen and legs.

Combination. SP.4, SP.8, ST.28, ST.40, ST.41, TE.6 Rd; CV.6 Rf M.

SP.9 yīn líng quán

Sea point, Water point.

General

SP.9 is one of the main points for resolving Damp, whether Damp Cold or Damp Heat, and especially Damp in the lower body, e.g. oedema. SP.9 can be used in combination with SP.6 to treat Damp-related disorders of the skin, the joints, the digestive, urinary and reproductive systems. Some examples are shown in Table 15.10.

Table 15.10 SP.6 + SP.9 combinations

Syndrome	Example	Combination
Damp Heat	eczema	SP.6, SP.9, GB.34, GB.39, TE.5 Rd
Damp Cold	arthritis of the knee	SP.6, SP.9, LR.7, ST.36, xī yǎn Rd M
Damp Cold	abdominal distension	SP.6, SP.9, CV.6, CV.9 Rd M
Damp	urinary dribbling	SP.6, SP.9, BL.23, BL.31 Rd; GV.4 Rf M
Damp Heat	leucorrhoea	SP.6, SP.9, CV.3 Rd; CV.6 E

Rd, Reducing method; Rf, Reinforcing method; E. Even method; M, moxa.

Common combinations of SP.9

Some common combinations with SP.9 are given in Table 15.11, in all these cases SP.6 can be added to the combination. SP.6 and SP.9 are used with Reducing method and the other points as indicated.

Table 15.11 Common combinations with SP.9

+ SP.15 Rd	Damp Heat in Intestine
+ ST.25 Rd	Damp Cold or Damp Heat in Intestine
+ ST.28 Rd	Damp in Lower Energizer, Stagnation of Qi in Kidney and Bladder
+ ST.36 Rf	Deficient Qi and Damp
+ ST.39 Rd	Damp Heat in Intestines
+ ST.40 Rd	Damp and Phlegm
+ GB.34 Rd	Damp Heat in Liver–Gallbladder
+ TE.6 Rd	Damp in Lower Energizer
+ GV.4 Rf M	Damp Cold and Deficient Kidney Yang
+ CV.3 Rd	Damp Heat
+ CV.4 Rf M	Damp Cold and Deficient Kidney Qi
+ CV.6 E	Damp and Stagnant Qi
+ CV.9 Rd	Damp Cold or Damp Heat
+ CV.12 Rf	Damp and Deficient Spleen Qi

Less common uses of SP.9

SP.9 can be used for palpitations, headache or vertigo, if these patterns are associated with Damp. SP.6, SP.9 and ST.40 are used with Reducing method to clear Damp and Phlegm, and BL.20 may be used with Reinforcing method and moxa. Other points are selected according to requirements.

SP.9, ST.36, PC.6 and CV.12 can be used with Reducing method for nausea and vomiting when this is due to Damp. In addition sìfèng can be pricked to remove food stagnation.

Syndromes

Skin disorders
Arthritis disorders
Digestive disorders due to Damp — see SP.6
Urinary disorders
Reproductive disorders

SP.10 xuè hǎi

General

SP.10 governs the Blood in three ways:

moves the Blood
cools the Blood
tonifies the Blood.

Moves the Blood

SP.10 is used with Reducing method to move the Blood in three main areas: uterus, leg, knee.

Moves the Blood in the uterus. SP.10 can treat amenorrhoea, irregular menstruation and dysmenorrhoea, but SP.4, SP.6, and SP.9 are more powerful in this respect, and SP.10 is usually used as a secondary addition to these primary points.

Moves the Blood in the leg. SP.10 can be used as part of a chain of Spleen points to move Qi and Blood in the leg to treat chronic psoriasis, varicose veins or poor circulation.

Moves Blood in the knee. SP.10 can be used with Reducing method, or bled and cupped for local knee injury or chronic arthritis of the knee.

Cools the Blood

SP.10 can be used in combination with SP.1, SP.2, or SP.6 with Reducing method or bleeding, to cool Heat in the Blood, to treat red, hot itchy skin disorders, or to treat menorrhagia.

Tonifies the Blood

Although SP.10 may be a less effective Blood tonic than SP.6, ST.36, BL.17, BL.20 or BL.43, it can be combined with these points, for example to moisten and nourish dry skin or to treat general anaemia. In this case the points are used with Reinforcing method, and perhaps moxa, in the absence of Deficient Yin.

Syndromes

Stagnant Blood
Heat in the Blood
Deficient Blood

Stagnant Blood

Pulse. Wiry, choppy.

Indications. Dysmenorrhoea, varicose veins, arthritis of the knee.

Example. Psoriasis due to Stagnant Blood.

Combination. SP.6, SP.10, LI.4, LI.10, BL.16, BL.17, BL.40 Rd.

Heat in the Blood

Pulse. Rapid, full, maybe wiry.

Indications. Menorrhagia, red skin lesions.

Example. Acute eczema with severe itching and dryness.

Combination. SP.6, SP.10, LI.4, HT.7 Rd; SP.1, PC.9, BL.40 B.

Deficient Blood

Pulse. Thin, choppy.

Indications. Blurred vision, dizziness, tiredness, insomnia.

Example. Dry, rough skin remaining after successful treatment of eczema due to Heat in the Blood.

Combination. SP.6, KI.6, ST.36, LI.4, BL.17, BL.20 Rf.

SP.15 dà héng

Point of Yin Link channel.

Channel

SP.15 is a point for abdominal problems, especially disorders of the Large Intestine. SP.15 has three main functions:

moves Qi
resolves Damp
tonifies Spleen Qi.

Moves Qi

Stagnation of Qi may arise in the abdomen from lack of exercise, poor posture, trauma, Cold and Damp, or Liver Qi Stagnation. This may result in abdominal distension and pain, and in constipation. By moving the Qi in the abdomen in general and the Intestines in particular, SP.15 can treat these conditions, often in combination with CV.6 and TE.6 with Reducing method.

Resolves Damp

Damp may be associated with Deficient Qi and Yang of the Spleen, and with Liver Qi Stagnation. It may show as Damp Cold or Damp Heat, loose stools, diarrhoea or

dysentery. SP.15 can be combined with SP.6 and SP.9 with Reducing method to remove the Damp.

Tonifies the Damp

If the Spleen and Large Intestine Qi is Deficient there may be chronic constipation, which can be treated with SP.15 combined with ST.36 and CV.6 with Reinforcing method. Since SP.15 tonifies Spleen Qi, it can be used, like SP.21 with Reinforcing method and moxa for cold weak limbs.

Syndromes

Stagnant Qi in the abdomen
Damp in the Intestine
Deficient Qi of the Intestines

Stagnant Qi in the abdomen

Pulse. Wiry, maybe slippery or flooding.

Indications. Abdominal distension and pain, constipation.

Example. Irritable bowel syndrome with colon pain.

Combination. SP.6, SP.15, LR.3, GB.27, CV.6, PC.6 E.

Damp in the Intestines

Pulse. Slippery, maybe wiry, flooding.

Indications. Abdominal distension, diarrhoea, dysentery.

Example. Indigestion and diarrhoea associated with food intolerance.

Combination. SP.6, SP.15, ST.36, LR.3, LR.13, LI.10 E.

Deficient Qi of the Intestines

Pulse. Empty or big, may be slippery.

Indications. Constipation, faecal incontinence.

Example. Chronic constipation, slow digestion and tiredness.

Combination. SP.15, ST.36, LI.10, CV.6, CV.12 E.

SP.21 dà bāo

Point of Great Spleen, Connecting Channel.

General

The main function of SP.21 is to move Stagnant Qi and Blood in the chest, since SP.21 controls the Great Spleen

Connecting channel which radiates through the chest. SP.21 is often combined with SP.4 for this purpose, since SP.9 is the opening point for the Thoroughfare channel, which flows through the three Energizers and can be used for Qi and Blood Stagnation in the chest. SP.1 is often added to the combination of SP.21 and SP.4, since, as the end point, and as the Well point of the Spleen it can move Stagnation anywhere on the channel.

SP.21, combined with either SP.1 or SP.4, or with both, can be used for heart and chest pain, hypochondriac pain, dyspnoea and asthma, and for depression and melancholy with feelings of fullness in the chest. In suitable combination, for example, with SP.1 and SP.6, it can be used for insomnia.

SP.21, as the point for the Great Connecting channel of the Spleen, can also be used for generalized aches and pains due to Stagnant Qi and Blood, not just in the chest, but in the whole body. In addition, if used with Reinforcing method, SP.21 can be effective in Deficiency conditions such as emaciation after long illness or weakness of the limbs.

Syndromes

Stagnant Qi and Blood in the chest
Stagnant Qi and Blood in the whole body

Stagnant Qi and Blood in the chest

Pulse. Wiry, maybe choppy, slow or irregular.

Indications. Hypochondriac pain, aches and pain, fullness in chest or heart.

Example. Depression and feeling of obstruction in the chest.

Combination. SP.1, SP.4, SP.21, PC.1, PC.6, CV.17 Rd.

Stagnant Qi and Blood in the whole body

Pulse. Hindered or wiry, full or empty maybe choppy.

Indications. General tiredness and weakness, aches in limbs.

Combination. SP.6, SP.21, ST.36, LI.4 Rf; SP.1 M.

Spleen point comparisons and combinations

The functions of the main poins of the Spleen channel are given in Table 15.12.

Table 15.12 Spleen point comparison

Point	Point type	Syndrome
SP.1	Well point	Stagnant Spleen Qi
	Wood point	Bleeding, psychological problems
SP.2	Spring point	Heat in Spleen and Stomach
	Fire Point	Deficient Spleen Yang
	Tonification point	
SP.3	Stream point	Deficient Spleen Qi and Yang
	Earth point	Damp and Phlegm
	Source point	Deficient Blood, psychological problems
SP.4	Connecting point	Stagnant Qi and Blood
	Opening point of Thoroughfare channel	in the legs, in the uterus, in the Lower Jiao
		in the Stomach, in the Heart and chest
		Deficient Qi of Kidneys and Spleen
SP.6	Meeting point of Spleen,	Deficient Qi and Blood
	Liver and Kidney channels	Sinking of Spleen Qi
		skin disorders, arthritis, circulatory disorders
		digestive disorders, urinary disorders
		reproductive disorders, psychological disorders
SP.8	Accumulation point	Stagnant Blood in the uterus
		Stagnant Qi and Blood in the legs
		Stagnant Qi in the abdomen
SP.9	Sea point	Damp
	Water point	skin disorders, arthritis, digestive disorders, urinary disorders,
		reproductive disorders
SP.10		Stagnant Blood, Heat in the Blood, Deficient Blood
SP.15	Point of Yin Link	Stagnant Qi in the abdomen
	channel	Damp in the Intestine
		Deficient Intestine Qi
SP.21	Point of Great Spleen	Stagnant Qi and Blood
	Connecting channel	in the chest, in the whole body
		Deficient Qi and Blood

Some common combinations of Spleen channel points with each other and with points from other channels are given in Tables 15.13 and 15.14 respectively.

Table 15.13 Combinations of Spleen points

Point	Combination	Syndromes	Example
SP.1	SP.2	Deficient Spleen Yang	poor peripheral circulation
SP.1	SP.3	Deficient Spleen Qi	slow digestion
SP.1	SP.4	Stagnant Spleen Qi	epigastric fullness and pain
SP.1	SP.6	Spleen not holding the Blood	bleeding haemorrhoids
SP.1	SP.8	Stagnant Blood	painful varicose veins
SP.1	SP.10	Heat in the Blood	acute eczema
SP.1	SP.21	Stagnant Qi and Blood	depression and chest pain
SP.2	SP.3	Deficient Spleen Qi and Yang	Cold Damp diarrhoea
SP.2	SP.10	Heat in the Blood	varicose inflammation
SP.2	SP.15	Deficient Spleen Qi and Yang	abdominal distension
SP.3	SP.9	Deficient Spleen Qi and Damp	feelings of lethargy and heaviness
SP.3	SP.10	Deficient Spleen Blood	anaemia
SP.3	SP.15	Deficient Intestinal Qi	constipation
SP.4	SP.8	Stagnant Blood	dysmenorrhoea
SP.4	SP.15	Stagnant Qi	abdominal distension and pain
SP.4	SP.21	Stagnant Qi and Blood	chest pain
SP.6	SP.8	Stagnant Qi and Blood	varicose veins
SP.6	SP.9	Damp Heat	arthritis
SP.6	SP.10	Heat in the Blood	psoriasis
SP.6	SP.15	Damp Heat in Intestines	diarrhoea
SP.6	SP.21	Deficient Spleen and Heart Blood	tiredness and palpitations
SP.8	SP.10	Stagnant Blood	knee trauma
SP.8	SP.15	Stagnant Qi and Blood	lower abdominal pain
SP.9	SP.15	Damp Heat in Lower Energizer	dysentery
SP.1	SP.2, 3	Stagnant Spleen Qi	overeating
SP.1	SP.2, 4	Stagnant Qi and Blood	poor peripheral circulation
SP.1	SP.2, 6	Stagnant Spleen Qi	insomnia
SP.1	SP.2, 10	Heat in the Blood	menorrhagia
SP.1	SP.4, 8	Stagnant Blood in the legs	varicose veins and poor circulation
SP.1	SP.4, 15	Stagnant Qi in the Intestines	abdominal distension and pain
SP.1	SP.4, 21	Stagnant Qi and Blood in the chest	chest pains and palpitations
SP.1	SP.6, 10	Stagnant Qi and Heat in the Lower Energizer	menorrhagia and dysmenorrhoea
SP.2	SP.3, 9	Deficient Spleen Qi and Yang with Damp	oedema
SP.6	SP.9, 15	Damp Heat in Intestines	irritable bowel syndrome
SP.6	SP.10, 21	Heat in the Blood and Deficient Heart Yin	eczema and insomnia
SP.1	SP.2, 4, 8	Stagnation of Blood in the legs	cold feet
SP.1	SP.2, 4, 12	Stagnation of Blood in the legs	Buerger's disease
SP.1	SP.2, 6, 21	Stagnation of Qi and Heat	restlessness and insomnia
SP.2	SP.6, 9, 10	Stagnation of Qi and Blood with Damp Heat	chronic psoriasis

Table 15.14 Combinations of Spleen and Stomach points

Spleen point	Stomach points	Syndrome	Example
SP.1	ST.45	Stomach Fire	gastritis with excessive appetite
		Stomach and Heart Fire	dream-disturbed sleep
		Heat in the Blood	blood in the stool
		Stagnant Spleen and Stomach Qi	mental congestion
		Stagnant Blood	cold feet and legs
SP.2	ST.44	Heat in Stomach and Intestines	gastritis and constipation
		Deficient Spleen Yang	coldness and exhaustion
		Stagnant Stomach Qi	epigastric pain and distension
SP.3	ST.36	Deficient Qi and Blood	muscular atrophy
		Deficient Spleen Qi	loss of appetite and loss of weight
		Damp and Phlegm	nausea and vomiting
SP.4	ST.21	Stagnant Stomach Qi and Rebellious Stomach Qi	epigastric pain and belching
SP.4	ST.30	Deficient Qi and Blood	lethargy and weak muscles
		Stagnant Qi and Blood	poor circulation in the legs
SP.4	ST.36	Deficient Qi and Blood of Heart and Spleen	palpitations and insomnia
		Deficient Qi of Spleen and Kidneys	fearful insecurity
SP.4	ST.40	Stagnation of Qi in Lower Energizer	abdominal distension and oedema
		Stagnation of Qi and Blood	chest pain following injury in the chest
SP.6	ST.2	Deficient Qi and Blood eye disorders	blurred vision
SP.6	ST.8	Hyperactive Liver Yang	headache
SP.6	ST.18	Deficient Qi and Blood	insufficient lactation
SP.6	ST.21	Deficient Stomach Yin	gastritis and restless exhaustion
SP.6	ST.25	Damp Heat in the Intestines	diarrhoea
SP.6	ST.28	Damp Heat in the Bladder	dysuria
SP.6	ST.29	Stagnant Blood in uterus	dysmenorrhoea
SP.6	ST.30	Sinking of Spleen Qi	uterine prolapse
SP.6	ST.36	Deficient Qi and Blood	emotional lability
		Sinking of Spleen Qi	stomach prolapse
		Deficient Blood	hair loss
		Deficient Blood of Heart and Spleen	worry and insomnia
		Deficient Stomach Yin	sore throat
		Deficient Lung Qi and Yin	cough and sore throat
		Deficient Spleen and Kidney Qi	oedema
		Liver invades Spleen and Stomach	nausea, belching and indigestion
SP.6	ST.37	Dryness in the Intestines	constipation
SP.6	ST.39	Damp Heat in Intestines	enteritis
SP.6	ST.40	Damp and Phlegm	cloudy urine
SP.6	ST.44	Deficient Stomach Yin	weight loss
SP.6	ST.45	Deficient Stomach and Heart Yin	restless insomnia
SP.8	ST.40	Stagnant Blood in legs	varicose veins
SP.9	ST.36	Deficient Spleen Yang	urinary retention
SP.9	ST.39	Damp Heat in Intestines	dysentery
SP.9	ST.40	Stagnant Qi and Damp in Lower Energizer	abdominal distension and oedema
SP.10	ST.36	Deficient Blood	dry rough skin
SP.10	ST.45	Heat in the Blood	eczema
		Stagnant Blood	psoriasis
SP.12	ST.30	Stagnant Blood	groin sprain
		Damp Heat	urinary retention
SP.15	ST.25	Heat in Stomach and Intestines	constipation
		Damp Heat in Intestines	diarrhoea
		Stagnant Qi in Intestines	abdominal distension and pain
SP.15	ST.36	Deficient Spleen Yang	feeling of cold and pain in the abdomen
SP.15	ST.37 or ST.39	Damp Heat in Intestines	diarrhoea
SP.15	ST.40	Stagnation of Qi and Damp in Lower Energizer	abdominal pain
SP.21	ST.16	Stagnant Lung Qi	asthma
SP.21	ST.36	Deficient Qi	emaciation from long illness
SP.21	ST.40	Stagnant Qi and Blood in chest	chest pain

Stomach 16

CHANNEL CONNECTIONS

MAIN CHANNEL PATHWAY

The main pathway starts lateral to the ala nasi, at LI.20, ascends to the inner canthus, at BL.1, and descends through ST.1, ST.2 and ST.3 to enter the upper gum at GV.26. Re-emerging, it curves over the lips to meet the Large Intestine channel at ST.4, before meeting under the lips at CV.24. It then goes back along the cheek through ST.5, ST.6 and ST.7, ascending through GB.3, GB.6 and GB.4, to meet the Gallbladder channel at ST.8.

From ST.5, a branch descends the throat through ST.9 and ST.10 to the supraclavicular fossa, with a connection to GV.14 at the base of the neck. From the supraclavicular fossa, an internal pathway passes through the diaphragm to connect with the Stomach and the Spleen. The superficial pathway from the supraclavicular fossa descends the chest and abdomen to ST.30 at the groin, where it meets the internal pathway descending from the Stomach.

From ST.30 the superficial pathway runs down the anteriolateral leg to ST.45 at the nailpoint of the second toe. A branch from ST.42 links with the Spleen channel at SP.1.

CONNECTING CHANNEL PATHWAY

Starting from ST.40, this pathway connects with the Spleen channel. A branch runs up the leg and body to converge with the other Yang channels at the back of the head and neck, and another branch connects with the throat.

Table 16.1 Crossing points on the Stomach channel

Point	Crossing
ST.1	Yang Heel
ST.2	Yang Heel
ST.3	Yang Heel
ST.4	Large Intestine, Yang Heel
ST.7	Gallbladder
ST.8	Gallbladder, Yang Link

RELATIONSHIP OF STOMACH TO SPLEEN

The Spleen and Stomach work together in the digestion of food, but the Spleen is also concerned with the conversion of the digestion products into Qi, Blood and body Fluids. Therefore Spleen points are generally more used for tonifying Qi and Blood, or for regulating body Fluids, than are Stomach points. There are exceptions to this, since ST.36 can be used for Deficient Qi and Blood, just as ST.40 can be used for Damp and Phlegm. Similarly, SP.4 can be used for epigastric pain, and SP.6 can be used to tonify Stomach Yin. However, most Stomach points are either used for problems of the stomach and intestine organs, or for problems along the course of the Stomach channel.

BRIGHT YANG RELATIONSHIP

The Stomach and Large Intestine channels are combined in the Bright Yang channel pair of the Six Divisions. This pair of channels controls the front of the body, especially the face, so that local and distal Stomach and Large Intestine points can be combined for problems of face, eyes, nose, sinuses, lips, teeth and gums.

The Bright Yang connection allows problems on the Large Intestine channel to be treated with Stomach points, e.g. ST.38 for shoulder sprain; or problems on the Stomach channel to be treated with Large Intestine points, e.g. LI.5 for ankle sprain in the area of ST.41.

The stomach and intestines are physically linked in the digestive system, so that the two organs are often simultaneously affected by general digestive problems such as Heat and Stagnation. Large Intestine and Stomach points can be used to treat such problems, e.g. LI.4 + ST.44 Rd for Heat in Bright Yang, or LI.10 + ST.37 for Stagnation of Qi with indigestion and constipation.

Also, traditionally, the Bright Yang channels are held to be rich in Qi and Blood, so that the famous combination of LI.4 and ST.36 can be used for general weakness and exhaustion due to Deficient Qi and Blood.

FUNCTIONS OF STOMACH POINTS

TREAT CHANNEL PROBLEMS

Stomach points can be used as local points to treat problems on the Stomach channel, e.g. ST.8 for frontal headaches, linked either to Deficient Blood or Damp, from Deficiency of Spleen and Stomach. Stomach points can also be used as distal points to treat problems on the Bright Yang channels, e.g. ST.45 + LI.4 for eye problems, or ST.44 + LI.5 for gingivitis. Pairs of points or chains of points on each of the Bright Yang channels can be used for this, e.g. LI.4, LI.20, ST.2, ST.45 for sinusitis, or LI.1,

LI.4, LI.20, ST.2, ST.44, ST.45 for allergic rhinitis and conjunctivitis.

TONIFY QI AND BLOOD

The Bright Yang combination of LI.4 + ST.36 is the most powerful for this purpose, and ST.36 is far more frequently used than the Source point ST.42. ST.36 may be combined with the Extra channel Opening points SP.4 and PC.6, and ST.30 added for Deficiency of Qi and Blood of Spleen and Heart, with weakness and insomnia.

TRANSFORM DAMP

ST.36 can reduce Damp and Phlegm by tonifying a Deficient Spleen, whilst ST.40 can relieve conditions of Excess accumulations of Damp and Phlegm. ST.8 can relieve Damp and Phlegm in the head, and points such as ST.43 and ST.44 can relieve local Damp Heat in arthritis.

REGULATE DIGESTION

Local points, such as ST.21, can be used for epigastric pain and discomfort, as can distal points like ST.44 and ST.45. CV.12 and PC.6 are often included in such combinations.

MOVE QI AND BLOOD

While Spleen points like SP.4, SP.6, SP.8 and SP.10 are more powerful for systemic Stagnation of Qi and Blood, points like ST.30, ST.31 and ST.41 can be used to treat poor circulation in the legs, and ST.29 and ST.30 can be used as local points for abdominal pain from Stagnant Blood.

CLEAR THE MIND AND CALM THE EMOTIONS

By providing sufficient Qi and Blood to nourish and stabilize the Heart Spirit, ST.36 can treat anxiety, restlessness and insomnia. By relieving Damp and Phlegm, points such as ST.8, ST.38 and ST.40 can treat hypertension, headache, mental confusion and mental dullness. By tonifying and regulating the Spleen, ST.36 can treat worry and insecurity. By moving Stagnation of Qi and by draining Heat, ST.41–45 can relieve mental congestion, disorientation, depression, mania, hysteria and dream-disturbed sleep.

STOMACH SYNDROMES

Stomach syndromes are summarized in Table 16.2.

Table 16.2 Point combinations for Stomach syndromes

Syndromes	Signs and symptoms	Pulse	Tongue	Point combinations
Deficient Stomach Qi	tiredness, lethargy, weakness, appetite problems, abdominal distension, loose stools, worry and insecurity	empty	pale and flabby, toothmarks	CV.12, ST.36, SP.3 Rf M
Deficient Stomach Yang	feeling of cold, cold limbs and abdomen, desire for warmth, exhaustion, oedema, undigested food in stools	empty, deep, slow maybe slippery	pale, moist, maybe swollen, white coat	CV.6, CV.12, ST.28, ST.36, KI.7 Rf M
Phlegm–Damp in Stomach	as Deficient Stomach Qi + feeling of heaviness in head, limbs or body, maybe nausea, white discharges or fluid-filled skin eruptions	empty, slippery	pale and flabby, toothmarks, moist greasy, white coat	CV.12, ST.36, SP.3 Rf M + CV.6, CV.9 M; SP.9 Rd
Cold invades Stomach	sudden epigastric pain and sensation of cold, preference for warm food and drink, usually following excess intake of cold food and drink	flooding or tight, maybe deep and slow	thick white greasy coat	CV.10, CV.13, ST.21, ST.36, SP.4 Rd M
Stagnant Stomach and Liver Qi	distending pain in epigastrium, nausea and maybe vomiting or sour belching, worse with worry, frustration or depression	hindered or wiry, maybe slippery	maybe purplish	CV.12, PC.6, LR.3, LR.13 Rd; ST.36 Rf
Rebellious Stomach Qi	epigastric discomfort with nausea, vomiting, belching or hiccup	maybe wiry or flooding	various	CV.10, CV.14, PC.6, SP.4, Rd
Retention of food	prolonged feeling of epigastric distension and discomfort, following excess or hurried eating	full or flooding slippery	thick greasy coat	CV.10, CV.13, PC.6, SP.4, LI.10 Rd
Fear and anxiety invades Stomach	epigastric discomfort or nausea, aggravated by fear and anxiety, maybe palpitations	maybe moving or irregular	maybe trembling	CV.14, PC.6, SP.4 Rd; CV.4, ST.36 Rf
Deficient Spleen and Stomach Qi and Hyperactive Liver Yang	gastritis with faintness, tiredness and irritability when the patient goes too long without eating	empty, wiry, maybe choppy	pale, maybe trembling	GV.20, CV.12, GB.34, LR.3 Rd; SP.3, ST.36 Rf
Deficient Stomach Yin	patient is tired but restless, discomfort and maybe burning sensation in epigastrium	rapid, thin	red, maybe peeled	CV.12, SP.6, ST.36 Rf; ST.44 Rd
Stomach Fire	burning sensation and pain in epigastrium, thirst, constant hunger, constipation, bad breath	rapid, full, maybe wiry	dark red, dry yellow coat	CV.12, PC.8, ST.21, ST.44 Rd; ST.45 B; SP.6 Rf
Stagnant Stomach Blood	severe stabbing pain in epigastrium, maybe worse after eating, maybe blood in stools	wiry, full, maybe choppy,	purple or purple spots	CV.12, PC.6, ST.21, ST.34, ST.36, SP.4 Rd

Rd, Reducing method; Rf, Reinforcing method; B, bleeding; M, moxa.

Stomach points

ST.1 chéng qì

Point of the Yang Heel channel.

General

This is a main point for all eye problems, from varying aetiologies, including Wind Cold, Wind Heat and Hyperactive Liver Yang. The extra point, qiú hòu, can be used as an alternative to ST.1 for eye problems. However, when using ST.1, qiú hòu, BL.1 and similar points adjacent to the eyeball, care should be taken to avoid puncturing small blood vessels, and the patient should be warned that bruising can occur.

ST.2 can be substituted for ST.1, just as BL.2 is an alternative for BL.1, and although the substitute points are less powerful the risk of 'black eyes' is far less. Consequently, ST.1 and BL.1 can be reserved for more serious conditions, when ST.2 and BL.2 have not been sufficiently effective.

ST.1 combinations

Owing to the wide application of ST.1 for eye problems it

can be combined with any of the points that treat eye problems, see Chapter 32. ST.1 can be used as part of a combination of points on the Stomach and Large Intestine Channels, for example ST.1, ST.2, ST.41, LI.1, LI.4, LI.14.

Syndromes: eye disorders

Pulse. Various.

Indications. All eye disorders, including early-stage cataract and glaucoma.

Example. Optic neuritis.

Combination. ST.1, BL.1, LI.4, LI.14, GB.20, LR.3 E; ST.36, KI.6 Rf.

ST.2 sì bái

Point of Yang Heel channel.

General

ST.2 can be used for all eye problems, like ST.1. It is generally less powerful than ST.1, but there is less risk of bruising with ST.2. Whilst ST.1 is only used for eye problems, ST.2 can also be used for facial paralysis, trigeminal neuralgia, allergic facial swelling, and for nasal problems, such as sinusitis and sinus headache.

Syndromes

Eye disorders
Nasal disorders

Eye disorders

Pulse. Various

Indications. All eye problems.

Example. Blurred vision, tiredness and headache.

Combination. ST.2, ST.8, LI.1, LI.4, GV.20 E; ST.36, SP.6 Rf.

Nasal disorders

Pulse. Slippery, maybe wiry or flooding.

Indications. Rhinitis, sinusitis, headache.

Example. Nasal catarrh and headache.

Combination. ST.2, ST.3, ST.40, ST.45, LI.1, LI.4, LI.20, GB.20 E.

ST.3 jù liáo

Point of Yang Heel channel.

General

ST.3 can be used for eye problems, but is less effective than ST.1 and ST.2. It is mainly used for facial and nasal problems, in similar combinations to ST.2 above.

Syndromes: nasal disorders

See ST.2.

ST.4 dì cāng

Crossing point with Large Intestine channel, point of Yang Heel channel.

General

ST.4 is a point to regulate the face and mouth.

Regulates the face

ST.4 can be used for facial paralysis, due to Wind Cold, or for trigeminal neuralgia associated with Hyperactive Liver Yang. Both these conditions may have an underlying Deficiency of Qi and Blood, for which ST.36 with Reinforcing method and moxa can be added to the combination.

Regulates the mouth

ST.4 can be combined with LI.4 to treat disorders of the lips and mouth due to Wind Cold, Wind Heat, Stomach Heat, Fire poison, Deficient Qi and Blood, as shown in Table 16.3.

Syndromes

Facial disorders
Mouth disorders

Table 16.3 Combinations of ST.4 for mouth problems

Syndrome	Example	Combination
Wind Cold	cracked lips and face pain	ST.4, LI.4, LI.20, GB.20 Rd
Stomach Heat	red, cracked lips	ST.4, ST.44, LI.4, LI.11 Rd
Fire poison	acne around mouth	ST.4, ST.45, LI.4, LI.11, LI.18, CV.24 Rd
Deficient Qi and Blood	mouth sore when tired	ST.4, LI.4, LI.11 E; ST.36, SP.6, Rf

Facial disorders

Pulse. Maybe wiry, empty.

Indications. Facial paralysis, trigeminal neuralgia, face pain.

Example. Facial paralysis.

Combination. ST.4, ST.6, ST.44, LI.4, LI.19, GV.26 E; ST.36 Rf M; points are needled on the affected side, with the exception of LI.4, which is needled on the opposite side and ST.36 which is used bilaterally.

Mouth disorders

Pulse. Various.

Indications. Mouth and lip ulcers, cracked or swollen lips, toothache.

Example. Hypersalivation.

Combination. ST.4, ST.40, LI.4, CV.24 Rd.

ST.6 and ST.7 jiá chē and xià guān

General

These are local points for problems of the teeth, jaw, face, neck and throat for which they are often combined with LI.4 and TE.17. Some examples are shown in Table 16.4. ST.6 is more for problems of the lower head, such as sore throat and voice loss, and ST.7 is more for problems of the ears.

Table 16.4 Combinations of ST.6 and of ST.7

Syndrome	Example	Combination
Wind Heat	temporomandibular arthritis	ST.6, ST.7, ST.44, LI.4 Rd
Wind Cold	ear ache	ST.7, LI.4, TE.3, TE.17, TE.21 Rd
Stomach Fire	toothache and gingivitis	ST.5, ST.6, ST.42, LI.4, LI.11 Rd

ST.8 tóu wéi

Crossing point with Gallbladder channel, point of Yang Link channel.

General

The main function of ST.8 is to treat headaches and its secondary function is to treat eye problems associated with Wind invasion, such as excessive lachrymation.

ST.8 and headaches

ST.8 can be used for any headaches in the area local to the point, for frontal headaches due to Wind invasion, for headaches associated with digestive problems, and for headache and dizziness associated with Damp and Phlegm in the head. Table 16.5 shows some examples.

Table 16.5 Combinations of ST.8 for headaches

Syndrome	Example	Combination
Stomach Fire	headache and gastritis	ST.8, ST.44, ST.45, LI.4, LI.11 Rd
Damp and Phlegm	headache and lethargy	ST.8, ST.40, ST.45, LI.1, LI.4 Rd; GV.20 yìn táng E
Phlegm obstructs head and Heart	headache and psychosis	ST.8, ST.40, SP.6, LR.3, KI.1, PC.6, LI.4 Rd
Hyperactive Liver Yang	migraine	ST.8, GB.14 E; GB.34, LI.4, LU.7 Rd
Deficient Qi and Blood	headache and blurred vision	ST.8, BL.2, E; LI.4, ST.36, SP.6, GV.20 Rf

Syndromes: Headaches

Pulse. Maybe wiry, slippery, flooding, empty, thin or choppy.

Indications. Headache and face pain, headache and dizziness, headache and visual problems.

Example. Headaches with tiredness.

Combination. ST.8, GV.20 E; ST.36, SP.6, LI.4, CV.4 Rf.

ST.9 rén yíng

Sea of Qi point.

General

The two main uses of ST.9 are to regulate the neck and throat and to regulate blood pressure. ST.9 can also be used to calm Rebellious Stomach Qi, as in hiccup, nausea and vomiting, or Rebellious Lung Qi, as in cough and asthma. ST.9 is recommended by some texts for acute lower back sprain, however, this author prefers to use other points for this purpose.

Caution

Some texts forbid both needle and moxa at this point, due to the proximity of the carotid artery. Needling may be safely performed providing precautions are observed, see David Smyth, *Journal of Chinese Medicine* 1992, **39**, 17–18. ST.9 should be used with caution if treating very high blood pressure, since blood pressure may rise for a few seconds after needling.

Regulates neck and throat

ST.9 is often combined with LI.4 to treat these problems, for example:

goiter	ST.9, ST.36, SI.17, LI.4, PC.6, KI.3, SP.6 E
painful obstruction of the throat	ST.9, SI.17, LI.4, CV.22, CV.23 Rd

Regulates blood pressure

ST.9 can regulate both low and high blood pressure:

low blood pressure	ST.9, LI.4 E; ST.36, GV.20, CV.4 Rf
high blood pressure	ST.9, ST.36, LI.4, LI.11, LR.3 E

Syndromes

Neck and throat disorders
Blood pressure disorders

Neck and throat disorders

Pulse. Maybe wiry, slippery or flooding.

Indications. Oesophageal constriction, sore throat, painful obstruction of the throat, thyroid swelling.

Example. Laryngitis.

Combination. ST.9, LI.1, LI.15, SI.1, SI.17 E; KI.6 Rf.

Blood pressure disorders

Pulse. Wiry, maybe rapid, full, flooding or empty.

Indications. High or low blood pressure, dizziness, flushed face.

Example. Acute hypertension.

Combination. ST.9, PC.6, KI.1 Rd.

ST.12 quē pén — ST.17 rǔ zhōng

General

The ST points 13–16 are level with CV and KI points shown in Table 16.6. All these points, due to their anatomical location, can be effective for respiratory problems, such as bronchitis and asthma, often combined with ST.40, and for pain in the chest or ribs, and feeling of fullness in the chest often combined with PC.6. In addition, ST.12 can be used for nervous anxiety and insomnia, associated with Heart and Stomach, and can be combined with SP.4, PC.6 and CV.14.

Table 16.6 Segmental locations of Stomach points

CV	KI	ST
21	27	13
20	26	14
19	25	15
18	24	16

Caution

ST.12 has straight insertion of 0.3–0.5 units, and ST.13–16 have slanted insertions of 0.5–0.8 units, avoiding deep insertion.

ST.18 rǔ gēn

General

This point can be used for lung and chest problems, like ST.12–16, but its main use is to regulate the breasts and to facilitate lactation.

Syndromes: breast disorders

Pulse. Maybe hindered or wiry, maybe rapid, slippery or flooding.

Indications. Mastitis, premenstrual breast swelling and discomfort, insufficient or excessive lactation.

Example. Mastitis with pus.

Combination. ST.16, ST.18, ST.39, KI.22, GB.41, LI.4, LI.11 Rd.

ST.21 liáng mén

General

ST.21 is mainly used for acute painful Excess Stomach problems with Reducing method. It can be used for Deficient patterns, but CV.12 and ST.36 are better for these. ST.21 can be an excellent point for patterns of Excess, Stagnation and Heat affecting the stomach and duodenum with epigastric pain and discomfort.

Syndromes

Stagnation of Cold in the Stomach
Stagnation of food in the Stomach
Stomach Fire
Liver invades Stomach

Stagnation of Cold in the Stomach

Pulse. Wiry, maybe full, slippery, deep or slow.

Indications. Epigastric pain or discomfort with feelings of fullness and cold.

Combination. ST.21, ST.36, CV.12, Rd M; LI.10 Rd.

Stagnation of food in the Stomach

Pulse. Wiry, slippery, full or flooding.

Indications. Epigastric distension and discomfort with nausea.

Combination. ST.21, ST.36, ST.39, CV.10, PC.6 Rd.

Stomach Fire

Pulse. Rapid, full or flooding.

Indications. Bad breath, gingivitis, cracked red lips, red eyes, headache, gastritis.

Example. Severe gastritis and restlessness.

Combination. ST.21, ST.39, ST.44, LI.4, LI.11, PC.3 Rd.

Liver invades Stomach

Pulse. Wiry, maybe full or flooding.

Indications. Epigastric pain or discomfort, abdominal distension, indigestion, vomiting, nervous tension.

Example. Severe epigastric pain.

Combination. ST.21, ST.34, LR.3, LR.13, PC.6 Rd.

ST.25 tiān shū

Alarm point of the Stomach channel.

General

While ST.21 is mainly for Excess conditions with epigastric problems, ST.25 is mainly for Excess abdominal disorders. That is, ST.21 is more for the Stomach and ST.25 is more for the Intestines. ST.25 can also be used for menstrual problems and urinary stones.

ST.25 and psychological disorders

Like ST.21, ST.25 can be used for disorders of the Stomach and Intestines, associated with the different types of emotional stress, and can be combined with appropriate points as shown in Table 16.7.

Syndromes

Deficiency and Cold in Spleen and Intestines

Table 16.7 Combinations with ST.25 for psychological disorders

Syndrome	Example	Combination
Stagnant Lung and Large Intestine Qi	constipation, grief, withdrawal	+ LU.7, CV.17 Rd
Heart and Stomach Fire	manic behaviour, severe gastritis and colitis	+ PC.3, ST.44 Rd
Deficient Heart and Stomach Yin	anxiety, worry, irritable bowel syndrome	+ PC.6, SP.4, CV.14 E
Stagnation of Life Qi	frustration, depression, abdominal distension	+ PC.6, LR.3, CV.6 E
Deficient Heart and Kidney Qi	fearful anxiety, colitis	+ HT.5, KI.7, CV.14 E

Damp Heat in the Intestines
Heat in the Stomach and Intestines
Stagnant Qi in the Intestines

Deficiency and Cold in Spleen and Intestines

Pulse. Maybe wiry, slippery, empty, deep or slow.

Indications. Abdominal distension and pain, diarrhoea.

Example. Chronic diarrhoea and tiredness.

Combination. ST.25, ST.37, CV.6 Rf M; CV.8 M (on ginger on salt).

Damp Heat in the Intestines

Pulse. Slippery, rapid.

Indications. Diarrhoea, dysentery.

Example. Acute diarrhoea.

Combination. ST.25, ST.37, ST.44, SP.9 Rd.

Heat in the Stomach and Intestines

Pulse. Rapid, full or flooding.

Indications. Gastric or duodenal ulcers, constipation.

Example. ST.25, ST.39, ST.44, LI.4, LI.11, TE.6 Rd.

Stagnant Qi in the Intestines

Pulse. Wiry, maybe full or flooding.

Indications. Acute intestinal obstruction, oedema, abdominal masses, pain or distension.

Example. Constipation and colon pain.

Combination. ST.25, ST.39, CV.12, CV.6, LI.4, TE.6 Rd.

ST.28, ST.29 and ST.30 shuǐ dào, guī lái and qì chōng

These three points are located on the lower abdomen as shown below.

CV.4	KI.13	ST.28
CV.3	KI.12	ST.29
CV.2	KI.11	ST.30

They have overlapping functions, in that all three can be used to:

move Stagnant Qi and Blood in the Lower Energizer
warm and tonify Deficient Qi and raise Sinking Qi in the Lower Energizer
clear Damp Heat in the Lower Energizer.

However, the three points can be differentiated:

ST.28 is mainly for regulating fluids
ST.29 is mainly for regulating menstruation
ST.30 is mainly for regulating groin and genital area, and for strengthening prenatal and postnatal Qi.

ST.28 shuǐ dào

General

This point is useful for fluid problems, especially for those associated with Excess and Stagnation, with pain or distension. In treating Fluid disorders, it is necessary to decide whether the principle of treatment is to tonify Deficiency, to move Stagnation, to drain Excess, or to combine these methods in the same treatment. Table 16.8 gives examples.

Syndromes: Fluid disorders

Pulse. Slippery, maybe, wiry, full or flooding.

Indications. Oedema, urinary retention, urinary stones.

Table 16.8 Combinations with ST.28 for Fluid disorders

Syndrome	Example	Method	Combination
Deficient Qi and Yang of Kidney and Spleen	oedema and exhaustion	tonify and warm	ST.28, ST.36, CV.4, CV.12 Rf M
Stagnant Qi and Damp in Lower Energizer	oedema and distension	move and drain	ST.28, ST.40, CV.6, SP.6, SP.9, TE.6 Rd
Damp Heat in Lower Energizer	dysuria	move and drain	ST.28, CV.3, CV.6, SP.6, SP.9 Rd
Damp Heat in Lower Energizer and Deficient Kidney Yin	recurring urinary infections	move and drain	ST.28, CV.3, SP.6, SP.9 Rd; KI.6 Rf

Example. Recurring urinary tract infections.

Combination. ST.28, CV.3, SP.6, SP.9, HT.5, KI.2 E.

Alternation: BL.23, BL.28, BL.32, GB.25, SP.6, SP.9, HT.5 E.

ST.29 guī lái

General

ST.29 can be used to warm the Lower Energizer, for example for uterine prolapse or for hernias due to cold. However, the main function of ST.29 is to move Stagnant Blood in the uterus, for which it is often combined with CV.3. ST.29 can be alternated for this purpose with zǐ gōng, which is one unit lateral to it. ST.29 can be combined with a variety of points for menstrual problems, including ST.25, SP.4, SP.6, SP.8 and LI.4.

Syndromes: Stagnant Blood in the uterus

Pulse. Wiry, maybe choppy.

Indications. Dysmenorrhoea, uterine fibroids.

Example. Irregular menstruation with dysmenorrhoea.

Combination: ST.29, CV.2, CV.3, SP.6, LI.4 Rd.

ST.30 qì chōng

Point of Thoroughfare channel, point of Sea of Food.

General

ST.30 has the following main functions:

moves Stagnant Blood in the uterus
regulates local groin and genital problems
raises Qi to treat prolapses
regulates the Thoroughfare channel.

Moves Stagnant Blood in the uterus

ST.30 resembles ST.29 in this function, the difference is that ST.30 is better for local genital problems, and better for infertility, due to its link with the Thoroughfare channel. ST.30 like ST.29, can be combined with CV.3 or CV.6, for conditions of Stagnant Blood in the uterus, but for genital problems it can be combined with CV.1, CV.2 or CV.3.

Regulates local groin and genital problems

ST.30 can be used for pain and swelling of the external genitals, for example combined with KI.2 or KI.8, it can also be used for groin sprain, combined with such points as ST.31, CV.2, SP.12 and LR.10–12. ST.30 can be used for cold, pain and swelling in the lower abdomen; for example, in combination with CV.2, CV.4, ST.29 and ST.36.

Raises Qi to treat prolapses

ST.28, ST.29 and ST.30 all have the function of treating uterine prolapse or intestinal hernias; for example, in combination with CV.4, ST.36, GV.20 and LI.4 with Reinforcing method and moxa.

Regulates the Thoroughfare channel

ST.30 can regulate the Thoroughfare channel in three main ways:

    tonifies Jing
    tonifies prenatal and postnatal Qi
    moves the Blood.

Tonifies Jing.　ST.30 can be used to treat infertility and impotence due to Deficient Jing; for example, in combination with CV.4 and zǐ gōng.

Tonifies prenatal and postnatal Qi.　As a point of the Sea of Food, ST.30 can strengthen the ability of the Spleen and Stomach to form Qi and Blood. As a point of the Thoroughfare channel, ST.30 can link the prenatal Qi of the Kidneys with the postnatal Qi of the Spleen, and hence strengthen the whole body. ST.30 can be combined with SP.4, PC.6 and ST.3 with the Reinforcing method and moxa.

Moves the Blood.　The Thoroughfare channel can move Stagnant Blood not only in the uterus but in the body in general. If SP.4, PC.6 and CV.6 are combined with ST.30 with Reducing method, this can help to improve circulation in the legs and feet especially, since ST.30 is at the junction of legs and body, where energy blockages can easily occur.

ST.31 bìguān

General

ST.31 strengthens and moves Qi and Blood to treat problems of the hip, groin and upper leg and knees. It can be used for spasm or atrophy of the muscles in these areas to treat groin sprain, lymphadenitis, hernia, hemiplegia and lateral knee problems. For example, use ST.31 in combination with ST.32, GB.29, GB.31 and GB.34, for spasm and pain in the hip and upper thigh. ST.31 has a stronger effect than ST.32 to help to lift the leg, when the leg is dragged as in hemiplegia. It can be used for blocked arterial circulation into the leg, when it can be combined with SP.4, PC.6, CV.6, ST.31, ST.36 and ST.41.

ST.34 liáng qiū

Accumulation point

General

ST.34 has two main functions. One is to move Stagnant Qi and Blood and remove Wind Cold and Damp, to treat local problems of knee and lower thigh. For this it can be combined with ST.35 and other local points. The other function is, as the Accumulation point, to treat acute Excess Stomach disorders; for example, vomiting and gastritis. It is especially useful for epigastric pain in combination with ST.21.

ST.35 dú bí

General

ST.35 is the lateral of the two xī yǎn points below the kneecap. These points are excellent for problems of the knees. For Wind Cold and Damp, they can be used with needle and moxa stick, or moxa on the needle. The xī yǎn points can be combined with others, according to the location of the problem. For example, ST.34, ST.35 and ST.36 can be combined for knee pain on the Stomach channel or the medial xī yǎn point can be combined with LR.8 and Ah Shi points for medial knee pain.

ST.36 zú sān lǐ

Sea point, Earth point, point of Sea of Food.

General

ST.36 is one of the most important points on the body. Its main function is to strengthen the Spleen and Stomach to make Qi and Blood and to resolve Damp. The functions of ST.36 are:

    tonifies Qi
    harmonizes Nutritive and Defensive Qi
    raises the Qi
    tonifies Blood
    disperses Damp
    stabilizes mind and emotions
    regulates Stomach Qi
    regulates the Intestines
    regulates blood pressure
    other functions.

Tonifies Qi

ST.36 by tonifying the Qi of the Spleen and Stomach strengthens the Qi of the entire body. It is the best point of all for general improvement of strength, health and resistance to diseases. It is specific to treat chronic lability due to illness, weak constitution, overwork or old age. It can be used by itself for this purpose or in combination with other points, such as the classic formulas ST.36 + LI.4 and ST.36 + SP.6 to tonify Qi and Blood.

Tonifies Spleen and Stomach Qi. By strengthening the rotting and ripening functions of the Stomach, and the transforming and transporting functions of the Spleen, ST.36 can tonify Qi and Blood and resolve Damp. For these purposes, ST.36 can be combined with points such as BL.20, BL.21, CV.12, SP.3 and SP.6.

It also has the specific function of strengthening digestion, improving appetite, relieving indigestion, treating weight loss and strengthening weak muscles. For example, to regulate weight loss; ST.36 could be combined with SP.1, SP.2, SP.3 and CV.12, all with Reinforcing method.

Tonifies Lung Qi. ST.36 can be used in combination with LU.9 and BL.13 to strengthen Deficient Lung Qi, to treat cough and bronchitis, for example. Also, since as discussed later, ST.36 harmonizes Defensive and Nutritive Qi, it can prevent recurring respiratory infections.

Tonifies Kidney Qi. The Kidneys store not only prenatal Qi, but also the postnatal Qi, made by the Spleen, Stomach and Lungs, from the energies of food and air. When ST.36 is combined with points such as KI.3, BL.23 or CV.4, it can treat such Kidney problems as exhaustion, weak will, weak back and kness and urinary problems.

Tonifies Heart Qi. When ST.36 is combined with such points as HT.7, BL.15 or CV.17, it can help to treat problems relating to Deficient Heart Qi, such as palpitations, and poor circulation. It can also help to stabilize the emotions as described later.

Harmonizes Defensive and Nutritive Qi

Wind Cold Invasion in the Greater Yang stage can be of two types: Excess type with no sweating and Deficiency type with sweating without relief of symptoms. The principle of treatment is to open the pores and induce sweating in the Excess type, but to stop sweating yet drive out the invading factor in the Deficiency type. ST.36, with Even method, can do this because by strengthening the Nutritive Qi it stops sweating and by strengthening the Defensive Qi it expels the invading factor. ST.36 can therefore be used for the common cold, influenza and all Wind Cold patterns of the Deficiency type.

However, this is only one aspect of the ability of ST.36 to increase the resistance of the body to invasion. It can be used to treat such varying disorders as allergies, cold sores and acute bacillary dysentery. It can be used both to prevent and to treat such conditions.

Raises the Qi

ST.36 can be combined with LI.4 and GV.20, with Reinforcing method and moxa, to treat prolapses. Other points can be added, depending on the organ. For example, CV.12 for stomach and CV.4 for uterus. However, where prolapses are associated with long chronic Deficiency, treatment may be prolonged and surgery may be required where appropriate.

Tonifies the Blood

ST.36 in combination with such points as LI.4, SP.6, SP.10, BL.43, BL.17, BL.18 or BL.20, can tonify the Blood of Spleen, Liver and Heart — it can therefore treat a wide range of symptoms, including amenorrhoea, palpitations, insomnia, tiredness, dizziness, headache, brittle nails and dry skin. One important aspect is vision problems due to Deficient Blood, especially in the elderly, when ST.36 and LI.4 can often be included in the combination.

Disperses Damp

ST.36 can be combined with such points as CV.12 or BL.20, with Reinforcing method and moxa, to strengthen the Spleen to transform Damp associated with Deficiency. This contrasts with combinations such as SP.6, SP.9, TE.6 and ST.40 with Reducing method to resolve Damp associated with Stagnation. There may, of course, be Damp due to other Deficiency and Stagnation, and a suitable combination might be ST.36, CV.6 Rf M; SP.6, SP.9, ST.28 Rd.

Stabilizes the mind and emotions

ST.36 and the mind. ST.36 generally clears and strengthens the mind by tonifying Qi and Blood and by resolving Damp. More specifically, ST.36 helps to tonify Kidney Qi and the Qi and Blood of the Heart and Spleen, and therefore strengthens mental processes.

ST.36 and the emotions. Emotional disorders can be associated with Excess, Deficiency, Stagnation or Irregularity of Qi. ST.36 is important where the emotional problem is associated with Deficiency, for example depression, or with Irregularity or Stagnation based on Deficiency such as emotional lability or blockage respectively. Table 16.9 shows some examples.

Table 16.9 ST.36 and emotional disorders

Type	Syndrome	Example	Combination
Deficiency	Deficient Kidney Qi	procrastination due to fear	ST.36, KI.3, BL.52 Rf M
	Deficient Spleen Qi	worry about not having enough, material insecurity	ST.36, SP.3, BL.49 Rf M
Irregularity based on Deficiency	Hyperactive Liver Yang with Deficient Qi	touchiness, hypersensitivity, insecurity	ST.36 Rf M; LR.3, BL.47 Rd
	Disturbance of Heart Spirit with Deficient Qi	emotional lability, overexcitability	ST.36 Rf; HT.7, BL.44 E
Stagnation based on Deficiency	Stagnant Lung Qi with Deficient Kidney Qi	holding on to the past, withdrawal from life	ST.36 Rf M; LU.7, BL.42 E M

Rf, Reinforcing method; Rd, Reducing method; E, Even method; M, moxa.

ST.36, by strengthening the Earth element, can increase the qualities of stability and solidity to stabilize the emotions, and to give the feelings of strength and security which are necessary before people begin to let go of emotional blocks. People often hold on to emotional blocks and to negative patterns of thought and behaviour, because of the fear of inner emptiness if there is nothing there to replace them. ST.36 is a key point to provide the abundance of energy and inner feelings of security that allow people to begin to let go. ST.36 Rf M is therefore an excellent point to use with LU.7 Rd, for example, to allow people to let go of the past and begin to feel connected with the present.

Regulates Stomach Qi

ST.36 can be used for patterns with Stagnant or Rebellious Stomach Qi, such as nausea, vomiting, belching and epigastric pain. It can be combined with CV.13 for vomiting, or with CV.10 when food is not passing from the stomach into the duodenum. It can be combined with CV.14 when indigestion and nausea are linked to nervous tension.

Regulates the Intestines

ST.36 can treat disorders of the Intestines associated with Deficient of Stagnant Qi. For example, it is specific for constipation linked to Stagnant Qi. ST.36 can be used for constipation linked to Stagnant Qi, but ST.39 is preferable. For constipation of either type, ST.36 can be combined with ST.25 or SP.15, and either of these combinations can also be used for lower abdominal pain and distension.

Regulates blood pressure

ST.36 can be used with Reducing method to reduce hypertension from Hyperactive Liver Yang, Heart Fire or Phlegm and Damp. It is often combined with LI.4, LI.11, PC.6, LR.3 and GV.20.

Other functions

Three other functions of ST.36 are:

regulates the breasts
regulates the knees
expels stones.

Regulates the breasts. ST.36 can be used with Reinforcing method for insufficient lactation due to Deficiency, and with Reducing method for breast abscess. This reflects the dual ability of ST.36 to tonify chronic Deficiency, or rapidly to increase the resistance of the body to reduce acute infection.

For example:

lactation insufficiency with Deficient Qi and Blood	ST.18, ST.36, LI.4, CV.12, CV.17, BL.20 Rf (moxa if required)
mastitis and breast abscess with Stagnation of Qi and Fire poison	ST.16, ST.18, ST.36, LR.3, LI.10, SI.1, PC.6, CV.17 Rd

ST.36 can similarly be used for masses such as enlarged spleen, abdominal masses and enlarged lymph nodes. It can be combined with such points as LI.4, LI.10 and LI.11.

Regulates the knees. ST.36 can be used with ST.35 and ST.34 for local knee problems, acute and chronic, since it both moves and tonifies Qi and Blood in the Stomach channel, which will help to expel Wind, Cold and Damp. It will also help to reduce acute local infection and inflammation.

Expels stones. ST.36 can be used with Reducing method to assist expulsion of gallbladder or kidney stones. For kidney stones, ST.36 can be combined with ST.25, ST.28 and GB.25. For gallstones ST.36, can be combined with GB.24 and dǎn náng.

Syndromes

Deficient Qi
Sinking of Spleen Qi
Deficient Blood
Damp and Phlegm
Psychological problems
Rebellious Stomach Qi

Intestinal disorders
Hypertension

Deficient Qi

Pulse. Empty, maybe choppy or changing.

Indications. Tiredness, weakness, chronic ill health, inability to concentrate, depression.

Example. Repeated respiratory infections.

Combination. ST.36, LU.9, KI.3, BL.13, BL.20, BL.23 Rf M.

Sinking of Spleen Qi

Pulse. Empty, maybe slow and deep.

Indications. Tiredness, weak muscles, lethargy, prolapse.

Example. Rectal prolapse with haemorrhoids.

Combination. ST.36, LI.4, GV.1, GV.20 Rf M.

Deficient Blood

Pulse. Thin, choppy, maybe empty, deep and slow, maybe rapid.

Indications. Tiredness, feeling of vulnerability, insomnia, dry skin, greying hair.

Example. Blurred vision and exhaustion.

Combination. GB.1, BL.2, GV.20, LI.4 Rf; ST.36, CV.4 Rf M.

Damp and Phlegm

Pulse. Slippery, maybe empty or full.

Indications. Lethargy, feeling of fullness or heaviness in abdomen, chest or head, catarrh.

Example. Mental sluggishness and obesity.

Combination. ST.36, ST.45, SP.1, SP.2, CV.12, LI.4, GV.20 Rf M.

Psychological problems

Pulse. Empty, maybe choppy, changing or slippery.

Indications. Depression, lack of ambition, mental or emotional instability.

Example. Material insecurity, fear of not having enough.

Combination. ST.36, SP.4, CV.4, GV.20, PC.6 E.

Rebellious Stomach Qi

Pulse. Wiry, maybe slippery or flooding.

Indications. Nausea, vomiting , belching, hiccups, indigestion.

Example. Stage fright with nausea and vomiting.

Combination. ST.36, KI.7, CV.14, GV.20, PC.6, PC.8 Rd.

Intestinal disorders

Pulse. Maybe empty, slippery, flooding or wiry.

Indications. Constipation, abdominal distention, borborygmus.

Example. Irritable bowel syndrome with worry and tiredness.

Combination. ST.25, ST.36, GB.28, CV.6 E M; PC.6, yìn táng E.

Hypertension

Pulse. Wiry, maybe slippery, rapid, full or flooding.

Indications. Headache, dizziness, mental congestion, feeling of fullness in chest or head.

Example. Hypertension with frustration and anger.

Combination. ST.36, LI.4, LR.3, KI.1, PC.6, GV.20 Rd.

ST.37 shàng jù xū

Lower Sea point of the Large Intestine channel, point of the Sea of Blood.

General

The main function of ST.37 is to regulate the Large Intestine. It is especially useful for acute or chronic Damp Heat diarrhoea, for which it can be combined with ST.25, see page 229. ST.37 is a point of the Sea of Blood, and classically can be combined with BL.11 and ST.39 to tonify Blood. However, in the clinic, ST.36 is more commonly used than ST.37 for this purpose. Similarly, ST.37 can be used for anorexia, gastritis and hemiplegia, but ST.36 is generally more effective. ST.36, ST.37 or ST.39 can be combined with ST.13–16 for asthma, but if there is much Phlegm, then ST.40 may be preferred.

Syndromes: Large Intestine disorders

Pulse. Maybe wiry, slippery, rapid, full or flooding.

Indications. Gastroenteritis, diarrhoea, constipation, appendicitis.

Example. Colon spasms from nervous tension.

Combination. ST.37, SP.4, SP.15, CV.6, CV.14, PC.6 E.

ST.38 tiáo kǒu

General

ST.38 is primarily for pain and stiffness of the shoulder. Usually, ST.38 is manipulated on the affected side while the patient moves the shoulder to its limits, and then local shoulder and distal arm points are used. Like ST.37 and ST.39, ST.38 can also be used for numbness, pain and stiffness of the leg, knee and foot.

ST.39 xià jù xū

Lower Sea point of the Small Intestine, point of the Sea of Blood.

General

The main function of ST.39 is to regulate the Small Intestine, especially to drain Damp Heat. It can be combined with SP.6, SP.9 and SP.15, with ST.25 and ST.37, or with BL.27, BL.29 and BL.31 for diarrhoea and dysentery.

Like ST.37, ST.39 can be used for anaemia, but ST.36 is more commonly used. ST.39 can be used in combination with ST.37 and ST.41 for pain, paralysis or atrophy of the leg muscles.

Syndromes: Small Intestine disorders

Pulse. Slippery, rapid, maybe wiry, full or flooding.

Indications. Acute intestinal obstruction, abdominal pain, diarrhoea.

Example. Acute dysentery.

Combination. ST.25, ST.39, ST.44, SP.1, LI.4, LI.11 Rd; CV.6 E.

ST.40 fēng lóng

Connecting point.

General

ST.40 is specific for Phlegm and Damp. Whilst other points, such as SP.6, SP.9 and CV.9 may be better for Damp, ST.40 is the best general point for Phlegm. This can be 'substantial Phlegm' as in catarrh, obesity or lumps in the abdomen or under the skin, or 'insubstantial Phlegm', as in hypertension, depression and mental confusion. In general, Phlegm and Damp obstruct the clear flow of Qi in the channels, leading to tiredness, lethargy, depression and a feeling of heaviness in head, chest, abdomen or limbs. Phlegm is associated with different symptoms according to the area of the body for which ST.40 may be combined with different local points.

Head

The main disorders are headache or dizziness (ST.40 + ST.8), sinusitis (ST.40 + LI.4, ST.2, ST.3) and catarrhal deafness (ST.40 + GB.20, TE.17).

Neck and throat

Here, the main problems are boils, throat and catarrh, and swellings of the salivary, lymph or thyroid glands (ST.40 + LI.18, ST.9, TE.17, SI.17, CV.23).

Upper Energizer

For substantial Phlegm in the Lungs, with asthma and bronchitis, ST.40 may be combined with LU.1, LU.2, ST.14–16, CV.17 or CV.22. For insubstantial Phlegm in the Heart, with palpitations and feeling of oppression in the chest, ST.40 can combine with CV.17, CV.22 or PC.1. If Stagnation of Liver Qi aggravates patterns of either substantial or insubstantial Phlegm in the chest, then ST.40 can combine with LR.14. Back points BL.13, BL.15, BL.42 and BL.44 can also be used with ST.40.

Middle Energizer

Phlegm and Damp may disturb the Stomach, with nausea, vomiting and indigestion (ST.40 + CV.12, LR.13).

Lower Energizer

ST.40 can be combined with CV.6 for oedema and abdominal distension and pain. For Phlegm in the Intestines, with mucus in the stools, it can combine with ST.25. Where infertility is associated with blockage of the tubes by Phlegm, ST.40 may be used with ST.29, ST.30 or zǐ gōng.

Psychological problems

Stagnation of Qi associated with Phlegm can cause depression, and ST.40 is combined with points relating to the main organ involved:

Stagnant Lung Qi with Phlegm	ST.40 + LU.1, 6, 7 or CV.17
Stagnant Heart Qi with Phlegm	ST.40 + PC.6, HT.6 or CV.17
Stagnant Liver Qi with Phlegm	ST.40 + LR.3, or LR.14.

However, Phlegm can also obstruct the regular flow of Qi and cause irregular, erratic, confused, disturbed or chaotic speech and behaviour. This can be associated with the combination of Phlegm with Heart Fire, or with Liver Fire, Yang or Wind:

| Heart Phlegm Fire | ST.40 + KI.1, PC.5, PC.6, HT.6, HT.7, HT.8 |
| Liver Fire and Wind with Phlegm | ST.40 + KI.1, LR.1, LR.3 |

| Hyperactive Liver Yang with Phlegm | ST.40 + LR.3, GB.20, GV.20. |

When Phlegm and Damp are associated with Deficient Spleen Qi, the symptoms may include mental dullness, inability to concentrate, worry and mental confusion. ST.40 can then be combined with such points as GV.20, yìn táng, CV.12, CV.6, ST.36, ST.45, SP.6, LI.1 and LI.4.

Chest pain

ST.40 can be used for pain or discomfort in the chest, for example, after injury, often in combination with PC.6. This combination can be used as an alternative to PC.6 + SP.4.

Table1 6.10 ST.40 combinations for Phlegm and Damp

Channel	Syndrome	Example	Points
CV	Stagnant Qi and Damp in Lower Energizer	abdominal distension	CV.6
	Stomach Phlegm and Damp	nausea and vomiting	CV.12
	Heart Phlegm	nervous anxiety	CV.14
	Heart Phlegm	feeling of fullness in chest	CV.17
	Stagnant Liver Qi and Phlegm	feeling of lump in throat	CV.22
	Heart Phlegm Fire	hysteria, voice loss	CV.23
	Stomach Phlegm and Damp	hypersalivation	CV.24
GV	Phlegm Damp in head	mental congestion	GV.14,15
	Deficient Spleen and Damp	mental confusion	yìn táng
	Wind Phlegm	facial paralysis	GV.26
KI	Wind Phlegm and Fire	hypertension	KI.1
	Phlegm in Lower Energizer	infertility	KI.13
BL	Lung Phlegm	bronchitis	BL.13, 42
	Heart Phlegm	depression	BL.15, 44
	Deficient Spleen and Phlegm	sinusitis	BL.20, 49
HT	Heart Phlegm	manic depression	HT.6,7,8
SI	Lung Phlegm	bronchiectasis	SI.15
PC	Heart Phlegm	speech disorders	PC.5, 6
	Lung Phlegm	asthma	PC.6
	Stagnant Liver Qi and Phlegm	vomiting	PC.6
TE	Stagnant Qi and Damp in Lower Energizer	oedema	TE.6
	Lung Phlegm	catarrhal deafness	TE.17
LR	Stagnant Qi and Damp	depression and lethargy	LR.3
	Stagnant Damp in Middle Energizer	indigestion	LR.13
	Stagnant Qi and Phlegm in chest	palpitations and depression	LR.14
GB	Lung Phlegm	catarrh in nose and throat	GB.20
SP	Phlegm in chest	chest fullness and pain	SP.4
ST	Phlegm Damp in head	headache	ST.8
	Lung Phlegm Heat	painful swollen throat	ST.9
	Lung Phlegm	bronchitis	ST.14–16
	Phlegm in Intestines	mucus colitis	ST.25
	Phlegm in Lower Energizer	infertility	ST.29, 30
	Phlegm Fire in Heart and Stomach	mental agitation	ST.44
LU	Lung Phlegm	bronchial asthma	LU.1, 5, 6, 7
LI	Lung Phlegm	nasal catarrh	LI.4, 20
	Stagnant Qi in Lower Energizer	abdominal distension and pain	LI.10
	Phlegm and Fire poison	boils	LI.4, 11, 18

Syndromes

Lung Phlegm
Heart Phlegm
Spleen and Stomach Phlegm and Damp

Lung Phlegm

Pulse. Slippery, maybe empty or flooding, maybe wiry.

Indications. Catarrh in lungs, throat and nose.

Example. Sinusitis with frontal headache.

Combination. ST.2, ST.8, LI.20, GB.14 E; ST.40, LI.4 Rd.

Heart Phlegm

Pulse. Slippery, maybe irregular, slow or rapid.

Indications. Palpitations, feelings of fullness in the chest, manic depression.

Example. Confused speech and behaviour.

Combination. ST.40, ST.45, PC.6, HT.5, CV.23, GV.15 E.

Spleen and Stomach Phlegm and Damp

Pulse. Slippery, maybe empty or flooding, maybe wiry.

Indications. Nausea, indigestion, worry and mental congestion.

Example. Tiredness, mental confusion and poor memory.

Combination. ST.40, ST.45, LI.1, LI.4, BL.10, BL.20, GV.20 Rf.

ST.41 jiě xī

River point, Fire point, Tonification point.

General

ST.41 is not generally used as a Tonification point; ST.36 is the main point to strengthen Stomach and Spleen. ST.41 can be used as a Fire point, to drain Stomach Fire to treat red eyes, headaches, vomiting, constipation, mania and agitation. However, ST.44, the Water point, is more frequently used for this purpose by many practitioners.

ST.41 is perhaps most commonly used as a River point to treat the ankle joint, for arthritis, pain, stiffness or weakness.

ST.42, chōng yáng

Source point.

General

ST.42 is little used as a Source point to tonify the Stomach, being overshadowed by the more powerful ST.36. It can be used as a Source point, however, in combination with LI.4 or TE.4, to strengthen Qi and stabilize the emotions. It can be used for lack of appetite and anorexia.

ST.44 nèi tíng

Spring point, Water point.

General

ST.44 is the most important point to drain Stomach Fire, for which the basic combination can be ST.44, LI.4, LI.11; points can be added to this formula depending on the body area affected by the Stomach Fire, as shown in Table 16.11.

Table 16.11 Additions to the basic combination for Stomach Fire

Area	Ailment	Modification
Head	headache	+ ST.8, tài yáng, GB.20
	sinusitis	+ ST.2, ST.3, LI.20
	trigeminal neuralgia	+ ST.4–7
	toothache, gingivitis	
Throat	blocked throat	+ ST.9
	sore throat	+ CV.23
	tonsillitis	+ SI.17
Abdomen	epigastric pain	+ ST.21
	diarrhoea	+ ST.25
	constipation	+ SP.15

Regulates the skin

Stomach Fire can contribute to skin rashes, acne and boils, and to the basic formula of ST.44, LI.4 and LI.11, such points as PC.9, SP.1, LR.1, GV.10 and BL.17 can be added.

Regulates mind and emotions

By dispersing Stomach Fire, ST.44 can treat mental restlessness and agitation and improve concentration and study. Since Stomach Fire may be associated with Heart Fire, ST.44 can be used for anxiety, hysteria, panic, mania and manic depression, often in combination with PC.3 and HT.5.

Stops bleeding

Stomach Fire can contribute to Heat in the Blood and this can cause bleeding from nose, stomach, intestines and urinary system. ST.44, LI.4 and LI.11 can combine to drain the Stomach Fire and other points can be added. For example, for epistaxis, add GV.23 and BL.40; for gastro-intestinal bleeding add SP.1 and PC.3; for haematuria, add HT.5 and CV.3.

Regulates the face

ST.44 has special effects on the face, and is often combined with LI.4 for facial disorders, not only from Stomach Fire, but also from Exterior to Interior Wind, such as facial paralysis.

Syndromes

  Stomach Fire
    Head and face disorders
    Stomach and Intestinal disorders
    Skin disorders
    Psychological disorders

Head and face disorders

Pulse. Rapid, full or flooding, maybe wiry or slippery.

Indications. Toothache, trigeminal neuralgia, headache.

Example. Sinusitis with purulent discharge.

Combination. ST.2, ST.40, ST.44, LI.4, LI.11, LI.20, GB.20, BL.13 Rd.

Stomach and Intestinal disorders

Pulse. Rapid, full or flooding, maybe wiry or slippery.

Indications. Gastritis, bad breath, constipation.

Example. Voracious appetite.

Combination. ST.21, ST.39, ST.44, LI.4, LI.10, PC.3, CV.14 Rd.

Skin disorders

Pulse. Rapid, maybe thin, choppy or full.

Indications. Eczema, dry skin.

Example. Acute, severe, red, itchy eczema.

Combination. SP.1, ST.45, LU.11, LI.1 B; ST.44, LI.4, LI.11 Rd.

Psychological disorders

Pulse. Rapid, maybe thin, full or flooding, maybe rapid or irregular.

Incications: Mania, epilepsy, schizophrenia, hysteria.

Example. Severe worry, agitation, restlessness and anxiety.

Combination. ST.37, ST.44, SP.1, SP.2, PC.3, PC.6, CV.14, GV.20 Rd.

ST.45 lì duì

Well point, Metal point.

General

The main function of ST.45 is to drain Stomach Fire, and like ST.44, it can treat Stomach Fire patterns of the eyes, nose, teeth, face, stomach and skin. Like ST.44, and often in combination with it, it can treat mental and emotional disorders associated with Stomach and Heart Fire; for example, disorientation, restless agitation and dream-disturbed sleep.

ST.45 as a Well point

ST.45 can also act as a Well point to invigorate not only the circulation of Qi and Blood in the Stomach channel, but also the mind. It can be used for arterial circulation in the feet, combined with SP.1 and SP.4 for varicose veins, with ST.40, ST.41 and SP.8. For mental dullness and congestion it can be combined with SP.1 and yìn táng, and for hangover it can be used with ST.40, LI.1 and LI.4.

Syndromes

  Stomach Fire — see ST.44
  Stagnant Qi in Stomach channel

Stagnant Qi in Stomach channel

Pulse. Hindered or wiry, maybe slippery or flooding.

Indications. Headache, mental congestion, poor circulation, hangover.

Example. Cold feet, tiredness, mental lethargy.

Combination. ST.45, SP.1 M; ST.40, LI.1, LI.4, GV.16, GV.20, yìn táng E.

Stomach point comparisons and combinations

The functions of the main points of the Stomach channel are listed in Table 16.12.

Table 16.12 Stomach point comparisons

Point	Point type	Syndrome
ST.1	point of Yang Heel channel	eye disorders
ST.2	point of Yang Heel channel	eye disorders
		nasal disorders
ST.3	point of Yang Heel channel	nasal disorders
ST.4	Crossing point with Large Intestine channel	facial disorders
	point of Yang Heel channel	mouth disorders
ST.8	Crossing point with Gallbladder channel	headaches
	point of Yang Link channel	
ST.9	Sea of Qi point	neck and throat disorders
		blood pressure disorders
ST.18		breast disorders
ST.21		Stagnation of Cold in Stomach
		Stagnation of food in stomach
		Stomach Fire
		Liver invades Stomach
ST.25	Front Collecting point	Deficiency and Cold in Spleen and Intestines
		Damp Heat in Intestines
		Heat in Stomach and Intestines
		Stagnant Qi in Intestines
ST.28		Fluid disorders
ST.29		Stagnant Blood in uterus
ST.30	point of Sea of Food	Stagnant Blood in uterus
	point of Thoroughfare channel	groin and genital disorders
		prolapse from Sinking Qi
		Thoroughfare channel disorders
ST.35		knee disorders
ST.36	Sea point, Earth point	Deficient Qi
	point of Sea of Food	Sinking Qi
		Deficient Blood
		Damp and Phlegm
		psychological disorders
		Rebellious Stomach Qi
		Intestinal disorders
		hypertension
ST.37	Lower Sea point of Large Intestine	Large Intestine disorders
	point of Sea of Blood	
ST.38		shoulder disorders
ST.39	Lower Sea point of Small Intestine	Small Intestine disorders
	point of Sea of Blood	
ST.40	Connecting point	Lung Phlegm
		Heart Phlegm
		Spleen and Stomach Damp and Phlegm
ST.41	River point, Fire point, Tonification point	ankle and foot disorders
ST.44	Spring point, Water point	Stomach Fire
		head and face disorders
		Stomach and Intestinal disorders,
		skin disorders
		psychological disorders
ST.45	Well point, Metal point	Stomach Fire

Some common combinations of Stomach points are summarized in table 16.13.

Table 16.13 Combinations of Stomach points

Point	Combination	Syndromes	Example
ST.1	ST.2	eye disorders	optic neuritis
ST.1	ST.44	Stomach Fire eye disorders	red, painful eyes
ST.2	ST.3	Lung Phlegm	sinus headache
ST.2	ST.36	Deficient Blood eye disorders	blurred vision
ST.2	ST.4	Stomach Fire	eye and face pain
ST.3	ST.40	Lung Phlegm	sinusitis
ST.3	ST.4	Wind Cold	facial paralysis
ST.4	ST.36	Deficient Qi	cold sores around the mouth
ST.4	ST.44	Stomach Fire	red, cracked lips
ST.8	ST.36	Deficient Qi and Blood	headache and tiredness
ST.8	ST.40	Damp and Phlegm	headache and mental dullness
ST.8	ST.44	Stomach Fire	headache and hot feeling in the head
ST.9	ST.44	Stomach Fire	sore throat
ST.18	ST.36	Deficient Qi and Blood	insufficient lactation
ST.18	ST.37	Fire poison	breast abscess
ST.21	ST.25	Stagnant Qi in Stomach and Intestines	epigastric and abdominal pain and distension
ST.21	ST.34	Stomach Fire	severe epigastric pain
ST..21	ST.44	Deficient Stomach Yin	burning sensation in epigastrium
ST.25	ST.36	Cold and Damp in Intestines	diarrhoea
ST.25	ST.37	Deficiency and Stagnation in Intestines	constipation
ST.25	ST.39	Damp Heat in Stomach and Intestines	gastroenteritis
ST.28	ST.36	Cold and Damp in Lower Energizer	oedema
ST.29	ST.30	Stagnant Blood in uterus	dysmenorrhoea
ST.30	ST.31	Stagnant Blood in leg	Buerger's disease
ST.30	ST.36	Deficient Qi and Blood	exhaustion
ST.31	ST.32	Wind Cold Damp in leg	thigh weakness
ST.31	ST.41	Stagnant Blood in leg	poor circulation
ST.34	ST.35	Wind Cold Damp	knee arthritis
ST.35	ST.36	Wind Heat Damp	knee arthritis
ST.36	ST.40	Deficient Spleen Qi and Phlegm	chronic asthma
ST.36	ST.44	Deficient Stomach Yin	restless exhaustion
ST.36	ST.45	Stagnant Stomach Qi	mental congestion
ST.37	ST.44	Heat in Stomach and Intestines	constipation
ST.39	ST.44	Damp Heat in Small Intestine	dysentery
ST.40	ST.44	Phlegm Fire in Heart and Stomach	mania
ST.40	ST.45	Heart Phlegm	speech disorders
ST.41	ST.43	Wind Heat Damp	foot arthritis
ST.44	ST.45	Heat in the Blood	eczema
ST.2	ST.3, 40	Lung Phlegm	sinus headache
ST.2	ST.40, 44	Phlegm Fire in Lungs and Stomach	sinusitis with yellow nasal discharge
ST.4	ST.5, 6	Hyperactive Liver Yang	trigeminal neuralgia
ST.4	ST.37, 44	Fire Poison	boils and acne
ST.5	ST.6, 7	Wind Cold	face pain
ST.6	ST.7, 8	Wind Heat Damp	temporomandibular arthritis
ST.8	ST.40, 44	Stomach Phlegm and Fire	headache, gastritis and nausea
ST.18	ST.37, 44	Fire poison	mastitis
ST.21	ST.25, 39	Damp Heat in Stomach and Intestines	gastroenteritis
ST.21	ST.34, 44	Stomach Fire and Stagnant Stomach Qi	epigastric distension and burning pain
ST.25	ST.37, 44	Heat in Large Intestine	colonic bleeding
ST.30	ST.31, 32	Stagnant Blood	sprain of groin and thigh
ST.2	ST.3, 40, 45	Phlegm Fire in Lungs and Stomach	sinusitis with purulent nasal discharge
ST.2	ST.8, 40, 45	Lung Phlegm and Phlegm Damp in head	sinusitis, frontal headache and dizziness
ST.30	ST.31, 36, 41	Deficient Qi and Stagnant Blood	poor circulation in legs
ST.32	ST.34, 35, 36	Stagnantion Qi and Blood with Wind Cold Damp	thigh and knee pain

Liver 17

Liver channel

CHANNEL CONNECTIONS

MAIN CHANNEL PATHWAY

Starting near LR.1 on the big toe, the superficial pathway ascends the medial leg, crossing the Spleen channel at SP.6 and then at SP.12 and SP.13 before curving around the genitals. It then runs up the abdomen crossing the Conception channel at CV.2, CV.3 and CV.4, to end at LR.14 in the sixth intercostal space. An internal pathway enters the body from LR.13 to curve around the stomach and connect with the liver and gallbladder before running up through the diaphragm into the chest. An internal pathway leaves LR.14 to run up through the hypochondriac region and chest, to the throat, nasopharynx and eye, before running upwards to meet the Governor channel at GV.20 at the vertex.

CONNECTING CHANNEL PATHWAY

The Connecting channel of the Liver starts from LR.5 and one branch connects with the Gallbladder channel and another branch runs up the leg to the genitals.

Table 17.1 Crossing points on the Liver channel

Point	Crossing	Other functions
LR.13	GB	Alarm point of Spleen
		Gathering point for the five Yin organs
LR.14	SP	Alarm point of Liver
		Point of Yin Link channel

ORGAN RELATIONSHIPS OF THE LIVER

The functions of the Liver points depend upon connections of the Liver channel, or the functions of the Liver and on its relationship with the other organs.

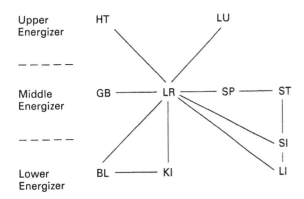

Fig. 17.1 Organ relationships of the Liver.

TERMINAL YIN RELATIONSHIP

The Liver and Pericardium channels are combined in the Terminal Yin channel pair of the Six Divisions. Pericardium points can be used for the results of Stagnant Liver Qi and Liver Fire in the Upper and Middle Energizers especially, in combination with Liver points. Table 17.7 shows combinations of Liver and Pericardium points for a variety of ailments, ranging from depression to fungal infections of the hands and feet.

LIVER AND CONCEPTION CHANNELS

Liver and Conception points both often have the function of moving Stagnant Qi. Liver and Conception points, used either separately or in combination can move Stagnant Qi, Stagnant Blood, Damp and Damp Heat in the Upper, Middle and Lower Energizers.

Table 11.8 shows some basic combinations of Conception and Liver points.

FUNCTIONS OF LIVER POINTS

REGULATE MIND AND EMOTIONS

Each individual has within them an inner potential that can unfold throughout their lives. When they are aware of that potential and in tune with it, they can see the path of their life unfolding before them so that they can act with certainty and confidence. Intuition is the ability to feel and to perceive that inner unfolding, and planning is external manifestation of intuition.

The problem for Wood-type personalities, as discussed in Chapter 4, is that if they lose contact with their intuition, their plans and decisions can become inappropriate, involving them in increasingly difficult life situations which may take many years to work out. Wood people then feel increasingly blocked and obstructed and

become easily frustrated, angry and depressed.

Liver points can help to relieve the inner pressure that derives from the conflict between a need for rapid decisions and actions, and inner uncertainty as to the right action to take. LR.1, LR.3 and LR.14, can relieve this inner pressure and move Stagnation. LR.2 can relieve the feeling of restless impatience that often pushes the Wood types into a succession of rapid unwise decisions. These points can be combined with GV.20 yìn táng, or other head points, to relieve the feeling of pressure and tension in the head to allow the person to view life with more patience, calmness and clarity.

However, the use of Liver points, or BL.18 and BL.47, the Back Transporting points for the Liver, may have no lasting effect for Wood types, unless they learn the lesson of patience, and learn to act from their intuition in stillness, not from a feeling of restlessness and pressure.

MOVE STAGNANT QI AND BLOOD

When people lose contact with the harmonious unfolding of their inner selves, they may feel increasingly hindered and blocked. The Stagnation of Qi that follows can result in headaches, muscular tension, breast problems, menstrual problems, or in Stagnation of Qi in Heart, Spleen, Lungs or Kidneys.

Liver, Pericardium and Conception points, especially, can be combined to treat many of these problems. For example, chest pain associated with suppressed anger and depression can be treated with CV.17, PC.1, PC.6, LR.3 and LR.14.

CALM HYPERACTIVE LIVER YANG AND WIND

Hyperactive Liver Yang can be associated either with the Excess patterns of Stagnant Liver Qi or Liver Fire, or with the Deficiency patterns of Deficient Qi, Deficient Blood or Deficient Yin. If GV.20, GB.20, LR.3 E is used as the basic formula for Hyperactive Yang, then LR.2, KI.1 Rd can be added for Liver Fire, or PC.6, LR.14 Rd added for Stagnant Liver Qi. Alternatively, CV.4 KI.3 Rf can be added for Deficient Kidney Qi, CV.12, ST.36 Rf for Deficient Spleen Qi, SP.6, SP.10, LR.8 Rf for Deficient Blood, or SP.6, KI.6 Rf added for Deficient Yin.

In addition to this, the basic formula can be modified according to which body area is affected by the Hyperactive Liver Yang:

+ GB.14, tài yáng E	for lateral headache
+ GB.1, TE.23 E	for conjunctivitis
+ GB.2, TE.17 E	for ear problems
+ GV.9, GV.16 E	for spinal stiffness
+ GB.21, GB.34 Rd	for general muscular tension
+ GB.34, BL.58 Rd	for calf spasm.

So, for example, a person with Hyperactive Liver Yang associated with Deficient Liver Blood, with dull generalized headache and blurred vision, could be treated with:

GV.20, yìn táng, GB.1, GB.40, SP.6, SP.10, LR.3 Rf.

CLEAR LIVER FIRE

Liver Fire associated with expressed and suppressed anger, impatience, irritability and resentment, can manifest in headache, skin rash, menorrhagia, or invade Heart, Stomach or Lungs. The Spring points (and Fire points) LR.2 and PC.8 can be combined to disperse Fire in Liver, Heart or Stomach. Bleeding the Well points, LR.1 and PC.9, can enhance this treatment. In addition, ST.45 can be bled for Liver Fire invading Stomach, and LU.11 can be bled for Liver Fire invading Lungs. For Liver Fire itself, tài yáng, yìn táng, or the apex of the ear can be bled to give relief, or LR.2 and PC.8 can be combined with GV.20 and KI.1 with Reducing method.

CLEAR LIVER–GALLBLADDER DAMP HEAT

Stagnation of Liver Qi may result in the accumulation of Damp and Heat. This can affect the head area with ear, eye or skin infections; the Middle Energizer with gastritis and cholecystitis; or the Lower Energizer with salpingitis, urethritis or genital itching, pain or discharge.

The Extra channel Opening points GB.41 + TE.5 can act as a basic combination for Liver–Gallbladder Damp Heat in the head area or Lower Energizer, and LR.5, the Connecting point can be added to this combination. For Damp Heat in the Middle Energizer, GB.34 + TE.6 is often a better combination, to which LR.3 + LR.14 can be added for cholecystitis, or LR.3 + LR.13 added for gastritis.

STRENGTHEN DEFICIENT LIVER BLOOD

LR.3 + LR.8 can be used for Deficient Liver Blood, in combination with ST.36 + SP.6. If Deficient Blood is associated with Deficient Kidney Jing, then CV.4 and KI.6 can be added. Tonification of BL.17, BL.18, BL.20 and BL.23 can be alternated with treatment on the front of the body. GV.20 and yìn táng can be added if Deficient Blood results in dizziness and generalized headache, or GB.34 + GB.40 can be added if Deficient Blood leads to weak muscles.

CLEAR COLD FROM THE LIVER CHANNEL

LR.5 can be combined with CV.3 and LR.10, LR.11 and LR.12 to remove Cold invading the Liver channel and causing genital pain. Much moxa should be used and such points as LR.1, CV.2, CV.6 and ST.30 may be added.

STRENGTHEN DEFICIENT LIVER FIRE

The Yin Wood types may lack the Liver Qi, Yang and Fire necessary to express their own personalities and assert themselves sufficiently to prevent them being dependent on, influenced by, or dominated by others. The Fire points LR.2 and GB.38 can be strengthened with needles and moxa, and this treatment stabilized with the Source points LR.3 and GB.40. The treatment should be discussed with the patient, since there may be a temporary increase in anger and irritability.

LIVER SYNDROMES

Liver syndromes are summarized in Table 17.2.

Table 17.2 Point combinations for Liver and Gallbladder syndromes

Syndromes	Signs & symptoms	Pulse	Tongue	Point combination
Stagnant Liver Qi	frustration, depression, feeling blocked and obstructed, feeling of distension in chest, hypochondrium or abdomen, sighing, headache	hindered or wiry	maybe purplish	PC.6, LR.3, LR.14 Rd
+ Stagnant Heart Qi	+ sadness and melancholy, maybe discomfort or pain in the chest, maybe poor peripheral circulation	+ maybe irregular	as above	+ CV.17, PC.1, SP.4 Rd
+ Stagnant Spleen Qi	+ worry and overconcern, abdominal distension and discomfort, borborygmus, irregular bowel movements	+ maybe slippery	+ greasy coat	+ CV.6, CV.12, SP.4, SP.15 Rd
+ Stagnant Stomach Qi	+ epigastric distension and discomfort, nausea, vomiting, hiccuping or sour belching	+ maybe slippery	+ greasy coat	+ CV.13, ST.21, ST.36, SP.4 Rd
+ Stagnant Lung Qi	+ suppressed anger and grief, holding on to past relationships, maybe feeling of pain, discomfort or fullness in chest	+ maybe flooding and deep	+ maybe swelling in Lung area	+ CV.17, LU.1, LU.7 Rd

Table 17.2 *(cont'd)*

Syndromes	Signs and symptoms	Pulse	Tongue	Point combination
+ Stagnant Kidney Qi	+ fear and resentment of change and of the developmental changes of life, e.g. menstruation, childbirth, midlife, maybe amenorrhoea or infertility	+ maybe deep and choppy	+ maybe swollen	+ CV.6, KI.8, KI.13 E
+ Stagnant Gallbladder Qi	+ hypochondriac pain, nausea, jaundice, e.g. cholecystitis	+ maybe slippery	+ maybe yellow greasy coat	+ dǎn náng, GB.24, GB.34 Rd
+ Stagnant Qi in muscles	+ muscle tension in legs, shoulders and neck especially, headache, suppressed anger	+ maybe full	+ maybe deviated	+ GB.21, GB.34 Rd
+ Stagnant Qi in chest or breasts	+ feeling of distension and pain in chest or breasts, worse with suppressed emotions or before menstruation, maybe feeling of obstruction in throat	+ maybe flooding	+ various	+ CV.17, SI.1, ST.18 Rd
+ Stagnant Qi and Damp in Lower Energizer	+ oedema and abdominal distension and pain, worse with suppressed emotion, feeling of heaviness and cold, maybe delayed menstruation	+ maybe slippery or empty	+ maybe moist greasy coat	+ CV.6, ST.28, SP.6, SP.9 E M
+ Stagnant Blood in Lower Energizer	+ dysmenorrhoea, endometriosis, irregular menstruation	+ maybe choppy	+ maybe red purple	+ CV.3, CV.6, ST.29, SP.6 Rd
Hyperactive Liver Yang	irritability, dizziness, headache	wiry	maybe normal	GV.20, GB.20, GB.34, SP.6, LR.3 R
+ Disturbance of Heart Spirit	+ restlessness, overexcitement or anxiety, insomnia	+ maybe irregular	+ maybe trembling	+ CV.14, HT.6, KI.6 E
+ Deficient Spleen Qi	+ tiredness, faintness, headache or empty feeling in head, worse if too long between meals	+ empty maybe choppy	+ pale, flabby	+ CV.12. ST.36, SP.3 Rf
+ Deficient Kidney Qi	+ tiredness, emotional lability, maybe tinnitus or empty headache, better with rest	+ deep empty, choppy	+ pale, flabby	+ CV.12, ST.36, KI.3 Rf
+ Deficient Kidney Yin	+ tired but hot and restless, maybe eye irritation or headache with sensation of Heat	+ thin, rapid	+ red, no coat	+ CV.4, KI.6 Rf; KI.2 Rd
Liver Wind	dizziness, loss of consciousness, tremors, numbness or paralysis of limbs; tics, spasms or deviation or mouth and face	wiry and various·	maybe moving or deviated + various	GV.16, GV.20, GB.20, LI.4, SP.6, LR.3 E
Liver Fire	expressed or suppressed anger, with headache, dizziness, feelings of heat, red face and eyes, maybe epistaxis	wiry, rapid full	dark red, yellow coat	GV.20, PC.8, KI.1, LR.3 Rd; SP.6 Rf
+ Heart Fire	+ overexcitement, excessive talking, mania or anxiety	+ maybe hasty	+ dark red tip, trembling	+ PC.9 B; HT.3 Rf
+ Lung Fire	+ coughing, fever, haemoptysis, maybe chest pain worse on coughing	+ maybe flooding	+ maybe greasy coat	+ LU.11 B; LU.10 Rd; LU.5 Rf
+ Stomach Fire	+ burning pain in epigastrium, thirst, bad breath, constipation, maybe haematemesis	+ maybe choppy	+ maybe deep centre crack	+ CV.12, ST.21, ST.44, ST.45 Rd
+ Heat in the Blood	+ menorrhagia or severe red, hot, itchy skin rash	full wiry, rapid	dark red, yellow coat	+ LI.4, LI.11, SP.10, LR.1 Rd
Liver-Gallbladder Damp Heat	feverishness, maybe bitter taste, maybe feeling of heaviness, maybe suppressed anger or resentment	wiry, rapid, slippery	red, greasy yellow coat	GB.34, SP.6 Rd
+ Damp Heat in head area	+ otitis media or conjunctivitis	wiry, rapid, slippery	red, greasy yellow coat	+ TE.3, TE.17, GB.1, GB.41, GB.44 Rd
+ Damp Heat in Middle Energizer	+ nausea, epigastric or hypochondriac pain, maybe jaundice	wiry, rapid, slippery	red, greasy yellow coat	dǎn náng, TE.6, GB.24, SP.9 Rd
+ Damp Heat in Lower Energizer	+ genital pain, itching and discharge	wiry, rapid, slippery	red, greasy yellow coat	+ CV.3, TE.5, GB.24, GB.41 Rd
Deficient Liver Blood	blurred vision, dull headache, tiredness, dizziness; weakness, numbness or tremors of muscles	thin, choppy	pale, thin	GV.20 E; LI.4, SP.6, ST.36, LR.8 Rf
+ Deficient Kidney Jing	+ poor memory, poor concentration, tinnitus, weak joints, lack of confidence and restricted mobility	+ deep	+ flabby	+ CV.4, KI.6, GB.39 Rf
Cold invades Liver channel	pain in lower abdomen and testes, with feeling of cold which is better with warmth	deep, wiry	maybe pale, and moist	CV.3, LR.1, LR.5, LR.11, ST.30 Rf M
Deficient Liver-Gallbladder Fire	lack of independence, assertion and anger, difficulty in saying no or preventing invasion of boundaries	empty, maybe deep and slow	maybe pale and flabby	CV.6, LR.2, GB.38 Rf M; LR.3, GB.40 Rf
Deficient Gallbladder and Kidney Qi	fearfulness, timidity, lack of confidence, self-doubt, uncertainty and indecision	empty, maybe hindered	maybe pale and flabby	CV.4, TE.4, GB.13, GB.40, KI.7 Rf M

Rd, Reducing method; Rf, Reinforcing method; E, Even method; B, bleeding; M, moxa.

Liver points

LR.1 dà dūn

Well point, Wood point.

General

LR.1 has three main functions:

invigorates the Liver
clears Liver Fire
regulates the Lower Energizer.

Invigorates the Liver

Like other Well points, LR.1 can stimulate the Liver channel and organ and move Stagnation of Qi. This can help physical aches and pains, emotional frustration and depression, or mental obstruction to the free-flow of plans and insights. For such mental problems, LR.1 can be combined with LR.14, to open the whole length of the channel, and with yìn táng to open the mind to clear visualization and intuition.

Clears Liver Fire

LR.1 is often combined with LR.2 to clear Liver Fire to treat hypertension, headache, eye inflammations, skin rashes, epilepsy, anger and irritability and extreme mental restlessness. As a Well point, LR.1 can be used for loss of consciousness and severe acute conditions, while LR.2, the Spring point, is used for both acute and chronic patterns of Liver Fire.

Regulates the Lower Energizer

LR.1 regulates the Lower Energizer in four main ways

clears Damp Heat
stops bleeding
moves Stagnant Qi and Blood
regulates muscle tone.

Clears Damp Heat. LR.1 clears Damp Heat from the bladder and urethra to treat cystitis and difficult urination and drains Damp Heat from the genitals to treat pain, inflammation, swelling, itching or discharge in the genital area.

Stops bleeding. By removing Liver Fire, LR.1 cools Heat in the Blood, which reduces bleeding of the Excess Heat type in the Lower Energizer, e.g. abnormal uterine bleeding or blood in urine or stool.

Moves Stagnant Qi and Blood. This function of LR.1 relieves pain in the genitals, uterus, urinary system, intestines or in the lower abdominal muscles, e.g. due to groin sprain or hernia.

Regulates muscle tone. In addition to reducing muscle tension to treat spasm in the muscles of the lower abdomen, LR.1 can also increase muscle tone to treat uterine prolapse or urinary incontinence.

Syndromes

Stagnation of Liver Qi
Liver Fire
Problems of the Lower Energizer
  Damp Heat
  Bleeding
  Stagnant Qi and Blood
  Reduced muscle tone

Stagnation of Liver Qi

Pulse. Wiry or hindered.

Indications. Mental congestion, depression, headache, hangover, breast pain, hypochondriac pain.

Example. Difficulty in visualizing or planning for future possibilities in life.

Combination. LR.1, GB.44 Rd; GB.13, GB.40, yìn táng E; KI.3 Rf.

Liver Fire

Pulse. Rapid, wiry, full or flooding.

Indications. Bursts of anger, hypertension, frustration, headache.

Example. Frustration of plans, dreams and creative energy, with anger and depression.

Combination. LR.1, LR.2, GB.38, TE.6 Rd.

Problems of the Lower Energizer

Damp Heat

Pulse. Rapid, slippery, wiry, maybe thin or flooding.

Indications. Cystitis, urethritis, leucorrhoea, scrotal or vaginal itching.

Example. Cystitis with restlessness and irritability.

Combination. LR.1, LR.5, CV.3, BL.66 Rd.

Bleeding

Pulse. Rapid, maybe wiry, thin or flooding.

Indications. Blood in urine or stool, abnormal uterine bleeding.

Example. Abnormal uterine bleeding due to Heat.

Combination. LR.1, SP.1, SP.10, CV.3, ST.36 E.

Stagnant Qi and Blood

Pulse. Wiry, maybe choppy, maybe deep and slow.

Indications. Dysuria, intestinal pain, dysmenorrhoea, scrotal pain, hernia pain.

Example. Groin sprain on right side.

Combination. LR.1, LR.12, SP.12, ST.30 on the right, CV.2 Rd M.

Reduced muscle tone

Pulse. Maybe empty, choppy or wiry.

Indications. Urinary incontinence, enuresis, uterine prolapse.

Example. Uterine prolapse and weak lower abdominal muscles.

Combination. LR.1, LR.8, ST.29, ST.36, CV.4, GV.20 Rf M.

LR.2 xíng jiān

Spring point, Fire point.

General

LR.2 has three main functions:

clears Liver Fire
clears Damp Heat
tonifies Liver Fire.

Clears Liver Fire

This has five main aspects:

clears Liver Fire and Liver Wind
clears Liver and Heart Fire
clears Liver and Lung Fire
clears Liver and Stomach Fire
clears Liver Fire and Heat in the Blood.

These aspects are discussed later as syndromes.

Clears Damp Heat

LR.2 is not a main point for Damp Heat; generally LR.5 is more specific for this pattern.

Tonifies Liver Fire

Like most Fire points, LR.2 can be used not only to drain Excess Fire but also to tonify Fire in patterns of Deficient Fire and Yang. For example, LR.2 can be used with Reinforcing method and moxa to increase self-confidence and self-assertion to help 'the human doormats', the people who let others walk all over them, intrude in their lives, dominate their personalities and stifle their creativity. LR.2 can be used in this way to help the people who 'can't say no', so that they can be firm and definite in restricting the influence of other people in their lives.

When LR.2 is used in this way, it is necessary to check pulse and tongue regularly for signs of excessive Heat, and to check with the patient that the balance has not swung too far from useful self-assertion into aggressive behaviour. The patient needs to be advised that there may be periods of irritability, intolerance, impatience or anger, whilst a new personal balance is achieved. This process can be more harmonious with suitable meditation techniques.

If the practitioner is not accustomed to helping patients deal with their emotions, it is best not to moxa LR.2 or GB.38.

Syndromes

Liver Fire
    Liver Fire and Liver Wind
    Liver and Heart Fire
    Liver and Lung Fire
    Liver and Stomach Fire
    Liver Fire and Heat in the Blood
Damp Heat
Deficient Liver Fire

Liver Fire and Liver Wind

Pulse. Wiry, rapid, full or flooding.

Indications. Hypertension, headache, vertigo, tinnitus, epilepsy, childhood convulsions.

Example. Bursts of violent anger with the feeling of sitting on an emotional volcano.

Combination. LR.2, LI.1, GV.20 Rd; LR.1 PC.9, tài yáng B.

Liver and Heart Fire

Pulse. Wiry, rapid, full or flooding.

Indications. Hypertension, insomnia, night sweats, nervous anxiety with palpitations.

Example. Easily frustrated, tense and angry when plans and enthusiasms seem blocked.

Combination. LR.2, KI.1, SP.6, BL.15, BL.18, BL.44, BL.47, HT.8 E.

Liver and Lung Fire

Pulse. Wiry, rapid, full or flooding, maybe slippery.

Indications. Sore throat, cough, bronchitis, chest pain.

Example. Sporadic, barking cough with sticky yellowish phlegm which is difficult to cough up, chest soreness on coughing.

Combination. LR.2, LR.14, CV.17, LU.10 Rd; LU.5, KI.6 Rf.

Liver and Stomach Fire

Pulse. Wiry, rapid, thin, full or flooding, maybe slippery.

Indications. Bad breath, gingivitis, toothache, headache, gastritis.

Example. Gastritis with extreme worry, nervous tension and irritability associated with work stress.

Combination. LR.2, LR.13, PC.7, CV.12, ST.21, ST.36, ST.44 Rd; SP.6 Rf.

Liver Fire and Heat in the Blood

Pulse. Wiry, rapid, full or flooding.

Indications. Epistaxis, abnormal uterine bleeding, haematuria, melaena aggravated by frustration and suppressed anger.

Combination. LR.2, PC.8, KI.1 Rd; LR.1, PC.9 B; GV.20 E.

Damp Heat

Pulse. Wiry, slippery, rapid, maybe full flooding or thin.

Indications. Cystitis, urethritis, genital itching.

Example. Leucorrhoea, irritability and impatience.

Combination. LR.2, LR.8, CV.3, PC.5 Rd.

Deficient Liver Fire

Pulse. Maybe wiry, empty choppy, deep or slow.

Indications. Headache, epigastric pain or distension, weakness or stiffness of muscles, self-doubt, lack of self-assertion.

Example. Lack of inner certainty and direction in life, so that personality projects only weakly into the environment.

Combination. LR.2, GB.38 Rf M; BL.18, BL.48, BL.52 Rf.

LR.3 tài chōng

Stream point, Source point, Earth point.

General

LR.3 is one of the most used points in acupuncture. It is mainly used in Excess conditions with Reducing or Even method to move Stagnation of Qi or Blood and to calm Hyperactive Liver Yang. The functions of LR.3 can be listed as:

moves Stagnant Qi and Blood
calms Hyperactive Liver Yang
clears Liver Wind and reduces spasms and pain
clears Liver–Gallbladder Damp Heat
tonifies Liver Blood
calms the Spirit
removes Cold in the Liver channel

Moves Stagnant Qi and Blood

This relates to the main function of the Liver to maintain a free flow of Qi and Blood everywhere in the body.

Physical problems. Figure 17.2 shows the main areas affected by Liver Qi stagnation. These depend on the areas adjacent to the superficial pathways of the Liver and Gallbladder channels and on the connections made with organs or body parts by the internal Liver channel pathways.

Emotional and mental problems. The Wood-type personality is more conscious of seeming obstructions to their plans, creativity and personal energy expression, than the other Five Element types. The Wood-type is more likely to react to seeming obstruction with frustration and anger or depression.

Calms Hyperactive Liver Yang

LR.3 is generally better to calm Hyperactive Liver Yang than any other Liver point, especially when it is associ-

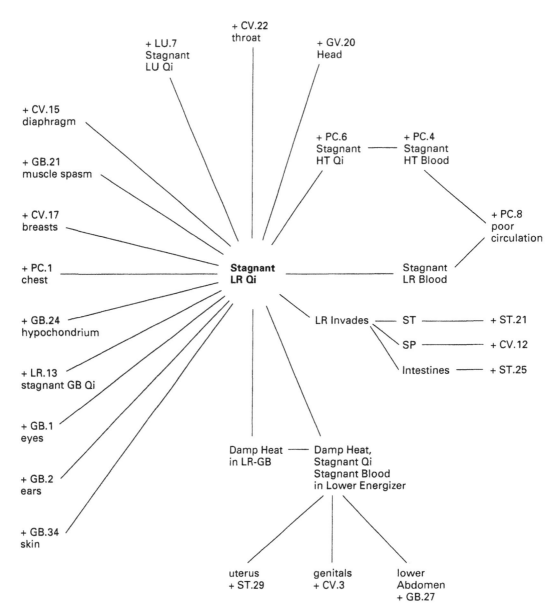

Fig. 17.2 Point combinations with LR.3 for Stagnant Qi (the points given are only examples, there are many other possibilities).

ated with Stagnant Liver Qi, for example, in premenstrual syndrome. LR.2 can sometimes be superior to LR.3 in treating Hyperactive Liver Yang, but only if it is associated with patterns of Liver Fire.

Clears Liver Wind and Reduces spasms and pain

Stagnant Liver Qi, Hyperactive Liver Yang and Liver Wind can all produce muscle spasms and pain, and all can be treated with LR.3. For spasm due to Stagnant Liver Qi and Hyperactive Liver Yang, LR.3 may best combine with GB.34 and SP.6. For spasms and convulsions due to Liver Wind, LR.3 may best combine with GB.20, GV.20 and LR.1.

Clears Liver–Gallbladder Damp Heat

LR.3 is not as effective for this function as LR.5 or GB.34, but is specifically indicated when the Damp Heat is associated with Stagnant Qi of Liver and Gallbladder. If the Damp Heat is more associated with Liver Fire, then it may be more effective to combine LR.5 with LR.2, or GB.34 with GB.38.

Tonifies Liver Blood

Liver Blood is necessary to nourish the eyes, muscles and tendons and to nourish and stabilize the Spiritual Soul. LR.3 or LR.8 can tonify Liver Blood, but in cases of Deficient Liver Blood are usually combined with points that tonify the capacity of the Spleen to produce Blood, e.g. SP.3, SP.6, SP.10 and ST.36. LR.3 can also be combined with BL.17, BL.18, BL.20 or BL.43 to tonify Liver Blood.

Calms the Spirit

Firstly, LR.3 is one of the main points on the body with a generalized calming effect and is often combined with LI.4 for this purpose. Second, since it is a Source point, LR.3 has specific calming and stabilizing effects on the Liver, partly by calming Liver Yang and Wind, and partly by tonifying Liver Blood.

Removes Cold in the Liver channel

This is a minor function of LR.3, important only when there is Cold invasion of the Liver channel, with genital pain in men, or white vaginal discharge in women. The principle of treatment is to warm and to move Stagnation in the channel with local and distal points.

Table 17.3 Comparison of LR.1, LR.2 and LR.3

Indications	LR.1	LR.2	LR.3
Loss of consciousness due to Liver Fire, Wind and Phlegm	X	–	–
Muscle spasm and pain due to Liver Wind or Stagnant Liver Qi	X	–	X
Deficient Liver Blood, e.g. tics, weak muscles, blurred vision	–	–	X
Bleeding due to Heat	X	X	–
Liver Fire			
acute	X	X	–
acute and chronic	X	X	X
Liver Fire and Stagnant Liver Qi	X	X	X
Liver Damp Heat			
with Liver Fire	X	X	–
with Stagnant Liver Qi	X	–	X
Hyperactive Liver Yang	X	X	X
Stagnation of Qi and Blood	X	–	X
Mental stagnation and depression			
acute	X	–	X
chronic	X	–	X
General calming	–	–	X
Calms the Spirit			
agitation due to Liver Fire	X	X	X
mood changes due to Hyperactive Liver Yang	–	–	X

Syndromes

Stagnant Qi and Blood
  Stagnant Liver and Heart Qi
  Stagnant Liver and Heart Blood
  Stagnant Liver and Lung Qi
  Breast problems
  Liver invades Spleen, Stomach or Intestines
  Stagnant Liver and Gallbladder Qi

  Stagnant Qi and Blood in the Lower Energizer
Hyperactive Liver Yang
Liver Wind, spasms and pain
Liver–Gallbladder Damp Heat
Deficient Liver Blood
Disturbance of Spirit
Cold in the Liver channel

Stagnant Liver and Heart Qi

Pulse. Hindered or wiry, empty or full, maybe deep.

Indications. Sadness, depression, pain or discomfort in the chest.

Example. Difficulties and frustrations in communication in a relationship.

Combination. LR.3, PC.6, CV.6, CV.17, CV.22 E.

Stagnant Liver and Heart Blood

Pulse. Wiry, choppy, maybe deep or flooding.

Indications. Chest pain, headache, poor circulation, depression.

Example. Cold hands and feet with feeling of congestion and heat in the chest.

Combination. LR.3, LR.14, PC.8, PC.1, CV.17 Rd; SP.6 E.

Stagnant Liver and Lung Qi

Pulse. Hindered or wiry, maybe slippery.

Indications. Restricted breathing, sighing, depression.

Example. Congested feeling in the chest, feelings of frustration and blockage, withdrawal from life.

Combination. LR.3, LR.14, CV.15, CV.17, LU.1, LU.7 Rd.

Breast problems

Pulse. Hindered or wiry, maybe flooding or rapid.

Indications. Insufficient lactation, mastitis, premenstrual syndrome.

Example. Mastitis and ulceration with discharge.

Combination. LR.3, LR.14, CV.17, PC.1, PC.8, local points Rd.

Note. Acupuncture must not be done unless there is first Western medical diagnosis. PC.1 and local points are used with horizontal insertion, subcutaneously only.

Liver invades Spleen, Stomach or Intestines

Pulse. Wiry, maybe empty or flooding, maybe slippery.

Indications. Epigastric or abdominal distension, discomfort and pain, nausea, constipation.

Example. Constipation with right-sided abdominal pain.

Combination. LR.3, GB.34, TE.6, CV.6 Rd; GB.28 on the right side Rd.

Stagnant Liver and Gallbladder Qi

Pulse. Hindered or wiry, maybe empty or flooding.

Indications. Indigestion, cholecystitis, hypochondriac pain, depression.

Example. Stiff, aching muscles, self-doubt and frustration, procrastination.

Combination. LR.3, GB.21, GB.34, SP.6, yìn táng E.

Stagnant Qi and Blood in the Lower Energizer

Pulse. Hindered or wiry, maybe thin, choppy flooding or full.

Indications. Lower back pain, lower abdominal pain, dysmenorrhoea, irregular menstruation, dysuria.

Example. Ovulation pain with depression at ovulation and menstruation.

Combination. LR.3, SP.6, LI.4, CV.3, zǐ gōng Rd.

Hyperactive Liver Yang

Pulse. Wiry, empty, changing, thin, flooding or full; maybe rapid.

Indications. Hypertension, migraine, dizziness, tinnitus, photophobia, muscle tension.

Example. Headache, nausea, mental confusion and emotional hypersensitivity.

Combination. LR.3, GB.20, tài yáng E; CV.4, KI.3 Rf.

Liver Wind, spasms and pain

Pulse. Wiry, jerky, maybe rapid.

Indications. Convulsions, epilepsy, hemiplegia, muscle tremors, muscles spasms and pain.

Example. Suppressed anger, with tremors, spasms and pain in the muscles.

Combination. LR.3, GB.20, GB.21, GB.34, sì shén cōng Rd.

Liver–Gallbladder Damp Heat

Pulse. Wiry, slippery, rapid, maybe thin, full or flooding.

Indications. Hepatitis, cholecystitis, cholelithiasis, eczema, leucorrhoea.

Example. Feeling of heaviness, restlessness and heat; nausea, headache and emotional bitterness and hatred.

Combination. LR.3, LR.14, LI.4, LI.11, SP.6, SP.9, GB.34 Rd.

Deficient Liver Blood

Pulse. Choppy, thin, maybe wiry.

Indications. Amenorrhoea, blurred vision, dizziness, headache, tiredness, muscular weakness.

Example. Insomnia, with an out-of-the-body sensation before falling asleep.

Combination. LR.8, SP.6, ST.36, Bl.47, yì míng Rf.

Disturbance of Spirit

Pulse. Various, maybe wiry, rapid, jerky or irregular.

Indications. Frustration, depression, irritability, impatience, intolerance, resentment, suppressed anger.

Example. Extreme generalized nervous tension.

Combination. LR.3, LI.4, GV.20 Rd.

Cold in the Liver channel

Pulse. Wiry, deep, slow.

Indications. Genital pain, leucorrhoea, hernia pain.

Example. Testis pain, aggravated by cold.

Combination. LR.3, LR.12, CV.2, CV.3, ST.30 Rd M; PC.6 E.

LR.5 lǐ gōu

Connecting point.

General

The main function of LR.5 as the Connecting point linking the Liver and Gallbladder channels, is to clear Damp Heat in the Lower Energizer, especially for genital problems. It has the secondary function of moving Stagnant Qi in the Lower Energizer. It is more limited in function than LR.3 which has the primary function of moving Stagnant Qi anywhere in the body, and the secondary function of clearing Damp Heat. LR.5 is said to firm Jing, so that it can be used for many sexual dysfunctions related to Liver and Kidney; for example, impotence, premature ejaculation, frigidity and sterility.

Syndromes

Damp Heat in the Lower Energizer
Stagnation of Qi in the Lower Energizer
Sexual problems

Damp Heat in the Lower Energizer

Pulse. Wiry, rapid, slippery, maybe thin, full or flooding.

Indications. Vaginal itching, leucorrhoea, abnormal urine bleeding, salpingitis.

Example. Scrotal inflammation, itching and pain.

Combination. LR.5, LR.11, CV.1, CV.3, ST.30, PC.8 Rd.

Stagnation of Qi in the Lower Energizer

Pulse. Wiry, maybe empty, choppy, full or flooding.

Indications. Lower back pain, lower abdominal pain, orchitis, hernia pain, dysuria, endometriosis.

Example. Irregular menstruation and dysmenorrhoea.

Combination. LR.5, CV.3, zǐ gōng, PC.5 Rd.

Sexual problems

Pulse. Wiry, maybe empty, choppy, thin or flooding; maybe slow or rapid.

Indications. Impotence, frigidity, sterility, depression, pain during or after intercourse.

Example. Difficulty to obtain or maintain an erection, skin rash, depression.

Combination. LR.5, CV.3, CV.14, CV.17, PC.6 Rd; CV.4 KI.6 Rf.

LR.8 qū quán

Sea point, Water point, Tonification point.

General

The main use of LR.8 is with Reducing method to drain Damp Heat in the Lower Energizer, especially for urinary

problems. LR.5 is more for genital problems and LR.8 is more for urinary problems. Also LR.8 can be used for Damp Cold. LR.8 can be used with Reinforcing method to tonify Liver Yin and Liver Blood, and to moisten dryness, reflecting its functions as a Water point and Tonification point. LR.8, the Water point, with Reinforcing method can be combined with LR.2, the Fire point, with Reducing method, to control Liver Fire. LR.8 can be used for Stagnant Liver Qi in the Lower Energizer, but is more commonly used for local knee problems.

Syndromes

Damp Heat in the Lower Energizer
Deficient Liver Blood — see LR.3
Deficient Liver Yin and Liver Fire
Local knee problems
Stagnation of Qi in the Lower Energizer — see LR.5

Damp Heat in the Lower Energizer

Pulse. Wiry, rapid, slippery, maybe thin.

Indications. Urinary retention, burning urination, diarrhoea, vaginitis.

Example. Dysuria.

Combination. LR.8, SP.6, CV.3, CV.6, TE.6.

Deficient Liver Yin and Liver Fire

Pulse. Thin, rapid, maybe choppy or wiry.

Indications. Dry rough skin, red skin rashes, dry red itchy eyes, sore throat.

Example. Vaginal dryness.

Combination. LR.8, KI.6, ST.36, CV.4 Rf; LR.2, KI.2 Rd.

Local knee problems

Pulse. Various, maybe wiry, slow or rapid.

Indications. Pain, stiffness or weakness in the knee.

Example. Weakness of knee, which can give way when standing or walking.

Combination. LR.4, LR.7, LR.8, LR.9, KI.10, BL.39, BL.40 Rf M.

LR.10–12 zú wǔ li, yīn lián, jí mài

LR.10–12 can be used as secondary, local points for Damp Heat, Damp Cold or Stagnation of Qi and Blood in the area of the upper thigh, groin and genitals. For example, they can be used for retention of urine, pain in the penis, scrotal inflammation, prolapsed uterus or hernia pain. They are often used in combination with CV.2 or CV.3, and in combination with distal Liver points.

LR.13 zhāng mén

Alarm point of the Spleen. Crossing point with Gallbladder channel, Gathering point for the five Yin organs.

General

LR.13 has three main functions:

moves Stagnant Liver Qi
harmonizes Liver and Spleen
clears Liver–Gallbladder Damp Heat

In addition, as the Alarm point of the Spleen, if used with Reinforcing method and moxa, it can tonify Yang of Spleen and Stomach, to treat lethargy, abdominal pain and distension, ascites and diarrhoea.

Syndromes

Stagnant Liver Qi
Liver invades Spleen and Stomach
Damp Heat in Liver–Gallbladder

Stagnant Liver Qi

Pulse. Wiry.

Indications. Chest or hypochondriac pain, enlarged spleen or liver, depression.

Example. Hypochondriac pain, headache and sciatica.

Combination. LR.13, LR.3, tài yáng, GB.21, GB.30, GB.34, TE.6 Rd.

Liver invades Spleen and Stomach

Pulse. Wiry, slippery, empty or full.

Indications. Belching, nausea, vomiting, pancreatitis, epigastric or abdominal distension or pain, borborygmus, constipation.

Example. Indigestion and flatulence aggravated by worry and depression.

Combination. LR.13, LR.3, CV.12, CV.14, ST.21, ST.36 E.

Damp Heat in Liver–Gallbladder

Pulse. Wiry, rapid, slippery, maybe thin or flooding.

Indications. Nausea, vomiting, indigestion with bitter taste, headache.

Example. Cholecystitis with irritability and right-sided hypochondriac and abdominal pain.

Combination. LR.13, GB.24, GB.27, dǎn náng Rd on the right; SP.6 E on the left.

LR.14 qí mén

Alarm point of the Liver, Crossing point of Spleen and Yin Link on the Liver channel.

General

LR.14 is primarily used to move Stagnant Liver Qi, and secondarily to clear Liver–Gallbladder Damp Heat. LR.14 is more used than LR.13 to treat mental and emotional congestion due to Stagnant Liver Qi. The two end points of the Liver channel, LR.1 and LR.14 are often combined to treat mental stagnation with difficulty in clear visualization of life possibilities, lack of sense of direction in life, and lack of flexibility in adapting preconceived plans to actual life situations. LR.13 and LR.14 are compared in Table 17.4. Note that LR.13 is the Front Collecting point for the Spleen and LR.14 for the Liver.

Table 17.4 Comparison of LR.13 and LR.14

	LR.13	LR.14
Stagnant Heart and Lung Qi	–	X
breasts	–	X
diaphragm	–	X
Gallbladder	X	X
enlarged Spleen and Liver	X	–
abdomen distension	X	–
worry	X	–
planning	–	X

Syndromes

Stagnant Liver Qi
Breast problems — see LR.3
Damp Heat in Liver–Gallbladder — see LR.13

Stagnant Liver Qi

Pulse. Hindered or wiry.

Indications. Chest pain, restricted breathing, cough, hypertension, sadness, depression.

Example. Headache, frustration and anger from lack of ability to adapt plans to changing conditions.

Combination. LR.14, LR.1, GV.20, yìn táng, TE.6, GB.37 Rd.

Liver point comparisons and combinations

The functions of the main points of the Liver channel are listed in Table 17.5.

Table 17.5 Liver point comparisons

Point	Point type	Syndromes

LR.1	Well point
	Wood point
		Stagnant Liver Qi
		Liver Fire
		Lower Energizer problems
		    Damp Heat
		    Stagnant Qi and Blood
		    bleeding
		    deficient muscle tone

LR.2	Spring point Fire point Sedation point	Liver Fire Damp Heat Deficient Liver Fire

LR.3	Stream point
	Source point
		Stagnant Qi and Blood
		    Stagnant Liver and Heart Qi
		    Stagnant Liver and Heart Blood
		    Stagnant Liver and Lung Qi
		    breast problems
		    Liver invades Spleen, Stomach and intestines
		    Stagnant Liver and Gallbladder Qi
		    Stagnant Qi and Blood in Lower Energizer
		Hyperactive Liver Yang
		Liver Wind, spasms and pain
		Liver–Gallbladder Damp Heat
		Deficient Liver Blood
		Disturbance of the Spirit
		Cold in the Liver Channel

LR.5	Connecting point	Damp Heat in the Lower Energizer Stagnant Qi in the Lower Energizer sexual problems
LR.8	Sea point Water point Tonification point	Damp Heat in the Lower Energizer Deficient Liver Blood Deficient Liver Yin and Liver Fire local knee problems Stagnant Qi in the Lower Energizer
LR.10–12		local thigh, groin and genital problems
LR.13	Spleen Front Collecting point, Meeting point of Liver and Gallbladder, Gathering point for five Yin organs	Stagnant Liver Qi Liver invades Spleen and Stomach Damp Heat in Liver–Gallbladder
LR.14	Liver Front Collecting point, Meeting point of Liver, Spleen and Yin Link	Stagnant Liver Qi Stagnant Liver and Heart Qi Stagnant Liver and Lung Qi breast problems Damp Heat in Liver–Gallbladder

Some common combinations of Liver points with each other and with other channel points are summarized in Table 17.6 and Tables 17.7 and 17.8 respectively.

Table 17.6 Combinations of Liver points

Point	Combination	Syndromes	Example
LR.1	LR.2	Liver Fire	acute red itchy eczema
LR.1	LR.3	Stagnant Liver Qi	mental congestion
LR.1	LR.8	Damp Heat in Lower Energizer	scrotal eczema
LR.1	LR.14	Stagnant Liver Qi	premenstrual syndrome
LR.2	LR.5	Liver Fire and Damp Heat	vaginal itching
LR.2	LR.8	Deficient Liver Yin and Liver Fire	chronic conjunctivitis
LR.3	LR.4	Liver Wind and Stagnant Qi and Blood	hemiplegia with foot contracture
LR.3	LR.5	Stagnant Liver Qi and Damp Heat	dysmenorrhoea and abnormal uterine bleeding
LR.3	LR.8	Deficient Liver Blood	early-stage cataract
LR.3	LR.13	Liver invades Spleen	irritable bowel syndrome
LR.3	LR.14	Stagnation of Liver Qi	frustration and depression
LR.5	LR.8	Deficient Liver Yin and Damp Heat	cystitis
LR.5	LR.13	Liver–Gallbladder Damp Heat	cholecystitis
LR.8	LR.7	Stagnation of Blood and Cold	knee problems
LR.8	LR.9–12	Stagnation in Liver channel	thigh and groin problems
LR.13	LR.14	Stagnation of Liver Qi	hypochondriac pain
LR.1	LR.2,LR.5	Liver Fire and Damp Heat	varicose eczema
LR.1	LR.3,LR.8	Stagnation of Qi and Blood in Liver channel	painful varicose veins
LR.1	LR.3,LR.12	Stagnation of Cold in Liver channel	orchitis
LR.1	LR.3,LR.13	Liver invades Spleen	overweight and depression
LR.1	LR.3,LR.14	Stagnant Liver Qi	suppressed anger and resentment
LR.3	LR.13,LR.14	Stagnant Liver Qi and Liver invades Stomach	oppressive feeling in chest and epigastric
LR.7	LR.8,LR.9	Stagnant Blood in Liver channel	distension knee pain

Table 17.7 Combinations of Liver and Pericardium points

Liver points	Pericardium points	Syndromes	Example
LR.1	PC.3	Heat in the Blood	diarrhoea with melaena
	PC.4	Stagnant Liver and Heart Qi	acute depression
	PC.9	Heat in the Blood	severe acute red eczema
LR.2	PC.3	Liver and Stomach Fire	gastritis
	PC.5	Liver and Heart Fire	hyperthyroidism
	PC.7	Heat in the Blood	acne
	PC.8	Damp Heat	fungal infection of hands and feet
	PC.9	Liver and Heart Fire	acute hypertension
LR.3	PC.1	Stagnant Liver and Heart Blood	angina pectoris
	PC.3	Stagnant Heart and Lung Qi	diaphragm spasm
	PC.4	Stagnation and Disturbance of Spirit	anxiety and depression
	PC.5	Liver Wind and Heart Phlegm	confused speech
	PC.6	Stagnant Liver and Lung Qi	sporadic painful cough
LR.5	PC.8	Damp Heat in the Lower Energizer	jaundice
LR.8	PC.5	Damp Heat in the Lower Energizer	irregular menstruation
LR.13	PC.3	Liver invades Stomach	vomiting and epigastric pain
	PC.6	Liver invades Spleen and Stomach	belching and flatulence
LR.14	PC.1	Stagnant Qi in breasts	mastitis
	PC.2	Stagnant Lung Qi	cough with stifling sensation
	PC.4	Stagnant Heart Blood	heart and chest pain
	PC.6	Stagnant Heart Qi	frustration in relationships
	PC.7	Stagnant Liver Qi	hypochondriac fullness and pain

NB. These are only examples, many other combinations can be made.

Table 17.8 Combination of Liver and Gallbladder points

Liver point	Gallbladder point	Syndrome	Example
LR.1	GB.1, GB.38, GB.44	Liver–Gallbladder Fire	conjunctivitis
	GB.26, GB.41	Liver–Gallbladder Damp Heat	vaginitis
LR.2	GB.20, GB.38	Liver–Gallbladder Fire	hypertension
	GB.38	Deficient Liver–Gallbladder Fire	lack of assertion
LR.3	GB.24, GB.34	Stagnant Gallbladder Qi	cholecystitis
	GB.21, GB.34	Stagnant Liver Qi	muscle spasm
	GB.28, GB.34	Liver invades Intestines	constipation
	GB.14, GB.20	Hyperactive Liver Yang	migraine
LR.5	GB.26, GB.34	Liver–Gallbladder Damp	irregular menstruation
LR.8	GB.1, GB.37	Deficient Liver Blood	blurred vision
LR.10–12	GB.26–28	Damp Heat in Lower Energizer	genital inflammation
LR.13	GB.24, GB.34	Liver invades Stomach	acid regurgitation
LR.14	GB.23, GB.24	Stagnant Liver Qi	hypochondriac pain

Gallbladder 18

Gallbladder channel

CHANNEL CONNECTIONS

MAIN CHANNEL PATHWAY

The main channel pathway starts at GB.1 at the outer canthus, crosses TE.22 at the temple, ascends to ST.8 on the forehead, then descends behind the ear, descending the neck to cross SI.17. From the shoulder, the channel connects with GV.14, descends the shoulder, crossing SI.12, to the supraclavicular fossa.

A branch of the main pathway starts behind the auricle, enters the ear at TE.17, emerges from the ear to cross SI.19 and ST.7, and terminates at the outer canthus. Another branch descends from the outer canthus to cross ST.5 on the jaw, returns to the eye region, and descends the neck to the supraclavicular fossa. An internal pathway from the supraclavicular fossa descends into the body connecting with the liver and gallbladder, descends to the genitals, connects with BL.31–34, and joins with GB.30 at the hip.

The superficial pathway descends from the supraclavicular fossa to descend the sides of the chest and abdomen, crossing the Liver channel at LR.13, before running down the lateral leg to end at GB.44 on the fourth toe. A branch from GB.41 joins with the Liver channel at LR.1.

CONNECTING CHANNEL PATHWAY

This leaves the main pathway on the thigh, crosses the hip joint, enters the pelvic region and converges with the Liver Divergent channel. Then it ascends the body and

Table 18.1 Crossing points on the Gallbladder channel

Point	Crossing
GB.1	TE, SI
GB.3,4,6	TE, ST
GB.7,8,10,11,12,30	BL
GB.13–21, GB.35	Yang Link
GB.15	BL, Yang Link
GB.26–28	Belt

connects with the liver and the gallbladder. Ascending, it crosses the heart and the oesophagus, disperses in the face, connects with the eye, and rejoins the main pathway at the outer canthus.

RELATIONSHIP OF GALLBLADDER AND LIVER

Although Liver and Gallbladder points can sometimes be used interchangeably, e.g. LR.3 for gallbladder problems, and GB.34 for Hyperactive Liver Yang, Gallbladder points are generally better for problems along the Gallbladder channel. For example, GB.21 is specific for trapezius spasm and GB.2 is specific for ear problems. Generally, Gallbladder points tend to have a more direct effect on Yang, for example by sinking Hyperactive Yang in the head, while Liver points can also have the effect of controlling Yang by nourishing Yin. Often, if Gallbladder points are used, SP.6, KI.6 or Liver points are added to give the treatment a better Yin–Yang balance.

LESSER YANG RELATIONSHIP

The Gallbladder and Triple Energizer channels form the Lesser Yang pair of the Six Divisions, which controls the side of the head, body and legs. The Lesser Yang pair can be balanced by pairs of points such as GB.41 + TE.5, or GB.34 + TE.6, to treat patterns simultaneously involving different areas on the sides of the body. For example, GB.41 + TE. 5 can be used for a combination of otitis media and itching rash on the sides of the legs due to Damp Heat, or GB.34 + TE.6 can be used for combination of lateral headaches and irritable bowel syndrome, due to Stagnant Liver Qi + Hyperactive Liver Yang. Another combination is TE.3 + GB.44 for conjunctivitis due to Liver–Gallbladder Fire. This combination could be balanced with KI.6, to nourish Yin.

Chains of points on both Lesser Yang channels can be used if there is a multiplicity of symptoms in different areas. For example TE.3, TE.5, TE.17 + GB.1, GB.2, GB.26, GB.41, for Liver–Gallbladder Damp Heat with eye and ear inflammation, and genital irritation and discharge. It is particularly important when using chains of points on Six Division Yang channel pairs, to balance Yin and Yang by adding Yin points, such as LR.5 and CV.3 in this instance.

In some cases, points on the Lesser Yang pair can be combined with points on the Terminal Yin pair. For example, depression with chest pain and nausea, due to Stagnant Liver Qi.

FUNCTIONS OF GALLBLADDER POINTS

TREAT CHANNEL PROBLEMS

One of the main uses of the Gallbladder points is to treat problems along the course of the channel. Local and distal Gallbladder points can be combined with local and distal Triple Energizer points, as described earlier. Use can be made of the points at which the Gallbladder channel crosses with other channels. For example:

GB.13 + ST.8	for upper lateral headaches
GB.20 + GV.14	for neck problems
GB.21 + SI.12	for shoulder problems
GB.24 + LR.13	for rib problems
GB.30 + BL.32	for sciatica.

MOVE STAGNANT LIVER QI

LR.1, LR.3, LR.14, CV.6 and PC.6 are better than most Gallbladder points for moving generalized Stagnant Liver Qi. Gallbladder points are better for moving Stagnant Qi in the muscles, e.g. GB.21 and GB.34, or in specific areas, e.g. GB.24 in the hypochondrium or GB.28 in the colon.

The general effect of the Liver points and the more local effect of the Gallbladder points can be combined. For example LR.1 can be combined with GB.27 for unilateral abdominal pain, or LR.3 can be combined with GB.25 for pain in the lower back and side.

TE.6 can be combined with GB.34 for generalized Stagnation of Liver Qi; for example, constipation or pain in chest and sides.

CALM HYPERACTIVE LIVER YANG

The most important consideration is the underlying cause of the Hyperactive Yang. For example, if the Hyperactivity originates in Deficient Kidney Qi, then not only can the Kidney Deficiency be treated with acupuncture, but the patient can be shown how changes in lifestyle can reduce the drain on Kidney Qi, and how to increase the Dan Tian energies with Qi Gong and meditation.

CLEAR LIVER–GALLBLADDER DAMP HEAT

Combinations from Damp Heat are discussed above in the section on the Lesser Yang relationship. It is important to establish the origins of the Damp Heat. For example, if chronic resentment and holding on to bitterness and hatred are contributing to the Damp Heat, then counselling and visualization techniques can be used to help to clear this aspect of the personality. Otherwise, acupuncture alone is generally not enough.

STRENGTHEN GALLBLADDER QI

The Source points GB.40 and TE.4 can be combined with CV.4 and KI.3, to strengthen Gallbladder and Kidney Qi, to help the person find their own inner strength and certainty, in order to treat indecision, lack of confidence and self-doubt. This treatment can be alternated with BL.19, BL.23, BL.48 and BL.52.

GALLBLADDER SYNDROMES

The Gallbladder syndromes are included in Table 17.2 on the Liver Syndromes.

Gallbladder points

GB.1 tóng zǐ liáo

Crossing point with Small Intestine and Triple Energizer channels.

General

The two main indications of GB.1 are eye problems and lateral headaches.

Eye problems

GB.1 can be used for all eye problems, but especially those with Liver, Gallbladder and Triple Energizer involvement (see Table 18.2).

Table 18.2 GB.1 and eye disorders

Syndromes	Example	Combination
Wind Heat	conjunctivitis	GB.1, BL.2 E; GB.43, TE.3 Rd
Liver–Gallbladder Fire	red, sore eyes	GB.1, BL.2 E; GB.38, LR.2 Rd or GB.1, BL.2 E; GB.41, TE.3 Rd
Hyperactive Liver Yang	photophobia	GB.1, GB.14 E; GB.34, LR.3 Rd
Deficient Kidney and Liver Yin	dry, itchy eyes	GB.1, BL.2 E; LR.2 Rd; SP.6, KI.6 Rf
Deficient Kidney Jing	early-stage cataract	GB.1, GB.20, BL.2, BL.62, KI.6 Rf
Deficient Liver Blood	blurred vision	GB.1, BL.2 E; LR.3, LR.8, GB.37, ST.36 Rf

Rd, Reducing method; Rf, Reinforcing method; E, Even method.

Lateral headaches

GB.1 can be used for lateral headaches and migraines associated with Liver Fire and Hyperactive Liver Yang (see Table 18.3).

Table 18.3 GB.1 and headaches

Syndromes	Example	Combination
Liver–Gallbladder Fire	migraine and hypertension	GB.1, tài yáng E; KI.1, LR.2, PC.8 Rd
Liver Fire and Deficient Kidney Yin	lateral headache	GB.1, GB.14 E; LR.2, GB.38, TE.5 Rd; SP.6, KI.6 Rf
Hyperactive Liver Yang and Deficient Kidney Qi	headache and eyestrain	GB.1, GB.20, TE.23 E; GB.34, LR.3, TE.3 Rd, KI.3 Rf
Hyperactive Liver Yang and Deficient Spleen Qi	headache and hypoglycaemia	GB.1, GB.20 E; GB.34, LR.3 Rd; LI.4, ST.36, Rf

Rd, Reducing method; Rf, Reinforcing method; E, Even method.

Syndromes

Eye problems
Headaches

Eye problems

Pulse. Various

Indications. Conjunctivitis, early-stage cataract or glaucoma, photophobia, blurred vision.

Example. Eyestrain, headache and muscle tension.

Combination. GB.1, GB.14, BL.2 E; GB.21, GB.34, LR.3, HT.7 Rd; SP.6 Rf.

Headaches

Pulse. Wiry, maybe rapid and superficial, thin or full.

Indications. Lateral headaches and migraine.

Example. Premenstrual headache and irritability.

Combination. GB.1, GB.41, tài yáng, TE.5 E; CV.4 Rf.

GB.2 tīng huì

General

The main indication of GB.2 is to treat all ear disorders. In addition to this it can treat local facial problems, e.g. toothache, facial paralysis or headache, whether due to Wind Cold, Wind Heat or other factors.

Ear problems

GB.2 can be used to treat all ear problems, although it is perhaps not quite so effective as TE.17 with which it is often combined (see Table 18.4).

Table 18.4 GB.2 and ear disorders

Syndrome	Example	Combination
Wind Cold	earache	GB.2, GB.20 E; TE.5, LI.4 Rd
Wind Heat	ear inflammation and sore throat	GB.2, SI.17 E; TE.5, SI.2 Rd
Liver–Gallbladder Damp Heat	otitis media	GB.2, TE.17 E; GB.34, LR.5, TE.3 Rd
Hyperactive Liver Yang and Deficient Kidney Qi	tinnitus	GB.2, GB.20, TE.17, GV.20 E; LR.3 GB.34 Rd; KI.3 CV.4 Rf

Rd, Reducing method; Rf, Reinforcing method; E, Even method.

Syndromes

Ear problems
Face problems

Ear problems

Pulse. Various.

Indications. Deafness, tinnitus, otitis media.

Example. Tinnitus worse with tiredenss.

Combination. GB.2, TE.17, SI.3, GV.20 E; BL.62, KI.6 Rf.

Face problems

Pulse. Various.

Indications. Hemiplegia, facial paralysis, temporomandibular arthritis, toothache, mumps.

Example. Lateral facial pain and headache.

Combination. GB.1, GB.2, GB.43, SI.2, SI.17, SI.18, LI.4 E.

GB.5–GB.12

The points GB.5–GB.12 can all be used for migraine, tinnitus, deafness and epilepsy when due to Liver Yang Fire, and Wind. For example, GB.7 or GB.8 can be used for neck pain, migraine or vomiting caused by alcohol. GB.5, GB.6 and GB.9 can also be used for disturbance of movement and speech originating in the central nervous system. GB.5 and GB.6 are close to the motor area and GB.8 and GB.9 are close to the lateral speech area of scalp acupuncture.

GB.6 and GB.9 can be used to calm the mind in serious mental disorders, often in combination with each other and with GB.34. GB.12 can also calm the mind to treat mania and insomnia, but in addition, can treat ear, neck and head problems from Wind Cold or from Heat.

GB.13 běn shén

Point of the Yang Link channel.

General

GB.13 is a main point for psychological disorders and can be combined with a variety of points depending on the pattern of disharmony; for examples see Table 18.5. GB.13 can also calm Interior Wind to treat epilepsy and hemiplegia, and calm Hyperactive Liver Yang to treat headache or vertigo.

Table 18.5 GB.13 and psychological disorders

Syndrome	Example	Combination
Heart and Gallbladder Fire	schizophrenia	GB.13, GB.38, ST.40, HT.5 Rd
Hyperactive Liver Yang and Heart Fire	hallucinations and insanity	GB.13, GB.40, GV.24, PC.5 Rd
Hyperactive Liver Yang	confusion and anger	GB.13, GB.34, GV.20, LI.4 Rd
Hyperactive Liver Yang and Deficient Spleen Qi	severe worry and confusion	GB.13, GB.34, ST.36, SP.6, yìn táng E
Deficient Kidney Qi	fear and suspicion	GB.13, GB.40, SI.3, BL.62 E

Rd, Reducing method; E, Even method.

Syndromes: psychological problems

Pulse. Maybe wiry, empty or full, choppy, changing, irregular or scattered.

Indications. Schizophrenia, hallucinations, mania, confusion, jealousy, suspicion, fear.

Example. Obsessive, repetitive thoughts and worry.

Combination. GB.13, ST.40, ST.45, SP.1, yìn táng, LI.4 Rd.

GB.14 yáng bái

Crossing with Stomach and Yang Link channels.

General

GB.14 has three main indications: eye problems and frontal headaches due to Liver Yang and facial problems due to Wind Cold.

Syndromes

Eye problems
Frontal headaches
Facial paralysis

Eye problems

Pulse. Maybe wiry, rapid and superficial, thin or choppy.

Indications. Lacrimation, twitching of the eyelids, ptosis of the eyelids, outer canthus pain.

Example. Photophobia and eyestrain.

Combination. GB.14, GB.20, GB.37, LR.3, LI.4, tài yáng E.

Frontal headaches

Pulse Wiry, maybe thin, empty, choppy, changing or rapid.

Indications. Frontal headache, supraorbital pain, eye pain, outer canthus pain, vertigo.

Example. Frontal headache and sinus pain.

Combination. GB.14, GB.20, BL.2, LI.4, ST.2, ST.40 E.

Facial paralysis

Pulse. Supperficial and tight, maybe empty or slow.

Indications. Facial paralysis.

Example. Facial paralysis with difficulty in frowning and in raising the eyebrows.

Combination. GB.14, BL.2, TE.23, LI.4 E.

GB.20 fēng chí

Meeting point with the Triple Energizer and Yang Link channels.

General

GB.20 is one of the main acupuncture points of the body. It is specific for eye, ear and sinus problems; for pain and stiffness of shoulder and neck, for generalized muscular aches and for occipital headaches.

GB.20 can disperse Wind Cold or Wind Heat to treat the common cold or influenza, and it can calm Interior Wind to treat vertigo, seizures and hemiplegia. It can be used to strengthen the brain to treat poor memory and concentration, and it can clear Liver Fire and Yang to treat hypertension, hyperthyroidism, anger and stressful hyperactivity.

Syndromes

Eye problems
Ear problems
Sinus problems
Wind Cold and Wind Heat
Head, neck and shoulder problems
Liver Fire and Hyperactive Liver Yang
Liver Wind
Mental problems

Eye problems

Pulse. Various.

Indications. Colour blindness, sudden blindness, early-stage cataract and glaucoma, conjunctivitis.

Example. Blurred vision, tiredness, weak muscles.

Combination. GB.1, GB.20, GB.37, LR.3, yìn táng, ST.36, SP.6 Rf.

Ear problems

Pulse. Various, maybe wiry.

Indications. Aural vertigo, deafness, tinnitus, earache.

Example. Catarrhal deafness.

Combination. GB.2, GB.20, TE.3, TE.17, SI.17, ST.40 E.

Sinus problems

Pulse. Slippery, maybe wiry.

Indications. Sinus congestion and pain, catarrhal deafness, frontal headache, heavy feeling in the head.

Example. Acute sinus infection with raised temperature.

Combination. GB.20, ST.3, ST.44, ST.45, LI.1, LI.4, LI.20 Rd.

Wind Cold and Wind Heat

Pulse. Superficial and tight or rapid.

Indications. Generalized body ache, ache in shoulders and neck, occipital headache, common cold.

Example. Influenza with chills and cough.

Combination. GB.20, LU.7, LI.4 Rd; BL.11, BL.13 Rd M.

Head, neck and shoulder problems

Pulse. Wiry, maybe empty, thin, choppy.

Indications. Neck trauma, torticollis, arthritis of neck and shoulders.

Example. Depression, tension with stiff neck and shoulders.

Combination. GB.20, GB.21, GB.34, BL.10, BL.11, BL.62, SI.3 E.

Liver Fire and Hyperactive Liver Yang

Pulse. Wiry, maybe rapid, thin or full.

Indications. Hypertension, headache, hyperthyroidism, vertigo, tinnitus, deafness.

Example. Hypertension with stressful, abrasive behaviour.

Combination. GB.20, GB.34, GV.20, tài yáng, LV.2, PC.8 Rd; LR.8, SP.6 Rf.

Liver Wind

Pulse. Wiry, maybe choppy, thin or full, rapid.

Indications. Muscle spasm, muscle tremors, vertigo, convulsions, mental confusion, epilepsy, hemiplegia.

Example. Ministrokes, with dizziness, mental confusion and temporary hemiplegia.

Combination. GB.20, GV.20, LR.3, KI.1, ST.40, PC.5 Rd; SP.6, KI.3 Rf M.

Mental problems

Pulse. Empty, thin, choppy, maybe deep or slow.

Indications. Poor memory, loss of concentration, mental tiredness.

Example. Mental confusion and mental cloudiness in the elderly.

Combination. GB.20, GB.39, GV.16, GV.20, BL.62, KI.6, SI.3 Rf.

GB.21 jiān jǐng

Meeting point with Triple Energizer and Yang Link channels.

General

The main function of GB.21 is to relieve tension in the muscles in general and in the muscles of the shoulders and neck in particular.

GB.21 and GB.20

GB.21 can be used like GB.20 to relieve hypertension due to Hyperactive Liver Yang with Stagnation of Liver Qi or with Liver Fire; indeed GB.20 and GB.21 are often used together. GB.20 is generally more effective for this purpose, but in those patients who have experienced aggravation of headache or faintness after use of GB.20, GB.21 may be preferable. However, it should be noted that some authors recommend caution in the use of GB.21 in pregnancy or with heart problems.

GB.21 in gynaecology and obstetrics

GB.21 can be used for abnormal uterine bleeding, difficult labour, retention of placenta, postpartum haemorrhage and sensation of cold after childbirth. It will also treat insufficient lactation and mastitis.

Syndromes

  Muscular tension
  Hyperactive Liver Yang
  Gynaecological and obstetric problems

Muscular tension

Pulse. Wiry, maybe empty, thin, choppy or full.

Indications. General muscular tension, muscle spasms in shoulders and neck, torticollis.

Example. Feeling of stiffness and numbness down left side of the body, aggravated by tension.

Combination. GB.21, GB.30, GB.34, GB.41, TE.5 Rd on the left; SP.6 Rf on the right.

Hyperactive Liver Yang

Pulse Wiry, maybe empty, thin or rapid.

Indications. Hypertension, headache, hemiplegia.

Example. Suppressed anger with aches in shoulders and grinding of teeth at night.

Combination. GB.21, GB.38, LR.2, BL.47, LU.7 Rd.

Gynaecological and obstetric problems

Pulse. Wiry, maybe choppy.

Indications. Difficult labour, retention of placenta, post-partem haemorrhage.

Example. Insufficient lactation.

Combination. GB.21, CV.17, ST.18, SI.1 E.

GB.24 rì yuè

Alarm point of Gallbladder.

General

GB.24 has two main functions, to clear Liver–Gallbladder Damp Heat and to move Stagnant Liver Qi, including Invasion of Stomach by the Liver, with such signs as gastric and duodenal ulcers, belching and vomiting. GB.24 is also a point to expel gallstones.

Syndromes

Damp Heat in Liver–Gallbladder
Stagnation of Liver Qi
Liver invades Stomach

Damp Heat in Liver-Gallbladder

Pulse. Wiry, slippery and rapid, maybe thin or flooding.

Indications. Cholecystitis, cholelithiasis, hepatitis.

Example. Acute cholecystitis.

Combination. GB.24, dǎn náng, LR.13, PC.6 Rd.

Stagnation of Liver Qi

Pulse. Hindered or wiry.

Indications. Difficulty in speaking, frequent sighing, intercostal pain, spasm of the diaphragm.

Example. Depression and withdrawal with tiredness and heavy sensation in the chest.

Combination. GB.24, GB.34, LR.3, LR.14, PC.6, LU.7 Rd.

Liver invades Stomach

Pulse. Wiry, maybe slippery, thin or flooding.

Indications. Nausea, vomiting, belching, hiccups, gastritis.

Example. Gastric ulceration with much work stress.

Combination. GB.24, GB.34, ST.21, ST.44, CV.12, PC.3 Rd.

GB.25 jīng mén

Alarm point of the Kidneys.

General

The most important function of GB.25 is that is can move Stagnant Qi in its surrounding area, which has three main aspects as shown in Table 18.6. If used with Reinforcing method and moxa in combination with BL.23 and KI.7, for example, GB.25 can tonify Kidney Qi and Yang, to treat Cold and Damp in the lower back or urinary system.

Table 18.6 Three functions of GB.25 to move Stagnant Qi

Example	Combination
Stagnant Intestinal Qi	lower abdominal pain, borborygmus, diarrhoea GB.25 + GB.27, SP.15
Stagnant Liver–Gallbladder Qi	Dyspnoea, intercostal or hypochondriac pain GB.25 + GB.24, LR.13
Stagnant Kidney Qi	dysuria, nephritis, lower back pain, stones in upper urinary tract GB.25 + BL.23, BL.52 or GB.25 + ST.28, CV.4

Syndrome: Stagnant Qi

Pulse. Wiry, maybe empty, thin, choppy or deep.

Indications. Lower abdominal pain and distension, intercostal pain, nephritis.

Example. Pain around Kidney area and in hypochondrium, with exhaustion and irritiblity.

Combination. GB.24, GB.25, GB.34 Rd; BL.22, BL.23 E M; KI.3 Rf M.

GB.26 dài mài

Crossing point with the Belt channel.

General

GB.26 regulates the Belt channel and has three main functions: it moves Stagnant Qi and Blood in the uterus to regulate menstruation; it transforms Liver–Gallbladder Damp Heat in the Lower Energizer; and it regulates Stagnation in the leg channels to move Stagnation of Qi in the lower body.

Table 18.7 Three functions of GB.26

Syndromes	Example	Combination
Stagnant Qi and Blood in uterus	irregular menstruation, dysmenorrhoea	GB.26 + GB.41, SP.6, CV.6
Damp Heat in Lower Energizer	leucorrhoea, cystitis, diarrhoea	GB.26 + GB.27, GB.41, LR.5, CV.6
Stagnant Qi in lower body	coldness or pain in lower abdomen, lower back, hip or legs	GB.26 + GB.28, GB.41, SP.4, ST.30, CV.6

Syndromes: Belt channel disharmonies

Pulse. Wiry, maybe slippery and rapid or slow.

Indications. Endometriosis, irregular menstruation, vaginal prolapse, hernia, cold legs and feet.

Example. Dysmenorrhoea with lower back pain.

Combination. GB.25, GB.26, GB.41, CV.6, SP.6, LI.4 E.

GB.27 and GB.28 wǔ shā and wéi dào

Crossing points with the Belt channel.

General

These points are similar in function to GB.26, but are more local in their effects. Like GB.26, as points on the Belt channel, they can regulate menstruation and clear Damp Heat in the Lower Energizer. However, GB.26 is better for hip and leg problems, while GB.27 and GB.28 are better for uterovaginal prolapse or hernia. These two points are especially useful when there is pain or discomfort of unknown origin in the right or left lower abdomen in a Wood-type patient, with a history of pain of varying location on the sides of the body. They can then be combined with GB.21, GB.25, GB.41 and TE.5 or TE.6.

GB.30 huán tiào

Crossing point with Bladder channel.

General

The main indication of GB.30 is for hip and leg problems, especially sciatica. Sciatica may involve pressure on and inflammation of the sciatic nerve or the spinal nerves leading into it. There may be unilateral pain in the lower back, hip and buttock, with radiation down the Gallbladder and/or Bladder channels on the leg, and sometimes radiation to the groin and the front of the thigh. GB.30 can also be used for arthritis of the hip, for atrophy of the muscles of hip and leg and for hemiplegia. The principal effect of GB.30 is to move Stagnant Qi and Blood in the Gallbladder and Bladder channels, and secondarily to remove Exterior Wind, Cold and Damp, to drain Damp Heat and to tonify Qi and Blood.

Combining points with GB.30

Points can be combined with GB.30 according to the locations of the pain and according to the syndromes of Chinese medicine involved. If no needle sensation is obtained with GB.30, zuǒ gǔ can be substituted. If the needle sensation at GB.30 reaches right to the foot, then either no other needle is necessary or perhaps just one other needle at the main site of pain on the leg. The further the needle sensation reaches down the leg from GB.30 the fewer points need be used.

Table 18.8 Combinations with GB.30 for problems associated with sciatica

Problems associated with sciatica	Combination with GB.30
Spinal nerve involvement	jiā jǐ points on the side and near the vertebrae affected
Deficient Kidney Qi	BL.23, KI.3 Rf
Deficient Kidney Yang with invasion of Cold and Damp	GV.4, BL.23, BL.60 Rf M
Damp Heat in Liver–Gallbladder	GB.41 Rd
Deficient Qi in Gallbladder channel	GB.40 Rf
Hyperactive Liver Yang and muscle tension	GB.21, GB.34 Rd
Stagnation of Qi with muscle spasm in upper hip and lateral thigh	GB.29, GB.31, Rd M
Pain and spasm in lateral knee and calf	GB.33, GB.39 Rd
Pain along Bladder channel from buttock to ankle	BL.54, BL.36, BL.37, BL.40, BL.57, BL.59 Rd
Pain in sacrum	BL.31–33 Rd
Pain radiating to groin and frontal thigh on Stomach channel	ST.30, ST.31, ST.41 Rd
Deficient Qi and Blood	ST.36 Rf M

Rf, Reinforcing method; Rd, Reducing method; M, moxa.

GB.30 and skin rashes

GB.30 and GB.31 may be used for Wind Heat skin rashes on the lower body, and may be combined with GB.20 if the rashes are also on the upper body. If Damp Heat is involved, then GB.30 and GB.31 can be combined with GB.41 and TE.5.

Syndromes: hip and leg problems

Pulse. Wiry, maybe empty, thin or choppy, maybe slow and deep or superficial and rapid.

Indications. Arthritis of the hip joint, sciatica, hemiplegia, leg muscles atrophy.

Example. Disc problems at right fifth lumbar vertebra with pain down Bladder and Gallbladder channels on the right leg.

Combination. GB.30, GB.34, GB.40, BL.36, BL.40, BL.64, jiā jǐ fifth lumbar, E; on the right side.

GB.31 fēng shì

General

This point can be used for hip and leg problems, usually in combination with GB.30 and distal Gallbladder points. It can also be used for Wind Heat or Damp Heat skin rashes, as described above.

GB.33 xi yáng guān

General

This is an important point for all knee problems involving the Gallbladder channel, whether due to Stagnation of Qi and blood following trauma, Damp Heat in arthritis, or Invasion of Wind, Cold and Damp associated with Deficient Qi in the Gallbladder channel. It can be combined with local and distal Gallbladder points or local knee points on other channels.

GB.34 yáng líng quán

Sea point, Earth point, Gathering point for sinews.

General

GB.34 is one of the most used points on the body and has the following main functions:

regulates muscles and tendons
regulates Gallbladder channel
moves Stagnant Liver and Gallbladder Qi
calms Hyperactive Liver Yang
calms Liver Wind
regulates mind and emotions
clears Damp Heat in Liver–Gallbladder
regulates the Intestines.

Regulates muscles and tendons

Along with GB.40, the Source point, GB.34, the Gathering point for the sinews, has a tonifying affect upon the Gallbladder channel and organ, and upon the muscles and tendons. It can therefore be used to strengthen or tone weak muscles just as much as it can be used to relax muscle spasms due to Stagnant Liver Qi, Hyperactive Liver Yang or Liver Wind. GB.34, with its main action on the muscles of the lower body, can be combined with GB.21, which has its main action on the upper body.

Regulates the Gallbladder channel

Whilst GB.34 can regulate the whole of the Gallbladder channel and can especially be used for head pain due to Hyperactive Liver Yang, its greatest effect is on the hypochondrium, hips, legs and knees.

Moves Stagnant Liver and Gallbladder Qi

While LR.3 can move Stagnant Liver Qi anywhere in the body, GB.34 is most effective in treating the effects of Stagnant Liver Qi on Gallbladder and Stomach.

Calms Hyperactive Liver Yang

GB.34 and LR.3 are the two points on the lower body most used to calm Hyperactive Liver Yang. They may be combined together and the points GB.20 and GV.20 added to the combination.

Polarity in combinations. The advantage of LR.3 and GB.34 over GV.20 and GB.20, is that since the leg points are at the opposite end of the body to the head, the main site of disturbance, they are often more effective in sinking the Hyperactive Yang. If the head points only were used, they might not be so effective, or might even aggravate the disturbed movement of Qi.

Origins of Hyperactive Liver Yang. Different points can be combined with GB.34, depending on the origin of the Hyperactive Yang:

Hyperactive Liver Yang and Deficient Kidney Yin	GB.34 + GB.38 Rd; SP.6, KI.6 Rf
Hyperactive Liver Yang and Deficient Kidney Qi	GB.34 + GB.40 E; KI.3 Rf
Hyperactive Liver Yang and Deficient Spleen Qi	GB.34 + GB.20 Rd; SP.3, CV.12 Rf
Hyperactive Liver Yang and Stagnant Liver Qi	GB.34 + LR.3, GV.20 E or Rd.

Calms Liver Wind

While GB.34 is not a main point to control Liver–Gallbladder Fire, it can calm the Liver Wind that may be associated with Liver Fire, Hyperactive Liver Yang or Deficient Liver Blood, to treat convulsions, vertigo, muscle spasms and tremors. It can be combined as follows:

Liver Wind associated with Liver Fire	GB.34 + KI.1, LR.2 Rd; tài yáng B
Liver Wind associated with Liver Yang	GB.34 + GB.20, GV.20, LR.3 Rd; KI.3 Rf
Liver Wind associated with Deficient Liver Blood	GB.34 + GV.20 Rd; ST.36, SP.6, LI.4 Rf.

Regulates mind and emotions

GB.34 does not have the strong effect of LR.3 in treating general pain or nervous tension, but it can be used for the effects of specific Liver and Gallbladder syndromes on the mind and emotions, as shown in Figure 18.1.

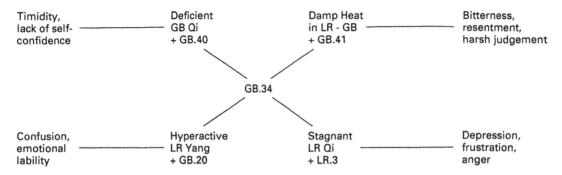

Fig. 18.1 GB.34 and psychological disorders

Clears Damp Heat in the Liver–Gallbladder

This is especially for Damp Heat in the Middle Energizer, with Stomach and Gallbladder symptoms.

Regulates the Intestines

GB.34 is an empirical point for chronic constipation.

Syndromes

  Muscle and tendon problems
  Gallbladder channel problems
  Stagnant Liver–Gallbladder Qi
  Hyperactive Liver Yang and Wind
  Psychological problems
  Damp Heat in Liver–Gallbladder
  Constipation

Muscle and tendon problems

Combination.   GB.21, GB.34, LR.3, PC.6 Rd; SP.6 Rf.

Gallbladder channel problems

Pulse.   Wiry, maybe empty, thin, choppy or full.

Indications.   Hemiplegia, sciatica, pain, stiffness or weakness of hip and lateral thigh, knee or calf.

Example.   Hypochondriac pain and calf spasm.

Combination.   GB.24, GB.34, BL.58, SP.6 Rd.

Stagnant Liver–Gallbladder Qi

Pulse.   Wiry, maybe empty or full, maybe slippery.

Indications.   Intercostal pain, hypochondriac pain, headache, oppressive feeling in chest.

Example.   Depression and frustration with much sighing, apparent tiredness and muscle stiffness.

Combination.   GB.21, GB.24, GB.34, TE.6, LR.3 E.

Hyperactive Liver Yang and Wind

Pulse.   Wiry, maybe empty, thin choppy or full, maybe rapid.

Indications.   Hypertension, hemiplegia, headache, tinnitus, deafness, muscle tremors.

Example.   Vertigo with frustration and suppressed anger.

Combination.   GB.34, GB.43, LR.3 Rd; KI.6, KI.10 Rf.

Psychological problems

Pulse.   Hindered or wiry, maybe slow or rapid, maybe empty, thin, choppy or full.

Indications.   Self-doubt, lack of assertion, indecision, mental confusion, mood changes, irritability.

Example.   Forgetfulness, disorientation, fearfulness and indecision.

Combination.   GB.13, GB.34, KI.3, HT.3 E.

Damp Heat in Liver–Gallbladder

Pulse.   Wiry, maybe slippery and rapid, maybe thin or flooding.

Indications.   Hepatitis, cholecystitis, nausea, indigestion.

Example.   Epigastric and hypochondriac discomfort and acid regurgitation.

Combination.   GB.34, LR.13, CV.12, ST.36, PC.6 E.

Constipation

Pulse. Hindered or wiry, maybe thin, empty or flooding.

Indications. Chronic constipation.

Combination. GB.28, GB.34, CV.6, LI.10, TE.6 Rd.

GB.37 guāng míng

Connecting point.

General

The main function of this point is to treat eye disorders of all kinds, for which it can be combined with GB.1, see page 259. It can also treat pain and spasm of the calf and foot.

Syndromes: eye problems

Pulse. Various.

Indications. All eye disorders.

Example. Degeneration of vision, weak legs and mental confusion in the elderly.

Combination. GB.1, GB.13, GB.37, SP.6, KI.3, TE.3 E.

GB.38 yáng fǔ

River point, Fire point.

General

This point can be used for Stagnation of Qi in the Gallbladder channel, with generalized muscle tension and hypochondriac pain, or it can be used for Damp Heat, but GB.34 is better for both functions. The main use of GB.38 is as the Fire point. GB.34 can be used with Reducing method to drain Gallbladder Fire to treat red eyes, gastritis, constipation, migraine and anger.

GB.38 can also be used with Reinforcing method and moxa to increase Fire in the Gallbladder, to help patients become more strongly individualized and to push out the boundaries of their personality and creativity with more confidence and assertion. For this it can be combined with LR.2 and BL.48.

Syndromes

Gallbladder Fire
Deficient Gallbladder Fire

Gallbladder Fire

Pulse. Wiry, rapid, maybe thin or full.

Indications. Migraine, conjunctivitis, indigestion with bitter taste.

Example. Headache with restlessness, feeling of heat in the head and chest, irritability.

Combination. GB.38, GB.43 tài yáng, TE.5 Rd; SP.6 Rf.

Deficient Gallbladder Fire

Pulse. Hindered or wiry, maybe empty, thin, choppy or deep.

Indications. Hesitation, procrastination, uncertainty, dithering.

Example. Always asking for advice but never acting on it.

Combination. GB.38 Rf M; CV.4, KI.4, SP.6, yìn táng Rf.

GB.39 xuán zhōng

Gathering point for the Marrow.

General

The most important function of this point is that it tonifies Kidney Jing and tonifies the Marrow so that it can be used for weakness and spasm of muscles, weakness, stiffness and inflammation of joints, for degeneration of the bones and for tinnitus and gradual hearing loss.

To tonify Kidney Jing, GB.39 can be combined with BL.62, SI.3 and KI.6. To strengthen the bones it can be combined with BL.11, BL.23 and GV.4. To regulate muscles and tendons to support the joints, GB.39 can be combined with GB.34 and GV.12. GB.39 is especially useful to treat old people with declining Jing, to treat weak limbs, tinnitus and deafness. GB.20 can be added to tonify the Marrow and improve mental clarity. If combined with SP.6 and KI.6 to tonify Kidney Yin, and LR.3 to reduce Interior Wind, GB.39 can help to prevent strokes.

Additional uses of GB.39

Like GB.34, GB.39 can be used for painful obstruction of the throat, and for cough with feeling of fullness and pain in the chest. Like GB.28, GB.34 and GB.38, GB.39 can be used for constipation, and it can also be used for dysuria, painful defecation and haemorrhoids. GB.39 can be used often in combination with GB.20 and GB.21, for lateral neck pain and stiffness.

Syndromes

Muscle, joint and bone problems
Chronic ear problems

Muscle, joint and bone problems

Pulse.   Empty, thin, choppy or deep, maybe wiry.

Indications.   Hemiplegia, arthritis, ankylosing spondylitis, weak legs in the elderly.

Example.   Weakness of the left knee.

Combination.   GB.33, GB.34, GB.39, BL.40, KI.3, KI.10 Rf on left side; SP.6 Rf on right side.

Chronic ear problems

Pulse.   Empty, thin, choppy or deep, maybe slow or fast.

Indications.   Gradually increasing deafness or tinnitus.

Example.   Chronic deafness and mental slowness and confusion.

Combination.   GB.2, GB.13, GB.39, GV.20, TE.3, HT.7, KI.6 Rf.

GB.40 qiū xū

Source point.

General

The main use of GB.40 is to tonify and move the Qi in the Gallbladder channel when there are problems along the path of the channel due to Deficiency and Stagnation of Qi, and to tonify Gallbladder Qi to treat indecision and timidity. In both cases GB.40 can be combined with GB.34.

To treat self-doubt and timidity due to Deficient Gallbladder Qi, GB.40 can be combined with KI.7 and with BL.48 and BL.52. To treat lack of confidence and lack of assertion due to Deficient Gallbladder Fire, GB.40 can be combined with GB.38, the Fire point.

Syndromes

Deficiency and Stagnation of Qi in the Gallbladder channel
Deficiency of Gallbladder Qi

Deficiency and Stagnation of Qi in the Gallbladder channel

Pulse.   Wiry and empty.

Indications.   Feeling of ache in hips and legs that can move about, often accompanied by feeling of coldness.

Example.   Weakness in lower back, hip and legs.

Combination.   GB.25, GB.30, GB.40, BL.23, BL.60 Rf M.

Deficiency of Gallbladder Qi

Pulse.   Hindered or wiry; empty, thin, choppy or deep.

Indications.   Headache, frustration, uncertainty, indecision.

Example.   Lack of sense of direction in life, postponement of decision, muddling along from day to day.

Combination.   GB.40, KI.7, GV.24, TE.4 Rf M; KI.1 M.

GB.41 zú lín qì

Stream point, Wood point, Opening point of the Belt channel.

Regulates menstruation

As the Opening point of the Belt channel, GB.41 has a strong regulating effect not only on the uterus, but also on the hormonal balance of the menstrual cycle. It can treat not only menstrual pain and irregularity, but also changes of mood during the cycle relating to Stagnation of Liver Qi and Hyperactive Liver Yang. It can treat premenstrual headaches and breast soreness and menstrual problems caused by the side-effects of the birth control pill; whether of starting or stopping the pill or of changing one type of pill for another. To regulate the hormonal balance of the menstrual cycle, GB.41 is best combined with TE.5, the Opening point of the Yang Link channel — see Chapter 10.

Clears Damp Heat

GB.41 is perhaps the main point on the Gallbladder channel to clear Damp Heat in the Lower Energizer and breasts, to treat leucorrhoea or cystitis, for example, while GB.34 is better to treat Damp Heat in the Middle Energizer, with cholecystitis. Either GB.41 or GB.34, when combined with TE.3 and TE.17, can treat otitis media due to Damp Heat.

Regulates the Liver

GB.41 can drain Liver Fire and treat conjunctivitis, move Stagnant Liver Qi and treat dyspnoea, chest pain and hypochondriac pain, and calm Hyperactive Liver Yang to treat headache.

Syndromes

Menstrual problems
Breast problems
Damp Heat in the Lower Energizer

Menstrual problems

Pulse. Wiry, maybe rapid, thin and choppy.

Indications. Premenstrual syndrome, irregular menstruation, lower back pain with menstruation.

Example. Headaches and depression as side-effects of the birth control pill.

Combination. GB.14, GB.20, GB.41, SP.6, CV.6, TE.5 E.

Breast problems

Pulse. Wiry, maybe slippery and rapid.

Indications. Sore breasts at menstruation, mastitis, breast abscess.

Example. Mastitis.

Combination. GB.21, GB.41, LR.3, CV.17, TE.6 Rd.

Damp Heat in the Lower Energizer

Pulse. Wiry, rapid, slippery, thin or full.

Indications. Genital eczema, leucorrhoea, cystitis, urethritis.

Example. Vaginal pruritis and discharge.

Combination. GB.26, GB.41, CV.3, SP.6, TE.5 E.

GB.43 xiá xī

Spring point, Water point, Tonification point.

General

This point is useful in treating problems in throat, ears, eyes and head, arising from Hyperactive Liver Yang and Liver Fire and is often combined with TE.3. It can also be used for anxiety, palpitations, hypertension and chest pain, combined with HT.3.

GB.44 zú qiào yīn

Well point, Metal point.

General

GB.44 is similar to GB.43 in treating problems of throat, ears, eyes and head due to Liver Fire and Yang, and it too can be used for hypertension and dream-disturbed sleep. GB.44 is perhaps better for eye problems and GB.43 for ear problems, but the two points have very similar functions. GB.44 can be reduced or bled.

Gallbladder point comparisons and combinations

The functions of the main points of the Gallbladder channel are listed in Table 18.9.

Table 18.9 Gallbladder point comparisons

Point	Point type	Syndromes
GB.1		eye problems lateral headaches
GB.2		ear problems face problems
GB.13		psychological problems
GB.14		eye problems frontal headache facial paralysis
GB.20		eye problems ear problems sinus problems Wind Cold and Wind Heat head, neck and shoulder problems Liver Fire and Hyperactive Liver Yang Liver Wind mental problems
GB.21		muscular tension Hyperactive Liver Yang gynaecological and obstetric problems
GB.24	Front Collecting point of Gallbladder	Damp Heat in Liver–Gallbladder Stagnation of Liver Qi Liver invades Stomach

GB.25	Front Collecting point of Kidney	Stagnant Qi
		  Intestinal
		  Liver–Gallbladder
		  Kidneys

GB.26	Meeting point with Belt channel	Belt channel disharmonies
GB.30	Meeting point with Bladder channel	hip and leg problems
GB.34	Sea point, Earth point, Gathering point for sinews	muscle and tendon problems Gallbladder channel problems Stagnant Liver–Gallbladder Qi Hyperactive Liver Yang psychological problems Damp Heat in Liver–Gallbladder constipation
GB.37	Connecting point	eye problems
GB.38	Fire point, Sedation point	Gallbladder Fire Deficient Gallbladder Fire
GB.39	Gathering point for marrow	muscle, joint and bone problems chronic ear problems
GB.40	Source point	Deficiency and Stagnation of Qi in Gallbladder channel Deficient Gallbladder Qi
GB.41	Stream point, Wood point, Opening point of Belt channel	menstrual problems breast problems Damp Heat in Lower Energizer
GB.43	Spring point, Water point, Tonification point	Hyperactive Liver Yang and Fire ear problems
GB.44	Well point, Metal point	Hyperactive Liver Yang and Fire eye problems

Some common combinations of Gallbladder points with each other are summarized in Table 18.10.

Table 18.10 Combinations of Gallbladder points

Point	Combination	Syndrome	Example
GB.1	GB.2	Hyperactive Liver Yang and Wind Cold	lateral headache and earache
GB.1	GB.14	Hyperactive Liver Yang	headache and photophobia
GB.1	GB.20	Deficient Qi and Blood	blurred vision
GB.1	GB.37	Deficient Blood and Jing	early-stage cataract
GB.1	GB.38	Liver Fire	red, sore, itchy eyes
GB.1	GB.44	Hyperactive Liver Yang	dream-disturbed sleep
GB.2	GB.20	Wind Heat and Phlegm	catarrhal deafness
GB.2	GB.34	Damp heat in Liver–Gallbladder	otitis media
GB.2	GB.39	Deficient Kidney Jing	failing eyesight in the old
GB.2	GB.43	Hyperactive Liver Yang	tinnitus
GB.13	GB.38	Liver Fire	schizophrenia
GB.13	GB.40	Deficient Gallbladder Qi	uncertainty and confusion
GB.14	GB.20	Hyperactive Liver Yang	headache and eyestrain
GB.14	GB.34	Hyperactive Liver Yang	frontal headache
GB.20	GB.21	Stagnation of Liver Qi	shoulder muscle tension
GB.20	GB.34	Hyperactive Liver Yang	vertigo and tinnitus
GB.20	GB.40	Deficient Kidney Qi and Hyperactive Liver Yang	dizziness, and empty moving sensation in the head
GB.21	GB.34	Stagnation of Liver–Gallbladder Qi	generalized muscular tension
GB.21	GB.41	Stagnation of Qi	breast problems
GB.24	GB.34	Liver invades Stomach	gastritis
GB.25	GB.34	Stagnant Qi in Gallbladder channel	hypochondriac pain and lower back pain
GB.26	GB.27	Damp Heat in Lower Energizer	leucorrhoea
GB.26	GB.41	Stagnant Qi in uterus	irregular menstruation
GB.30	GB.31	Stagnant Qi and Blood	trauma to hip and thigh
GB.30	GB.34	Deficient and Stagnant Qi in Gallbladder channel	weakness and ache in leg muscles
GB.30	GB.39	Deficient Kidney Jing and Liver Blood	weakness in hip and knee joints ·
GB.30	GB.40	Stagnation of Qi and Blood	sciatica
GB.34	GB.39	Stagnant Liver Qi and Kidney Jing and Yin	hemiplegia
GB.34	GB.40	Deficient Gallbladder Qi	indecision
GB.34	GB.41	Stagnation and Damp Heat in Liver–Gallbladder	gastritis and eczema
GB.34	GB.39	Damp Heat	varicose eczema
GB.40	GB.41	Stagnant Blood	ankle sprain
GB.41	GB.44	Liver Fire	headache and eye inflammation
GB.1	GB.14, 20	Hyperactive Liver Yang	hypertension and headache
GB.1	GB.38, 44	Liver–Gallbladder Fire	early-stage glaucoma
GB.2	GB.20, 34	Hyperactive Liver Yang	tinnitus, worse with stress
GB.14	GB.20, 34	Hyperactive Liver Yang	migraine
GB.20	GB.21, 34	Stagnant Liver Qi and Hyperactive Liver Yang	headache and generalized muscle tension
GB.24	GB.27, GB.34	Stagnant Liver–Gallbladder Qi	epigastric and lateral abdominal pain
GB.29	GB.30, 40	Stagnation of Qi and Blood	sciatica
GB.30	GB.31, 33	Stagnation of Qi and Blood	hip and knee pain
GB.30	GB.34, 39	Deficient Jing and Stagnation of Qi	stiff, weak hips and legs in the elderly
GB.30	GB.34, 41	Damp Heat and Stagnation of Qi	arthritis of the hip
GB.31	GB.34, 41	Damp Heat and Wind Heat	eczema of the legs
GB.3	GB.14, 20, 34	Hyperactive Liver Yang	migraine and hypertension
GB.2	GB.8, 20, 41	Damp Heat in Liver–Gallbladder	unilateral skin rash in ear, temple and mastoid area
GB.21	GB.25, 27, 34	Stagnation of Qi in Gallbladder channel	unilateral pain in neck, back and lower abdomen
GB.29	GB.30, 31, 40	Wind Cold and Stagnation of Qi and Blood	sciatica with hip muscle spasm
GB.30	GB.33, 34, 40	Stagnation of Qi and Blood	sciatica and knee pain

Heart 19

Heart channel

CHANNEL CONNECTIONS

MAIN CHANNEL PATHWAY

Originating in the heart, one branch of the channel descends through the diaphragm and connects with the small intestine. A second branch emerges from the heart and ascends to the throat and eye. A third branch from the heart connects with the lungs and emerges at the axilla, running down the arm as the superficial pathway, along the medial arm to the medial tip of the little finger.

CONNECTING CHANNEL PATHWAY

Starting at HT.5, it connects with the Small Intestine channel. A second branch follows the main channel to the heart before ascending to the tongue and eye.

CROSSING POINTS ON THE HEART CHANNEL

There are no Crossing points on the superficial channel, but the following channels have deep pathway connections with the heart:

  Main channels: SI, SP, KI
  Divergent channels: SI, BL, ST, GB
  Connecting channel: PC
  Extra channel: GV

THE HEART ORGAN SYSTEM AND THE ENERGY CENTRES

THE HEART CENTRE

If linked to the energies of the higher self, the Heart centre is the focus for the energies of selfless love and compassion; if linked to the lower self, the Heart centre can be disturbed by the emotions of selfish love, passion, fear and a confused mixture of affection and hatred. These emotions can disturb the Heart organ system and lead to a Deficiency, Stagnation or Irregularity of Heart Spirit. The points relating to the Heart centre, CV.17, GV.11, BL.15 and BL.44, can be used to treat these problems.

HEART AND HEAD CENTRES

If mental confusion is combined with emotional disturbance, and either mental worries affect the flow of love in the Heart centre, or selfish passion clouds thinking, yìn táng or GV.20 can be combined with CV.17.

HEART AND THROAT CENTRE

The Throat centre governs communication of ideas and feelings through speech. If a person cannot express their needs in a relationship, and emotional pressure builds up causing throat or chest problems, CV.23 can be combined with CV.17. If the person thinks and feels too much without being able to express or clear the pressure of their thoughts and feelings GV.24 can be added to CV.23 and CV.17.

HEART AND SOLAR PLEXUS CENTRE

If the Solar Plexus centre is too open and sensitive to the emotional environment, then the Heart centre may be affected with insomnia, palpitations and anxiety. CV,17 can then be combined with CV.14 or CV.15. If the person is a Yang Water type, with great internal stress from fear of losing control and the constant effort of trying to dominate, then CV.14 may be combined with GV.20 and KI.1 or KI.7. If the person is a nervous and fearful TV + Yin Link personality type, then SP.4 and PC.6 may be added to CV.14.

HEART AND DAN TIAN

If the Dan Tian energy is weak then either the Spirit may be Deficient, and the person depressed, or the person may not have enough Qi to hold the emotions stable. In either case, CV.4 can be combined with CV.17.

Qi Gong and meditation techniques focusing on the Dan Tian and KI.1 centres, can calm, stabilize and strengthen by taking people out of the disturbance of the Head and Heart centres, down into the physical body.

HEART AND REPRODUCTIVE CENTRE

Sex and reproduction can be closely linked with both love

and creativity. Problems of Heart and Reproductive centres together may lead to chronic depression, feelings of loneliness and lack of fulfilment, or to breast and uterine carcinomas. CV.17 can be combined with CV.3, and with LU.7 + KI.6.

BALANCING HEAD, HEART AND BODY CENTRES

The ideal for a human being is to create an harmonious balance between the centres of Head, Heart and body, between wisdom, love and strength. While point combinations based on GV.20, CV.17 and CV.4 may assist this, it can only be realized by a continuous daily discipline, working with the energy centres of the body. The first step is generally to strengthen the Dan Tian centre to give strength and stability, and then later to calm the Head and Heart centres, and finally to balance these three main centres together.

RELATIONSHIP OF HEART WITH OTHER ORGANS

HEART AND PERICARDIUM

The relationship between heart and pericardium is discussed in Chapter 23 and the functions of Heart and Pericardium points compared in Table 23.1.

HEART AND SMALL INTESTINE

The Heart–Small Intestine relationship is more between Yin–Yang paired channels and not so much between the two organs, as discussed in Chapter 20.

HEART AND KIDNEYS

Heart and Kidneys are linked by the Control cycle of the Five Elements, in which there is an evolving balance between Water and Fire. The expansive energies of the spirit, of love, are balanced by the concentrative energies of will and limitations, joy is controlled by fear.

Also, the Heart needs the stored energy of Kidneys in order to function, and this is supplied by the Spleen. CV.4, CV.12 and CV.17 can be combined to strengthen Spleen, Kidneys and Heart. The Heart and Kidney channels are combined as the Lesser Yin pair of the Six Divisions, and these two channels are linked and balanced through the Extra channel system of Conception, Thoroughfare and Yin Link.

FUNCTIONS OF HEART POINTS

TREAT CHANNEL PROBLEMS

This function is not so important in this case. The Heart points are more used for systemic problems. However, they have their local use, e.g. HT.8 for palmar eczema or Dupuytren's contracture. Heart and Pericardium points may be combined for local problems, e.g. fungal infection of the palm, or carpal tunnel syndrome; or Heart and Small Intestine points may be combined for injuries of the ulnar side of the wrist.

REGULATE HEART SPIRIT

HT.7 can tonify Qi and Blood to stabilize the Spirit; HT.6 can move Stagnant Qi and move depression and Stagnation of the Spirit; HT.5 can move Phlegm in the Heart and treat confusion; HT.3 or HT.8 can clear Fire and calm the Spirit, as in mania and insomnia.

When Stomach Phlegm or Fire disturbs the Spirit, Stomach points such as ST.8, ST.40, ST.44 and ST.45 can be combined with Heart and Pericardium points. When Stagnant Liver Qi, Hyperactive Liver Yang or Liver Fire disturbs the Spirit, LR.3, GB.34 or LR.2, respectively, can be added. To balance Heart and Kidney, HT.7 and KI.3 can be combined for Deficient Heart and Kidney Qi; HT.6 and KI.6 for Deficient Heart and Kidney Yin; and HT.8 and KI.2 for Heart and Kidney Fire. HT.6 + KI.6 can be used for nervous sweating and HT.7, KI.3, CV.4, CV.14 can be used for nervous trembling.

Table 19.1 relates Heart syndromes to mental, emotional and speech problems.

TREAT MENTAL DULLNESS

The Well points HT.9 and PC.9 can be combined with the Source points HT.7 and PC.7 to treat mental dullness, and CV.4 and GV.4 can be added. If there is Phlegm clouding the mind, ST.8 and ST.40 can be added.

TREAT SPEECH DISORDERS

The combination of PC.5, HT.5, CV.23 and GV.15 can be used as a basis for speech problems, adding ST.40 and CV.22 for Phlegm, or KI.2 and HT.8 for stammering due to Heart–Kidney Deficiency Fire.

DISPERSE HEART FIRE

Heart Fire, resulting in hypertension, headaches, mania, or burnout, can be treated by simultaneously reinforcing the Water points HT.3, PC.3, KI.10 and reducing the Fire points HT.8, PC.8, KI.2. Alternatively, the Well and Spring points can be combined with Reducing method, HT.9 + HT.8, PC.9 + PC.8 or KI.1 + KI.2.

Table 19.1 Heart syndromes and behavioural problems

Syndrome	Mental problem	Emotional problem	Speech problem
Deficient Heart Yang	mental exhaustion, severe lack of mental interest and clarity	apathy, depression, deep introversion	silent or little speech, dull, boring and lacking interest
Deficient Heart Qi	mental tiredness, difficulty holding attention steady	lack of joy and liveliness or emotional lability	wandering from one subject to another, or lacking interest
Deficient Heart Blood	mental tiredness, poor memory	feeling emotionally weak and vulnerable	forgetting what they were going to say
Deficient Heart Yin	mental tiredness and restlessness	emotionally labile, difficult to feel at peace, overenthusiasm	talking rather too fast, talking is tiring, maybe stammering
Deficient Heart Fire	mental agitation, concentration difficult due to restlessness	overenthusiasm, overexcitement, hyperactivity	talking too much and too fast, talking in abrupt bursts
Excess Heart Fire	severe mental agitation, excessive, intense and fiery mental activity	mania, manic depression, severe exhausting hyperactivity	rapid, very forceful speech, perhaps alternating with periods of silence
Stagnant Heart Qi	thoughts and ideas not flowing freely, thinking seems blocked	sadness, frustration and feeling of blockage, especially in relationships	silence, perhaps alternating with enthusiastic speech in a social situation
Phlegm obstructs Heart	feelings of mental dullness, slowness, heaviness, obstruction or confusion	maybe lethargy and slow emotional response and bursts of anger and excitement	aphasia or slurred or confused speech

MOVE STAGNANT HEART QI AND BLOOD

The Accumulation points, HT.6 and PC.4, can be combined with the Alarm points CV.14 and CV.17 and with the Back Transporting points BL.15 and BL.14, to treat chest pain or poor peripheral circulation due to Stagnant Heart Qi and Blood. LU.7 can be added for Stagnant Lung Qi, LR.3 and LR.14 for Stagnant Liver Qi, or PC.6 + SP.4 can be combined with CV.4 to make use of the TV + Yin Link pair.

CV.4, KI.2 and KI.7 Rf M can be added if there is underlying Deficiency of Heart and Kidney Yang, as in angina with exhaustion and cyanosis of lips and nails.

DISPERSE HEART FIRE MOVING DOWNWARDS

HT.5, HT.8, SI.2 and SI.5 can combine to clear Heart Fire when it moves down the body to affect the Lower Energizer with such problems as genital inflammation and irritation, or cystitis. CV3 and SP.6 may be added to the Heart and Small Intestine points.

HEART SYNDROMES

The Heart syndromes are summarized in Table 19.2.

Table 19.2 Point combinations for Heart syndromes

Syndrome	Signs and symptoms	Pulse	Tongue	Point combinations
Deficient Heart Qi	worse with exertion, tiredness, palpitations; lack of joy or emotional lability	empty, maybe changing or flooding	hollow or crack in Heart area	CV.4, CV.17, ST.36, KI.3 Rf M; HT.7 Rf
Deficient Heart Yang	exhaustion, pallor, maybe cyanosis, cold extremities, feeling of cold, palpitations, maybe chest pain	empty to minute, deep, slow	pale, swollen, moist	GV20, CV.4, CV.6, CV.17, HT.8, KI.2 Rf M
Deficient Heart Blood	tiredness, dizziness, insomnia, palpitations, poor memory, pallor	thin, choppy	pale, thin, maybe dry	CV.4, CV.17, ST.36, SP.6, SP.10 Rf M; HT.7, PC.7 E
Stagnant Heart Qi	sadness and depression improved by exercise or social stimulation, maybe pain or oppressive feeling in chest	hindered, maybe irregular	maybe slightly purple	CV.6, CV.17, LU.7, PC.6, SP.6, LR.3 E
Stagnant Heart Blood	pain and discomfort in heart area, maybe radiating down left arm, maybe cyanosis of lips and nails	wiry, maybe choppy or irregular	purple	CV.14, CV.17, PC.1, PC.6, SP.4, SP.21 Rd + CV.4, KI.7 Rf M for Deficient Kidney Yang
Deficient Heart Yin	restless anxiety and insomnia, palpitations, feelings of heat, malar flush, perspiration, dry mouth	thin, rapid, maybe irregular	red, especially at tip, thin, dry, maybe crack to tip, no coat	CV.14, CV.17, HT.7 E; HT.3, SP.6, KI.6 Rf
Heart Fire	overexcitement, overenthusiasm, hectic, rushed hyperactivity, excessive talking, mania and maybe severe depression, maybe whole face red, feelings of heat	full, rapid, maybe irregular	dark red, especially at tip, yellow coat	CV.14, PC.8, KI.1 Rd; KI.6, SP.6 Rf + LR.1, LR.2 Rd for Liver Fire + LI.11, ST.45 Rd for Stomach Fire
Heart Fire moving downward	restlessness and agitation, maybe feelings of heat and discomfort in chest, thirst, maybe tongue ulcers, maybe burning urination or haematuria	rapid, flooding	red with dark red tip, yellow coat	HT.5, HT.8, SI.2, SI.5, ST.39 Rd + CV.3, SP.6 for cystitis + CV.23, CV.24, ST.4, ST.45 Rd for tongue ulcers
Kidney fear invades Heart	fearful jumpiness and apprehension, fear of loss of control of emotions or of a situation, maybe feeling of shakiness or actual trembling	empty or thin, maybe moving or irregular	maybe trembling	GV.20, CV.14, KI.1 E; CV.4, HT.7, KI.3, ST.36 Rf
Heart Phlegm	depression, mental confusion or dullness, maybe confused or reduced speech, lethargy, maybe feeling of oppression or dull pain in chest	slippery, maybe wiry or hindered	maybe swollen, maybe pale, thick greasy coast	CV.17, BL.15, HT.5, HT.9, PC.5, ST.40 Rd; CV.12 Rf M
Heart Phlegm Fire	mental and emotional restlessness, confusion or disturbance which may be severe, maybe incoherent speech, insomnia or palpitations	full or flooding, rapid	red or dark red with thick yellow greasy coat	GV.20, GV.24, BL.15, HT.5, PC.5, KI.1, ST.40 Rd; HT.9, PC.9 B

Rf, Reinforcing method; Rd, Reducing method; E, Even method; M, moxa; B bleeding.

Heart points

HT.3 shào hǎi

Water point of Heart channel.

General

The two main functions of HT.3 are:

cleans Excess or Deficiency Heart Fire, e.g. eczema or insomnia
moves Stagnation in the Heart channel, e.g. pain in arm or chest.

There are two main traditions of needling method for HT.3, one tradition is of using HT.3 with Reducing method, the other of using this point with Reinforcing method.

HT.3 with Reducing method

HT.3 is used with Reducing method to clear Excess or Deficiency Fire or to move Stagnation in the Heart channel. For example, HT.3 can be reduced to treat red, hot, itchy eczema with mental agitation. If the condition is very acute and severe, then HT.3 can be combined with HT.9, the Well point, and both points can be needled with Reducing method or bled.

If the condition is relatively superficial or physical, for example skin irritation or feverishness, Pericardium points may be preferred to Heart points, e.g. PC.3 and PC.9. If the condition is relatively deeper or emotional, for example extreme agitation and desperation, Heart points may be preferred to Pericardium points.

HT.3 with Reinforcing method

HT.3 is used as the Water point, according to Five Element theory, with Reinforcing method to control Heart Fire by strengthening Water.

Reinforce the Water Point, reduce the Fire Point

The effect of the Water point to control the Fire can be emphasized by simultaneously reducing the Fire point:

HT.3 Rf   +   HT.8 RD
Water Point   Fire Point

This technique can be used to treat either Excess or Deficiency Fire of one organ, in this case the Heart.

Treating Fire in two organs

If there is Excess or Deficiency Fire in two organs at the same time, this can be treated by reinforcing the Water point and reducing the Fire point of each organ. For example, if there is both Heart and Liver Fire and the person is both aggressive and overenthusiastic, the point combination could be:

Water points   Fire points
Rf   Rd
HE.3 + LR.8   +   HE.8 + LR.2

Or if there is simultaneous Heart and Kidney Fire and the person has insomnia, restlessness and cystitis, the point combination could be:

Water points   Fire points
Rf   Rd
HE.3 + KI.10   +   HE.8 + KI.2

Strengthening Kidney Water to control Heart Deficiency Fire

In some patterns of Heart Deficiency Fire where there is no simultaneous Kidney Fire but there is Deficient Kidney Yin. Since Kidney Yin can be the source of the Yin of other organs, strengthening Kidney Yin can tonify Heart Yin and thus help to control Heart Fire. So to the combination of HE.3 Rf + HE.8 Rd, can be added KI.6 Rf.

Deficient Heart Yin predominates

In cases where Heart Deficiency, especially Deficient Heart Yin is more important than Deficiency Heart Fire, the emphasis is more on tonification and less on clearing Heat. For example, if the patient is tired and restless but the pulse is more thin than rapid. In this case a suitable combination could be:

HT.3 Water point Rf to control any Fire	HT.7 Source point Rf to tonify Qi	KI.3 Source point Rf to tonify Yin and Qi

Sequence of combinations as treatment progresses

As treatment progresses, it may be necessary to shift emphasis of treatment from an acute effect to a more long-standing underlying cause. For example, a patient might come initially with an acute Excess Heart Fire condition, such as severe eczema with extreme itching and agitation and desperation. In this acute phase the method of reducing or bleeding HT.3 would be best:

HT.3 B + HT.9 B.

If on a subsequent visit, the severity of the signs were reduced, and the pulse had changed from rapid, full and wiry to rapid and thin, the method of reinforcing HT.3, to treat Heart Deficiency Fire, might be used:

HT.3 Rf + HT.8 Rd.

With more treatment, the Heart Fire might further reduce, and the pulse become less rapid, revealing an underlying deficiency of Heart and Kidney Yin. The point combination might then be changed to:

HT.3 + HT.6 + KI.6 Rf.

Syndromes

Excess Heart Fire
Heart Deficiency Fire

Excess Heart Fire

Pulse. Rapid, full or flooding, maybe wiry.

Indications. Extreme restlessness, agitation or insomnia, severe acute eczema with emotional distress.

Example. Overenthusiastic manic hyperactivity.

Combination. HT.3, HT.9, KI.1 Rd.

Heart Deficiency Fire

Pulse. Thin, rapid.

Indications. Restless enthusiasm alternating with tiredness, night sweats, palpitations, anxiety.

Example. Insomnia.

Combination. HT.3, HT.6, KI.6, KI.10 Rf; HT.8 Rd.

HT.5 tōng lǐ

Connecting point of Heart channel.

General

HT.5 can be used to tonify Heart Qi, for example, to treat symptoms of tiredness, blurred vision, chest pain and sensation of heaviness in the body. However, HT.5 also has two other specific functions:

regulates communication
clears Heart Fire draining downward.

HT.5 regulates communication

HT.5 regulates communication in three ways: it clears the mind; it calms the mind and emotions; and it regulates the tongue.

HT.5 clears the mind. Since HT.5 tonifies Heart Qi, it strengthens the ability of the spirit to vitalize and activate the mind, so that clear and rapid thinking can form the basis of efficient communication. For this purpose HT.5 can be combined with other points to strengthen and clear the mind, e.g. BL.10, BL.44, BL.52, BL.64, BL.67 and KI.3 Rf.

HT.5 calms the mind and emotions. If the mind and emotions are agitated, thinking becomes confused and erratic. By tonifying Heart Qi and by clearing Heart Fire, HT.5 calms the mind and allows clear thought and speech. Here, HT.5 can be combined with other points to calm disturbance of Heart Spirit, e.g. PC.6, CV.14, CV.24 Rd; KI.6 Rf.

HT.5 regulates the tongue. The feelings of the Heart or the ideas of the mind can only express in speech through the tongue. HT.5 can treat sequelae of cerebrovascular accident or head injuries which affect the speech and tongue. HT.5 can combine with other points to increase the freedom of movement of tongue and fluency of speech, e.g. CV.23, GV.15, ST.40 E.

HT.5 clears Heart Fire draining downward

Since HT.5 is the Connecting point linking the Heart and Small Intestine channels, it can be used to clear Heart Fire which has moved downwards, through the Small Intestine and Bladder channels, into the Lower Energizer to cause abnormal uterine bleeding, cystitis or vaginitis.

Syndromes

Communication problems
Heart Fire draining downwards

Communication problems

Pulse. Various.

Indications. Hemiplegia with aphasia, depression or hysteria with aphasia, stammering, sudden loss of voice and confused speech.

Example. Transposing of words or syllables when tired.

Combination. HT.5, CV.4, CV.17, ST.36, KI.3 Rf.

Heart Fire draining downward

Pulse. Rapid, maybe full or thin, maybe wiry.

Indications. Hypertension, tongue ulcers, sweating, insomnia, menorrhagia.

Example. Cystitis with feverish restlessness.

Combination. HE.5, HE.8, SI.5, CV.3, ST.39 Rd.

HT.6 yīn xì

Accumulation point of the Heart channel.

General

The two main functions of HT.6 are that it tonifies Heart Yin and moves Stagnant Qi and Blood in the Heart channel. It can also clear Heart Deficiency Fire occurring with Deficient Heart Yin.

HT.6 as an Accumulation point

This point can be used for acute painful conditions of the Heart or Heart channel, for example, involving Stagnation of Qi, Blood or Phlegm, and so can be used for pain and stiffness along the Heart channel and pain or oppressive feeling in the chest and heart. Which points are combined with HT.6 will depend on the type of Stagnation, for example:

Stagnant Qi   HT.6 + CV.17, PC.6, CV.6, LR.3
Stagnant Blood   HT.6 + CV.17, PC.4, PC.2, SP.4
Stagnant Phlegm HT.6 + CV.17, PC.6, GV.15, ST.40.

The use of HT.6 to tonify Yin and drain Deficiency Fire

HT.6 is the point of choice to tonify Heart Yin. HT.3 and HT.7 can also tonify Heart Yin, but HT.3 is more to strengthen Water to control Fire and HT.6 may be combined with KI.6 and/or SP.6 to tonify Heart Yin, since these points can tonify the Kidney Yin on which Heart Yin is based. HT.7 is more to tonify Qi. HT.3 and HT.8 used together, may be better than HT.6 to clear Heart Deficiency Fire, and if Heart Deficiency Fire drains downward, then HT.5 or HT.8 may be more efficient than HT.6.

Syndromes

Stagnation of Qi and Blood in Heart channel
Deficient Heart Yin

Stagnation of Qi and Blood in Heart channel

Pulse. Hindered or wiry, maybe empty or full.

Indications. Pain or stiffness along arm, pain or oppressive feeling in heart or chest.

Example. Angina pectoris.

Combination. HT.6, PC.4, SP.4, CV.14, CV.17 Rd.

Alternation. HT.6, PC.4, SP.4, BL.15, BL.17 Rd.

Deficient Heart Yin

Pulse. Thin, rapid, maybe choppy or irregular.

Indications. Palpitations, anxiety, restlessness, insomnia.

Example. Night sweats.

Combination. HT.6 + KI.7 E.

HT.7 shén mén

Source point, Earth point and Sedation point of the Heart channel.

General

HT.7 is the most used point on the Heart channel and one of the most important points on the body. It is the most widely used point for Disturbance of the Spirit and is specific for Heart pattern emotional problems with underlying chronic Deficiency. HT.7 is compared with HT.5 and HT.6 in Table 19.3.

Table 19.3 Comparison of HT.5, HT.6 and HT.7

Syndrome	HT.5	HT.6	HT.7
Deficiency Heart Qi	x	-	X
Deficiency Heart Blood	-	-	x
Deficiency Heart Yin	-	X	x
Deficiency Heart Fire	x	x	x
Excess Heart Fire	X	-	x
Heart Fire drains downward	X	-	x
Stagnation in Heart channel	x	X	x
Phlegm obstructs Heart	x	x	x
Mental dullness	x	x	x
Disturbance of Spirit	x	x	X
Speech problems	X	x	x

X, primary use; x, secondary use.

HT.7 and Five Element theory

According to Five Element theory, HT.7 is the Sedation point of the Heart channel because it is the Earth point. Excess Heart conditions are treated by sedating HT.7 to move the Excess energy and around the Five Element promotion cycle from Heart to Spleen, from Fire to Earth.

Clinical use of HT.7 for Excess Heart syndromes

In clinical practice, HT.7 is commonly reinforced since it is the Source point and is capable of tonifying Heart Qi, Blood and Yin. HT.7 is listed for three main types of Excess Heart pattern:

278 POINT COMBINATIONS FOR THE MAIN ACUPUNCTURE POINTS

Stagnation of Qi, Blood or Phlegm in Heart channel
Excess Heart Fire
acute nervous tension and anxiety.

In the clinic, HT.6 is often preferable for Stagnation and HT.3, HT.8 or HT.9 more effective for Excess Heart Fire. The main clinical use of HT.7 for Excess conditions is to calm acute severe nervous tension with anxiety. For this it is often combined with PC.6.

HT.7 as a Source point

The Source point of the Yin organs are excellent neutral points which can tonify the organ and balance Yin and Yang. Points like HT.7, PC.7, LU.9 and KI.3 are mainly used to strengthen and stabilize, as discussed on page 61. Not only can HT..7 strengthen Heart function by tonifying Heart Qi, and to a lesser extent, Heart Blood and Yin, but HT.7 is excellent to treat emotional lability by stabilizing the Spirit. For this purpose, HT.7 can be combined:

Front treatment   HT.7 + CV.4, CV.17, ST.36, SP.6, KI.3 Rf

Back treatment   HT.7 + BL.15, BL.44, ST.36. SP.6, KI.3 Rf.

HT.7 clears the mind

HT.7 can strengthen and clear the mind by strengthening and regulating the Spirit which vitalizes mental activity.

The role of Heart and Spleen. HT.7 tonifies the Qi which provides the energy and the Blood which provides the material substratum for mental activity. HT.7 can be combined with SP.3, ST.36 and BL.20 to tonify the ability of the Spleen to provide the Heart with Qi and Blood, in order to strengthen memory.

The role of Heart and Kidney. HT.7 can also be combined with CV.4, KI.3 and BL.64 to tonify the ability of the Kidneys to provide the Heart with Qi and Yang, in order to strengthen the ability of the mind to focus and concentrate on a task or theme with steadiness and endurance.

HT.7 and the Well points. The Well points, especially BL.67, ST.45 and LI.1, can invigorate the mind, but they do not tonify it. Their effect is more a quick stimulation by moving of Stagnation, rather than a lasting tonification of chronic Deficiency. However, a combination of the Well points with points such as HT.7, BL.64, KI.3 and ST.36, give the mind simultaneous stimulation and tonification; for example, for mental stagnation and tiredness after long work or study.

HT.7 calms the mind and emotions

HT.7, like LI.4 and LR.3, can relieve generalized nervous tension, whether acute or chronic, but it is specifically indicated for nervous tension associated with anxiety, overexcitement, overenthusiasm and the other emotional imbalances associated with the Heart organ system.

Heart and Kidneys. Many of the indications for emotional problems associated with Heart points in general and HT.7 in particular, relate to the balance between Heart and Kidneys. For example, impotence associated with anxiety and fear of failure, fearful overexcitement, laughing and joking in an attempt to suppress fear, or restless sleep with frightening dreams. For these conditions, HT.7 can be combined with KI.3, the Source point of the Kidneys, and with the inner and outer Bladder line points, BL.15 and BL.23, and BL.44 and BL.52.

Heart and other Yin organs. Although the combination of anxiety and fear, of Heart and Kidneys may be predominant, other organ combinations are found in the clinic, as shown in Table 19.4.

Table 19.4 HT.7 and the treatment of the Five Emotions

Source points	Back points	Emotions
HT.7 + KI.3	BL.15, BL.44 + BL.23, BL.52	anxiety + fear
HT.7 + LR.3	BL.15, BL.44 + BL.18, BL.47	anxiety + anger
HT.7 + SP.3	BL.15, BL.44 + BL.20, BL.49	anxiety + worry
HT.7 + LU.9	BL.15, BL.44 + BL.13, BL.42	anxiety + withdrawal

The range of Heart emotions and behaviour

The list of adjectives below describes a range of Heart behaviour going far beyond mere anxiety or the excess or lack of joy.

compassionate	expansive	vulnerable
charming	larger-than-life	disorientated
warm	theatrical	confused
fiery	colourful	panicky
feverish	spontaneous	hysterical
passionate	impulsive	burned-out
intense	erratic	bored
manic	unstable	serious
hyperactive	foolish	depressive
enthusiastic	immature	selfish

HT.7 can treat a variety of Heart syndromes, and their associated behavioural problems, depending on the other points with which HT.7 is combined.

Syndromes

Deficient Heart Qi
Deficient Heart Qi and Blood
Deficient Heart Qi and Yang
Instability of Heart Yin–Yang Balance
Deficient Heart Qi and Yin
Deficient Heart Qi and Heart Deficiency Fire
Acute severe nervousness

Deficient Heart Qi

Pulse.   Empty, maybe choppy, changing or irregular.

Indications.   Physical and mental tiredness, emotional lability, palpitations, asthma.

Example.   Tired of talking, avoiding social situations.

Combinations.   HT.7, CV.4, CV.17, ST.36, KI.3 Rf.

Deficient Heart Qi and Blood

Pulse.   Thin or empty, choppy.

Indications.   Insomnia, poor memory, thoughts drifting, dizziness, headache.

Example.   Tired and tearful with feelings of vulnerability.

Combination.   HT.7, BL.20, BL.44, BL.49, SP.6, SP.10, ST.36 Rf.

Deficient Heart Qi and Yang

Pulse.   Empty, slow, deep.

Indications.   Cold hands and feet, chest pain, exhaustion, depression, lack of sexual interest.

Example.   Mental exhaustion, dullness, slowness and lack of interest.

Combination.   HT.7 Rf; GV.4, GV.11, GV.14, GV.20, KI.3 Rf M.

Instability of Heart Yin–Yang balance

Pulse.   Empty or thin, maybe irregular or rapid on occasion.

Indications.   Sometimes warm and sometimes cold, sometimes hypoactive and sometimes hyperactive, sometimes manic and sometimes depressed.

Example.   Menopausal syndrome with mood swings.

Combination.   HT.7, KI.3, BL.42, BL.52, SP.6, ST.36 E.

Deficiency of Heart Qi and Yin

Pulse.   Empty or thin, slightly rapid, maybe irregular.

Indications.   Restlessness, tiredness, emotional lability, insomnia, palpitations.

Example.   Restless nervous anxiety, longing for peace and quiet.

Combination.   HT.7, HT.3, KI.3, KI.10, CV.4, CV.14, GV.20E.

Deficient Heart Qi and Heart Deficiency Fire

Pulse.   Thin, maybe choppy or empty, rapid or hasty.

Indications.   Feverish sensation in chest, overexcitable, talking, talking too much and too fast.

Example.   Nervousness, stammering and feeling embarrassment in social situations.

Combination.   HT.7, KI.3, CV.4 Rf; HT.8, KI.2, CV.14 Rd.

Acute severe nervousness

Pulse.   Thin, rapid, maybe moving or hasty.

Indications.   Painful, jumpy, anxious, tense, easily upset.

Example.   Extreme emotional hypersensitivity.

Combination.   HT.7, PC.6, LR.3, KI.1, GV.20 Rd.

HT.8 shào fǔ

Fire point and Spring point of the Heart channel.

General

The functions of HT.8 are those of a Fire point. HT.8 can be reduced to clear Excess Fire, Deficiency Fire, Phlegm Fire or Downward Draining Fire from the Heart channel. On the other hand, HT.8 can also be used with Reinforcing method and moxa to tonify Heart Yang and Heart Fire. However, the main use of HT.8 is with Reducing method to clear all types of Excess Heart Fire. It can also be used, with points such as GV.10, GV.12 and BL.40 to clear Fire poison and treat boils.

HT.8 and HT.7

HT.8 and HT.7 can be used together, both with Reducing method to calm extreme acute nervous anxiety. Alternatively, HT.8 can be reduced to clear Heart Deficiency Fire, while HT.7 is reinforced to tonify the underlying pattern of Deficient Heart Qi and Yin. Thirdly, if HT.8 is used with Reinforcing method and moxa to tonify Heart Fire, HT.7 can be reinforced, as the Source point, to stabilize the treatment to prevent overexcitement of the Spirit.

However, generally HT.8 is used with Reducing method for acute Excess Heart Fire conditions with severe mental and emotional fiery restlessness and agitation, while HT.7 is used to tonify Heart Qi and Blood to stabilize less severe symptoms of chronic emotional lability and stress.

Syndromes

Heart Deficiency Fire
Excess Heart Fire
Heart Fire draining downward
Heart Phlegm Fire
Deficient Heart Yang
Local hand problems

Heart Deficiency Fire

Pulse. Thin, rapid maybe hasty.

Indications. Feverish sensation in palms and chest, arrythmia, sore throat, eye irritation.

Example. Constant tiredness from restless overenthusiasm.

Combination. HT.8, KI.2, CV.14 Rd; HT.6, KI.6, CV.4 Rf.

Excess Heart Fire

Pulse. Full or flooding, rapid, maybe wiry.

Indications. Haemoptysis, fevers, hyperthyroidism, hypertension and headaches.

Example. Eczema with intense itching and distress.

Combination. HT.8, PC.8, HT.9, PC.9, KI.1, GV.20 Rd.

Heart Fire draining downwards

Pulse. Full or flooding, rapid, maybe wiry.

Indications. Melaena, haematuria, menorrhagia, cystitis, feverishness, tongue ulcers.

Example. Vulvar pruritis.

Combination. HT.5, HT.8, CV.2, CV.3, LR.5, KI.2 Rd.

Heart Phlegm Fire

Pulse. Full, slippery, rapid, maybe irregular.

Indications. Chaotic, confused or disorientated thinking, speech or behaviour with sudden irritability and rage.

Example. Confused behaviour with sudden irritability and rage.

Combination. HT.5, HT.8, GB.13, GB.34, ST.40, GV.20 Rd.

Deficient Heart Yang

Pulse. Empty to minute, deep, slow.

Indications. Slow dull thinking, hypoactivity, cold extremities, hypersomnia.

Example. Boredom, apathy, depression.

Combination. HT.8, HT.9, SI.1, SI.5. BL.64, KI.3 Rf M.

Local hand problems

Pulse. Various.

Indications. Dupuytren's contracture, skin disorders of the palm, injuries and arthritis of hand and palm.

Example. Eczema of the palm with irritation and exudation.

Combination. HT.7, HT.8, PC.7, PC.8, SP.6, SP.9, ST.44 E.

HT.9 shào chōng

Well point, Wood point and Tonification point of Heart channel.

HT.9 as a Well point

Like all Well points, HT.9 can be used to clear extreme Heat and Interior Wind for severe fevers, delirium, seizures and loss of consciousness. As a Well point of the Heart channel, when bled or reduced, it can clear Excess Heart Fire and Heat in the Blood to treat extreme severe acute conditions, affecting both physical body and emotions, such as severe anxiety with feeling of fullness in the heart region, eczema with extreme agitation and mania and hysteria with violent palpitation.

HT.9 as a Tonification point

Since HT.9 is the Wood point, then according to the Five Element system, it is the Tonification point of the Heart channel. However, in clinical practice, while HT.9 can be used together with HT.8 to tonify Heart Yang, it is not so much used to tonify Heart Qi, Blood or Yin.

Syndromes

Loss of consciousness
Excess Heart Fire
Deficient Heart Yang

Loss of consciousness

Pulse. Maybe minute or wiry.

Indications. Seizures, apoplexy, fainting, sunstroke.

Example. Sunstroke and sunburn.

Combination. HT.9 and GV.26 E to restore consciousness then HT.9, HT.3, GV.14, LI.4 E once consciousness is properly restored.

Excess Heart Fire

Pulse. Full or flooding, rapid, maybe wiry.

Indications. Face and neck red and hot, discomfort and heat sensations in the chest, extreme restlessness.

Example. Hypertension, headache and eye irritation.

Combination. HT.3, HT.9, KI.1, BL.66, GV.20 Rd; BL.2 E.

Deficient Heart Yang

Pulse. Empty to minute, slow deep.

Indications. Exhaustion, depression, cold extremities.

Example. Severe depression, chest pain, numbness in the arm and finger.

Combination. HT.9, HT.6, GV.14, GV.20, PC.6, ST.36, KI.2 Rf.

HT.9 is compared with HT.3, 5, 6 and 8 in Table.19.5.

Table 19.5 Comparison of HT.3, 5, 6, 8 and 9 in regulating Fire

Syndrome	HT.3 Water point	HT.5 Connecting point	HT.6 Accumulation point	HT.8 Fire point	HT.9 Well point
Deficient Heart Yang	-	-	-	X	x
Deficient Heart Yin	x	-	X	-	-
Deficiency Heart Fire	X	x	x	X	-
Excess Heart Fire	X	x	x	X	X
Heart Fire moving downward	-	X	-	x	-
Heart Phlegm Fire	-	x	x	x	–

X, primary use; x, secondary use.

Heart point comparisons and combinations

The functions of the main points of the Heart channel are compared in Table 19.6.

Table 19.6 Heart point comparisons

Point	Point type	Syndromes
HT.3	Water point	Excess Heart Fire
Heart Deficiency Fire
Stagnation in Heart channel
HT.5	Connecting point	Communication problems
Heart Fire draining downward
HT.6	Accumulation point	Stagnation in Heart channel
Deficient Heart Yin
HT.7	Source point	Deficient Heart Qi
Instability of Heart Yin–Yang balance
Acute nervousness
HT.8	Fire point	Heart Deficiency Fire
Excess Heart Fire
Heart Fire draining downward
Heart Phlegm Fire
Deficient Heart Yang
local hand problems
HT.9	Well point	loss of consciousness
Excess Heart Fire
Deficient Heart Yang

Some common combinations of Heart points with each other and with other channel points are summarized in Tables 19.7 and 19.8 respectively.

Table 19.7 Combinations of Heart points

Point	Combination	Syndromes	Example
HT.3	HT.6	Deficient Heart Yin and Heart Deficiency Fire	tiredness, restlessness and insomnia
HT.3	HT.7	Deficient Heart Qi and Deficient Heart Yin	emotional lability and restless anxiety
HT.3	HT.8	Heart Deficiency Fire	excessive talking and easily tired
HT.3	HT.9	Excess Heart Fire	severe eczema
HT.5	HT.8	Heart Phlegm Fire	confused speech and behaviour
HT.6	HT.2	Stagnation in Heart channel	pain in arm and chest
HT.7	HT.8	Deficient Heart Yang	tiredness and impotence
HT.7	HT.9	Deficiency and Stagnation of Heart Qi	difficulty in expressing feelings
HT.8	HT.9	Excess Heart Fire	feverish manic excitement

Table 19.8 Combinations of Heart and Other Points

HT point	HT point type	KI point	GV point	CVpoint	Function of CV point
HT.3	Water point	KI.10	–	CV.14	Disturbance of Spirit
HT.5	Communication point	–	GV.15	CV.23	communication problems
HT.6	Accumulation point	KI.6	GV.11	CV.17	Stagnation in Heart channel
				CV.14	Disturbance of Spirit
HT.7	Source point	KI.3	GV.11	CV.14	Disturbance of Spirit
				CV12	Deficient Heart + Spleen Blood
				CV.4	Deficient Heart + Kidney Qi
HT.8	Fire point	KI.2	GV.14	CV.14	Disturbance of Spirit
				CV.4	Deficient Heart Yang
HT.9	Well point	KI.1	GV.26	CV.1	loss of consciousness

Small Intestine 20

Small Intestine channel

CHANNEL CONNECTIONS

MAIN CHANNEL PATHWAY

From the ulnar side of the little finger, the main channel pathway runs up the posterior arm to the shoulder joint. It circles round the scapula, crossing the Bladder channel at BL.36 and BL.11, and the Governor channel at GV.14, then runs forward over the shoulder, down into the supraclavicular fossa and into the body. This internal branch connects with the heart, passes along the oesophagus, connects with the stomach and small intestine and meets the Conception channel at CV.13 and CV.14. A branch from the small intestine descends the leg to meet the Stomach channel at ST.39, the Lower Sea point of the Small Intestine.

From the supraclavicular fossa, the superficial pathway runs up the neck and divides on the cheek. One branch goes up the outer canthus, meets the Gallbladder channel at GB.1 and runs back across the temple to enter the ear at SI.19. The other branch ascends the cheek to the inner canthus to meet the Bladder channel at BL.1.

CONNECTING CHANNEL PATHWAY

Running from SI.7, one branch connects with the Heart meridian and another branch runs up the arm to connect with LI.15.

Table 20.1 Crossing points on the Small Intestine channel

Point	Crossing
SI.10	Yang Link, Yang Heel
SI.12	GB, TE, ST, LI
SI.18	TE
SI.19	GB, TE

FUNCTIONS OF SMALL INTESTINE POINTS

Most of the indications for the Small Intestine points are for Small Intestine channel problems either as local or distal points – see Table 20.2. For example SI.17 and SI.1 are local and distal points for sore throat, and SI.19 and SI.3 are local and distal points for tinnitus. The other main functions of the Small Intestine points are to calm Heart Spirit when it is disturbed by Heart Fire and to regulate the Governor channel. SI.3 is the Opening point for the Governor channel, which itself can regulate the spine and calm or stimulate Heart Spirit.

One of the functions of the Small Intestine organ is to receive the material from the Stomach, resulting from the processing of food and drink by the Spleen, and to separate this into its more and less useful components to pass on the wastes to the Large Intestine and to absorb the purer products for transportation by the Spleen.

While the solids and some of the fluids pass from the Small to the Large Intestine, most of the impure fluids are passed from the Small Intestine to the Bladder. These processes of digestion, absorption and elimination are powered by Spleen and Kidney Yang. However, Small Intestine points are rarely used for Small Intestine organ problems, such as enteritis or lower abdominal pain. The main points for this are from the Stomach and Spleen channels, e.g. ST.25 and ST.39 and SP.15.

Similarly, Small Intestine points are rarely used to regulate fluid metabolism. SI.2 can be used for burning urination, but this is mainly for Heart Fire moving downward. So on the physical level, Small Intestine points are not much used for separation of the pure from the impure.

CLEARS THE MIND

Parallel to the material sorting of solid and fluid components by the Small Intestine, is the digesting and sifting of information and ideas. This involves absorption of the useful and its integration into the stored and working concept systems of the brain and the letting go of rubbish, that which is not useful or that which is no longer useful. The mental role of the Small Intestine is therefore intermediate between Spleen and Large Intestine, and the aspect of sorting between the more and less useful is similar to the Gallbladder function of deciding between possible options.

Points such as SI.1 and SI.3 can be used to aid the Governor channel and the brain, and can be useful points to treat mental congestion and tiredness.

CALM HEART SPIRIT

There is not a close clinical relationship between Heart and Small Intestine, although they are paired Fire organs with a deep Small Intestine channel connection to the Heart. The main use of Small Intestine points for Heart problems is of SI.3, 4, 5 and 7 to calm disturbance of the Spirit, mainly associated with Heart Fire. SI.3 has the dual function of calming the Spirit to treat anxiety and mental restlessness and of regulating the Governor channel to clear the mind and strengthen concentration. SI.2 can be used with HT.8 to treat Heart Fire draining downward, but there are few other examples of Small Intestine points used for Heart problems.

REGULATE THE GOVERNOR CHANNEL

SI.3 is the Opening point for the Governor channel, and in combination with BL.62 can regulate the spine, neck, shoulders and legs (see Chapter 10). In addition, the combination of Small Intestine and Bladder channels represents the Greater Yang pair of the Six Divisions. Owing to the Extra channel and Six Divisions relationships, chains of points on the Small Intestine and Bladder channels can be combined to treat problems on the back of the body; for example, SI.3, SI.12, SI.15 with BL.10, BL.23 and BL.62 for multiple sclerosis (see Chapter 27).

SMALL INTESTINE SYNDROMES

Point combinations for syndromes of Small and Large Intestines are given together in Table 22.2.

Table 20.2 Problems treated with Small Intestine points

Channel problems	Local points	Distal points
fingers	SI.1–3	–
wrist and hand	SI.3–5	–
forearm	SI.6–7	SI.3–5
elbow	SI.8	SI.3,6,7
shoulder and neck	SI.9–15	SI.3–6
spine and Governor channel	SI.15	SI.3
respiration	SI.15	–
throat	SI.16, 17	SI.1–5
jaw, teeth, cheek, nose	SI.18	SI.2, 5
ears	SI.19	SI.1–3, 5
eyes	–	SI.1–6
head	–	SI.1–5
Other problems		
Governor channel (e.g. spinal problems)	SI.10, 14, 15	SI.3
Disturbance of Spirit (e.g. due to Heart Fire)	SI.16	SI.3–5, 7
breasts	–	SI.1, 11
urination	–	SI.2
digestion	–	SI.4, 8

Small Intestine points

SI.1 shào zé
Well point, Metal point.

General

SI.1 as a Well point

Acute conditions. As a Well point, SI.1 can treat severe acute Excess conditions of Heat and Internal Wind with fever or loss of consciousness.

Chronic physical conditions. SI.1 can also be used as a Well point for conditions of chronic Deficiency and stagnation of Qi to invigorate the Small Intestine channel. For example, it can be used as part of a chain of Small Intestine points to treat stiffness of the shoulder and upper arm, such as SI.1, SI.9, SI.10 and SI.12 with Reducing method and moxa.

Chronic mental conditions. SI.1 can be used as a Well point to invigorate the mind and stimulate the ability to digest and assess ideas, separating the useful from the dross. It can be combined with BL.67 to stimulate the mind, and further combined with SI.3 and BL.62 for a deeper tonifying effect on the mind.

SI.1 to clear Wind Heat

Like the other Small Intestine points on the lower arm, SI.1 can be used to clear Wind Heat, especially for sore throat and acute tonsillitis, in combination with SI.17.

SI.1 to treat Small Intestine channel problems

Again like the other lower arm Small Intestine points, SI.1 can be used to treat chronic Small Intestine channel problems from finger pain to ear ache.

SI.1 to treat breast problems

An important empirical use of SI.1 is to treat mastitis and insufficient lactation, especially when due to Excess or Stagnation.

Syndromes

Small Intestine channel problems
Heat and Wind Heat
Breast problems
Mental congestion

Small Intestine channel problems

Pulse. Empty or full, maybe wiry, maybe superficial.

Indications. Headache, chronic neck stiffness, deafness, tinnitus, posterior lateral arm problems.

Example. Acute torticollis.

Combination. SI.1, SI.3, SI.15, BL.66 Rd.

Heat and Wind Heat

Pulse. Superficial, rapid.

Indications. Tonsillitis, sore throat, headache, epistaxis, conjunctivitis.

Example. Conjunctivitis.

Combination. SI.1, BL.2, BL.67, TE.3, GB.1 E.

Breast problems

Pulse. Various, maybe wiry.

Indications. Mastitis, insufficient lactation.

Example. Premenstrually sore breasts

Combination. SI.1, ST.18, CV.17, LR.3, LR.14, PC.6 Rd.

Mental congestion

Pulse. Hindered, maybe empty or choppy.

Indications. Difficulty in separating more suitable information from less suitable information.

Example. Mental congestion and tiredness following excessive study.

Combination. SI.1, BL.67, ST.36, ST.45, LI.1, yìn táng E.

SI.2 qián gǔ
Spring point, Water point.

General

As a Spring point and a Water point, SI.3 can be used to clear Heat and Wind Heat. Owing to the relationship of Small Intestine and Bladder in fluid metabolism, SI.2 as the Water point can treat burning urination, especially in cases of downward movement of Heart Fire. Like all the Small Intestine points from SI.1 to SI.8, SI.2 can treat problems of the Small Intestine channel from arthritis of the fingers to otitis media and conjunctivitis.

Syndromes

Heat and Wind Heat in Small Intestine channel
Heat in the Bladder

Heat and Wind Heat in Small Intestine channel

Pulse. Superficial, rapid or full, rapid, maybe wiry.

Indications. Pain and swelling in the jaw, sore throat, headache, fever, ear problems.

Example. Arthritis of the hand with heat and swelling.

Combination. SI.2, SI.3, SI.5 Rd; BL.66, KI.6 Rf.

Heat in the Bladder

Pulse. Rapid, wiry, maybe thin or full.

Indications. Burning urination, haematuria, feverishness, insomnia.

Example. Cystitis with restlessness at night.

Combination. SI.2, HT.8, CV.3, SP.6 E.

SI.3 hòu xī

Opening point of Governor channel, Wood point of Small Intestine channel, Tonification point.

General

This is the most important point on the Small Intestine channel. While the other Small Intestine points on the lower arm can treat problems of the Small Intestine channel, SI.3 can also treat Governor channel problems, especially those of the upper body. If SI.3 is combined with BL.62, this combination can treat problems of the entire spine and both arms and legs.

Heat and Wind Heat

SI.3 treats Heat and Wind Heat, both because it is a Small Intestine point on the lower arm and because SI.3 regulates the Governor channel which regulates Heat. SI.3 can therefore be used to treat fevers, common cold and influenza, for example, often in combination with GV.14.

Small Intestine and Governor channel problems

SI.3 can treat problems of the areas covered by these two channels, whether due to Wind Cold, Wind Heat, Deficiency, Excess or Stagnation. This includes pain or stiffness of upper back, spine, shoulders, arms, neck or headache

and also problems of Interior Wind in the Governor channel such as dizziness, tremors, epilepsy or convulsions.

Neck problems

In addition to treating hand, arm, ear and eye problems like other lower arm Small Intestine points, SI.3 is specific for acute or chronic neck problems. It can either be used as part of a chain of Small Intestine points or, for acute neck sprain, it can first be used by itself, manipulating the needle while the patient moves their neck.

Calms the Spirit

Like SI.5 and SI.7, SI.3 can calm the Heart Spirit, due to the internal connections of both the Small Intestine channel and the Governor channel with the Heart. The Small Intestine is an organ belonging to the Fire element, and SI.3 can clear Heart Fire associated with mania, hysteria, agitation, restlessness and insomnia with dream–disturbed sleep and night sweating.

Regulates the Mind

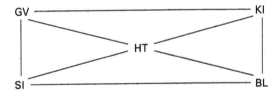

Fig. 20.1

In addition to the role of SI.3 in linking Governor, Small Intestine and Heart to clear Heart Fire and calm the Spirit, when SI.3 is combined with BL.62, the Kidneys and the Bladder channel are brought into the relationship. The Kidneys and the Governor and Bladder channels nourish and regulate the brain. SI.3 and BL.62 can be used with Reinforcing method to treat mental exhaustion and loss of the ability to assess and sort ideas, or to give some mental strength, structure and 'back bone' to help to face the problems and choices of life. SI.3 and BL.62 can be used with Even or Reducing method to treat mental and physical rigidity and inflexibility and the reluctance to assimilate new ideas, partly due to fear of letting go of old structures.

Syndromes

Heat and Wind Heat
Small Intestine and Governor channel problems
Neck Problems
Problems of mind and Spirit

Heat and Wind Heat

Pulse. Rapid, superficial or full, maybe wiry.

Indications. Conjunctivitis, epistaxis, fever, arthritis of hand, arm, elbows or shoulder.

Example. Sore throat, dry mouth, feverishness.

Combination. SI.3, SI.17, GV.14 Rd; KI.6 Rf.

Small Intestine and Governor channel problems

Pulse. Various

Indications. Pain or stiffness in spine, upper back, shoulders, arms, neck, headache, dizziness and tremors.

Example. Arthritis of shoulders, spine and legs with inflammation and tiredness.

Combination. SI.3, SI.10, BL.11, BL.62, GV.3, GV.14 E.

Neck problems

Pulse. Various, maybe wiry.

Indications. Acute or chronic neck problems.

Example. Acute neck sprain.

Combination. SI.3, SI.15, BL.66, GV.13, GV.14 Rd.

Problems of mind and Spirit

Pulse. Various

Indications. Mental agitation, mental inflexibility, mental exhaustion, inability to discriminate.

Example. Spineless character, lacking mental clarity and resolve.

Combination. SI.1, SI.3, BL.62, BL.67, GV.4, GV.24, KI.7 Rf.

SI.4 wàn gǔ

Source point.

General

SI.4 is mainly used for local problems of wrist, hand or fingers, and also for distal Small Intestine channel problems, e.g. elbow, neck or head pain. The points SI.1–8 can all clear Heat and Wind Heat and SI.4 can treat fevers without sweating, sore throat, mumps and childhood convulsions. Although SI.4 is the Source point of the channel, it is not much used to tonify or regulate the Small Intestine organ. Indeed as discussed on page 284, the Small Intestine points in general are not the main points used to treat the Small Intestine as an organ, but rather as a channel.

SI.4 can be used to treat problems of the Middle Energizer, for example vomiting, gastritis, diabetes and Gallbladder Damp Heat problems such as jaundice, cholecystitis and hypochondriac pain. The internal pathway of the Small Intestine passes along the oesophagus, through the diaphragm, to connect with stomach and small intestine.

Syndromes

The main syndromes for which SI.4 is used are Small Intestine channel problems.

Pulse. Various.

Indications. Hand, elbow and neck pain, painful throat and headache.

Example. Arthritis of wrist and fingers with inflammation and heat.

Combination. SI.3, SI.4, SI.5, LI.4 Rd; shí xuān fifth finger, bā xié between fourth and fifth fingers B; SP.6, KI.6 Rf.

SI.5 yáng gǔ

Fire point.

General

SI.5 has the usual functions of a Small Intestine point on the lower arm to treat Small Intestine channel problems and to clear Heat and Wind Heat. It is especially useful as a local point for problems of the wrist, including arthritis. The other main use of SI.5 relates to its functions as a Fire point on a Fire channel. It can be used to clear Heart Fire and to calm the mind and emotions, and for this purpose can be combined with HT.8, both with Reducing method. By clearing Heat and calming the Heart Spirit, SI.5 can allow the patient to assess in calmness the various possibilities open to them in their lives. Often, a Fire-type personality is feeling too rushed, tense and agitated to assimilate information properly and to discriminate between suitable and unsuitable possibilities.

Syndromes

Small Intestine channel problems – as for SI.4
Disturbance of Heart Spirit

Disturbance of Heart Spirit

Pulse. Rapid, thin or full, maybe wiry or irregular.

Indications. Fear and agitation in children, mania, depression, restlessness and anxiety, incoherent speech.

Example. Feeling too rushed and pressurized to separate the important and unimportant aspects of a situation in calmness.

Combination. SI.5, BL.60 Rd; HT.6, KI.6 Rf; yìn táng E.

SI.6 yǎng lǎo

Accumulation point.

General

SI.6, as the Accumulation point of the channel, is used for pain or stiffness along the course of the channel, especially involving stiffness in the tendons and joints restricting movement of elbow, shoulder and neck. This includes lower back pain and hemiplegia. The other main use of SI.6 is to treat eye pain or problems of vision relating to Small Intestine, Bladder or Heart channels.

Syndromes

Small Intestine channel problems
Eye problems

Small Intestine channel problems

Pulse. Wiry, empty or full.

Indications. Restriction of movement in elbow, shoulder or neck, arthritis, hemiplegia.

Example. Stiffness of whole spine and back.

Combination. SI.6, SI.10, BL.11, BI.59, GV.12 Rd.
Note. SI.6 is Accumulation point of Small Intestine, SI.10 is Crossing point of Yang Heel and Small Intestine, BL.59 is Accumulation point of Yang Heel.

Eye problems

Pulse. Various.

Indications. Eye pain, blurred vision, feeling of congestion or heaviness of the eyes.

Example. Dull pain in the eyes and blurred vision worse with tiredness.

Combination. SI.1, SI.6, BL.2, BL.62, BL.67 E.

SI.7 zhī zhèng

Connecting point. SI.7 can treat Small Intestine channel problems, especially pain in the forearm and elbow, and, since it is the Connecting point, can also be used to calm the Heart Spirit. Syndromes treated are similar to those of SI.5.

SI.8 xiǎo hǎi

Earth point.

General

The main use of this point is for elbow problems. It can also treat the usual Small Intestine channel symptoms and calms Heart Spirit. Syndromes treated are similar to those of SI.5.

SI.9 jiān zhēn

SI.9 is an excellent point for shoulder problems, when the point is painful on palpation, even when the Small Intestine channel is not the main channel involved. SI.9 can also be used for excessive underarm perspiration.

SI.10 nào shū

Meeting point of Yang Heel, Yang Link and Small Intestine channels.

General

SI.10 is very similar in use to SI.9, and is especially useful in that it can be combined with BL.57 or BL.62, the Accumulation and Opening points respectively, for the Yang Heel channel, for problems of shoulders, back and spine. SI.10 can be used either for restricted shoulder movement, often in combination with SI.9, or it can be used in combination with SI.3 and BL.62 for generalized stiffness of shoulders and spine. SI.10 is also indicated for acute and chronic throat swelling, such as parotitis and lymphadenitis, for which it can be combined with SI.8.

Syndromes

Restricted shoulder movement
Generalized spinal stiffness

Restricted shoulder movement

Pulse. Maybe wiry, maybe empty or flooding.

Indications. Acute or chronic restriction of shoulder movement.

Combination. ST.38 with manipulation of needle while patient moves shoulder; then, SI.9 and SI.10 Rd if these points are tender on palpation, and finally LI.4, LI.10, LI.15 Rd or other relevant points.

Generalized spinal stiffness

Pulse. Maybe wiry, maybe thin, empty or choppy.

Indications. Chronic rigidity of neck, shoulders and upper and lower spine.

Combination. SI.3, SI.10, SI.15, BL.10, BL.11, BL.62, GV.12, GV.14 E.

SI.11 tiān zōng

General

This point resembles SI.9 and SI.10 in that it is often tender on palpation during shoulder problems and can be used as a local point. It can also be used with PC.6 for pain or fullness in the chest and ribs, with SI.1 for mastitis, with SI.15 for cough and asthma, with BL.17 for painful hiccups, and with SI.18 for swelling in cheek and jaw.

SI.12–SI.15 bǐng fēng, qū yuán, jiān wài shū, jiān zhōng shū

These points can all be used for shoulder and neck problems. SI.15 is more specifically for the neck and combined with GB.20 and GB.21, TE.15 and TE.16, BL.11 and BL.10 or with GV.14, GV.15 or GV.16 for neck problems. SI.15 can also be combined with BL.13 for bronchitis.

SI.16 tiān chuāng

Window of Heaven point.

SI.16 and SI.17 are listed as Window of Heaven points, in fact the name tiān chuāng means 'heavenly window'. Heaven can mean the upper third of the body, so that Window of Heaven points can open blocks to energy flow between head and body, to relieve symptoms of sense organs, neck and head. For example, SI.16 can be used when the patient feels overloaded with information and feels depressed, pressurized or confused because of lack of time and peace of mind to digest the information and separate useful from useless. This feeling of pressure and stress may be associated with Heart Fire and Fire poison in the neck and head region, for example acne and boils.

Syndromes

Mental congestion and depression
Heart Fire and Fire poison

Mental congestion and depression

Pulse. Hindered, maybe slippery.

Indications. Mental congestion, confusion, depression.

Example. Feeling of heaviness, sluggishness and fullness in the head with confusion over correct course of action.

Combination. SI.1, SI.3, SI.16, BL.67, BL.62 E.

Heart Fire and Fire poison

Pulse. Rapid, thin or flooding, maybe wiry or slippery.

Indications. Nervous tension, insomnia, difficult concentration, red skin eruptions on neck and face.

Example. Severe acne, aggravated by stress.

Combination. SI.5, SI.16, LI.5, LI.18, ST.40, HT.8 Rd.

SI.17 tiān róng

Window of Heaven point.

General

SI.17 can be used as a Window of Heaven point by itself or in combination with SI.16. Both these points can also be used for throat problems due to Damp Heat and Fire poison; for example, parotitis or pain and swelling of the throat, in combination with SI.2 or SI.5. Tiān róng is specific for severe acute tonsillitis, especially in combination with ST.1 or LU.11.

Syndromes

SI.17 is mainly used to treat throat problems.

Pulse. Rapid or normal, maybe thin or flooding, maybe slippery.

Indications. Pain or difficulty swallowing, parotitis, tonsillitis, pharyngitis.

Example. Catarrhal deafness with blockage of Eustachian tubes following sinusitis and sore throat.

Combination. SI.2, SI.17, TE.17, GB.20, LI.4, ST.40 Rd.

SI.18 quán liáo

Crossing point of Small Intestine and Triple Energizer channels. SI.18 is mainly used as a local point for facial problems to clear Wind, Cold or Heat, e.g. for trigeminal neuralgia, facial paralysis, tics, toothache, swelling of the jaw, swelling or burning sensation of the cheeks. For these problems SI.18 can be combined with SI.2 or SI.5.

SI.19 tīng gōng

Meeting point of Gall Bladder, Triple Energizer and Small Intestine channels.

General

The main use of this point is to treat ear disorders, for which it can be combined with SI.1, SI.2 or SI.5, especially if there are signs of Heat or Wind Heat. For ear disorders more related to Deficiency, SI.19 is better combined with SI.3 and BL.62. A secondary function of SI.19 is to calm the Heart Spirit to treat insanity or auditory hallucinations.

Syndromes: ear disorders.

Pulse. Rapid or normal, thin or flooding, maybe wiry or slippery.

Indications. Deafness, tinnitus, otitis media, pain in the ear, face and head.

Example. Earache and headache from Wind Heat invasion.

Combination. SI.5, SI.19, BL.60, GB.20 Rd.

Small Intestine point comparisons and combinations

The functions of the main points of the Small Intestine channel are given in Table 20.3.

Table 20.3 Small Intestine point comparisons

Point	Point type	Syndromes
SI.1	Well point Metal Point	Small Intestine channel problems Wind Heat Breast problems Mental congestion
SI.2	Spring point, Water point	Heat and Wind Heat in Small Intestine channel Heat in Bladder
SI.3	Opening point of GV, Wood point, Tonification point	Small Intestine channel problems Heat and Wind Heat Governor channel problems Disturbance of Spirit mental congestion
SI.4	Source point	Small Intestine channel problems
SI.5	Fire point	Small Intestine channel problems Disturbance of Spirit
SI.6	Accumulation point	Small Intestine channel problems (acute pain) eye problems
SI.8	Earth point	Small Intestine channel problems
SI.9		shoulder problems
SI.10	Crossing point of Small Intestine, Yang Heel, Yang Link	shoulder problems spinal problems
SI.11–15		local problems of shoulder and neck SI.11 and SI.15 can also treat cough and asthma
SI.16	Window of Heaven point	mental congestion and depression Heart Fire and Fire poison
SI.17	Window of Heaven point	throat problems
SI.18	Crossing point of Small Intestine and Triple Energizer	facial problems
SI.19	Crossing point of Small Intestine, Triple Energizer, Gallbladder	ear problems

Some common combinations of Small Intestine channel points with each other and with Bladder points are shown in Tables 20.4 and 20.5 respectively.

Table 20.4 Small Intestine point combinations

Point	Combination	Syndromes	Example
SI.1	SI.3	Deficient and Stagnant Small Intestine Qi	mental congestion
SI.1	SI.6	Deficient and Stagnant Small Intestine Qi	eye problems
SI.1	SI.17	Heat and Wind Heat	tonsillitis
SI.1	SI.18	External Wind and Stagnant Qi	facial pain
SI.1	SI.19	Deficient and Stagnant Small Intestine Qi	tinnitus
SI.2	SI.5	Heart Fire	cystitis and restlessness
SI.2	SI.17	Wind Heat	pharyngitis
SI.2	SI.19	Wind Heat, Damp Heat	ear infection
SI.3 4 or 5	SI.2	Damp Heat	arthritis of hand and wrist
SI.3	SI.8	Stagnation of Qi and Blood	elbow problems
SI.3 SI.3	SI.10 } SI.15 }	Stagnant Qi in Small Intestine and GV channels	shoulder, neck and upper back problems
SI.4	SI.5 or 6	Stagnant Qi or Damp Heat in Small Intestine channel	wrist problems
SI.5	SI.16	Heart Fire and Fire poison	acne
SI.5	SI.17	Wind Heat and Fire poison	parotitis
SI.6	SI.8–15	Stagnation of Qi and Blood	local problems
SI.7	SI.8	Stagnation of Qi and Blood	elbow problems
any combination of two SI.9–SI.15		Stagnation of Qi and Blood Wind Invasion	local shoulder, neck or upper back problems
SI.11	SI.15	Stagnation of Lung Qi	respiratory problems
SI.16	SI.17	Stagnation of Small Intestine Qi	depression and mental congestion
SI.17	SI.19	Stagnant Qi and Phlegm	catarrhal deafness

The main function of Small Intestine points is to treat problems on the superficial pathway of the channel from finger to ear. Pairs of SI points can be two local points, e.g. SI.1 and SI.2 for a finger problem, or one local plus one distal point e.g. SI.6 and SI.10 for a shoulder problem. Chains of three or more Small Intestine points can also be three local points, e.g. SI.3, 4 and 5 for a hand and wrist problem or mixed local and distal points, e.g. SI.5, 17 and 19 for a throat and ear problem due to Wind Heat. Chains of points of three or more can also be used for problems involving different areas of the Small Intestine channel, e.g. SI.5, 8, 10 and 15 for arthritis of the wrist, elbow, shoulder and neck.

Table 20.5 Combinations of Small Intestine and Bladder points

SI points	BL points	Syndromes	Example
SI.1	BL.67	Stagnation of Qi	mental congestion
SI.2	BL.66	Wind Heat or Bladder Heat	headache and stiff neck, cystitis
SI.3	BL.62	Deficient Jing and Qi	blurred vision
SI.5	BL.60	Heart Fire	agitation and anxiety
SI.15	BL.11	Stagnant Qi and Blood	neck and upper back problems
SI.16	BL.40	Fire poison	acne

Lung 21

Lung channel

CHANNEL CONNECTIONS

MAIN CHANNEL PATHWAY

Starting in the Middle Energizer, the internal pathway descends to connect with the large intestine, before ascending to the stomach and passing through the diaphragm to connect with the lungs. It then ascends to the throat, before emerging at LU.1. The superficial pathway runs down the medial arm from LU.1, to end at the medial nail point of the thumb, LU.11.

CONNECTING CHANNEL PATHWAY

This channel separates from the main pathway at LU.7 and connects with the Large Intestine channel. Another branch flows from LU.7 to disperse through the thenar eminence.

FUNCTIONS OF LUNG POINTS

TREAT CHANNEL PROBLEMS

Lung points can be used to treat local channel problems, e.g. LU.1 and LU.2 for shoulder problems or LU.5 for elbow problems. These local points can be combined with LU.7 as a distal point. Since LU.7 connects with the Large Intestine channel, and since the Muscle Region of this channel goes over the neck and head, LU.7 can be used for neck and head pain. Also, as the Connecting point, LU.7 can be used on the opposite side, to balance a chain of Large Intestine points on the affected side, e.g. LI.4, 10, 14 and 15 for shoulder spasm.

TONIFY LUNG QI AND LUNG YIN

LU.9, ST.36 and KI.7 can be combined to tonify both Deficient Lung Qi and deficient Defensive Qi, to prevent recurring infections. This combination can be alternated with

293

BL.13, BL.20 and BL.23. LU.5, LU.9, ST.36 and KI.6 can be combined to tonify Lung Yin and moisten dryness. If Lung Yin is associated with Lung Fire, then KI.2 and LU.10 can be reduced.

DISPERSE EXTERIOR WIND

LU.7 + LI.4 is the basic combination to disperse Exterior Wind Cold or Wind Heat. Back points such as GV.14, GV.15, GV.16, BL.11, BL.12, BL.13 or GB.20 can be added.

DISPERSE RETAINED PHLEGM IN LUNGS

The basic points are LU.1, LU.6 and LU.7, which can be combined with BL.13, CV.17, PC.6 and ST.40, all with Reducing method. LU.10 or LU.11 can be reduced also, if there is Phlegm Heat. For Phlegm Cold, the basic points are needled with moxa, and if the Cold is based on Deficient Spleen and Kidney Yang, then CV.6, CV.12 Rf M can be added.

MOVE STAGNANT LUNG QI

LU.1, LU.2, LU.6 and LU.7 can all move Stagnant Lung Qi, whether this is associated with suppressed grief or with lack of exercise and poor posture. LU.7 is usually the most effective for loosening emotional blocks. CV.3, CV.6, CV.12, CV.17, CV.22 or CV.23 can be added depending on which energy centres are involved in the Stagnation. GV.12, BL.13 and BL.42 can be used as an alternative, combined with GV.9, BL.17 and BL.46, if there is dyspnoea from Stagnation at the Solar Plexus centre. If other organ systems are involved in the emotional Stagnation then appropriate points can be added as shown in Table 21.1.

LUNG SYNDROMES

Lung syndromes are summarized in Table 21.1.

Table 21.1 Point combinations for Lung syndromes

Syndromes	Signs and symptoms	Pulse	Tongue	Point combination
Deficient Lung Qi	bright pale face, easy to catch colds, weak voice, weak cough, watery phlegm	empty	pale	CV.4, CV.17, LU.9, ST.36 Rf M
+ Spleen Damp	+ much phlegm, lethargy, feeling of heaviness, abdominal distension, loose stools	+ slippery	+ greasy coat	+ CV.12, LU.6, ST.40 Rd M
Deficient Lung Yin	tired but restless, malar flush, dry sore throat, dry cough with little phlegm, hoarse voice	thin, rapid	red, thin, dry, no coat	CV.4, CV.17, LU.5, LU.9, KI.6, ST.36 Rf; LU.10, KI.2 Rd
Wind invasion of Lungs	chills and fever, itchy throat cough, nasal obstruction, body aches	superficial	thin coat	LU.7, LI.4, BL.12 Rd
+ Wind Cold	+ chills predominant, aversion to cold, sneezing, clear watery mucus	+ tight	+ white coat	+ moxa on basic points
+ Wind Heat	+ fever predominant, thirst, painful red sore throat, maybe yellow nasal mucus	+ rapid	+ red dots on sides or tip	+ GV.14, TE.5, LI.11 Rd (no moxa)
+ Wind Dryness	+ dry nose, throat and lungs, often after acute or long–term exposure to smoke or dry central heating	superficial	thin coat	+ LU.5, KI.6 Rf
Stagnant Lung Qi	feeling of blockage in chest, dyspnoea, suppressed grief, depression and difficulties in letting go of the past	hindered, maybe slippery and flooding	normal or swollen in Lung area	CV.6, CV.17, LU.1, LU.7, KI.6 E or Rd
+ Stagnant Heart Qi	+ maybe palpitations or chest pain, difficulties in expressing feelings in a close relationship	+ maybe irregular	+ maybe uneven in Heart area	+ CV.23, PC.6 Rd
+ Stagnant Spleen Qi	+ clinging overconcern and possessiveness through insecurity, maybe with indigestion	+ maybe wiry	+ maybe swollen in Spleen–Stomach area	+ CV.12, PC.6, ST.40 Rd
+ Stagnant Kidney Qi	+ fear of being alone, fear of change, fear of the unknown, maybe breast or uterine carcinoma	+ maybe deep	+ pale	+ CV.3, LU.6, KI.8, KI.13, KI.25 E
+ Stagnant Liver Qi	+ suppressed anger, resentment and bitterness at changes in life or relationships	+ wiry	+ purple	+ PC.6, LR.3, LR.14 Rd
Retention of Phlegm in Lungs	chronic bronchitis with feeling of fullness in the chest	slippery, full	thick, greasy coat	CV.17, BL.13, LU.1, LU.6, ST.40 Rd
+ Cold	+ profuse white phlegm, maybe feelings of cold	+ maybe tight	+ pale, white coat	+ moxa on basic points
+ Heat	+ harsh cough, with yellow or green phlegm which may be sticky or difficult to expectorate, maybe feverish	+ rapid	+ red + yellow coat	+ LU.10 Rd; LU.11 B

Rf, Reinforcing method; Rd, reducing method; E, Even method; M, moxa; B, bleeding.

Lung points

LU.1 zhōng fǔ

Alarm point, Crossing point of Lungs and Spleen.

General

The main use of LU.1 is with Reducing method for Excess or Stagnation patterns, especially for acute conditions or for the acute phases of chronic illnesses.

Stagnation of Lung Qi

LU.1 can be used for Stagnant Lung Qi, whether this is associated with grief, trauma or Retention of Phlegm. For example, LU.1 is often combined with LU7 and CV.17 to open up the chest energy centre for depression, melancholy, bronchitis and other conditions associated with blocked grief.

Local Stagnation of Qi and Blood

Since the Muscle Region of the Lungs branches over the chest and shoulder, LU.1 can be used, especially with LU.7 or LU.6 to treat aches, pain and stiffness of chest, heart, throat, neck, shoulder and upper back. Local points, especially from the Large Intestine channel, can be added.

Retention of Phlegm

LU.1 can help to disperse accumulated Phlegm in the Lungs, especially Phlegm Heat. It can be combined with LU.6 and BL.13 in acute cases, such as bronchitic asthma, and CV.17, PC.6 and ST.40 can be added to clear chest Phlegm.

Heat in the Lungs

LU.1 can be used to clear Phlegm Heat in the Lungs, or it can treat acute Lung Heat conditions such as pneumonia, whooping cough or tonsillitis. LU.1 can then be combined with LU.5, LU.10 or LU.11, and with LI.4, LI.11 or GV.14.

Deficient Lung and Spleen Qi

LU.1 is the Crossing point of Lung and Spleen channels, so it can be used to treat cough due to accumulation of Phlegm associated with Deficient Lung and Spleen Qi. It can be combined with LU.9, ST.36 and BL.13 for this purpose.

Comparison of LU.1 with other points

LU.1 has some similar functions to LU.5, LU.6 and BL.13, and is often combined with these points.

LU.1 and LU.5. Both these points can be used with Reducing method, to treat Lung Heat and Retention of Phlegm Heat in the Lungs, but LU.1 can also treat Stagnation of Lung Qi and local problems of neck, shoulders and upper back. LU.5, used with Reinforcing method can tonify Deficient Lung Yin and moisten Dryness.

LU.1 and LU.6. Both these points can treat severe acute Excess conditions, such as asthma, but LU.6 is the stronger of the two, and can also stop bleeding due to Lung Heat.

LU.1 and BL.13. LU.1 is more for acute Excess patterns and is better to treat pain, while BL.13 is more for chronic Deficiency conditions, or for acute Wind Invasion. LU.1 is not usually used for Exterior Wind Cold or Wind Heat; LU.7, LI.4, BL.11 or BL.13 are better for this purpose. LU.1 is better for deeper, more severe, conditions, or for Stagnation or Qi of the chest due to emotional blockage.

LU.1 and LU.2. LU.2 is similar to LU.1 but less powerful.

Syndromes

Stagnation of Lung Qi
Local Stagnation of Qi and Blood
Retention of Phlegm
Heat in the Lungs

Stagnation of Lung Qi

Pulse. Hindered or wiry, full or flooding, maybe slippery.

Indications. Blocked grief, bronchitis, dyspnoea.

Example. Depression and occasional sobbing and feeling of fullness in the chest.

Combination. LU.1, LU.7, CV.17, KI.6 Rd.

Local Stagnation of Qi and Blood

Pulse. Wiry.

Indications. Stiffness, ache or pain in chest, neck, shoulders or upper back.

Example. Stiffness and pain in shoulder and upper arm.

Combination. LU.1, LU.3, LU.6, LI.15, LI.16, ST.38 Rd.

Retention of Phlegm

Pulse. Slippery, full or flooding, maybe wiry.

Indications. Asthma, bronchitis, dyspnoea, cough.

Example. Acute phase of bronchial asthma.

Combination. LU.1, LU.6, CV.17, BL.13, dìng chuǎn, ST.40 Rd; KI.3 Rf.

Heat in the Lungs

Pulse. Fast, full or flooding, maybe wiry.

Indications. Whooping cough, pneumonia, tonsillitis.

Example. Acute bronchitis with fever.

Combination. LU.1, LU.5, LI.4, ST.36 Rd.

LU.3 tiān fǔ

Window of Heaven point.

General

As a Window of Heaven point, LU.3 can be used for psychological disorders associated with the Metal element; for example, when a person feels locked inside themselves, withdrawn from life and relationships, or unable to let go of old fears and negative patterns of feelings and behaviour. LU.3 can be combined with LI.18, LU.1 or LU.7 to relieve depression and phobias.

Syndrome: Stagnation of Lung Qi

Pulse. Hindered or wiry, maybe deep or flooding.

Indications. Blocked grief, agoraphobia, claustrophobia.

Example. Fear of windows, depression and bronchitis.

Combination. LU.1, LU.3, LU.7, LI.4, LI.18, CV.14 Rd; KI.7 Rf.

LU.5 chǐ zé

Sea point, Water point, Sedation point.

General

LU.5 is the Water point of the Lung channel and is mainly used to cool Heat, tonify Yin and moisten dryness. The three main syndromes treated by LU.5 are Lung Heat, Retention of Phlegm Heat in the Lungs and Deficient Lung Yin.

Lung Heat

LU.5 can be used with Reducing method or bleeding for acute Lung Heat conditions such as acute bronchitis or tonsillitis. It may be combined with LU.1, LU.6, LU.10 or LU.11. LU.1 is more for Heat with Stagnation of Lung Qi; LU.6 is more for Phlegm Heat with bleeding or with asthma; LU.10 is more for dry cough and sore throat with chronic Heat signs; and LU.11 is more for severe acute fever.

Retention of Phlegm Heat in the Lungs

LU.5 can be used for Retention of Phlegm in the Lungs, using Reducing method. Although it is especially effective for Phlegm Heat it can also be used for Phlegm Cold. For these patterns, LU.5 can be combined with ST.40.

Deficient Lung Yin

LU.5 can be used with Reducing method to tonify Lung Yin, either in a chronic Deficiency situation, or after Lung Yin has been damaged by a severe fever. If there is some Deficiency Fire, LU.5, the Water point, used with Reinforcing method can be combined with LU.10, the Fire Point, with Reducing method. If there is Dryness, for example dry throat or dry skin, LU.5 can be combined with SP.6 and KI.6 all with Reinforcing method.

Syndromes

Lung Heat
Retention of Phlegm Heat in the Lungs
Deficient Lung Yin

Lung Heat

Pulse. Fast, full or flooding, maybe wiry.

Indications. Pneumonia, tonsillitis, acute bronchitis.

Example. Chronic bronchitis plus acute Wind Heat Invasion.

Combination. LU.5, LI.4, LI.11, GV.14 Rd; LU.11 B.

Retention of Phlegm Heat in the Lungs

Pulse. Slippery, rapid, full or flooding, maybe wiry.

Indications. Bronchiectasis, bronchitic asthma.

Example. Chronic bronchitis plus acute Wind Heat invasion.

Combination. LU.2, LU.5, LU.7, LI.4, CV.17, CV.22, ST.40 Rd.

Deficient Lung Yin

Pulse. Thin, rapid.

Indications. Chronic laryngitis, dry cough.

Example. Chronic bronchitis with afternoon fever.

Combination. LU.5, HT.6, KI.6, SP.6 Rf; KI.2, LU.10 Rd.

LU.6 kǒng zuì

Accumulation point.

General

LU.6 is mainly used as the Accumulation point for severe acute conditions of Excess and Stagnation.

Syndromes

Stagnant Lung Qi
Lung Heat, especially with bleeding
Retention of Phlegm Heat in the Lungs

Stagnant Lung Qi

Pulse. Wiry, full or flooding, maybe slippery.

Indications. Asthma, bronchitis.

Example. Severe cough with chest pain.

Combination. LU.6, LR.3, LR.14, CV.17, CV.22, ST.40 Rd.

Lung Heat

Pulse. Rapid, full or flooding, maybe wiry.

Indications. Acute phase of pulmonary tuberculosis or bronchitis.

Example. Acute bronchitis with feverishness.

Combination. LU.6, LU.10, BL.13 Rd; KI.6 Rf.

Retention of Phlegm Heat in the Lungs

Pulse. Rapid, slippery, full or flooding, maybe wiry.

Indications. Bronchitis, bronchiectasis.

Example. Acute phase of bronchitis with painful unproductive cough.

Combination. LU.1, LU.6, PC.6, CV.17, ST.40 Rd; KI.6 Rf.

LU.7 liè quē

Connecting point, Opening point of Conception channel.

General

This is perhaps the most frequently used point on the Lung channel. LU.7 can be used to treat problems along the course of the Lung, Large Intestine and Conception channels. As a Lung point it can be used to treat problems of the lungs, chest and throat. As the Connecting point between the Lung and Large Intestine channels, it can be used to treat Large Intestine channel problems, such as hemiplegia, arthritis of the shoulder, stiff neck, lock jaw, toothache, facial paralysis, nasal problems, trigeminal neuralgia and facial tics. Because the Muscle Region of the Large Intestine crosses over the head, it can also be used for frontal and lateral headaches.

As the Opening point of the Conception channel it can be used to treat Conception channel disorders, mainly in the Upper Energizer and the Lower Energizer, and usually in combination with KI.6.

LU.7 and Exterior Wind

LU.7 is one of the main points for expelling Exterior Wind from the body. It can be used for both Wind Cold and Wind Heat, but is most effective for Wind Cold, especially in the early stages of invasion. It strengthens the dispersing function of the Lungs to circulate Defensive Qi through the surface of the body, opening the pores, stimulating sweating and expelling the invading factor.

LU.7 can therefore be used for common cold or influenza, not only with cough and sore throat, but also with nasal discharge or obstruction, headache and aches in the muscles of neck and shoulders. For this LU.7, the connecting point of the Lung channel, is often combined with LI.4, the Source point of the Large Intestine channel.

LU.7 and Large Intestine channel problems

Through its link with the Large Intestine channel, LU.7 can treat affections of shoulder and arm, neck, head and face and nose.

Shoulder and arm problems. LU.7 can be used as a distal point for shoulder and arm problems of the Large Intestine channel; for example, hemiplegia, arthritis or 'frozen shoulder'. LU.7 is used with Reducing method on the opposite side to the problem.

Neck problems. LU.7 can be used for Wind Cold invasion of the neck in combination with LI.4, BL.10 and BL.11 with Reducing method and moxa. LU.7 can also be used with Reducing method for neck and shoulder problems on the Large Intestine channel, when it can be combined with points such as LI.4, LI.15, LI.16 and LI.18. For these affections, LU.7 can be used on the same or the opposite side to the problem, as preferred.

Head and face problems. LU.7 can be used with Reducing method for head and face problems involving the Large Intestine channel, in combination with the appropriate Large Intestine and Stomach points. In this case, LU.7 is usually used on the same side as the problem. For example, for frontal head and face pain following exposure to Wind Cold, LU.7 might be combined with LI.4, LI.20 and BL.2.

Nasal problems. LU.7 can be used in combination with LI.4 and LI.20 and BL.2 for nasal discharge and obstruction associated with Wind Cold or Wind Heat, for example common cold, allergic rhinitis, sinusitis. LU.7 is mainly used for acute Wind invasion nasal problems, and not so much for chronic conditions of retention of Phlegm.

LU.7 and Stagnant Lung Qi

LU.7 is not only for acute Wind invasion. It can also treat chronic conditions of Stagnation or Rebellion of Lung Qi, e.g. asthma or cough, by strengthening both the dispersing and descending functions of the Lungs.

LU.7 and the energy of the breath

Breathing is the act by which the energy of air is taken into the body, becoming the energy of the breath, to catalyse the energies of the body in the performance of their various functions. The act of breathing can be restricted by various emotions, such as worry, fear, grief, sadness, frustration and depression, so that the intake of air is reduced, and the energy of the body is correspondingly less. Tiredness resulting from this Stagnation of Qi of the chest can be treated by use of LU.7 with Reducing method. It must be differentiated from simple Deficiency of Lung Qi, which is treated by LU.9 with Reinforcing method.

LU.7 and the emotions

LU.7 is especially for emotional stagnation related to the Lungs and the Metal element – suppressed or incompletely expressed grief, with sadness, depression and withdrawal. Tears often follow the use of this point in such cases and patients can be told that this may happen. The release of emotion may be immediately after needle sensation or may occur in the week following the treatment.

LU.7 may be combined with LU.1, LU.3, BL.13, BL.42 or CV.17 for this purpose, usually with Reducing method. However, LU.7 may be combined with other points when the Qi of the chest has become Stagnant due to other emotions, as shown in Table 21.2.

Table 21.2 Combinations with LU.7 for emotional problems

Organs	Emotions	Back points	Distal points	CV points
Lungs	grief	BL.13, BL.42	–	CV.17, CV.22
Heart	sadness	BL.15, BL.44	PC.6	CV.17, CV.22
Diaphragm	various	BL.17, BL.46	various	CV.14
Liver	frustration	BL.18, BL.47	LR.3	CV.14, CV.17
Spleen	worry	BL.20, BL.49	SP.6	CV.12, CV.14
Kidneys	fear	BL.23, BL.52	KI.3	CV.6, CV.14

LU.7 and the Conception channel

The Extra channels can each be activated by either their own Opening point by itself, or by the combination of their own Opening point with the Opening point of the paired channel. Of all the eight Extra channels, the Conception channel is the one that is most usually activated by both Opening points in combinations; LU.7 and KI.6, rather than by LU.7 alone. The Conception channel is founded in the Kidneys and the Lower Energizer, and requires KI.6 for full activation. When combined with KI.6, LU.7 can treat Conception channel disharmonies in the Upper Energizer, such as asthma, or weak breathing in the elderly, and in the Lower Energizer, such as infertility, fibroids and menopausal problems.

LU.7 and water metabolism

LU.7 can be used for oedema of the Excess type, due to Exterior Wind invasion, since it enhances the dispensing and descending functions of the Lungs. LU.7 can then be combined with LI.4, BL.13, BL.22 and SP.9, all with Reducing method. However, LU.7 can also be used for chronic oedema of the Deficiency type, often associated with tiredness or old age. Here the Opening points for the Conception and Yin Link channels, LU.7 and KI.6, with Even method, are used together, often with CV.6 or CV.9 with Reducing method and moxa.

The combination of LU.7 and KI.6 strengthens the communication between Lungs and Kidneys both in breathing and in water metabolism, and can be alternated or combined with BL.13 and BL.23.

LU.7 and skin disorders

LU.7 can be used for two main types of skin disorders: those associated with Wind invasion, such as urticaria; and those associated with Conception channel problems, such as pain and itching on the anterior midline of abdomen and chest. For urticaria, LU.7 can be combined with LI.4, BL.12 and BL.13 with Reducing method. For Conception channel skin problems, LU.7 and KI.6 can be combined with appropriate local Conception points, with Reducing method.

Syndromes

External Wind
Large Intestine channel problems
Psychological problems
Conception channel problems
Water retention
Skin disorders

External Wind

Pulse. Tight, superficial, maybe rapid.

Indications. Common cold, influenza.

Example. Wind Cold invasion of occipital area and neck.

Combination. LU.7, LI.4 Rd; BL.10, BL.11, GV.16 Rd M.

Large Intestine channel problems

Pulse. Wiry

Indications. Problems of arms, shoulder, neck, head, face and nose.

Example. Acute Wind Cold invasion on chronic condition of sinusitis.

Combination. LU.7, LI.4, LI.20, ST.2, ST.3, ST.40 Rd.

Psychological problems

Pulse. Hindered or wiry.

Indications. Grief or other emotions congesting Qi in the chest with feelings of fullness in the chest.

Example. Fear and worry restricting breathing, with tiredness and bronchitis.

Combination. LU.7, CV.14, CV.17, BL.42 Rd; ST.36 Rf M.

Conception channel problems

Pulse. Empty or full, maybe wiry or slippery.

Indications. Asthma, oedema, itching, infertility, menopausal problems, tiredness, depression.

Example. Impotence associated with depression and stress.

Combination. LU.7, KI.6, CV.6, CV.14, yìn táng E.

Water retention

Pulse. Empty or flooding, slippery – maybe deep and slow.

Indications. Oedema, urinary retention.

Example. Oedema with depression and tiredness.

Combination. LU.7, KI.6 E; BL.23, BL.22, BL.13 Rf M.

Alternation. LU.7, KI.6 E, CV.4 Rf M; CV.8 M (on ginger on salt).

Skin disorders

Pulse. Superficial, tight, rapid.

Indications. Eczema, urticaria.

Example. Recurring acute allergic eczema.

Combination. LU.7, LI.4, ST.36, ST.44 Rd.

LU.9 tài yuān

Stream point, Earth point, Tonification point, Source point, Gathering point for the blood vessels.

General

The main function of LU.9 is to tonify Lung Qi and it is the best point on the Lung channel for this purpose. LU.9 can tonify both Lung Qi and Lung Yin, but LU.9 is most effective for Deficient Lung Qi, while LU.5 is most effective for Deficient Lung Yin. As the Source point, LU.9 strengthens the Lungs by making available the Source Qi, and LU.9 can therefore be combined with CV.4.

As the Earth point, LU.9 links Earth and Metal, Spleen and Lungs, in the production of body energy from air and food. Because of this special relationship, LU.9 is effective as a Tonification point for Deficient Qi, unlike some other Tonification points, such as SP.2.

Since Earth is the mother of Metal, points like SP.3 and ST.36 are among the most effective for strengthening Lung Qi, more effective in fact, than any other point on the Lung channel than LU.9.

Comparison of points to tonify Lung Qi

LU.9, BL.13 and ST.36 are perhaps the most effective points for Deficient Lung Qi.

LU.9, BL.13, ST.36. LU.9 is specifically for chronic Lung Deficiency and acts directly on the Lung organ and channel. ST.36 is equally effective, but acts more indirectly by strengthening the energy of the Spleen and

Stomach and of the body generally. BL.13 has a more specific effect on the Lung organ, but can also be used for a mixture of Lung Deficiency and Wind invasion.

Other points. LU.7 can tonify Defensive Qi and strengthen the dispersing function of the Lungs to expel Exterior invasion, but it is not much used for tiredness arising from chronic Lung Deficiency. GV.12 can tonify Lung Qi, but this is only one of the many functions of this point, which also include expelling Wind Heat, moving Stagnant Lung Qi and calming the Spirit. CV.17 can be used to tonify Heart and Lung Qi, but its more important function is to move Stagnant Heart or Lung Qi. However, when CV.17 is combined with CV.4, this combination can strongly tonify Heart and Lung Qi, especially when there is a foundation of Deficient Kidney Qi.

LU.9 as the Gathering point of the blood vessels

Classically, LU.9 is recommended to strengthen the blood vessels, for example for poor circulation or varicose veins. It could then be combined with CV.4, CV.17 and HT.7, all with Reinforcing method.

LU.9 combinations

LU.9 may be combined with BL.13 and ST.36 to tonify Lung Qi, or it may be used in the combinations shown in Table 21.3, when Deficiency of the Lungs is combined with Deficiency of other organs. All the points can be used with Reinforcing method and with moxa if there is no concurrent Deficient Yin, whereas LU.7 is used with Reducing method for Excess cough from either Exterior Wind invasion or Interior Stagnation of Lung Qi. For example:

cough due to Deficient Lung Qi	LU.9, BL.13, ST.36 Rf
cough due to Exterior Wind Cold	LU.7, LI.4, BL.11, BL.13 Rd
cough due to Stagnant Lung Qi	LU.7, PC.6, CV.17 Rd.

LU.7 and LU.9 can both be used for tiredness, but LU.9 would be used with Reinforcing method for tiredness due

Table 21.3 Combinations with LU.9 for deficient Qi

Deficient Qi of Lungs and:	Problem	Source point	Back points	CV points
Heart	respiratory and circulatory weakness	HT.7	BL.13 + BL.15	CV.17
Spleen	respiratory and digestive weakness	SP.3	BL.13 + BL.20	CV.12
Kidneys	respiratory and urinary weakness	KI.3	BL.13 + BL.23	CV4

to Deficiency with empty pulse, while LU.7 would be used with Reducing method for tiredness due to obstruction of the free movement of Qi in the chest, with hindered or wiry pulse. LU.9 could be combined with CV.4 to tonify Source Qi, while LU.7 could be combined with CV.6 to move Stagnant Qi associated with depression.

Syndromes

Deficient Lung and Heart Qi
Deficient Lung and Spleen Qi
Deficient Lung and Kidney Qi

Deficient Lung and Heart Qi

Pulse. Empty, maybe changing, maybe irregular.

Indications. Asthma, bronchitis or dyspnoea with palpitations or poor circulation.

Example. Tiredness, depression, cough and cold extremities.

Combination. LU.9, HT.7, CV.4, CV.17, ST.36 Rf M.

Deficient Lung and Spleen Qi

Pulse. Empty, maybe slippery.

Indications. Slow digestion, loose stools, tiredness, bronchitis.

Example. Chronic bronchitis with much white sputum, nausea and indigestion.

Combination. LU.1, LU.9, SP.3, ST.40, CV.17, CV.12 Rf M.

Deficient Lung and Kidney Qi

Pulse. Empty, slippery, deep, maybe slow or flooding.

Indications. Exhaustion, feelings of insecurity, indigestion, fluid retention.

Example. Shortness of breath and oedema.

Combination. LU.7, LU.9, CV.4, CV.12, ST.40, SP.9 Rf M.

LU.10 yú jì

Spring point, Fire point.

General

The specific function of LU.10 is to remove Lung Heat. It

can be used with Reducing method to remove Lung Heat in both acute and chronic situations. LU.10 is not effective for Retention of Phlegm Heat, for which LU.1, LU.5 or LU.6 would be more appropriate. Also, LU.10 is not effective for Lung Dryness or Lung Deficiency Fire based on Deficient Lung Yin, unless it is combined with points such as LU.5 or KI.6 with Reinforcing method to tonify Lung Yin. For severe, acute, painful conditions of Lung Heat with fever, LU.11 with bleeding gives quicker and more powerful results than LU.10.

We can summarize:

severe acute tonsillitis with fever	LU.11 B
acute or chronic sore throat from Lung Heat	LU.10 Rd
chronic sore throat from Lung Heat and Deficient Lung Yin	LU.10 Rd; LU.5 Rf
chronic dry throat from Deficient Yin	LU.5 + KI.6 Rf

Syndrome: Lung Heat

Pulse. Rapid, thin or full, maybe wiry.

Indications. Pneumonia, haemoptysis, sore throat, mastitis, chest pain, nervous anxiety with palpitations.

Example. Chronic sore throat with restlessness, feverishness and insomnia.

Combination. LU.10, CV.23 Rd; HT.6, SP.6, KI.6 Rf.

LU.11 shào shāng

Well point, Wood point.

General

In addition to the usual indications for a Well point, LU.11 is specific for acute severe throat conditions where Wind Heat is turning to internal Heat in the Lungs. In these cases, for example severe acute tonsillitis, LU.11 can be bled to effect rapid relief. LU.11 can also be bled to relieve skin conditions where the Heat in the Blood is associated with Lung Heat. For this, LU.11 can be combined with LU.5.

Syndrome: Wind Heat and Lung Heat

Pulse. Rapid, full, maybe wiry.

Indications. Mumps, tonsillitis, eczema, heatstroke.

Example. Swollen painful throat.

Combination. LU.11 B; LI.4, LI.18, SI.17 Rd.

Lung point comparisons and combinations

The functions of the main points of the Lung channel are given in Table 21.4.

Table 21.4 Lung point comparison

Point	Point type	Syndromes
LU.1	Alarm point Crossing point of Lungs and Spleen	Stagnation of Lung Qi local Stagnation of Qi and Blood Retention of Phlegm Heat in the Lungs
LU.3	Window of Heaven point	psychological disorders
LU.5	Sea point, Water point, Sedation point	Lung Heat Retention of Phlegm Heat in the Lungs Deficient Lung Yin
LU.6	Accumulation point	Stagnant Lung Qi Lung Heat Retention of Phlegm Heat in the Lungs
LU.7	Connecting point, Opening point of Conception channel	External Wind Large Intestine channel disorders psychological disorders Conception channel disorders water retention skin disorders
LU.9	Earth point, Tonification point, Source point, Gathering point for the blood vessels	Deficient Lung Qi
LU.10	Spring point, Fire point	Lung Heat
LU.11	Well point, Wood point	Wind Heat and Lung Heat Heat in the Blood

Some common combinations of the Lung points with each other are shown in Table 21.5.

Table 21.5 Combinations of Lung Points

Point	Combination	Syndrome	Example
LU.1	LU.3	Stagnation of Lung Qi	depression and withdrawal
LU.1	LU.6	Retention of Phlegm in Lungs	painful cough with sticky sputum
LU.1	LU.7	Stagnation of Lung Qi	unexpressed grief
LU.1	LU.9	Deficient Lung Qi with Retention of Phlegm	chronic bronchitis
LU.1	LU.10	Heat in the Lungs	acute lung infections
LU.3	LU.7	Stagnation of Lung Qi	claustrophobia
LU.5	LU.9	Deficient Lung Qi and Yin	recurring bronchitis
LU.5	LU.10	Deficient Lung Yin and Lung Heat	chronic dry cough
LU.5	LU.11	Heat in the Blood	acute eczema
LU.6	LU.7	Stagnant Lung Qi and Retention of Phlegm	acute asthma
LU.6	LU.10	Heat in the Lungs	haemoptysis
LU.10	LU.11	Wind Heat and Heat in the Lungs	tonsillitis and fever
LU.1	LU.3,7	Stagnant Lung Qi	loneliness, living in the past
LU.1	LU.6, 7	Stagnant Lung Qi and Retention of Phlegm	asthma with much sputum

Large Intestine 22

Large Intestine channel

CHANNEL CONNECTIONS

MAIN CHANNEL PATHWAY

Starting at LI.1, at the tip of the index finger, the Large Intestine channel ascends the lateral anterior arm to the shoulder, running via SI.12 to meet GV.14, before running over the neck to the supraclavicular fossa. The internal pathway descends from the supraclavicular fossa to connect with the lungs and the large intestine. The superficial pathway runs up the neck to enter the gums of the lower teeth, and circle the lips, crossing through ST.4, CV.24 and GV.26. From the philtrum the pathways from right and left cross, and the pathway from the right arm goes to the left of the nose, and the pathway from the left arm goes to the right of the nose. The pathway ends at LI.20, where it meets the Stomach channel.

CONNECTING CHANNEL PATHWAY

From LI.6, a branch connects with the Lung channel, and another branch runs along the main channel through the shoulder to the teeth. At the jaw, another branch enters the ear.

Table 22.1 Crossing points on the Large Intestine Channel

Point	Crossing
LI.14–16	Yang Heel
LI.20	ST

ORGAN RELATIONSHIPS OF THE LARGE INTESTINE

The Bright Yang relationship of the Large Intestine and Stomach is discussed in Chapter 16, and combinations such as LI.10, ST.25 and ST.37 can be used for Large Intestine problems. There is not a strong clinical link between Lungs and Large Intestine, and Lung points are not generally used to treat colon problems. The exception is LU.7, when grief is causing Stagnant Qi in the intestines.

There is a much stronger relationship between the Large Intestines and the Spleen and Stomach. Indeed, most of the points used to treat Small Intestine and Large Intestine organ problems are from the Spleen and Stomach channels. For example, SP.1, SP.4, SP.6, SP.9, SP.15, ST.25, ST.36, ST.37, ST.39, ST.40, ST.44 and ST.45. Small Intestine points are rarely used for Small or Large Intestine problems, and have their main clinical use for Small Intestine channel problems on the upper body.

FUNCTIONS OF THE LARGE INTESTINE POINTS

TREAT CHANNEL PROBLEMS

Large Intestine points can be used as local points to treat channel problems. For example, LI.20 for sinusitis, LI.18 for acne of the neck, LI.16 for shoulder problems, and so on. LI.4 is the most frequently used distal point in combination with such local points, but other distal points can be used, e.g. LI.1 for sinusitis and mental dullness.

Chains of Large Intestine points can be used, e.g. LI.4, 10 and 11 for shoulder problems, and can often be combined with chains of points on the Stomach channel, e.g. LI.14 and LI.20, with ST.37, ST.44 and ST.45, for sinusitis linked with Heat in the Bright Yang channels. Chains of Large Intestine points on the affected side, in a unilateral condition, may be combined with LU.7 on the healthy side to give a Yin–Yang balance. Large Intestine points for shoulder and arm problems may be combined with GV.14 and SI.12, since the main pathway crosses these points, and Large Intestine points for face problems may be combined with GV.26, CV.24 and ST.4 for the same reason.

CALM AND CLEAR THE MIND

LI.1, especially in combination with ST.45, can help to clear the mind, for example to treat hangover or mental congestion after too much study or mental work. LI.4, especially in combination with LR.3, can help to calm generalized emotional stress, especially associated with Hyperactive Liver Yang.

CLEAR WIND COLD AND WIND HEAT

The points of the Large Intestine channel can help to clear the local effects of the Exterior Wind Invasion, but LI.4, in combination with LU.7 or TE.5, can be used as a systemic point for Exterior Wind.

CLEAR HEAT IN STOMACH AND INTESTINES

Large Intestine and Stomach points can be combined to treat Heat in the Large Intestine and Stomach organ systems. For example, LI.11, ST.25, ST.37 and ST.44 can be reduced for constipation, and LI.1 and ST.45 can be added to this treatment for gingivitis. In addition, ST.4 could be added for cracked and bleeding lips.

CLEAR HEAT IN THE BLOOD

Combinations such as LI.4, LI.11, SP.6, SP.10 Rd can be used for hot, red, itching skin rashes due to Heat in the Blood. In severe acute cases, before using this combination, BL.40, PC.3 and PC.9 can first be bled.

MOVE STAGNANT QI AND BLOOD

LI.4 is one of the most powerful points for pain from systemic or local conditions of Stagnant Qi and Blood. It can be combined with SP.6 to facilitate childbirth, with ST.29 for dysmenorrhoea, with PC.6 for pain in the throat or epigastrium, with LU.7 for neck pain, and so on. LI.10 is useful for lower abdominal pain and distension, for example, in combination with such points as CV.6, TE.6, GB.34, ST.25, ST.37 and SP.15.

TONIFY DEFICIENT QI AND BLOOD

LI.4 is the only point on this channel that can have a strong effect to tonify Qi and Blood, and is usually combined with ST.36 to do this.

LARGE INTESTINE SYNDROMES

Large Intestine and Small Intestine syndromes are summarized in Table 22.2.

Table 22.2 Point combinations for intestine syndromes

Syndrome	Signs and symptoms	Pulse	Tongue	Point combinations
Deficient Intestine Yang	feeling of cold, cold limbs and abdomen, desire for warmth, exhaustion, oedema, undigested food in stools	empty, deep, slow, maybe slippery	pale, moist, maybe swollen, white coat	CV6, CV.12, ST.28, ST.36, KI.7 Rf M
Cold invades Intestines	acute abdominal pain and diarrhoea, with feeling of cold, following exposure of abdomen to Exterior Cold	maybe deep, wiry	maybe thick white coat	CV.6, LI.10, ST.25, ST.27, ST.37 Rd M
Large Intestine Dry (Deficient Blood and Yin)	constipation with dry stools, maybe thin body and dry mouth, e.g. in elderly or after severe blood loss in pregnancy	thin, maybe choppy	red or pale, thin dry, no coat	CV.4, TE.6, ST.36, SP.6, KI.6 Rf
Damp Heat in Intestines	diarrhoea or dysentery, maybe with abdominal pain, mucus or blood in the stools, offensive odour of stools or anal burning pain	slippery, rapid, maybe flooding	red, greasy, yellow coat	LI.11, ST.25, ST.37, ST.44 SP.6, SP.9 Rd
Heat in Small Intestines	restlessness and agitation, maybe feelings of heat and discomfort in chest, thirst, maybe tongue ulcers, maybe burning urination or haematuria	rapid, flooding	red with dark red tip, yellow coat	HT.5, HT.8, SI.2, SI.5, ST.39 Rd + CV.3, SP.6 Rd for cystitis + CV.23, CV.24, ST.4, ST.45 Rd for tongue ulcers
Heat in Large Intestines and Stomach	constipation with thirst, bad breath, feelings of heat and often with epigastric discomfort	rapid, full	red, thick, dry yellow to brown coat	LI.11, ST.25, ST.37, ST.44 ST.44 Rd; CV.6 E; SP.6, KI.6 Rf
Stagnant Qi in Intestines	constipation or irregular bowel movements, with abdominal distension and discomfort, maybe worse after emotional upset or suppression	hindered or wiry, maybe flooding	various	CV.6, TE.6, LI.10, ST.25, ST.37, GB.34 Rd
+ Stagnant Liver Qi	+ suppressed anger, frustration or depression, maybe headache	+ wiry	+ purplish	+ LR.3, LR.14 Rd
+ Stagnant Lung Qi	+ suppressed grief, maybe feeling of fullness in the chest	+ maybe deep	+ maybe uneven in Lung area	+ CV.17, LU.7 Rd
+ Stagnant Stomach Qi (retention of food)	+ prolonged epigastric distension and discomfort after eating or overeating, maybe after emotional upset or worry	+ slippery	+ thick greasy coat	+ CV.10, PC.6, ST.21 Rd
Obstructed Qi of Small Intestine	acute intestinal obstruction, with violent pain, maybe no passage of gas or faeces, maybe vomiting, perhaps of faecal matter	wiry, maybe slippery and flooding	thick coat	serious condition requiring immediate Western medical treatment CV.6, CV.12, PC.6, ST.25, ST.29, LR.3 Rd
Fear and anxiety invade Intestine	abdominal distension and irregular bowel movements associated with fear and anxiety	maybe rapid, irregular	maybe trembling	CV.14 Rd; CV.12, PC.6, anxiety ST.25, ST.37, SP.4 E; CV.4 Rf

Rf, Reinforcing method; Rd, Reducing method; E, Even method; M, moxa.

Large Intestine points

LI.1 shāng yáng

Well point, Metal point.

General

The main functions of LI.1 relate to its status as a Well point:

  clears Wind Heat and Lung Heat

moves Stagnant Qi and Blood

clears the mind.

Clears Wind Heat and Lung Heat

LI.1 can be used as a Well point in acute conditions, with Reducing method or bleeding, to remove external Wind Heat or internal Lung Heat, for example for sore throat, mumps and tonsillitis. However, bleeding LU.11 is more effective for acute tonsillitis, and LI.1 is more useful for fevers, such as pleurisy or influenza, when there is absence of sweating. LI.1 can also be used, with the other Well points, to clear Heat and Interior Wind in acute conditions.

Regulates the Large Intestine channel

As the end point of the channel, LI.1 can be used to move Stagnant Qi and Blood anywhere along the channel pathway, for example, for numbness of the fingers, shoulder pain or toothache. LI.1 can expel Wind Heat, for example acute conjunctivitis, or Wind Cold, for example arthritis of the shoulder. In the latter case when Wind Cold aggravates the Stagnation of Qi and Blood, LI.1 can be warmed with small cones of moxa. When used as a distal point, LI.1 can be combined with a local point on the Large Intestine channel, or indeed with a chain of Large Intestine points; for example, LI.1, LI.4, LI.15, LI.16 for restricted movement of the shoulder.

Clears the mind

LI.1 with Reducing method can be used to clear the mind, as in mental congestion or hangover. It is more effective combined with ST.45, to utilize the Bright Yang relationship, and this combination can be used in three main ways:

LI.1 + ST.45 B	clears Bright Yang Heat	e.g. mental restlessness
LI.1 + ST.45 Rd	moves Stagnant Qi	e.g. mental congestion
LI.1 + ST.45 M	tonifies Bright Yang	e.g. mental tiredness.

In each of these three situations, other Bright Yang points can be added to the combination. If there is chronic mental exhaustion with Deficiency of Qi and Blood, then ST.36 and LI.4 should be added.

Syndromes

  Wind Heat and Lung Heat
  Stagnant Qi and Blood
  External Wind
  Mental disorders

Wind Heat and Lung Heat

Pulse. Full, rapid, maybe wiry.

Indications. Fever with no sweating, mumps, pleurisy.

Example. Influenza with sore throat.

Combination. LI.1, LI.4, SI.17, GV.14 Rd.

Stagnant Qi and Blood

Pulse. Wiry.

Indications. Cough with shoulder pain, cough with feeling of fullness in the chest, toothache.

Example. Numbness of the fingers.

Combination. LI.1, LI.4, GV.14 Rd.

External Wind

Pulse. Superficial, maybe rapid.

Indications. Arthritis of hand and shoulder, facial pain.

Example. Acute conjunctivitis.

Combination. LI.1, LI.4, BL.62 Rd; BL.2, GB.1 E.

Mental Disorders

Pulse. Hindered, maybe empty, thin or choppy.

Indications. Hangover, mental restlessness, mental congestion, mental tiredness.

Example. Mental confusion and inability to concentrate.

Combination. LI.1, GB.13, GV.24, BL.2, BL.62 E.

LI.2 èr jiān

Spring point, Water point, Sedation point.

General

LI.2 is of less importance than LI.1. As a Spring point and as a Water point it clears Heat from the Large Intestine channel and organ, and can be used, for example, for arthritis of the fingers or for constipation with dry stools.

LI.3 sān jiān

Stream point, Wood point.

General

The main use of LI.3 is as a local point for arthritis of the hand. If the arthritis is of the first finger and thumb, then LI.3 can be combined with LI.1, LI.2, LI.4 or LI.5. If the arthritis is across the four metacarpal phalangeal joints, then LI.3 and SI.3 can be used, with the needles inserted towards each other, each to a depth of 1–1.5 units. LI.3 can also be used to clear Wind Heat; for example, for acute eye inflammations.

LI.4 hé gǔ

Source point.

General

LI.4 is one of the great points of acupuncture, with a wide range of actions:

clears Exterior Wind
regulates the Large Intestine channel
regulates the Large Intestine organ
clears Heat and Summer Heat
relaxes muscular tension
moves masses
moves Stagnant Blood in the uterus
relieves pain
calms Hyperactive Liver Yang and Interior Wind
calms the mind
relieves skin disorders
tonifies Qi and Blood

Clears Exterior Wind

LI.4 with Reducing method can clear both Wind Cold and Wind Heat, indeed LI.4 is the most effective point on the body to expel Wind Heat. LI.4 strengthens the dispersing action of the Lungs, and is often combined with LU.7 to expel external Wind invading the body with such signs as sneezing, nasal discharge, stiff neck and shoulders, as in the common cold or influenza. LI.4 can be combined with KI.7 to regulate sweating. This combination can be used when there is excessive sweating, as in Wind Heat or Deficiency, or to induce sweating to expel Wind Cold.

Regulates the Large Intestine channel

LI.4 can treat pain, inflammation or loss of function anywhere on the Large Intestine channel. For example, it can be used to treat arthritis of fingers, hand, wrist, elbow or shoulder, whether the arthritis is aggravated by Wind, Cold, Heat or Damp.

Arms. LI.4 can be included in a chain of points to treat fingers, hand, wrist, forearm, elbow, upper arm or shoulder. Reinforcing method, Reducing method, moxa, cupping or electricity can be used depending on the aetiology.

Neck, throat and tongue. LI.4 can be combined with LI.17, LI.18 and other local points to treat pain or stiffness of the neck, soreness or swelling of the throat, or pain and stiffness of the tongue. For example, LI.4, HT.5, KI.1 Rd for aphasia.

Face and head. LI.4 can be used for facial paralysis, trigeminal neuralgia, toothache, lockjaw and headaches at the front or side. For example, LI.4, LU.7, tài yáng, ST.40 for temporal headache.

Nose. LI.4 is the most important distal point for nose problems, such as rhinitis, allergic rhinitis, sinusitis and epistaxis. It is usually combined with LI.20, and often also with BL.2, yìn táng, GV.23, ST.3, BL.10 and GB.20.

Eyes. LI.4 can be used not only for acute eye problems associated with Wind Heat, but also with chronic eye disorders such as early-stage glaucoma or cataract, and blurred vision. For example, LI.1, LI.4, BL.2, GB.1, GB.20, ST.36 E for blurred vision.

Regulates the Large Intestine organ

LI.4 can be used for infantile diarrhoea, dysentery, constipation and abdominal pain. However, for chronic constipation LI.10 is more commonly used.

Clears Heat and Summer Heat

LI.4, LI.11 and GV.14 is one of the commonest combinations for fevers, when Wind Heat has turned to internal Heat. LI.4 with LI.11 can also be used for Heat in the Blood for acute red skin disorders, and the same combination can be used for sunburn or sunstroke due to Summer Heat. In this case, LI.1 with bleeding, may be added to the combination.

Relaxes muscular tension

Related to the ability of LI.4 to move Stagnant Blood, relieve pain, calm Hyperactive Liver Yang and calm the mind, is its capacity to relax muscular tension. In hemiplegia the ability to relax muscle spasm is combined with the function of LI.4 to strengthen weak and atrophied muscles by moving and tonifying the Blood. In hemiplegia LI.4 is often combined with LI.10 can release muscular tension in the forearm.

Moves masses

LI.4 can be used with Reducing method to move hard masses such as swellings of the lymph or salivary glands, or the thyroid. When combined with points that control the Lower Jiao such as SP.4 or SP.6, LI.4 can help to move masses in the abdomen or uterus.

Moves Stagnant Blood in the uterus

LI.4 is one of the main points for dysmenorrhoea, difficult or delayed childbirth or retained placenta, usually in combination with SP.4, SP.6 or SP.8 with Reducing method or electricity.

Relieves pain

LI.4, in suitable combination, is an excellent general point for relieving pain, especially of face, arms, intestine or uterus.

Calms Hyperactive Liver Yang and Interior Wind

LI.4 and LR.3, known as the Four Gates, is one of the most famous point combinations. It has an excellent general calming and analgesic effect and specifically calms Hyperactive Liver Yang and Interior Wind. This combination can therefore be used for hypertension with dizziness, headache and aggressive behaviour. For greater effect, LI.4 and LR.3 can be combined with GV.20 and KI.1, which is effective for acute, severe hypertension.

Calms the mind

The 'Four Gates' combination is excellent as a general initial treatment to calm the mind, indeed it is notorious as a symptomatic substitute for intelligent treatment. There are many effective formulas, involving LI.4, to calm the mind, which may be selected or modified according to the patient's need; for example:

LI.4 + LR.3
LI.4 + LR.3 + KI.1
LI.4 + LR.3 + GV.20
LI.4 + LR.3 + KI.1 + GV.20
LI.4 + LR.3 + SP.6
LI.4 + LR.3 + PC.6
LI.4 + LR.3 + SP.6 + PC.6
LI.4 + GB.20 + GB.34.

An important principle in using these combinations is polarity; the practitioner must decide whether to calm the disturbed energy in the upper body by using points on the head itself, or drain the energy down by using points on the feet, or both.

Relieves skin disorders

LI.4, usually in combination with LI.11, can be used to treat skin disorders due to Wind Heat, Heat in the Blood, Stagnant Blood, Fire poison, Damp Heat or Deficient Blood. Common combinations are:

LI.4 + LI.11 + SP.6 + SP.9   Damp Heat
LI.4 + LI.11 + SP.6 + SP.10   Heat in the Blood
LI.4 + LI.11 + GB.20 + GB.31   Wind Heat
LI.4 + LI.11 + BL.40 + GV.14   Summer Heat
LI.4 + LI.11 + BL.17 + GV.12   Fire poison
LI.4 + LI.11 + SP.8 + PC.4   Stagnant Blood
LI.4 + LI.11 + ST.36 + SP.6   Deficient Blood.

Tonifies Qi and Blood

LI.4 is commonly combined with ST.36 to tonify Qi and Blood, since the Bright Yang pair should be 'rich in Qi and Blood'. This combination can be used as a basis for muscular weakness, blurred vision, tiredness and Defi-

cient Blood skin disorders. Points such as BL.17, BL.18 and BL.43 can be added to the basic combination.

Syndromes

External Wind
Large Intestine channel disorders
Heat and Summer Heat
Muscular tension and pain
Stagnant Blood in the uterus
Hyperactive Liver Yang
Psychological disorders
Skin disorders

External Wind

Pulse. Superficial, tight, maybe rapid.

Indications. Common cold, influenza.

Example. Acute bronchitis.

Combination. LI.4, LU.7, BL.13, ST.36 Rd.

Large Intestine channel disorders

Pulse. Wiry, empty or full, slow or rapid.

Indications. Arthritis, hemiplegia, nasal disorders, facial paralysis, trigeminal neuralgia.

Example. Sore painful throat with difficulty swallowing.

Combination. LI.1, LI.4, LI.18, ST.9, ST.44 Rd.

Heat and Summer Heat

Pulse. Rapid, full or flooding.

Indications. Eczema, fever, diarrhoea, tonsillitis.

Example. Heatstroke.

Combination. LI.4, GV.14 Rd; LI.1, BL.40 B.

Muscular tension and pain

Pulse. Wiry, maybe choppy, maybe flooding.

Indications. Hemiplegia, trigeminal neuralgia, lockjaw, headache.

Example. General muscular tension and nervousness.

Combination. LI.4, GV.21, GB.34, GV.20, LR.3, SP.6 Rd.

Stagnant Blood in the Uterus

Pulse. Wiry, maybe choppy.

Indications. Endometriosis, dysmenorrhoea, pain in childbirth.

Example. Dysmenorrhoea with back pain.

Combination. LI.4, SP.6, BL.24, BL.31 Rd.

Hyperactive Liver Yang

Pulse. Wiry.

Indications. Hypertension with headache or dizziness, nervous tension.

Example. Headache and eye pain.

Combination. LI.4, GB.20, LR.3 Rd; GB.1, GB.14, SP.6 E.

Psychological disorders

Pulse. Hindered or wiry.

Indications. General nervous tension, hypersensitivity, suppressed grief.

Example. Withdrawal and depression.

Combination. LI.4, LI.18, LU.7. BL.42, SP.6 Rd.

Skin disorders

Pulse. Various.

Indications. Urticaria, acute red eczema, acute sunburn, weeping eczema, psoriasis, acne, boils.

Example. Acne on the back and neck.

Combinations. LI.4, LI.18, GV.10, GV.12, GV.14, BL.17, BL.40 Rd.

LI.5 yáng xī

River point, Fire point.

General

LI.5 has similar functions to LI.4, but it is not as powerful. LI.5 is mainly used with Reducing method as a Fire point, to remove Wind Heat, Heat, Damp Heat or Heat in the Blood, associated with problems such as arthritis, constipation, skin rashes and inflammation of eyes, teeth or throat. Some combinations of LI.5 are:

LI.5 + LI.2	constipation
LI.5 + LI.2	inflammation of teeth and throat
LI.5 + SI.5	redness and swelling of the eyes
LI.5 + LI.15	rash from Heat in the Blood
LI.5 + LU.7	arthritis of the wrist
LI.5 + LU.10	arthritis of the thumb

LI.5 + LI.3,4,6 arthritis of fingers, hand and wrist.

The commonest use of LI.5 is for arthritis of wrist and hand, especially when there is inflammation associated with Heat.

Syndrome

Arthritis of wrist and hand

Pulse. Maybe rapid and wiry, maybe thin or flooding.

Example. Acute rheumatoid arthritis of the wrist.

Combination. LI.4, LI.5, SI.4, SI.5, ST.41, ST.44, SP.6, GV.14 Rd.

LI.6 piān lì

Connecting point.

General

LI.6 is mainly used either as a local point for problems of the wrist and forearm, or to assist the Lungs to regulate water metabolism, to reduce oedema in the upper body. For oedema, it can be combined with LU.7. Also, LI.6 can be used, either as an alternative to LU.7 or in combination with it to treat psychological problems related to the Lungs.

LI.7 wēn liū

Accumulation point.

General

LI.7 can be used as an alternative to LI.4, or in combination with it, for severe acute painful conditions of either the Large Intestine channel or organ.

LI.10 shǒu sān lǐ

General

LI.10 has three main functions:

regulates Large Intestine channel disorders
moves Stagnation in Stomach and Intestines
softens masses.

Regulates Large Intestine channel disorders

LI.10 can treat problems anywhere on the channel, but is especially effective for problems of pain, spasm or atrophy in the muscles of the lower arm, for example, hemiplegia, arm injury, or arm problems due to repetitive use. LI.10 both moves and tonifies Qi and Blood and is often combined with LI.4 and LI.15. LI.10 is particularly important in hemiplegia, to release spasm in the muscles of the forearm.

Syndromes

Large Intestine channel disorders

Pulse. Wiry, maybe empty, thin or flooding.

Indications. Toothache, arm cramps, arm injury, atrophy of arm muscles, hemiplegia.

Example. Inability to extend the elbow.

Combination. LI.4, LI.10, LI.11, LI.12, Ah Shi points, ST.36 on opposite side Rd.

Stagnant Qi in Stomach and Intestines

Pulse. Hindered or wiry, maybe empty, slippery or flooding.

Indications. Indigestion, oedema, abdominal distension, faecal incontinence.

Example. Borborygmus, flatulence and abdominal discomfort.

Combination. LI.10, TE.6, CV.6, GB.27, GB.34 Rd.

Masses

Pulse. Maybe hindered or wiry, maybe slippery or flooding.

Indications. Breast lumps and abscesses, goiter, mumps, swelling of the lymph nodes and salivary glands.

Example. Breast abscess.

Combination. LI.4, LI.10, SI.1, ST.18, ST.36, CV.17 Rd.

LI.11 qū chí

Sea point, Earth point.

General

LI.11 resembles LI.4, in that it is one of the great points of acupuncture, with powerful effects and a wide range of actions. The list of actions of LI.11 resembles that of LI.4, but there are important differences.

expels Exterior Wind
clears Heat
regulates the Large Intestine channel
regulates the Large Intestine organ
relaxes muscular tension and relieves pain
moves masses
calms Hyperactive Liver Yang and clears Liver Fire
relieves skin disorders.

Expels Exterior Wind

LI.11 can be used to expel Wind Heat, like LI.4, but not so much for the early stage of Wind Heat Invasion, more for when Wind Heat is moving towards Bright Yang Heat, or Heat in the Blood, as in some skin rashes. Also, LI.11 is not used for Wind Cold, as in LI.4.

Clears Heat

LI.11 if often used with LI.4 and GV.14 for acute fever conditions, and in extreme cases the Well points can be bled in addition. LI.11 and LI.4 are very similar in their use for Summer Heat and Heat in the Blood. LI.11 is perhaps slightly more effective for Damp Heat, especially when associated with Stagnation in the Bright Yang organs. Both LI.4 and LI.11 can be used for Fire poison, especially for boils or throat swellings.

Regulates the Large Intestine channel

Both LI.4 and LI.11 are very effective for this purpose, but LI.4 is specific for the face and for the hands, while LI.11 is specific for the elbow and forearm.

Regulates the Large Intestine organ

LI.11 is perhaps more effective than LI.4 for Stagnation of Qi, Heat and Damp Heat in the Intestines. However, for Stagnation of Qi in the Intestines with constipation, distension and pain LI.10 is the point of choice.

Relaxes muscular tension and relieves pain

LI.11 is effective for this purpose in the shoulder, elbow and arm, but does not have the powerful general effect that LI.4 possesses, nor is it so effective for Stagnant Blood in the uterus, or for psychological problems.

Moves masses

While LI.4 can move masses both in the upper and lower body, LI.11 is mainly for masses in the back and upper body only, such as goiter and boils.

Calms Hyperactive Liver Yang and clears Liver Fire

Like LI.4, LI.11 can relieve Liver Yang, Fire and Wind to treat hypertension, allergies and menopausal flushes.

Relieves skin disorders

LI.4 and LI.11 are very similar in function in this case and are often used together. LI.4 is rather better for Wind Heat skin disorders and LI.11 is preferred for skin rashes related to Bright Yang Fire or Liver Fire.

Syndromes

  Large Intestine channel disorders
  Heat, Summer Heat
  Hyperactive Liver Yang
  Skin disorders

See LI.4 page 308 for a discussion of these syndromes.

LI.14 bì nào

Crossing point with Yang Link channel.

General

LI.14 is mainly used as a local point for problems of the upper arm and shoulder, often as part of a chain of points such as LI.4, LI.11, LI.14, LI.15, LI.16. Alternatively, LI.14 may be used as part of a group of local points for shoulder problems, such as jiān nèi líng, LU.2, LI.14, LI.15, TE.14, GV.14. LI.14 can also be used for eye problems; for example, in combination with LI.1 and LI.4.

LI.15 jiān yú

Crossing point with the Yang Heel channel.

General

LI.15 is mainly used as a local point for all problems of the shoulder and upper arm, including hemiplegia, arthritis, bursitis and injury. It is usually used as part of a chain or group of points, as described for LI.14. It is often used as a second phase of treatment for 'frozen shoulder', after use of ST.38. LI.15 is usually used with Reducing method, and moxa or electricity may be added where appropriate.

Other functions of LI.15

LI.15 can also be used as a secondary or a local point for skin rashes, often in combination with LI.4 and LI.11. For excessive sweating LI.15 can be combined with LI.4 and KI.7 and with SI.9 for excessive underarm perspiration.

Correct differentiation

It is most important to ascertain the main channel or channels involved in shoulder problems by asking the patient to locate the painful or restricted areas on moving the shoulder. The treatment will not be effective if LI.15 is used when the restriction is on the Lung or Small Intestine channel, and not on the path of the Large Intestine.

LI.16 jù gǔ

Meeting point with the Yang Heel channel.

General

While LI.16 can be used for such varied symptoms as cough, haemoptysis, goiter and fear in children, its main use is for shoulder problems, and to a lesser degree, problems of the arm and neck. Some combinations are:

LI.16 + LI.4, LI.14, LI.15	problems of shoulder and arm
LI.16 + TE.14, TE.15, SI.10, SI.12	shoulder problems
LI.16 + LI.4, LI.17, LI.18	neck and shoulder problems.

LI.18 fú tù

Window of Heaven point.

General

LI.18 has two main functions:

  regulates psychological balance
  regulates neck and throat.

Regulates psychological balance

LI.18 is a Window of Heaven point on the neck, where obstructions can arise to the free flow of energy between head and body. LI.18 especially relates to the free flow and free expression of the energies of the Lungs, the energies concerned with human bonding, the forming and breaking of relationships, with letting go, and with grieving and bereavement. LI.18 can be used for people who have suffered loss, who feel lonely and shut off, but who cannot easily break out of that self–imposed prison, who cannot easily shake off the darkness and heaviness of their depression, to find again a lightness and pleasure in being alive. For this purpose, LI.18 can be combined with BL.42, LU.7 and LI.4, or with LI.6, LU.1, CV.17 and CV.22 for example.

Regulates neck and throat

LI.18 can be used with LI.4 for neck sprain, but it is more used for problems of the throat and vocal cords, such as sore throat, asthma, dyspnoea, phlegm in the throat, difficulty in swallowing, nodules on the vocal cords, aphasia or hypersalivation. LI.18 can be combined with such points as LI.4, LU.7, HT.5, ST.40, SI.17, ST.9, CV.22, CV.23 or GV.15 as appropriate.

LI.18 can also be used for skin rashes, acne or boils on the neck, usually in combination with LI.4, LI.11, BL.17 and GV.12.

Syndromes

Psychological disorders

neck and throat disorders

Psychological disorders

Pulse. Hindered, maybe flooding or deep.

Indications. Loneliness, inability to express grief, avoidance of relationships.

Example. Feeling shut in but unable to break out of the withdrawn state.

Combination. LI.18, LU.7, KI.6, BL.42, BL,52 E.

Neck and throat disorders

Pulse. Maybe wiry, maybe slippery, maybe flooding.

Indications. Neck sprain, neck tension, loss of voice, phlegm in the throat, boils.

Example. Feeling of tension in the neck and throat, fear of loss of voice.

Combination. LI.4, LI.18, PC.6, CV.22, CV.23, LR.3 E.

LI.20 yíng xiāng

Crossing point with Stomach channel.

General

The main function of LI.20 is to clear the nose. In addition, LI.20 can be used for pain, swelling, itch or rashes of the face, especially local to the nose and mouth.

Clears the nose

The basic combination can be LI.20 with LI.4, BL.2 and LU.7. LI.20 is inserted 0.5 unit up towards bítōng, and BL.2 is inserted under the skin almost to BL.1. BL.2 is not then manipulated, but if the nose does not clear, then LI.20 can be manipulated periodically. In stubborn cases of chronic nasal congestion, LI.20 can be connected to LI.4 with electricity. LU.7 and LI.4 are used with Reducing method. The basic formula can be modified accord-

ing to the syndrome, as shown in Table 22.3.

Table 22.3 Combinations of LI.20 for nasal disorders

Syndrome	Addition to basic formula
Wind Cold	+ BL.10, BL.13 Rd M
Wind Heat	+ TE.5, LI.11 Rd
Deficient Lung Qi	+ LU.9, BL.13, ST.36 Rf
Deficient Spleen Qi with Phlegm	+ ST.40 Rd; ST.36 Rf M
Phlegm Cold in Lungs	+ LU.6, ST.40 Rd; BL.13 Rf M
Phlegm Heat in Lungs	+ LU.6, LU.10, ST.40, GB.20 Rd
Stomach Fire	+ ST.2, ST.3 E; ST.44, LR.2 Rd

Rd; Reducing method; Rf, Reinforcing method; E, Even method; M, moxa.

Regulates the face

While LI.4 can treat pain at any part of the face, LI.20 is more restricted to the area of nose, mouth and chin. This is due to the channel connections between LI.20, ST.4, GV.26 and CV.24. Also, LI.20 is especially for problems involving Deficiency, Stagnation or Heat in the Large Intestine and Stomach channels. For example:

cracked lips with Stomach Fire	LI.4, LI.11, ST.44 Rd; LI.20, ST.4 E
sores around mouth with Deficient Qi	LI.4, LI.20, ST.4 E; ST.36, SP.6 Rf
acne around nose, chin and throat	LI.4, LI.18, ST.44 Rd; LI.20, GV.26, CV.24 E

Syndromes

Nasal disorders

Facial disorders

Nasal disorders

Pulse. Various, maybe slippery.

Indications. Rhinitis, nasal polyps, loss of sense of smell.

Example. Allergic rhinitis and eczema of the face.

Combination. LI.4, LI.11, LI.20, ST.44 Rd; ST.3 E; LR.1, PC.1 B.

Facial disorders

Pulse. Various.

Indications. Trigeminal neuralgia, acne, eczema, facial paralysis, epistaxis.

Example. Facial pain.

Combination. LI.20, ST.5 El; LI.4, LR.3 Rd.

Large Intestine point comparisons and combinations

The functions of the main points of the Large Intestine channel are given in Table 22.4.

Table 22.4 Large Intestine point comparisons

Point	Point type	Syndromes
LI.1	Well point, Metal point	Wind Heat and Lung Heat; Large Intestine channel problems; mental disorders
LI.4	Source point	External Wind; Large Intestine channel disorders Heat and Summer Heat; muscular tension and pain Stagnant Blood in uterus; Hyperactive Liver Yang; psychological disorders; skin disorders
LI.5	River point, Fire point	arthritis of wrist and hand
LI.10		Large Intestine channel disorders; Stagnant Qi in Stomach and Intestines; masses
LI.11	Sea point, Earth point	Large Intestine channel disorders; Heat, Summer Heat, Damp Heat, Heat in the Blood; Hyperactive Liver Yang and Fire; skin disorders
LI.14	Crossing point with Yang Link	arm and shoulder disorders
LI.15	Crossing point with Yang Heel	shoulder disorders
LI.16	Crossing point with Yang Heel	shoulder and neck disorders
LI.18	Window of Heaven point	psychological disorders; neck and throat disorders
LI.20	Crossing point with Stomach	nasal disorders; facial disorders

Some common combinations of Large Intestine points with each other and with points from the Stomach channel are listed in Tables 22.5 and 22.6 respectively.

Table 22.5 Combinations of Large Intestine points

Point	Combination	Syndromes	Example
LI.1	LI.4	Stagnant Qi and Blood	mental congestion
LI.1	LI.5	Damp Heat	arthritis of the hands
LI.1	LI.15	Stagnant Qi and Blood	shoulder stiffness
LI.2	LI.5	Heat in Bright Yang	constipation with dry stools
LI.3	LI.4	Stagnant Qi and Blood	pain in thumb and index finger
LI.4	LI.5	Deficient Qi and Blood	atrophy of hand muscles
LI.4	LI.10	Stagnant Qi and Blood	hemiplegia
LI.4	LI.11	Damp Heat	eczema
LI.4	LI.14	Hyperactive Liver Yang	early-stage glaucoma
LI.4	LI.15	Stagnant Qi and Blood	pain in shoulder and arm
LI.4	LI.18	Fire poison	boils on the neck
LI.4	LI.20	Wind Heat	allergic rhinitis
LI.5	LI.11	Heat in the Blood	eczema with great restlessness
LI.6	LI.18	Stagnant Lung Qi	depression
LI.10	LI.11	Stagnant Blood	pain in forearm and elbow
LI.11	LI.12	Stagnant Blood	restricted elbow movement
LI.11	LI.14	Stagnant Blood	pain in elbow and upper arm
LI.14	LI.15	Stagnant Blood	pain in shoulder and upper arm
LI.15	LI.16	Stagnant Blood	pain in shoulder
LI.16	LI.18	Stagnant Blood	pain in shoulder and neck
LI.18	LI.20	Fire poison	acne of neck and face
LI.1	LI.2, 3	Damp Heat	arthritis of index finger
LI.1	LI.4, 18	Stagnant Qi	mental congestion and depression
LI.1	LI.4, 20	Stagnant Qi and Blood	nasal congestion and pain
LI.3	LI.4, 5	Wind Cold and Stagnant Qi	arthritis of hand
LI.4	LI.11, 15	Cold, Damp and Stagnation of Qi and Blood	stiffness of shoulder and arm
LI.4	LI.11, 18	Heat in Bright Yang	acne and boils
LI.4	LI.18, 20	Wind Cold	stiff neck and shoulder
LI.4	LI.18, 20	Wind Heat	pain in throat and face
LI.4	LI.11, 14, 15	Stagnant Qi and Blood	pain in arm and shoulder
LI.4	LI.14, 15, 16	Stagnant Qi and Blood	pain in arm and shoulder
LI.4	LI.11, 18, 20	Damp Heat	eczema of head and neck

Table 22.6 Combinations of Large Intestine and Stomach Points

LI point	ST points	Example
LI.1	ST.45	mental congestion
LI4	ST.1, 2	eye problems
	ST.2.3	sinusitis and frontal headache
	ST.4	cracked or sore lips
	ST.5, 6, 7	face pain and toothache
	ST.8	headache
	ST.18	mastitis
	ST.29, 30	dysmenorrhoea
	ST.36	tiredness with blurred vision
	ST.44	urticaria
LI.5	ST.41	headache with restless hyperactivity
	ST.44	toothache with gingivitis
LI.10	ST.40	abdominal distension
LI.11	ST.37	diarrhoea
	ST.44	psoriasis
LI.15	ST.38	shoulder pain
LI.18	ST.4	acne
	ST.9	oesophageal constriction
	ST.40	phlegm in the throat
	ST.44	boils
LI.20	ST.2,3	sinusitis
	ST.4	cracked lips
	ST.36	frequent rhinitis
	ST.40	phlegm in the sinuses
	ST.44	purulent nasal discharge
	ST.45	epistaxis

Pericardium 23

Pericardium channel

CHANNEL CONNECTIONS

MAIN CHANNEL PATHWAY

This channel begins in the chest where it is connected to the pericardium. One branch of the internal pathway descends through the chest and diaphragm to the abdomen, connecting with the Upper, Middle and Lower Energizers. The other branch of the internal pathway crosses the chest to emerge at PC.1 and descend the medial arm to end at the tip of the middle finger. A branch from PC.8 runs along the ring finger to join the Triple Energizer channel at TE.1.

CONNECTING CHANNEL PATHWAY

From PC.6, this channel runs up the arm to the chest to connect with pericardium and heart. The Divergent channel separates from the Main channel at the axilla, enters the chest to join with the Triple Energizer and runs up the throat to emerge behind the ear, where it links with the Triple Energizer channel.

A branch of the Pericardium Muscle Region enters the chest below the axilla and spreads over the chest and diaphragm.

PC.1 is the Crossing point of the Pericardium and Liver channels.

RELATIONSHIPS OF THE PERICARDIUM

The pericardium organ is closely integrated with the Heart. The Pericardium channel is linked with the Triple Energizer as a Yin–Yang channel pair, and is also linked to the Liver, according to the classification of the Six Divisions, as the Terminal Yin pair. These relationships are summarized in Figure 23.1.

PERICARDIUM–HEART RELATIONSHIP

The Pericardium is of secondary importance to the Heart, and assists the Heart functions of regulating the Spirit, ruling the Blood and mediating the domain of

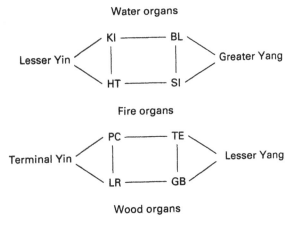

Fig. 23.1 Relationships of the Pericardium and Heart

communication, social behaviours and relationships. Heart and Pericardium points can be used for many similar indications; for example, heart pain and arrhythmias and emotional problems such as anxiety and mania. However, there are important differences as summarized in Tables 23.1 and 23.2.

Table 23.1 Comparison of point functions of Heart and Pericardium

Functions	Heart points	Pericardium points
Chronic/acute	more for chronic	more for acute/severe
Excess/Deficiency	more for chronic Deficiency e.g. of Heart Qi, Blood or Yin	more for acute Excess, e.g. Heart Fire or Phlegm, Stagnant Heart Qi and Blood
Fire	Heart Excess and Deficiency Fire; Heart Fire drains downward, e.g. cystitis, pruritis	Heart Excess Fire, high fever, delirium, mania
Chest	more for chest pain associated with Stagnant Heart Blood	also for chest pain from trauma or Stagnation of Lung or Qi
Lungs	more for Deficiency, e.g. Deficiency Heart and Lung Qi or Yang or sore throat due to Heart Deficiency Fire	more for Stagnant Lung Qi, e.g. asthma, cough or chest pain
Diaphragm	more for diaphragm spasm from Heart anxiety and Kidney fear	also for diaphragm spasm from Stagnation of Lung or Liver Qi, i.e. Rebellious Stomach Qi, e.g. dyspnoea, hiccups
Spleen or Stomach	more for chronic Heart–Spleen Deficiency, especially Deficiency Heart and Spleen Blood, e.g. insomnia	more for acute Stomach Stagnant or Rebellious Qi, e.g. nausea, vomiting epigastric pain

Table 23.2 Comparison of equivalent Pericaridium and Heart points

Point Type	PC point	HT point	Comparison
Water point	PC.3	HT.3	Both PC.3 and HT.3 can be used for Excess Heart Fire. PC.3 is better for Summer Heat and Heat in the Blood, HT.3 is better for Deficiency Heart Fire
Accumulation point	PC.4	HT.6	Both PC.4 and HT.6 can be used for acute painful patterns of Stagnant Heart Blood. HT.6 can also be used to tonify Heart Yin
Connecting point	PC.6	HT.5	Both PC.6 and HT.5 calm the Spirit, but HT.5 is more to improve communication and to clear downward moving Heart Fire, while PC.6 is more for Stagnation of Qi and Blood. PC.6 is also an Opening point for the Yin Link channel
Source point Earth point	PC.7	HT.7	Both PC.7 and HT.7 can stabilize Heart Qi, but HT.7 is better to tonify Heart Qi and Blood, while PC.7 is better for Stomach problems and for Damp Heat skin disorders
Spring point	PC.8	HT.8	Both PC.8 and HT.8 can drain Excess Heart Fire, but HT.8 can also treat Deficiency Heart Fire and Heart Fire draining downward. HT.8 is also better to tonify Heart Fire. PC.8 is better for Damp Heat. HT.8 is better for Heart and Kidney Fire, PC.8 is better for Heart, Liver and Stomach
Well point	PC.9	HT.9	Both PC.9 and HT.9 can act as Well points to clear Heat and Wind in acute fever or loss of consciousness. Again, PC.9 is more combined with LR.1 and HT.9 with KI.1. HT.9 is better for extreme emotional agitation due to Heart Fire and PC.9 is better for fevers or Summer Heat

PERICARDIUM–TRIPLE ENERGIZER RELATIONSHIP

Although Pericardium and Triple Energizer are Yin–Yang paired channels and both are Fire element systems, they have very little in common. While the Triple Energizer points mainly treat channel problems, the Pericardium points mainly treat the organs. The differences between the two systems are summarized in Table 23.3.

Table 23.3 Comparison of point functions of Pericardium and Triple Energizer

Function	Pericardium points	Triple Energizer points
Level of action	Internal – organ problems	External – channel problems
Organs	Heart, Liver, Stomach	Gallbladder
Body areas	chest, hypochondrium diaphragm, epigastrium	eyes, ears, sides of head, neck, throat, shoulders, arms
Heat patterns	Excess Heat, Excess Heart Fire, Summer Heat	Wind Heat, Damp Heat in Liver–Gallbladder
Skin problems	eczema from Heat in the Blood or Damp Heat	urticaria from Wind Heat or eczema from Liver–Gallbladder Fire and Damp Heat

PERICARDIUM–LIVER RELATIONSHIP

The Pericardium and Liver channels are combined in the Terminal Yin pair of the Six Divisions. PC.6 or PC.1 can be used for Stagnation of Liver Qi, especially if this invades the Heart, Lungs or Stomach. PC.8 can be used for Liver Fire, especially when this is combined with Fire of the Heart, Lungs or Stomach.

FUNCTIONS OF PERICARDIUM POINTS

MOVE STAGNANT QI AND BLOOD

Pericardium points are especially for moving Stagnant Qi of Liver, Heart, Lungs or Stomach, or moving Stagnant Heart Blood. For example:

PC.6 + LR.3	for depression from Stagnant Liver Qi
PC.6 + CV.17	for melancholy from Stagnant Heart Qi
PC.6 + LU.7	for dyspnoea from Stagnant Lung Qi
PC.6 + ST.21	for epigastric pain from Stagnant Stomach Qi
PC.4 + HT.6	for angina from Stagnant Heart Blood.

MOVE PHLEGM

Pericardium points can help to disperse Phlegm. For example:

PC.5 + HT.5	for chest pain from Heart Phlegm
PC.6 + LU.6	for bronchitis from Lung Phlegm
PC.6 + ST.40	for nausea from Stomach Phlegm
PC.6 + ST.8	for mental confusion from Phlegm in the head.

DISPERSE HEAT

Pericardium points can help to disperse Heat. For example:

PC.9 + BL.40	for sunburn and sunstroke from Summer Heat
PC.9 + PC.3	for acute red skin rash from Heat in the Blood
PC.8 + HT.8	for mania from Heart Fire
PC.8 + LR.2	for headache from Liver Fire
PC.8 + ST.44	for gastritis from Stomach Fire.

CALM REBELLIOUS QI

PC.6 can be combined with CV.22 for cough from Rebellious Lung Qi, or with CV.13 for nausea from Rebellious Stomach Qi.

REGULATE EMOTIONS

As mentioned above, pericardium points, especially PC.6, can treat depression, melancholy and grief associated with Stagnant Qi; and can treat mental and emotional confusion, disturbance and mania associated with Fire, Phlegm and Interior Wind. PC.6 is an important point for general emotional stress, whether connected with Heart anxiety, Kidney fear, Liver anger or Spleen worry. It can be combined with SP.4 in the TV + Yin Link Extra channel pair, to treat the emotions, since this pair treats the organ group Kidneys, Heart and Spleen. PC.6 + SP.4 can be combined with CV.14, to treat any disturbance of the Solar Plexus energy centre.

TREAT PAIN AND SHOCK

PC.9 can be combined with GV.26 for loss of consciousness; PC.6 can be combined with KI.3 and HT.7 for shock and postoperative recovery; and PC.6 can be used as an analgesic point during operations, especially of the upper abdomen, chest and throat.

PERICARDIUM SYNDROMES

The Pericardium points are largely used to treat the Heart syndromes, which are summarized in Table 19.2. General uses of the Pericardium points are given in Table 23.4.

Table 23.4 Syndromes treated with Pericardium points

Syndromes	Example	Points
Stagnant Lung Qi	asthma	PC.1,6
Retention of Phlegm in Lungs	bronchitis	PC.6
Rebellious Lung Qi	cough	PC.1,6
Stagnant Heart Qi	depression	PC.1,4,6,9
Stagnant Heart Blood	angina pectoris	PC.1,4,6
Heart Phlegm	mental confusion	PC.5,6
Disturbance of Spirit	anxiety	PC.1-9
Stagnant Liver–Gallbladder Qi	hypochondriac pain	PC.1,6,7,8,9
Stagnant + Rebellious Stomach Qi	nausea	PC.6
Diaphragm problems	restricted breathing	PC.4,6
Breast problems	premenstrual syndrome	PC.6
Pain and trauma	broken ribs	PC.6
Heart Fire	insomnia and mania	PC.3-9
Heat in the Blood	acute eczema	PC.3,8,9
Summer Heat	sunstroke and sunburn	PC.3,7,8,9
Damp Heat	eczema of the palms	PC.7,8
Stomach Fire	gastritis, bad breath	PC.3,5,7,8,9
Liver Fire and Wind	hypertension	PC.6,8,9
Loss of consciousness	sunstroke	PC.9
Yin Link patterns	palpitations	PC.6
Wrist and hand problems	carpal tunnel syndrome	PC.6,7,8

Pericardium points

PC.1 tiān chí

Crossing point of Pericardium and Liver channels, Window of Heaven point.

General

Like most Pericardium points, PC.1 can move Stagnant Qi of Heart, Liver and Lungs, and Stagnant Blood of the Heart. It is mainly used for local chest problems. Although this point is indicated for breast problems, it may not be suitable to use on women due to its proximity to glandular tissue. In men it can be useful for treating angina and other heart problems with pain or discomfort in the chest, especially when related to depression. PC.1, as a Window of Heaven point, can move Stagnant Qi of Heart and Liver, so that the patient can feel a stronger connection to life and a greater love for themselves and others.

Some combinations of PC.1 to move Qi in the chest are:

PC.1 + PC.4, PC.9

PC.1 + PC.6, SP.1, SP.4, SP.21
PC.1 + PC.6, LR.1, LR.3, LR.14.

CV.17, KI.23 and KI.24 may be added to these combinations.

Syndrome: Stagnant Qi and Blood in the chest

Pulse. Wiry, maybe choppy.

Indications. Pain or discomfort in the chest, restlessness or depression.

Example. Angina pectoris and arteriosclerosis with pain in the left chest and thigh.

Combination. SP.4, ST.40 Rd on the right; PC.1, PC.6, CV.17, KI.24, ST.30, ST.31 Rd on the left.

PC.3 qū zé

Water point.

General

As a Water point, PC.3 resembles HT.3 in that both can be used with Reducing method to treat acute Excess Heart Fire. Also, both points can be used to treat such problems as rheumatic heart disease, myocarditis, chest pain, pain in arm and elbow and tremors of hand and arm. However, as shown in Table 23.5, there are significant differences in the use of PC.3 and HT.3 to treat Heart Fire syndromes. Also, PC.3 can be used for problems of Stagnant Lung Qi, e.g. cough and bronchitis; diaphragm problems, e.g. dyspnoea; and Stomach disorders, e.g. stomach ache and vomiting.

Table 23.5 Comparison of the use of PC.3 and HT.3 for Heat disorders

Disorder	PC.3	HT.3
Summer Heat, e.g. sunstroke and sunburn	X	X
Heat in the Blood, Fire poison, e.g. febrile skin eruptions, acute eczema	X	X
Heat in the Blood with Stagnant Blood, e.g. abnormal uterine bleeding	X	–
Excess Heart Fire, e.g. severe restlessness and anxiety	X	X
Deficiency Heart Fire, especially with Deficient Kidney Yin, e.g. insomnia	–	X
Damp Heat in Stomach and Intestines, e.g. acute gastroenteritis	X	–

Syndromes

Summer Heat
Heat in the Blood
Excess Heart Fire

Summer Heat

Pulse. Superficial, rapid, flooding.

Indications. Sunburn, sunstroke.

Example. Sunstroke with gastroenteritis.

Combination. PC.3, PC.6, LI.4, ST.39 Rd; GV.20 E.

Heat in the Blood

Pulse. Rapid, maybe full or flooding, maybe wiry.

Indications. Febrile eruptions, acute, red, hot, itchy skin disorders.

Example. Acute eczema with restlessness and irritability.

Combination. PC.3, PC.9, LR.1 B; LI.4, LI.11, SP.6, SP.10 Rd.

Excess Heart Fire

Pulse. Rapid, full, maybe wiry.

Indications. Mania, manic depression, menopausal, hyperactivity, hypertension, headache.

Example. Hypertension and great overexcitement.

Combination. PC.3, PC.6, LR.3, GV.20, KI.1 Rd.

PC.4 xì mén

Accumulation point.

General

Like PC.1, PC.4 can treat a variety of heart problems, e.g. rheumatic heart disease, myocarditis and angina pectoris. Since it is the Accumulation point, it is especially useful for acute and painful conditions due to Stagnant Heart Qi and Blood. Also, it can regulate heart rhythm to treat palpitation and the arrhythmias, and can calm the Spirit to treat mania, hysteria and depression. While PC.4 can treat skin conditions due to heat in the Blood, it is most useful where there is also Stagnation of Blood as in boils. PC.4, like PC.1, can be used to treat spasms of the diaphragm and Rebellious Qi of Lungs or Stomach.

Syndromes

Stagnation of Heart Qi and Blood
Disturbance of Spirit
Problems of the diaphragm and of Rebellious Qi

Stagnation of Heart Qi and Blood

Pulse. Wiry, maybe choppy.

Indications. Feeling of fullness or pain in the chest, myocarditis, rheumatic heart disease.

Example. Angina pectoris.

Combination. PC.4, PC.7, HT.6, CV.14, CV.17, SP.4 Rd.

Disturbance of Spirit

Pulse. Maybe irregular, rapid, jerky, thin or choppy.

Indications. Nervousness with palpitations, fear of strangers, anxiety, mania and depression.

Example. Fear of meeting people, panic attacks in crowded places.

Combination. PC.4, HT.5, CV.14 Rd; SP.6, ST.36, KI.3 Rf.

Problems of the diaphragm and of Rebellious Qi

Pulse. Maybe irregular, jerky or wiry.

Indications. Cough, dyspnoea, restricted breathing, nausea, vomiting.

Example. Chest pain with vomiting.

Combination. PC.4, ST.36, CV.13, CV.17 Rd.

PC.5 jiān shǐ

Metal point.

General

Perhaps the most distinctive function of PC.5 is that it transforms Heart Phlegm. It can therefore be used to treat epilepsy, apoplexy, aphasia, childhood convulsions, manic depression and mental confusion. PC.5 also clears Fire and can be used to treat tonsillitis with fever, insomnia and hyperthyroidism. It is an empirical point for malaria, and like PC.4 can calm the Spirit, move stagnant Qi and Blood, and calm Rebellious Stomach Qi.

Syndromes

Phlegm obstructs the Heart
Disturbance of Spirit
Problems of the diaphragm } see PC.4
and of Rebellious Qi

Phlegm obstructs the Heart

Pulse. Slippery, maybe irregular, wiry, jerky or flooding.

Indications. Confusion of mind or speech, manic depression, hallucinations, aphasia.

Example. Mental vagueness and incoherence of speech that comes and goes.

Combination. PC.5, PC.9, ST.40, ST.45, yìn táng, GV.20, BL.62, BL.67 E.

PC.6 nèi guān

Connecting point, Opening point of Yin Link channel.

General

The main functions of PC.6 are to move Stagnation of Qi, Blood and Phlegm, and to calm Irregularity of Qi. PC.6 is not much used to tonify Deficiency, and although it can be used for Excess conditions such as heart Fire, it is generally only used for Excess when this is associated with Stagnation, e.g. Retention of Phlegm in the Lungs due to Stagnation of Lung Qi.

PC.6 and the treatment of Stagnant and Rebellious Qi

The main areas of action of PC.6 are summarized in Figure 23.2. For example, PC.6 can be used to treat Stagnant Gallbladder Qi with hypochondriac pain, cholecystitis or gallstones, or Rebellious Stomach Qi with morning sickness or epigastric pain or discomfort.

PC.6 mainly treats Stagnation of Qi in the Upper and Middle Energizers. It is only used for Stagnation in the Lower Energizer when combined with other points which have specific action on the lower abdomen, for example SP.4.

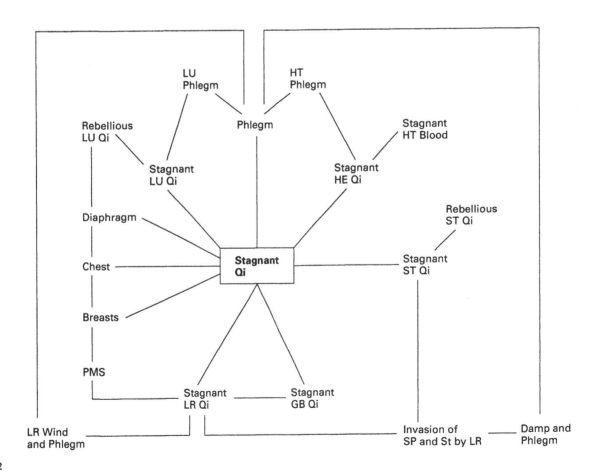

Fig. 23.2

Combining PC.6 with Conception or Liver channel points

PC.6 can be combined with points from the Conception or Liver channels especially, since these two channels are also involved with maintaining a free-flow of Qi. Some possible combinations of PC.6 with Conception points are:

Upper Energizer	+ CV.24	calms
	+ CV.17	moves and calms
Middle Energizer	+ CV.14	calms
	+ CV.12	moves and calms
Lower Energizer	+ CV.6	moves.

and with Liver points:

+ LR.14   problems of breasts, chest, ribs, diaphragm
+ LR.13   problems of hypochondrium, Spleen, Stomach and Gallbladder
+ LR.3   all problems of Stagnant Liver Qi, including hypertension and headache
+ LR.1   breast pain, genital pain, lower abdominal pain.

PC.6 for pain and shock

PC.6 can be used during surgery to counteract pain and shock, or after surgery or accident. It helps to prevent Stagnation of Qi and Blood and also has a strong calming effect. While it can be used for trauma on any area of the body, it is especially useful for thoracic injuries, such as broken ribs. PC.6 can be combined with other major points such as LI.4, SP.6, LR.3 or HT.7 to calm and move Qi, for example for pain or hypertension.

PC.6 to calm the spirit

PC.6 has an indirect calming effect on the Spirit by moving Stagnant Liver, Heart, Lung and Stomach Qi. In addition to this, it has a direct calming effect on the Heart and is often combined with HT.7, CV.17 or CV14 for this purpose. Compared with HT.7, it is more used for acute Excess conditions, especially those relating to Heart Phlegm, while HT.7 is more related to Deficient Heart Qi and Blood or Heart Deficiency Fire. PC.6 is mainly used to calm in chronic situations when combined with SP.4 as part of Extra channel treatment.

PC.6 as an Extra channel point

While PC.6 has its main action on the Upper and Middle Energizers, the combination of PC.6 and SP.4, by using the Yin Link and Thoroughfare channels as a pair can treat problems of the whole body by linking Kidneys, Spleen and Heart (see page 113). Conception points such as CV.4, 12, 14 or 17 are often added to the basic PC.6–SP.4 combination as follows:

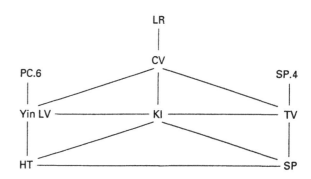

Fig. 23.3 PC.6 and the Extra channels.

PC.6 + SP.4 + CV.4	for exhaustion and poor peripheral circulation with Deficient Kidney Qi
PC.6 + SP.4 + CV.12	for worry, tiredness and epigastric discomfort with Deficient Spleen and Stomach Qi
PC.6 + SP.4 + CV.14	anxiety, insomnia and chest pain with Deficient Heart Yin
PC.6 + SP.4 + CV.17	sadness, depression, palpitations and obstructed feeling in the chest with Stagnant Heart Qi.

Syndromes

Stagnant Heart Qi
Stagnant Heart Blood
Heart Phlegm
Stagnant Lung Qi
Retention of Phlegm in the Lungs
Rebellious Lung Qi
Stagnant and Rebellious Stomach Qi
Stagnant Liver and Gallbladder Qi
Disturbance of Spirit
Pain, shock and trauma
Extra channel problems

Stagnant Heart Qi

Pulse.   Hindered or wiry, maybe empty or full.

Indications.   Sadness, depression, pain or discomfort in chest or heart.

Example.   Pain and closed–in feeling around heart after ending a difficult relationship.

Combination.   PC.6, CV.14, CV.17 Rd; SP.6, ST.36 Rf.

Stagnant Heart Blood

Pulse.   Wiry, maybe choppy, full or irregular.

Indications. Angina pectoris, chronic heart disease.

Example. Chest pain following cardiac bypass operation.

Combination. PC.6, PC.1, SP.4, SP.21, local chest points Rd; ST.36, KI.3 Rf.

Heart Phlegm

Pulse. Slippery, maybe hindered, wiry or irregular.

Indications. Mental slowness, dullness or confusion, erratic behaviour, confused or slurred speech.

Example. Hypertension with dull, heavy feeling in head, congested feeling in chest, depression and irritability.

Combination. PC.6, ST.40, LR.3, GV.20, CV.17 Rd.

Stagnant Lung Qi

Pulse. Hindered or wiry, maybe flooding, big empty, or slippery.

Indications. Chest pain, constrained or full feeling in chest, grief or depression, cough.

Example. Suppressed grief and withdrawal from life and relationships.

Combination. PC.6, LU.7, KI.6, CV.6, CV.17, yìn táng E.

Retention of Phlegm in the Lungs

Pulse. Slippery, maybe flooding, full or wiry, rapid or slow.

Indications. Cough, bronchitis, asthma.

Example. Painful cough with much sticky phlegm and tight chest.

Combination. PC.6, CV.17, CV.22, ST.16, ST.40, LR.3 Rd.

Rebellious Lung Qi

Pulse. Wiry, maybe slippery.

Indications. Cough, dyspnoea, spasm of the diaphragm.

Example. Cough in spasms with restricted breathing.

Combination. PC.6, KI.4, BL.13, BL.17, BL.46 Rd.

Stagnant Rebellious Stomach Qi

Pulse. Wiry, maybe slippery.

Indications. Epigastric discomfort or pain, nausea, vomiting, hiccup, belching, morning sickness.

Example. Nausea and epigastric distension following overeating.

Combination. PC.6, ST.21, ST.36, CV.13 Rd.

Stagnation of Liver and Gallbladder Qi

Pulse. Wiry or hindered, maybe choppy, slippery or empty, slow or rapid.

Indications. Hypertension, headache, nausea, premenstrual syndrome, hypochondriac pain, cholecystitis, depression.

Example. Prolonged frustration in execution of plans, with chest pain and headache.

Combination. PC.6, PC.1, LR.3, LR.14, CV.17, GV.20, yìn táng, tài yáng Rd.

Disturbance of Spirit

Pulse. Various

Indications. Extreme anxiety, panic, hysteria, mania, delirium, insomnia, palpitations.

Example. Panic attacks.

Combination. PC.6, CV.14, CV.17, CV.24, KI.1 Rd. CV.4, KI.3 Rf.

Pain, shock and trauma

Pulse. Maybe wiry, maybe empty or minute.

Indications. Trauma during or after surgery, injuries.

Example. Broken fifth and sixth right ribs.

Combination. PC.6, CV.16, ST.18, LR.3, LR.14 on the right Rd.

Extra channel problems

Pulse. Maybe wiry, choppy, thin or irregular.

Indications. Tiredness, worry, anxiety, insomnia, palpitations, menstrual problems, indigestion, chest pain.

Example. Exhaustion, poor appetite, indigestion, palpitations and nervousness.

Combination. PC.6, SP.4, CV.14 E; ST.36, CV.4 Rf.

PC.7 dà líng

Source point, Earth point.

General

The main functions of PC.7 are to calm the Spirit, to treat local hand and wrist problems, and to treat skin disorders due to Heat in the Blood and Damp Heat.

Table 23.6 Comparison of PC.7, PC.6 and HT.7

Disorder	PC.6	PC.7	HT.7
Stagnant Heart Blood	x	-	
Stagnant Heart Qi	x	x	x
Heart Phlegm	x	x	x
Stagnant Liver Qi	x	-	-
Stomach problems	x	x	-
Deficient Heart Qi	-	-	x
Heart Deficiency Fire, e.g. throat problems	-	x	x
Skin problems with Heat and intense itching	-	x	x
Skin problems with Damp	-	x	-
Heart and Kidney problems, e.g. fear and anxiety	-	x	x

PC.7 and tonification

PC.8 and PC.9, like HT.8 and HT.9, can be used with Reinforcing method and moxa to tonify Heart Fire, but apart from this, Pericardium points do not have much tonifying function. PC.7, as the Source point, can be used like HT.7 to stabilize a treatment; for example, PC.7 can be combined with PC.8 to stabilize tonification or sedation of Heart Fire. However, PC.7 is less effective than HT.7 to tonify Heart Qi and Blood.

PC.7 and the regulation of Qi

PC.7 can move Stagnant Heart or Stomach Qi, but is less effective for this than PC.6, which has the additional function of moving Stagnant Qi of Lungs, Liver and Gallbladder.

PC.7 calms the Spirit

PC.7, PC.6 and HT.7 can all be used in severe acute cases of Disturbance of the Spirit, but PC.6 is better when there is involvement of Liver Wind, and PC.7 and HT.7 are better in cases of Heart Fire. HT.7 is better to calm the Spirit when it is necessary to tonify Heart Qi and Blood, although both HT.7 and PC.7 can both calm the Spirit by stabilizing Heart Qi. HT.7 is best when there is Deficiency of Heart and Kidney, e.g. Deficient Heart and Kidney Yin, with fear, anxiety and restlessness.

PC.7 and PC.6 are not usually combined for organic problems, only as part of a chain of points to treat local problems, e.g. PC.7, PC.6 to treat carpal tunnel syndrome. PC.7 and HT.7 are often combined to stabilize and tonify Heart Qi and calm the Spirit.

Syndromes

Disturbance of Spirit
Wrist and hand problems
Skin disorders

Disturbance of Spirit

Pulse. Maybe irregular, wiry, hindered, thin, rapid or slow.

Indications. Insomnia, palpitations, anxiety, emotional lability, panic, hysteria, fright.

Example. Anxiety and mood changes due to Deficient Heart Qi and Heart Deficiency Fire.

Combination. PC.7, HT.7, SP.6, CV.17 E; CV.4 Rf.

Wrist and hand problems

Pulse. Maybe wiry.

Indications. Trauma, carpal tunnel syndrome.

Example. Dupuytren's contracture.

Combination. PC.7, PC.6, PC.8, HT.8, HT.7, TE.5, LR.3 E.

Skin disorders

Pulse. Rapid, maybe thin, flooding, slippery or wiry.

Indications. Eczema, scabies, acne.

Example. Weeping cracks on palms and fingers associated with Damp Heat.

Combination. PC.7, PC.8, PC.3, HT.8, SP.6. SP.9, LR.5 Rd.

PC.8 láo gōng

Fire point, Spring point.

General

PC.8 is mainly used as a Fire point and Spring point to drain Heart Fire. It can be used for patterns of chronic Heart Fire, such as mouth and tongue ulcers or incoherent speech, or acute fevers or heat stroke. It can be combined with LR.2 to treat Heart and Liver Fire, or with ST.44 to treat Stomach Fire with gastritis and foul breath.

PC.8 can be used with moxa to tonify Heart Fire, but HT.8 is more used for this, since in general the Heart channel is better for Deficiency and the Pericardium channel is better for Excess. PC.8 is most important as a local point for pain or stiffness of the hand, fungal infections, excessive sweating of the palms, or poor peripheral circulation.

Syndromes

Heart Fire
Local problems

Heart Fire

Pulse. Rapid, maybe flooding, full or wiry.

Indications. Fever, heatstroke, headache, hysteria, incoherent speech, chest pain.

Example. Hypertension with violent anger.

Combination. PC.8, LR.2, GV.20, KI.1 Rd; PC.9, LR.1 B.

Local problems

Pulse. Various.

Indications. Carpal tunnel syndrome, Dupuytren's contracture, eczema, fungal infections.

Example. Cold hands.

Combination. PC.8, PC.6, SP.4, CV.4 Rf M.

PC.9 zhōng chōng

Well point, Wood point.

General

The main function of PC.9 is to clear Heat in acute conditions. It can restore consciousness, especially when loss of consciousness follows Liver Wind, Phlegm and Fire, fever or heatstroke.

Syndromes

Heat
Skin disorders — see Heat
Loss of consciousness — see HT.9

Heat

Pulse. Rapid, full and flooding, maybe wiry.

Indications. Severe fever, delirium, heatstroke, cardiac pain and palpitation, swelling of the tongue.

Example. Acute eczema with feelings of desperation.

Combination. PC.9, PC.3, LR.1 B; KI.1, GV.20 Rd.

Pericardium point comparisons and combinations

The functions of the main points of the Pericardium channel are given in Table 23.7.

Table 23.7 Pericardium point comparisons

Point	Point type	Syndromes
PC.1	Window of Heaven point	Stagnant Qi and Blood in chest
PC.3	Water point	Heat in the Blood
		Excess Heart Fire
PC.4	Accumulation point	Stagnant Heart Qi and Blood
PC.5	Metal point	Heart Phlegm
PC.6	Opening point of Yin Link channel	Stagnant Heart Qi
	Connecting point	Stagnant Heart Blood
		Heart Phlegm
		Stagnant Lung Qi
		Rebellious Stomach Qi
		Retention of Phlegm in the Lungs
		Stagnant Liver and Gallbladder Qi
		Disturbance of Spirit
		pain, shock and trauma
		Extra channel problems
PC.7	Source point	Disturbance of Spirit
	Earth point	wrist and hand problems
		skin disorders
PC.8	Fire point	Heart Fire
	Spring point	local problems (including skin)
PC.9	Well point	Heat
	Wood point	skin disorders
		loss of consciousness

Some common combinations of Pericardium channel points with each other are given in Table. 23.8.

Table 23.8 Combinations of Pericardium points

Point	Combination	Syndrome	Example
PC.1	PC.4	Stagnant Heart Blood	angina pectoris
PC.1	PC.6	Heart Phlegm	oppressive feeling in chest
PC.1	PC.9	Stagnant Heart Qi	chest pain and depression
PC.3	PC.8	Heart Fire	eczema
PC.3	PC.9	Summer Heat	sunburn and sunstroke
PC.4	PC.7	Stagnant Heart Qi and Deficient Heart Qi	unstable moods and chest pain
PC.4	PC.1	Stagnant Heart Blood and Heart Fire	chest pain, hypertension
PC.5	PC.8	Heart Phlegm Fire	mania and confused speech
PC.6	PC.7	Stagnant Blood	wrist problems
PC.7	PC.8	Damp Heat	eczema of hand
PC.8	PC.9	Heart Fire	extreme overexcitement and agitation

Triple Energizer 24

Triple Energizer channel

CHANNEL CONNECTIONS

MAIN CHANNEL PATHWAY

Starting from the ulnar side of the tip of the fourth finger, the Triple Energizer channel runs up the lateral aspect of the arm to the shoulder, where it crosses the Small Intestine channel at SI.12 and the Governor channel at GV.14. It then goes forward over the shoulder, crossing the Gallbladder channel at GB.21, to enter the supraclavicular fossa.

An internal branch goes down into the chest, connects with the pericardium, and descends through the diaphragm to connect the Upper, Middle and Lower Energizers. A division of this internal branch runs down to connect with BL.39, the Lower Sea point of the Triple Energizer. Another internal branch runs up the chest from the pericardium to emerge at the neck and travel up behind the ear, crosses the Gallbladder channel at GB.6 and GB4, and descends the cheek to meet SI.18. A division of this branch enters the ear, emerges in front of the ear to join SI.19 and then GB.3, to terminate at TE.23 at the outer canthus.

CONNECTING CHANNEL PATHWAY

This starts at TE.5 and runs up to the chest to join the Pericardium channel. The Muscle Region of the Triple Energizer has a connection with the root of the tongue.

Table 24.1 Crossing points on the Triple Energizer channel

Point	Crossing
TE.17	GB
TE.20	GB,LI
TE.22	GB,SI

FUNCTIONS OF TRIPLE ENERGIZER AS AN ORGAN SYSTEM

This topic is controversial and can be summarized as three main theories:

Triple Energizer as the regulator of digestion and fluid metabolism
Triple Energizer as the distribution system for Source Qi
Triple Energizer as the Three Divisions of the body (three Energizers).

Table 24.2 Problems treated with Triple Energizer points

Channel problems	Local points	Distal points
Fingers	TE.1–4	–
Wrists and hands	TE.4–5	–
Forearms	TE.5–9	TE.3,4
Elbows	TE.10–11	TE.3,4,9
Shoulders	TE.12–15	TE.1,4,7
Neck	TE.15,16	TE.1,5
Ears, throat, face, jaw, tongue	TE.17,21	TE.1–5,10
Eyes	TE.23	TE.1–5
Head	TE.23,22	TE.1–3,5
Gallbladder channel	TE.17–23	TE.3,5,6
Skin		TE.6,7,10
Large Intestine	–	TE.6
Urination, oedema	–	TE.6
Digestion	–	TE.6,7

These three theories are not mutually exclusive and overlap in function. However, most of the functions of the Triple Energizer points are not so much related to these three theories, but to the treatment of Triple Energizer and upper Gallbladder channel problems.

There are few exceptions to this. TE.5 can be used for urinary incontinence; TE.4 can be used to tonify Source Qi and TE.6 can be used to move Stagnant Qi in each of the three Energizers. BL.39 and BL.22 the Lower Sea and Back Transporting points of the Triple Energizer respectively do influence fluid metabolism, but then both these points are on the Bladder channel. BL.40 can treat similar urinary problems to BL.39, and the indications of BL.20 and BL.23, are similar, relating to anatomical position on the back.

TRIPLE ENERGIZER ORGAN RELATIONSHIPS

TRIPLE ENERGIZER AND THE FIVE ELEMENT SYSTEMS

The Triple Energizer points are not much used for problems of the Pericardium, Heart or Small Intestine systems; they are more used for channel problems of the Triple Energizer and upper Gallbladder channels.

TRIPLE ENERGIZER AND GALLBLADDER RELATIONSHIP

These two channels combine in the Lesser Yang pair of the Six Divisions, so that, TE and GB points can be combined to treat problems on the sides of the head and body. For example, TE.3, TE.17, GB.2, GB.43 for ear problems. In addition, GB.41 + TE.5 are the Opening points for the Belt + Yang Link Extra channel pair. For example, GB.41 + TE.5 can be combined with GB26 and CV.3 for leucorrhoea.

FUNCTIONS OF TRIPLE ENERGIZER POINTS

TREAT CHANNEL PROBLEMS

Triple Energizer points can be used for local problems, such as TE.17 for deafness, or TE.23 for conjunctivitis. Triple Energizer points can be combined with Gallbladder points for such problems, e.g. TE.17 + GB.2, or TE.23 + GB.1. Chains of Triple Energizer points on the affected side, in a unilateral problem, can be balanced with PC.6 on the healthy side, just as chains of Gallbladder points can be balanced with LR.3 on the opposite side.

DISPERSE WIND HEAT

The Triple Energizer points can disperse Wind Heat in their local areas, and TE.5 can disperse Wind Heat systemically; for example, in combination with LI.4, or GB.20, or GB.41.

DISPERSE DAMP HEAT

TE.5 in combination with GB.41 can disperse systemic Damp Heat, and local points can be added, e.g. GB.2 for otitis media. SP.6 can be added to balance this rather Yang treatment.

CALM HYPERACTIVE YANG

TE.5 can combine with GB.41, TE.6 with GB.34, or TE.4 with GB.40, to calm Hyperactive Liver Yang, as in headaches, dizziness or tinnitus. Local points such as GB.20 or GB.2 can be added.

MOVE STAGNANT QI

TE.6 can move Stagnant Qi in the lower abdomen, e.g. in constipation, in combination with GB.34, or in oedema, in combination with ST.40.

COMPARISON OF SMALL INTESTINE AND TRIPLE ENERGIZER POINTS

The main function of most of the points on both these channels is to treat local or distal problems on the same channel. Both channels can treat problems of fingers, hand, wrist, forearm, elbow, shoulder, neck, throat, ears and eyes. Owing to the Greater Yang relationship of Small Intestine and Bladder, Small Intestine points can treat more the back of the body, whereas, due to the Lesser Yang relationship of Triple Energizer and Gallbladder, Triple Energizer points can treat more the sides of the body.

Although both channels can treat eye and ear problems due to Heat and Wind Heat, Small Intestine points are slightly better for eye and ear problems due to Kidney Deficiency, whereas Triple Energizer points are slightly better when these problems are due to Hyperactive Liver Yang, Liver Fire or Liver–Gallbladder Damp Heat.

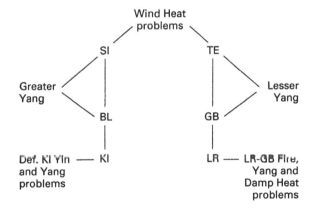

Fig. 24.1 Comparison of Triple Energizer and Small Intestine eye and ear problems.

TRIPLE ENERGIZER SYNDROMES

No point combination table is given for Triple Energizer syndromes, since this system is not generally associated with syndromes of its own.

Table 24.3 Comparison of Triple Energizer and Small Intestine functions

Function	SI	TE
Governor channel and spine	X	–
Back of body (Greater Yang)	X	–
Sides of body (Lesser Yang)	–	X
Gallbladder–Liver Yang, Fire or Damp Heat	–	X
Greater Yang stage invasion	X	X
Lesser Yang stage invasion	x	X
Stagnant Qi in the Triple Energizer	–	X
Liver depression and moodiness	–	X
Disturbance of Spirit	X	x
Skin	–	X
Large Intestine	–	X
Breasts	X	x
Urination, oedema	x	x
Respiration	x	x
Digestion	x	x

X, primary use; x, secondary use.

Triple Energizer points

TE.1 guān chōng

Well point, Metal point.

TE1 as a Well point

TE.1 can be used like other Well points of the hands to treat severe acute Excess conditions of Heat and Interior Wind, such as fevers, heatstroke and loss of consciousness. However, PC.9 is more used for this.

TE.1 to clear Wind Heat

All the Triple Energizer points on the lower arm, from TE.1 to TE.10, can be used to clear Wind Heat and Heat. TE.1 is especially for severe acute conditions.

TE.l to treat Triple Energizer channel problems

TE.1–10 can be used to treat either local or distal problems on the channel, including disorders of throat, jaws, face, ears, eyes and head. TE.1 is used in preference to SI.1, when the problem is more related to Gallbladder–Triple Energizer Damp Heat/Liver Heat/Wind Heat rather than Bladder–Small Intestine Deficiency/Wind Cold/Wind Heat. Also, SI.1 is better than TE.1 for treating mental congestion.

Bleeding TE.1

TE.1 is perhaps the least used of the six Well points of the hand. Nevertheless, it can be bled to relieve eye or ear problems associated with Wind Heat or Heat, or shoulder problems associated with Stagnation of Qi and Blood, if these problems involve the Lesser Yang channels and if it is combined with other Lesser Yang points.

Syndromes

Triple Energizer channel problems
Heat and Wind Heat

Triple Energizer channel problems

Pulse.   Maybe rapid, maybe wiry.

Indications.   Headache, neck pain, blurred vision, deafness, tinnitus.

Example.   Stiffness of the tongue.

Combinations.   TE.1, PC.9, CV.23 Rd.

Heat and Wind Heat

Pulse.   Rapid, superficial or full.

Indications.   Conjunctivitis, tonsillitis, headache.

Example.   Sore dry lips, mouth and throat.

Combination.   TE.1, TE.4, KI.6, SP.6, ST.36 E.

TE.2 yè mén
Spring point, Water point.

General

TE.2 like TE.1 can treat Triple Energizer channel problems and as the Spring point and Water point, like SI.2, it can remove Heat and Wind Heat. It is specifically used to treat arthritis of the fingers, ear problems due to Liver–Gallbladder Fire or Damp Heat, and to generate fluids to moisten dryness and soreness of throat and mouth.

Syndrome: Heat and Wind Heat in Triple Energizer channel

Pulse.   Rapid, superficial or full.

Indications.   Headache, vertigo, conjunctivitis, ear infections.

Example.   Arthritis of the fingers and hand.

Combination.   TE.1, TE.2, TE.3, TE.4, GB.43 Rd; KI.6 Rf.

TE.3 zhōng zhǔ
Wood point, Tonification point.

General

TE.3 is the main point on the arm for eye and ear problems. It has the usual lower arm Yang channel functions of clearing Heat and Wind Heat, and of treating both local and distal channel problems. Like other Triple Energizer points it also moistens dryness. However, its special qualities are based on its ability to treat eye and ear disorders of the Yang channel related to Heat or Damp Heat in the Liver and Gallbladder. In addition, TE.3 has the secondary function of moving Stagnant Liver Qi and calming Hyperactive Liver Yang, to treat eye pain, headache, dizziness, tinnitus, intercostal neuralgia, depression and mood swings. To treat these problems, TE.3 can be combined with such points as LR.2, LR.3, GB.20, GB.37, GB.38 and GB.41. Kidney points, such as KI.3 or KI.6 may be added if the Hyperactive Yang is associated with Deficient Kidney Qi or Yin.

Syndromes

Triple Energizer channel problems
Eye problems
Ear problems

Triple Energizer channel problems

Pulse.   Rapid or wiry or hindered.

Indications.   Intercostal neuralgia, shoulder pain, headache, vertigo.

Example.   Ache and stiffness in shoulder and neck.

Combination.   TE.3, TE.15, TE.16, GB.20, GB.21, GB.40 Rd; KI.3 Rf.

Eye problems

Pulse.   Various

Indications.   Conjunctivitis, blurred vision, corneal opacity.

Example.   Conjunctivitis.

Combination.   TE.3, TE.23, GB.37 E; KI.6, SP.6 Rf.

Ear problems

Pulse.   Various

Indications.   Deafness, tinnitus, otitis media.

Example.   Herpes zoster extending over the mastoid towards the ear.

Combination.   TE.3, TE.17, GB.3, GB.20, GB.34, LR.5 Rd.

TE.4 yáng chí

Source point.

General

The Triple Energizer points are mainly used to clear Excess Wind and Heat or to move Stagnation of Qi from the Triple Energizer channel. They are not usually used for tonification. However, according to the theory of Source points. TE.4 can be used to tonify Deficiency, especially Deficiency of Kidney Qi, for example in tinnitus or deafness. This is because one theory of the function of the Triple Energizer suggests that it is the pathway through which the Source Qi from the Kidney reaches the body in general and the Source points in particular. According to this theory, TE.4 can be combined with CV.4 and BL.64 to treat oedema due to Kidney Deficiency, or TE.4 can be combined with CV.12 and ST.42 to treat weak digestion and lethargy.

Syndromes

Triple Energizer channel problems
Deficient Kidney Qi and Yin

Triple Energizer channel problems

Pulse. Hindered or wiry, maybe empty.

Indications. Pain in wrist, arm, shoulder or chest, common cold, sore throat.

Example. Arthritis of the right wrist.

Combination. TE.4, TE.5, SI.4, SI.5 on right Rd; GB.40, BL.62 on the left Rd.

Deficient Kidney Qi and Yin

Pulse. Empty, maybe choppy, changing and deep.

Indications. Blurred vision, deafness, tinnitus, sore throat, thirst.

Example. Dry sore throat, irritation in the ears, tiredness.

Combination. TE.4, TE.17, KI.6, SP.6, ST.36 Rf.

TE.5 wài guān

Connecting point, Opening point of Yang Link.

General

TE.5 is the most important point on the channel and one of the most used points on the body. It is mainly for treating Exterior or channel problems rather than problems of the Yin organs or the psyche. It has only little use as the point connecting with the Pericardium channel, but extensive use as the Opening point of the Yang Link channel which integrates the Triple Energizer and Gallbladder channels and regulates the sides of the head, limbs and body.

Concept of Lesser Yang and the Yang Link channel

The integration of Triple Energizer and Gallbladder channels is strengthened when Yang Link and Belt channels are used together (see Fig. 24.2).

Functions of TE.5

TE.5 has the following main functions:

  treats Triple Energizer channel problems
  treats Gallbladder channel problems
    Stagnation of Liver–Gallbladder Qi
    Hyperactive Liver–Gallbladder Yang
    Liver–Gallbladder Damp Heat
  clears Wind Heat in Greater Yang stage
  regulates Lesser Yang
    regulates the sides of the body
    clears pathogens in Lesser Yang stage
    regulates Lesser Yang constitution.

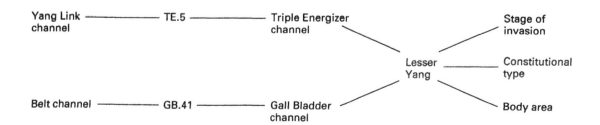

Fig. 24.2

Triple Energizer channel problems

TE.5 can be used for channel problems, e.g. arthritis, especially when this is of the Wind type. Both TE.3 and 5 can be used for ear problems, but TE.5 is especially useful when there is Liver–Gallbladder Damp Heat, Fire or Hyperactive Yang.

Gallbladder channel problems

Because it is the opening point of the Yang Link channel, TE.5 can treat both Triple Energizer and Gallbladder channel problems on the upper body, for example:

Stagnation of Liver–Gallbladder Qi	chest and hypochondriac pain, nausea, vomiting
Hyperactive Liver–Gallbladder Yang	headache, migraine, hypertension, muscular tension
Liver–Gallbladder Damp Heat	otitis media, conjunctivitis, bitter taste, nausea.

Most of these symptoms are channel and Yang organ problems, rather than Yin organ or psyche disorders.

Greater Yang Stage Wind Heat

TE.5 is a major point to clear Wind Heat when there are Greater Yang signs such as rapid superficial pulse, sore throat and fever predominant to chills. TE.5 can be used for Wind Cold but is more effective for Wind Heat. It is also said to tonify Defensive (Wei) Qi, but TE.4 in combination with KI.3 and ST.36 would be better for this, while TE.5 is more for acute Wind invasion.

Lesser Yang problems

Regulates the sides of the body. Combined with GB.41, TE.5 can be excellent to regulate problems on the sides of the body or on one side only. By itself, TE.5 can only treat the top half of the body while the combination of TE.5 plus GB.41 can treat from head to toe. These problems can involve feelings of ache, pain, numbness, heaviness, emptiness in the side of the head, limbs or body, which can occasionally be associated with feelings of alienation, unreality or uncertainty, for which GB.13 can be added to assist treatment.

Clears pathogens in the Lesser Yang stage. TE.5 can clear pathogens in the Lesser Yang stage, with signs of rapid wiry pulse, bitter taste and alternation of chills and fever. However, if these signs change to rapid flooding pulse with fever predominant, this is the Bright Yang stage and TE.5 should be changed to LI.4 and LI.11.

Regulates Lesser Yang constitution. As distinct from acute signs of pathogen invasion, ongoing possession of such signs as thin rapid wiry pulse, bitter taste, nausea, hypochondriac pain, headaches, muscular tension, irritability and impatience can be linked to the Lesser Yang constitution. An effective basis for harmonizing this constitution is TE.5 plus GB.41. It may also be necessary to tonify Kidney Qi and Yin for this constitution so that a basis for a point combination might be TE.5, GB.41 Rd; KI.6, SP.6 Rf.

Syndromes

Triple Energizer channel problems
Wind Heat
Gallbladder channel problems
Problems of the sides of the body
Lesser Yang constitution problems

Triple Energizer channel problems

Pulse. Hindered or wiry, maybe rapid.

Indications. Eye or ear problems, parotitis, trigeminal neuralgia, hemiplegia.

Example. Arthritis of wrist, elbow and shoulder.

Combination. TE.3, TE.5, TE.10, TE.14 Rd; SP.6 Rf.

Wind Heat

Pulse. Superficial, rapid.

Indications. Common cold, influenza, sore throat.

Example. Influenza with feverishness and headache.

Combination. TE.5, LI.4, GB.20, GV.14.

Gallbladder channel problems

Pulse. Wiry, maybe rapid and thin or full.

Indications. Migraine, earache, tinnitus, irritability.

Example. Hypertension, headache and muscular tension.

Combination. TE.5, GB.20, GB.21, GB.34, LR.3 Rd.

Lesser Yang constitution problems

Pulse. Wiry, thin, rapid, maybe empty in Kidney position.

Indications. Touchy, tense, irritable, impatient person with tense muscles and headaches.

Example. Premenstrual syndrome with gastritis and bitter taste.

Combination. TE.5, GB.21, GB.41, ST.36, SP.6 E.

Problems of the sides of the body

Pulse. Wiry or hindered, maybe empty thin, choppy or changing.

Indications. Problems involving symptoms along one or both sides of the body.

Example. Feeling of ache and emptiness on left calf, hip and temple.

Combination. TE.5, GB.1, GB.30, GB.34, GB.41 E on the left; KI.3 Rf on the right.

TE.6 zhī gōu

Fire point.

General

TE.6 is of almost equal importance to TE.5, but TE.6 treats on a slightly deeper energy level. It can be used like TE.5 to treat Wind Heat and channel problems, but is more important to clear Wind Heat combined with Heat in the Blood, and to move Stagnant Qi in each of the three Energizers.

TE.6 to treat skin problems

Because it not only clears Wind Heat and moistens dryness like other Triple Energizer points, but also clears Heat in the Blood and moves Stagnant Qi, TE.6 can treat a variety of skin disorders including urticaria, eczema, psoriasis and herpes zoster.

This is partly due to TE.6 being the Fire point of the channel, so that it clears Heat at a deeper level than TE.5. TE.6 can also be used to clear Heat in menopausal syndrome, as the Fire point on a Fire channel, and because it regulates the Qi of the chest.

TE.6 moves the Qi

TE.6 can regulate Stagnation of Qi in each of the three Energizers.

- Upper Energizer: angina pectoris, pleuritis, chest pain or feeling of constriction in the chest, intercostal pain, insufficient lactation.
- Middle Energizer: hypochondriac pain, belching, vomiting, pain of cholecystitis.
- Lower Energizer: oedema, constipation, painful defecation.

The Stagnation of the Qi can be due not only to Liver but also to Heart, Lungs, Stomach or Bladder.

Syndromes

Triple Energizer channel problems — see TE.5
Skin problems
Stagnant Qi
  in Upper Energizer
  in Middle Energizer
  in Lower Energizer
    constipation
    oedema

Skin problems

Pulse. Maybe wiry, rapid and thin or flooding.

Indications. Urticaria, eczema, psoriasis, herpes zoster.

Example. Psoriasis in chronic phase, resistant to treatment.

Combination. TE.6, LI.4, LI.11, SP.6, SP.10 Rd.

Stagnant Qi in Upper Energizer

Pulse. Wiry or hindered.

Indications. Pleuritis, myocarditis, angina pectoris.

Example. Ache in chest and upper back during influenza with cough.

Combination. TE.3, TE.6, GB.21, GB.39 Rd.

Stagnant Qi in Middle Energizer

Pulse. Wiry, maybe slippery and flooding.

Indications. Cholecystitis, hypochondriac pain, vomiting.

Combination. TE.6, GB.34, CV.12, ST.21.

Stagnant Qi in Lower Energizer: constipation

Pulse. Maybe wiry, thin or empty.

Indications. Abdominal distension, constipation, pain on defecation.

Example. Constipation in the elderly.

Combination. TE.6, LI.10, GB.34 Rd; CV.6 E; KI.6 Rf.

Stagnant Qi in Lower Energizer: oedema

Pulse. Maybe wiry, slippery, flooding or empty.

Indications.   Oedema, abdominal distension.

Example.   Oedema of abdomen and legs.

Combination.   TE.6, LI.10, ST.40, SP.8, CV.6, CV.9 E.

TE.7 huì zōng

Accumulation point.

General

As an Accumulation point, TE.7 can be used in acute severe Excess conditions to relieve pain, e.g. painful skin conditions, pain in the arm, pain in and around the ear.

TE.8 sān yáng luò

Crossing point of TE, SI, LI.

General

As the Crossing point of the three arm Yang channels, TE.8 can be used for problems affecting more than one channel on the arm or shoulder. It can also clear the senses and treat deafness, vertigo, lassitude and sudden hoarseness or loss of voice.

TE.10 tiān jǐng

Earth point, Sedation point.

General

TE.10 can be used for Triple Energizer channel problems, especially of the elbow. The other main use of TE.10 is to clear Damp Heat, Phlegm and Fire poison to treat skin problems and inflammation of the tonsils and lymph glands. A secondary use is to regulate the Heart Spirit and Stagnant Liver Qi to treat anxiety, hysteria, depression and moodiness.

Syndromes

  Elbow problems
  Skin problems
  Throat and lymph gland problems

Elbow problems

Pulse.   Wiry, maybe empty.

Indications.   Lower arm, elbow and upper arm pain.

Example.   Stiffness of elbow joint and tension of muscles of forearm.

Combination.   TE.8, TE.10, TE.11 Rd M.

Skin problems

Pulse.   Superficial and rapid or slippery and rapid.

Indications.   Urticaria, eczema.

Example.   Urticaria.

Combination.   TE.6, TE.10, LU.7, GB.31 Rd.

Throat and lymph gland problems

Pulse.   Slippery, maybe fast and flooding, maybe hindered or wiry.

Indications.   Tonsillitis, painful blockage of the throat, cough with pus and blood, goitre.

Example.   Painful cough with obstructed throat and swollen neck glands.

Combination.   TE.1, TE.10, SI.17, ST.40 Rd.

TE.14 and TE.15 jiān liáo and tiān liáo

These two points are mainly for shoulder problems involving the Triple Energizer channel, as opposed to the Large or Small Intestine channels. However, TE.14 can be combined with LI.15 or SI.10 for general shoulder problems involving more than one channel. TE.14 and TE.15 can each be used as part of a chain of points to treat problems involving arm, shoulder and upper back, e.g. TE.4, 10, 14 and 15. TE.14 can be used with SI.9 and HT.6 for excessive underarm perspiration, or with TE.6 and TE.10 for urticaria of the upper body.

TE.17 yì fēng

Crossing point with Gallbladder channel.

General

TE.17 is the most used and most generally effective local point of all types of ear problems, including pain radiating from the ear into the facial and mastoid areas, aural vertigo and auditory hallucinations. It can also treat a variety of facial problems especially when these are due to Exterior Wind. For example:

parotitis	TE.17, SI.17, TE.6, LI.4 Rd
facial paralysis	TE.17, ST.4, LI.4, LI.20 E
mandibular arthritis	TE.17, ST.7, ST.44 E
sudden voice loss	TE.8, TE.17, HT.5 E
aural vertigo	TE.8, TE.17, GB.20, GV.15, PC.6, LR.3 E.

Syndromes

Ear problems due to Excess
Ear problems due to Deficiency

Ear problems due to Excess

Pulse. Rapid, maybe wiry, slippery, full or flooding.

Indications. Hypertension, headache, ear infection, fever, irritability, restlessness.

Example. Otitis media due to Liver–Gallbladder Damp Heat

Combination. TE.5, TE.17, GB.34, LR.5 Rd.

Ear problems due to Deficiency

Pulse. Empty or thin, maybe deep and choppy in Kidney position.

Indications. Deafness, tinnitus, dizziness.

Example. Recurring low-grade ear infections.

Combination. TE.3, TE.17, GB.2, GB.34 E; ST.36, KI.3 Rf.

TE.21 ěr mén

General

This is a local point with similar functions to TE.17, but less powerful in effect. It is rather more for ear problems with headache due to Hyperactive Liver–Gallbladder Yang and less for throat problems than TE.17. It can be combined with TE.23 for headache or with TE.17 for ear problems.

TE.23 sī zhú kōng

General

This is a local point for eye and facial problems, whether due to Wind invasion or to Liver Yang and Fire.

Syndromes

Hyperactive Liver Yang
Eye problems

Hyperactive Liver Yang

Pulse. Wiry, maybe empty, thin or full.

Indications. Temporal headache, migraine, trigeminal neuralgia.

Example. Headache with eyestrain and muscular tension.

Combination. TE.23, GB.20, GB.21, GB.34 Rd; SP.6, KI.3 Rf.

Eye problems

Pulse. Superficial and rapid, or wiry and various.

Indications. Corneal opacity, conjunctivitis, hysteria with loss of vision, ingrown eyelash, blurred vision.

Example. Redness, itching and swelling of the eyes.

Combination. TE.23, BL.2, GB.44 E; KI.6 Rf.

Triple Energizer point comparisons and combinations

The functions of the main points of the Triple Energizer channel are given in Table 24.4.

Table 24.4 Triple Energizer points comparison

Point	Point type	Syndrome
TE.1	Well point	Triple Energizer channel problems
	Metal point	Heat and Wind Heat
TE.2	Spring point	Heat and Wind Heat in Triple Energizer channel
	Water point	
TE.3	Wood point	Triple Energizer channel problems
	Tonification point	eye and ear problems
TE.4	Source point	Triple Energizer channel problems
		Deficient Kidney Qi or Yin
TE.5	Connecting point	Triple Energizer channel problems
	Opening point of Yang Link	Wind Heat (Greater Yang stage)
		problems of the sides of the body
		Lesser Yang constitutional problems
TE.6	Fire point	Triple Energizer channel problems
		skin problems
		Stagnant Qi
TE.10	Earth point	Triple Energizer channel problems (especially elbow)
	Sedation point	throat and lymph gland problems
TE.14 }		shoulder problems
TE.15 }		
TE.17	Meeting point with Gallbladder	ear problems
TE.23		Hyperactive Liver Yang
		eye problems

Some common combinations of Triple Energizer points with each other and with Gallbladder points are shown in Tables 24.5 and 24.6 respectively.

Table 24.5 Combinations of Triple Energizer points

Point	Combination	Syndromes	Example
TE.1	TE.3	Heat and Wind Heat	eye or ear problems
TE.1	TE.14	Stagnant Qi and Blood	shoulder problems
TE.1	TE.10	Fire poison and Wind Heat	throat problems
TE.1	TE.17	Heat and Wind Heat	ear problem
TE.2	TE.23	Wind Heat	conjunctivitis, headache
TE.3	TE.17	Various	all ear problems
TE.3	TE.23	Wind Heat, Liver Fire,	eye problems and headache
		Liver Yang, Liver–Gallbladder Damp Heat	
TE.4	TE.10	Stagnant Qi and Blood	elbow problems
TE.4	TE.14	Deficient and Stagnant Qi	shoulder pain and fatigue
TE.5	TE.17	Liver–Gallbladder Damp Heat	otitis media
TE.5	TE.23	Hyperactive Liver Yang	migraine
TE.6	TE.10	Wind Heat	urticaria
TE.6	TE.17	Liver–Gallbladder Fire and Damp Heat	herpes zoster (local)
TE.10	TE.17	Retention of Phlegm or Fire poison	parotitis
TE.17	TE.21	Various	all ear problems
TE.2	TE.17,23	Wind Heat	sore throat and conjunctivitis
TE.3	TE.17,23	Hyperactive Liver Yang	tinnitus and headache

In addition, chains of three or more Triple Energizer points can be used to treat channel problems, e.g. TE.1, 14 and 15 for shoulder problems, or TE.4, 10 and 11 for elbow problems.

Table 24.6 Combinations of Triple Energizer and Gallbladder points

TE point	GB point	Syndrome	Example
TE.1	GB.44	Wind Heat, Liver Fire	conjunctivitis
TE.2	GB.43	Liver Fire and Hyperactive Yang	migraine
TE.3	GB.37	Various	all eye problems
TE.4	GB.40	Deficient Gallbladder Qi	indecision, uncertainty
TE.5	GB.41	Yang Heel and Belt channel	headaches as side effect of birth control pill
TE.6	GB.34	Stagnation of Qi in Lower Energizer	constipation
TE.10	GB.31	Wind Heat/Heat in the Blood	urticaria
TE.15	GB.21	Stagnant Qi and Blood	shoulder problems
TE.17	GB.20	Stagnant Qi and Phlegm	catarrhal deafness
TE.17	GB.2	Various	all ear problems
TE.23	GB.14	Hyperactive Liver Yang	headache and photophobia, eye problems

Point combinations for diseases

Part III gives point combinations for some of the main diseases treated by acupuncture. Each chapter is usually divided into sections on different disorders. Each section gives aetiology, syndromes and treatment for the disorder as briefly as possible. In a final summary table, the key signs, pulse and tongue, are given for each syndrome of the disorder to help differentiation. Point combinations are given for each syndrome, and where appropriate, modifications of the basic combinations are also given. More detailed discussion of aetiology is given for disorders for which there has previously been little information available, for example the psychological disorders.

Respiratory syndromes 25

Common cold and influenza syndromes

Acupuncture is not so much used in the West to treat acute colds and influenza. It is more commonly used to treat the pattern of reduced body resistance with recurring colds or influenza, especially where these are likely to progress to asthma, bronchitis or other syndromes. Acupuncture can also be used to treat the persisting debility that sometimes follows influenza.

There are two main aspects of treatment, firstly, in the acute phase to expel the invading Wind Cold or Wind Heat, and secondly, between attacks, to strengthen Deficiency.

AETIOLOGY

In Chinese medicine colds and influenza are patterns of invasion by Wind Cold or Wind Heat. Invasion may follow exposure to Wind, Cold or Damp, and these may convert in the body to the pattern of Wind Heat.

DEFICIENT YIN AND DEFICIENT YANG

Invasion is predisposed by Deficiency of Defensive Qi. Also, Deficient Yang constitutions will tend to give a Wind Cold reaction to invasion by Wind, while Deficient Yin constitutions tend to give a Wind Heat reaction in the body, even though Wind Cold was the external climate. Malnutrition, physical overwork and living and working in cold, damp environments will tend to produce Deficient Yang and a Wind Cold reaction. Smoking, emotional stress and living and working in dry, hot environments, such as those produced by central heating and air conditioning, will tend to produce Deficient Yin and a Wind Heat reaction.

PSYCHOLOGICAL FACTORS

Factors that tend to create Deficiency or Stagnation of Qi will tend to impair the circulation of Lung Qi and Defensive Qi which is necessary to prevent invasion. Kidney fear, Liver anger, Heart anxiety and Spleen worry can all result in Deficiency

341

of Qi. Stagnation of Qi can result from Lung grief, Liver depression and Heart melancholy. All these psychological factors can contribute to reduce resistance to invasion.

THE FUNCTION OF COLDS AND INFLUENZA

One function is that these illnesses indicate Deficiency of Defensive Qi, that the system is weak and needs to rest. Many people ignore these warning signs. They work through the influenza making it worse, and by establishing a pattern of chronic tiredness, predispose the body to future illness.

A second function may be that colds and influenza, and fevers in general, act as a release for accumulated psychological tension from the continuous everyday stresses of life. They may also be a periodic cleansing process where the accumulated toxins are metabolized with release of Heat. If this is the case, then the suppression of this process will lead to retention of Heat and Damp Heat within the body, which can later manifest as illness.

Where colds and influenza indicate Deficient Defensive Qi, this must be tonified, and where they indicate accumulation of Interior Heat, this must be released. In Deficiency, the pulse will be empty, and where there is Interior Heat, the pulse may be rapid and flooding.

SYNDROMES

Acute
Wind Cold
Wind Heat

Underlying Patterns
Deficient Defensive Qi
Deficient Yang
Deficient Yin
Retained Interior Heat

TREATMENT

In the acute phase, use Reducing method to clear Wind Cold or Wind Heat. Between attacks, tonify the underlying Deficiency of Defensive Qi, Yang or Yin, or clear Deficiency Fire or Retained Interior Heat.

The syndromes of cold and influenza are shown in Table 25.1.

POST-INFLUENZA EXHAUSTION

Influenza is sometimes followed by protracted exhaustion and debility. In some of these cases, there may be recurring bouts of the initial symptoms of feverishness and muscular ache. This pattern may merge into that of myalgic encephalomyelitis, see page 448. Rest is essential, especially during recurrence of feverishness. Treatment in the chronic phase is according to which of the four underlying patterns is present. During acute phase, the Exterior or Retained pathological factor must be expelled.

Example

A man of 40 had occasional severe colds or bouts of influenza, between which he felt tired and debilitated, and sometimes restless, hot, irritable, heavy and uncomfortable without any other signs of cold or flu. His pulse was usually deep, empty and choppy, but when he felt hot and restless, was slightly rapid, flooding and wiry. His tongue was pale, with red spots on the edges and a yellowish greasy coat.

The diagnosis was an underlying pattern of Deficient Kidney and Lung Qi, with Retained pathological factor of Damp Heat, perhaps as a result of previous infections which had not been expelled from the body. During the bouts of influenza, point combinations for Wind Heat were used, e.g. GV.14, LU.7, LI.4, TE.5 Rd. In his chronic tired phase the combination was LU.7, ST.36, KI.7 with Reinforcing method to tonify Defensive Qi Heat. During the times of heat and irritability, when the Damp Heat was manifesting but not clearing from the system, TE.5, LI.10, GB.34, GB.41, SP.6 and SP.9 were used with Reducing method.

Table 25.1 Cold and influenza syndromes

Syndrome	Signs and symptoms	Pulse	Tongue	Point combination
Acute				
Wind Cold	acute sneezing, nasal obstruction with copious clear discharge, muscle aches, chills more than fever, aversion to Wind and Cold	superficial tight	normal or pale, thin white coat	LU.7, LI.4 Rd; BL.11, BL.13 Rd M + GB.20 Rd M for headache + SI.3, BL.63 Rd M for ache in neck and shoulders + LI.20 Rd for rhinitis
Wind Heat	acute sore throat, nasal obstruction maybe with yellow phlegm, fever more than chills	superficial rapid	normal or red, thin yellow coat	GV.14, LI.14, LI.11, TE.5 Rd + LU.10, SI.17 Rd for sore throat.
Underlying patterns				
Deficient Defensive Qi	easy to catch colds or flu, which easily progress to bronchitis or other chronic conditions, chronic tiredness	empty, maybe deep	pale, flabby	LU.7, ST.36, KI.7 Rf M alternate BL.13, BL.20, BL.23 Rf M
Deficient Yang	cold limbs and body, exhaustion, maybe depression, frequent colds or flu of Wind Cold type	slow, empty deep	pale, flabby, moist white coat	GV.4, GV.14, LU.7, ST.36, KI.7, BL.13, BL.23 Rf M + CV.4, CV.17, KI.27 Rf M for chronic cough and asthma
Deficient Yin	frequent colds or flu of Wind Heat type, tired, restless, feverish, chronic sore throat or dry cough	thin, rapid	red, no coat	CV.4, LU.7, ST.36, KI.6 Rf + KI.2, LU.10 Rd for Deficiency Fire + CV.23 or SI.17 for sore throat + CV.22 Rd; LU.5 Rf for cough
Retained Interior Heat	recurring colds or flu with Heat signs, chronic restlessness, feeling of Heat in the body, worse with emotional stress	rapid, thin or flooding	red, maybe swollen	LU.7, LI.10, TE.6, ST.37, ST.44 Rd alternate GV.14, BL.13, BL.17, BL.40 Rd + LR.3 Rd for Stagnant Liver Qi + CV.17 Rd for Stagnant Lung or Heart Qi.

Rd, Reducing method; Rf, Reinforcing method; M, moxa.

Asthma syndromes

The Western syndrome of asthma approximates to the Chinese syndrome Xiao Chuan, which means wheezing and difficult breathing. If the attack is very severe, then acupuncture is not appropriate and the asthma should be treated with Western medicine. Asthma can be treated either during attacks, when the principle of treatment is mainly to remove spasm, or between attacks when the principle of treatment is both to treat the underlying causes and to remove spasm.

AETIOLOGY

The three main aetiological factors in asthma are Deficiency, Wind Invasion and emotional stress.

DEFICIENCY

Three main organ system Deficiencies can predispose to asthma:

Deficient Lungs
Deficient Kidneys

Deficient Spleen.

Deficient Lungs

Deficient Lungs may facilitate Wind Cold Invasion, or may fail to disperse phlegm, so that it accumulates, aggravating asthma.

Deficient Kidneys

Deficient Kidneys may fail to hold down the breath properly, with shortness of breath, or may contribute to weak Defensive Qi and repeated respiratory infection.

Deficient Spleen

If Spleen is not transforming Damp properly and Phlegm accumulates in the body, it may obstruct the air passages, aggravating asthma.

WIND INVASION

The concept of Wind Invasion in Chinese medicine includes asthma precipitated by actual cold wind, acute infections, or by allergic responses to airborne allergens or to allergens in food and drink.

PSYCHOLOGICAL FACTORS

In addition to Deficiency and Wind Invasion, asthma may also be originated by emotional stresses, such as Kidney fear or Heart anxiety and overexcitement. Treatment in these cases would aim at stabilizing Kidney or Heart.

SYNDROMES

During an attack
Retention of Phlegm and Cold in the Lung
Retention of Phlegm and Heat in the Lung
Retention of Phlegm in the Lung and Deficiency of Lung and Kidney

Between Attacks
Deficient Lung Qi and Deficient Defensive Qi
Deficient Lung Qi and Deficient Lung Yin
Deficient Spleen Qi and Accumulation of Phlegm
Deficient Lung Qi and Deficient Kidney Qi

During or between attacks
Stress from Kidney fear
Stress from Heart anxiety
Allergy

TREATMENT

BASIC POINT COMBINATION

The basic point combination for all the asthma syndromes listed in Table 25.2 is:

dìng chuǎn, CV.17, BL.13, LU.6, PC.6, ST.40 Rd; KI.3 Rf

During an attack, strong Reducing method can be used on all points except KI.3, and between attacks, Even method can be used. If these points are insufficient, LU.1 and LU.7 can be added with Reducing method.

Caution

This combination, which involves Reducing method on points on arms, legs, back and front, may be too strong for patients with Deficient Qi of Lungs and Kidneys, who are tired, weak and fearful, especially on a first treatment. They may faint with this combination, and a modification for this group, during an attack, could be:

CV.17, LU.6, PC.6, ST.40 Rd; KI.3 Rf

This treatment can be done with the patient lying down. KI.1 can also be massaged if the patient is very fearful. Further points can be added, if required at subsequent treatments.

CHILDREN

For young children, LU.6, PC.6, ST.40 Rd may be enough during a moderate attack. Between attacks, the combination of BL.13, BL.20 and BL.23 can be used with moxa, to strengthen Defensive Qi to prevent the respiratory infections which often trigger asthma attacks. These three points can be used with moxa as a preventive treatment in late summer, to reduce the frequency of respiratory infections in autumn and winter.

MODIFICATIONS OF BASIC POINT COMBINATIONS

The basic combination may be modified for each different asthma syndrome as shown in Table 25.2. For example, during an attack aggravated by anxiety and overexcitement, CV.14 and HT.7 with Even method can be added to the basic combination.

Example

A woman of 50 had continual asthma which was mostly low-grade but with occasional severe attacks which were worse with tiredness and fearful insecurity. She had an occasional cough with white phlegm, a pulse which was slippery and empty especially in the Lung and Kidney positions, and a pale tongue with deep tooth marks, a hollow in the Lung area, and a thick slippery, moist, greasy white coat. These symptoms indicate the asthma syndrome of Retention of Phlegm and Deficient Lung and Kidney Qi with Kidney fear.
Points selected could be:

dìng chuǎn, CV.17, CV.14, BL.13, PC.6 Rd; LU.9, ST.36, KI.3 Rf
alternate dìng chuǎn, GV.14, BL.13 E; GV.4, BL.23 Rf

Table 25.2 Asthma syndromes: basic combination is dìng chuǎn, CV.17, BL.13, LU.6, PC.6, ST.40 Rd; KI.3 Rf

Syndrome combination	Signs and symptoms	Pulse	Tongue	Modifications to basic combination
During				
Retention of Phlegm Cold in Lung	acute asthma, much white phlegm, feelings of cold	slippery, wiry	pale, thick greasy white coat	+ M on BL.13, ST.40, KI.3
Retention of Phlegm Heat in Lung	acute asthma, sticky yellow phlegm, feelings of heat	slippery wiry, rapid	red, thick greasy yellow coat	+ GV.14, LI.11 Rd
Retention of Phlegm + Deficient Lung and Kidney Qi	acute asthma, chronic tiredness and shortness of breath	slippery, wiry, empty	pale, flaccid, white greasy coat	+ LU.9, ST.36 Rf (-ST.40)
Between				
Deficient Lung Qi + Deficient Defensive Wei Qi	easy to get colds, which then progress to asthma and bronchitis	empty, especially at superficial level	pale	+ LU.7, ST.36, KI.7 Rf M (-ST.40, KI.3)
Deficient Lung Qi + Deficient Lung Yin	chronic asthma, chronic dry cough, tiredness, restlessness	thin, maybe rapid	pale with red tip	+ LU.9, KI.6 Rf (-KI.3)
Deficient Spleen + Phlegm	chronic asthma, low appetite, tiredness, cough with much phlegm	empty, slippery	pale, flaccid, greasy white coat	+ CV.22 Rd; CV.12 Rf M
Deficient Lung Qi + Deficient Kidney Qi	chronic asthma and shortness of breath, tiredness, maybe lower back and urinary problems.	empty, slippery,	pale, flaccid maybe deep	+ LU.9, KI.27 Rf M
During or between				
Kidney fear	asthma especially aggravated by fear, maybe lower back pain	empty, thin or choppy	pale, flaccid	+ CV.14 Rd; KI.1 M
Heart anxiety	asthma especially aggravated by anxiety or over excitement, unstable moods	maybe irregular	maybe red at tip, maybe trembling	+ CV.14, HT.7 E
Allergy	asthma especially aggravated by certain food or drinks, or by airborne allergens	maybe wiry, thin, rapid	maybe red, maybe yellow coat	+ LI.4, ST.44, LR.2 Rd (-KI.3) for food + LU.7, LI.4, LI.20 Rd (-LU.6, KI.3) for airborne allergens

Rd, Reducing Method; Rf, Reinforcing Method; E, Even method; M, moxa.

Cough and bronchitis syndromes

In Chinese medicine, cough is a sign of many Lung disorders, mild or serious, acute or chronic, of Cold or Heat, Deficiency or Excess, Interior or Exterior. The Western category of bronchitis may also be subdivided into Chinese syndromes.

AETIOLOGY

Cough may occur independently of bronchitis and has a wider aetiology. Bronchitis is an Interior condition involving Retention of Phlegm, whereas cough may be Exterior or Interior and does not necessarily involve Retention of Phlegm. Cough may be due to the Exterior factors of Wind Cold, Wind Heat or Wind Dryness. These Exterior invasions can be predisposed by chronic Deficiency of Defensive Qi associated with Deficiency of Lungs, Kid-

neys and Spleen. Deficient Spleen Qi can result in Phlegm which may be retained in the Lungs, and become Phlegm Cold or Phlegm Heat, depending on whether the invasion was of Wind Cold or Wind Heat, and on whether the person is constitutionally Deficient Yang or Deficient Yin.

Deficient Lung and Kidney Yin can lead to a chronic dry cough, or can develop into Lung Heat, especially if there is also Liver or Heart Fire. Lung Heat may cause haemoptysis, or may combine with Phlegm to give Retention of Phlegm Heat as in acute and chronic bronchial infections.

PSYCHOLOGICAL FACTORS

Stagnation of Lung Qi due to recent or long-accumulated suppressed grief, can weaken the dispersing function of the lungs and cause Retention of Phlegm. Suppressed excitement or suppressed anger can turn to Heart or Liver Fire respectively, and contribute to Lung Heat. Chronic general stress can lead to Deficient Qi or Yin of Kidneys and Lungs, and chronic fearfulness can lead to restriction of breathing.

SYNDROMES

Exterior
Wind Cold
Wind Heat
Wind Dryness

Interior Excess
Retention of Phlegm Cold
Retention of Phlegm Heat

Interior Deficiency
Deficient Lung Qi
Deficient Kidney Qi
Deficient Spleen with Phlegm
Deficient Lung and Kidney Yin

TREATMENT

There is no basic combination for all the cough and bronchitis syndromes, as with asthma, as all the syndromes have their individual combinations as shown in Table 25.3.

Example

A man of 65 had continuous asthma and bronchitis with periodic aggravations. During the aggravations there was much sticky yellow-green phlegm and a raised temperature. He also had sinusitis. His pulse was flooding, slippery and rapid, and his tongue was red with a dry, greasy, yellow-brown coat.

The diagnosis was Retention of Phlegm Heat in the Lungs with periodic Lung Fire. The point combination was:

dìng chuǎn, CV.17, CV.22, LU.1, LU.6, ST.40, ST.44 Rd

GV.14 and LI.11 Rd were added for Lung Fire during acute aggravations, and LI.4, LI.20, and ST.3 Rd added for sinusitis when necessary.

Table 25.3 Cough and bronchitis syndromes

Syndromes	Signs and symptoms	Pulse	Tongue	Point combination
Exterior				
Wind Cold	common cold with acute cough, with white sputum, and chills predominant	superficial, tight	thin white coat	CV.22 Rd; LU.7, LI.4, BL.13 Rd M
Wind Heat	common cold with acute cough, with sore throat, and fever predominant	superficial, rapid	red tongue, thin yellow coat	GV.14, CV.22, LU.7, LI.4, TE.5 Rd
Wind Dryness	acute, dry cough, with dry nose and throat, but not necessarily any signs of Heat	superficial	thin, dry, white or yellow coat	LU.7, LI.4 Rd; LU.5, KI.6 Rf
Interior Excess				
Retention of Phlegm Cold in Lungs	cough with much white phlegm, feelings of cold	slippery, full	pale tongue, thick white coat	CV.17, CV.22, BL.13, LU.1, LU.6, ST.40 Rd M
Retention of Phlegm Heat	cough with sticky yellow sputum, feelings of heat	slippery, full, rapid	red tongue, yellow greasy coat	CV.17, BL.13, LU.1, LU.6, LU.10, ST.40 Rd + GV.14, LI.11 Rd for Lung Fire + LU.5, KI.6 Rf for Deficient Lung and Kidney Yin
Interior Deficiency				
Deficient Lung Qi	chronic weak cough, weak voice, easy to get colds	empty	pale, maybe hollow behind tip	CV.17, BL.13, LU.9, ST.36 Rf
Deficient Kidney Qi	weak cough, easily tired, back pain, urinary frequency	empty, deep	pale, thin white coat	CV.4, CV.17, LU.9, KI.3, ST.36 Rf
Deficient Spleen Qi with Phlegm	chronic phlegmy cough, poor appetite, loose stools, tiredness	empty, slippery	pale tongue thick greasy white coat.	CV.17, CV.22, ST.40 Rd M; CV.12, SP.3 Rf M
Deficient Lung and Kidney Yin	chronic dry cough with tiredness and restlessness	thin rapid	red, no coat	CV.22 or CV.23 Rd; CV.4, LU.7, KI.6 Rf + LU.10, LI.2 Rd for Lung Heat and haemoptysis

Rd, Reducing Method; Rf, Reinforcing method; M, moxa

Rhinitis and sinusitis syndromes

Rhinitis refers to infections of the mucus membranes of the nose, and sinusitis refers to infections of the mucus membranes of the nasal sinuses. Rhinitis is generally more acute, linked with Wind Cold or Wind Heat invasion in Chinese medicine. Sinusitis is generally more chronic, sometimes a progression of rhinitis, and is linked with Retention of Phlegm Cold and Retention of Phlegm Heat.

AETIOLOGY

Factors resulting in weakened Defensive Qi and Deficient Lung Qi can predispose to Wind Invasion. These factors include weak constitution and the constant physical and emotional stresses of life. There may be an inherited tendency to nasal and respiratory problems, and any factors that increase Phlegm, such as Deficient Spleen, Deficient Lungs, or unwise diet, can aggravate this tendency. Allergic responses involving the respiratory system are included in the category of Wind Invasion in Chinese medicine. These include both responses to airborne allergens such as dust, mites and pollen and to allergens in food and drink. These responses may involve rhinitis, sinusitis or asthma, and are discussed in greater detail in Chapter 28.

Sinusitis may be associated with facial pain, headache, earache, otitis media and acute or chronic bronchitis, and may be linked with Retention of Phlegm Heat in the Lungs, Stomach Fire or Liver Fire.

SYNDROMES

Exterior
Wind Cold
Wind Heat

Interior Excess
Retention of Phlegm Cold in Lungs
Retention of Phlegm Heat in Lungs
Stomach Fire

Interior Deficiency
Deficient Lung Qi
Deficient Spleen Qi with Phlegm

TREATMENT

Treatment of rhinitis and sinusitis can involve combination of local and distal points on the same channels, eg.:

Local point	Distal point
LI.20	LI.4
ST.2 or 3	ST.45
BL.2	BL.67

The main local point is LI.20, which can be inserted under the skin towards bí tōng. Supplementary local points are bí tōng, yìn táng, GV.25, BL.2, ST.2 and ST.3. Adjacent points are GV.23, GV.24, BL.7, BL.10 and GB.20. Distal points can be selected according to function:

Distal point	Function
LU.7	Wind Invasion
LU.9	Deficient Lung Qi
LI.4	all nasal problems
TE.5	Wind Heat
ST.36	Deficient Defensive Qi
ST.40	Retention of Phlegm
ST.44	Stomach Fire
ST.45	Stomach Fire
LR.2	Liver Fire
KI.7	Deficient Defensive Qi
BL.67	nasal obstruction and discharge

In addition, BL.13 can be used to disperse Wind or to strengthen the Lungs, BL.20 to strengthen the Spleen and clear Phlegm, and BL.13, BL.20 and BL.23 together to tonify Defensive Qi.

The main syndromes of rhinitis and sinusitis are shown in Table 25.4.

Example

A man of 35 had nasal obstruction and discharge which was sometimes white and copious, and sometimes yellow and sticky. He usually felt cold, but when the discharge was yellow, often had a flushed face and bad breath. The pulse was empty and slippery, but thin and wiry in the Stomach position. The tongue was pale with some red spots, the coat was greasy and usually white, but sometimes yellow and dry. The diagnosis was Deficient Spleen Qi with Retention of Phlegm in the nose with occasional Stomach Fire.

The basic combination was LI.4, LI.20, ST.40 Rd; ST.2 E; BL.13, ST.36 Rf M. When the Phlegm was yellow, LU.10, ST.44 and ST.45 were added with reducing method, and BL.13 and ST.36 were omitted.

Table 25.4 Rhinitis and sinusitis syndromes

Syndrome	Signs and symptoms	Pulse	Tongue	Point combination
Exterior				
Wind Cold	acute rhinitis with clear mucus, sneezing, chills predominant	superficial, tight	thin white coat	LI.4, LI.20, LU.7 Rd; BL.2 E; BL.11, BL.13 Rd M
Wind Heat	acute rhinitis with itchy sore throat and eyes, signs of Heat	superficial, rapid	red tongue, thin yellow coat	LI.4, LI.20, LU.7, TE.5, LI.11 Rd; BL.2 E
Interior Excess				
Retention of Phlegm Cold in Lung	chronic sinusitis with much white mucus, maybe cough with much white phlegm	slippery, full	pale tongue, thick white greasy coat	LI.4, LI.20, LU.6, ST.40 Rd; BL.2 E; BL.13 Rf M
Retention of Phlegm Heat in Lung	chronic sinusitis with purulent yellow phlegm, signs of Heat	slippery, full, rapid	red tongue, thick greasy yellow coat	bí tōng, LI.4, LI.20, LU.10, ST.40, GB.20, BL.13 Rd
Stomach Fire	sinusitis with purulent yellow phlegm, aggravated by food allergies, indigestion, bad breath	slippery, full, wiry	red tongue, thick, dry, yellow coat	LI.4, LI.20. ST.44, ST.45, LI.2 Rd; ST.2 E
Interior Deficiency				
Deficient Lung Qi	chronic sinusitis, easy to get colds, weak cough, white phlegm	empty	pale tongue, white coat	LI.4, LI.20 Rd; BL.2 E; LU.9, BL.13, ST.36 Rf; alternate BL.13, BL.20, BL.23 Rf M
Deficient Spleen with Phlegm	chronic sinusitis, easily tired, poor appetite, much phlegm	empty, slippery	pale tongue, thick greasy white coat	LI.4, LI.20, ST.40 Rd; BL.2 E; SP.3, ST.36 Rf M

Rf, Reinforcing method; Rd, Reducing method; E, Even method; M, moxa

Sore throat and loss of voice syndromes

Sore throat and loss of voice can be presenting symptoms, but are often secondary aspects of a variety of syndromes. Some of these are serious, for example, carcinoma of the lungs and vocal cords, and must be excluded from the diagnosis.

AETIOLOGY

In Chinese medicine the aetiologies of sore throat and loss of voice are similar, and are discussed together here. Although hoarseness of voice can be due to Wind Cold Invasion, the main syndromes are those of Heat and Dryness; specifically, Wind Heat, Lung Fire, Stomach Fire and Deficiency Fire of Kidneys and Lungs. The strength of the voice depends on the strength of Lung and Kidney Qi, and the lubrication of the throat and vocal cords on Lung and Kidney Yin.

If the constitution is weak, or if Lung and Kidney Yin are weakened by illness, overwork, lack of sleep and emotional stress, then sore throat and hoarse voice may occur. Life style is most important in this case, and smoking, living and working in dry, dusty, smoky or polluted environments, and exposure to allergens, may all aggravate throat conditions. Also, any factor that increases Stomach Fire, such as alcohol, spicy, greasy food and irregular eating habits, may contribute to inflammation and soreness in the throat.

LOSS OF VOICE

The Lungs rule the vocal cords and the voice, and the Heart rules the tongue and speech, but there is some overlap between the two. Hoarseness may result from Lung syndromes, or it may result from the dry mouth of acute stage fright or the chronic stress of fear and anxiety, associated with Deficient Yin of Heart and Kidneys.

SYNDROMES

Exterior
    Wind Heat
    Wind Dryness

Interior Excess
    Lung Fire
    Stomach Fire

Interior Deficiency
    Deficient Lung and Kidney Yin

TREATMENT

LOCAL AND DISTAL POINTS

The principle of combination of local and distal points on the same channel can be used, for example:

Local point	Distal point
LI.18	LI.4
SI.17	SI.2
ST.9	ST.44
CV.23	CV.4

Combinations can be chosen according to location of the discomfort, organs affected, or the type of syndrome. For example, for Deficiency Fire of Kidneys, CV.4 Rf + CV.23 Rd may be a useful combination to tonify Kidney Qi and to relieve local inflammation.

KIDNEY POINTS

KI.6 is specific for sore throat or hoarseness due to Deficient Kidney Yin, and can be combined with LU.5, the Water point, to moisten the throat. KI.2, the Spring point and Fire point, can be reduced to drain Deficiency Fire of the Kidneys, and can be combined with LU.10, the Fire point of the Lungs, for Lung and Kidney Fire. KI.3 can be combined with LU.9 to strengthen the voice in loss of voice due to weak Qi of Lungs and Kidneys. Either CV.4 can be added to enhance this, or BL.13 + BL.23.

EXTRA CHANNELS

The Extra channels combination of LU.7 + KI.6 can be excellent for sore throat or hoarseness due to underlying chronic Deficient Yin with acute Wind Heat Invasion. LU.7 is reduced to clear Wind Heat, KI.6 is reinforced to tonify Yin, and CV.23 may be reduced to clear local Heat and soreness.

WELL POINTS AND SPRING POINTS

Well and Spring points may be used in acute severe sore throat or tonsillitis, either separately or combined. For example, LU.10 + LU.11 or ST.44 + ST.45. Well points may be bled in acute cases, the classic case being LU.11 for acute tonsillitis, which can be effective within minutes in reducing heat, pain and swelling.

LOSS OF VOICE DUE TO STRESS

Where anxiety, fright and apprehension, associated with Deficient Heart and Kidney Yin, contribute to loss of voice, PC.5 or HT.5 can be added with Even or Reducing method. HT.5, the Connecting point, can be combined with SI.2 and SI.17 on the paired channel.

Example

A girl of 10 had chronic mild sore throat with restlessness and malar flush. She had occasional severe tonsillitis with high fever and painful swollen throat. Her pulse was normally thin and rapid, but full and rapid during tonsillitis. Her tongue was normally red with no coat, but dark red during tonsillitis.

The diagnosis was chronic Deficient Yin of Lungs and Kidneys with Deficiency Fire, and occasional Lung Fire during tonsillitis. The basic combination was LU.5, KI.6 Rf; LU.10, KI.2 Rd. During tonsillitis, first LU.11 was bled, and then LI.4 and SI.17 were reduced. As she improved the Deficiency Fire signs reduced, and the basic combination was changed to LU.5, KI.6, ST.36 Rf.

Table 25.5 Sore throat and loss of voice syndromes

Syndrome	Signs and symptoms	Pulse	Tongue	Point combination
Exterior				
Wind Heat	acute sore throat or hoarseness with cold or influenza, signs of Heat	superficial, rapid	red tongue, thin yellow coat	TE.3, TE.5, LU.7, LI.4 Rd or SI.2, SI.17, LI.4 Rd
Wind Dryness	acute or chronic dry sore throat and hoarseness, often from dry environment	maybe thin	maybe normal or slightly red	LU.7, LI.4 Rd; LU.5, KI.6 Rf
Interior Excess				
Lung Fire	acute tonsillitis, severe pain and swelling	full, rapid	dark red tongue	LU.11 B; LI.4, SI.17 Rd
Stomach Fire	red sore throat, bad breath, gingivitis, gastritis	full, rapid, wiry	dark red tongue, dry yellow coat	LI.4, LI.18, ST.43, ST.45 Rd; SP.6 Rf + CV.22, ST.40 Rd for Phlegm
Interior Deficiency				
Deficient Lung and Kidney Yin	chronic hoarseness and dry sore throat, tired but restless	thin, rapid	red tongue, no coat	CV.4, LU.5, KI.6 Rf + CV.23, LU.10, KI.2 Rd for Deficiency Fire + CV.23, CV.14, HT.5 Rd for fear and anxiety

Rd, Reducing method; Rf, Reinforcing method; B, bleeding

Circulatory and related 26 syndromes

Headaches and hypertension syndromes

In both Chinese and Western medicine, headache and migraine are merely presenting symptoms, the manifestations of underlying syndromes. Essential hypertension, otherwise known as primary hypertension, may be asymptomatic, or headache and dizziness may be the commonest symptoms. Although headache and hypertension do not always occur together, they have been dealt with together in this section, since their Interior aetiology and syndromes are very similar.

Since headaches may be associated with serious conditions, such as cerebral tumour or haemorrhage, it is best to obtain Western medical diagnosis before giving acupuncture for any undiagnosed acute headache, or for any chronic headache that is steadily or suddenly increasing in severity.

AETIOLOGY

In Western medicine, the origin of both headache and primary hypertension is largely unknown. In Chinese medicine, these symptoms mainly relate to Liver syndromes. There may be inherited tendencies to headache and to hypertension which are activated by a variety of factors, including tiredness, overwork, irregular hours, lack of sleep, illness, malnutrition, unwise eating habits, allergic reactions, drugs, medication, trauma and emotional stress. The most important factor is probably emotional stress.

THE FUNCTION OF HEADACHES

Headaches may have two main functions. The first being a relatively safe way of 'letting off steam', of releasing the pressure of suppressed emotions. Many people not only live their lives in such a way as to create emotional stress, but also are unable to process and resolve these stresses within themselves. Illnesses, such as headaches, fevers, or skin rashes, may give a form of release to accumulated stress and suppressed emotion.

The second function of headaches may be as a warning from the body to the person that all is not well, and that they need firstly to rest, and secondly to examine their lives and to correct negative patterns of behaviour, before a more serious illness develops.

After all, if the headache is an indication of hypertension, two very common progressions are myocardial infarction or cerebrovascular accident, two of the commonest causes of death.

PSYCHOLOGICAL TYPES

Headaches may be associated with the worry, mental congestion and mental overstrain of the Spleen type. They may relate to the anxiety, panic, expressed mania, or suppressed overexcitement of the Fire type. However, probably the most common cause of headaches and migraines is suppressed irritation and anger. It is not only the Yang Liver types, energetic, aggressive, assertive and extrovert, who suffer from headaches, but also the Yin Liver type. While the Yang type is more likely to express irritation and anger, the Yin type is more likely to suppress it. Yin people may not feel confident or strong enough to express their anger, or they may feel frightened or disgusted by it, and may try to maintain a pleasant submissive persona by suppressing their emotions.

EXTERIOR PATTERNS

Exposure to Wind Cold can create acute headaches, either as a single symptom or as part of a pattern of common cold or influenza. LU.7 and LI.4 with Reducing method, can be combined with GB.20 and GB.21, with BL.10 and BL.11, or with GV.14 and GV.15, depending on the channels affected, and Reducing method can be used on these points with moxa or cupping as preferred.

Allergic responses with rhinitis or sinusitis, seen in Chinese medicine as Wind Heat, may involve acute frontal headaches, which can be treated by combining LU.7 and LI.4 with local points on the Bright Yang channel, such as LI.20, ST.2 and ST.3. For headache over the eyes, BL.2 and BL.67 can be added.

Most commonly, Wind Cold is merely an aggravating factor to an existing chronic pattern of headache and neck pain due to Deficiency and Stagnation of Qi and Blood. This is often associated with chronic arthritis or sequelae of neck injury. SI.3 and BL.62 are the basic distal points, to which selected local points, such as GV.13, GV.14, GV.15, GV.16. BL.10, BL.11 or BL.12, can be added with Even method, and with moxa if there are no heat signs.

INTERIOR EXCESS

The main patterns of Interior Excess are those of Hyperactive Liver Yang with Stagnant Liver Qi, and of Liver–Gallbladder Fire. These patterns are especially related to the pressure of the emotions of anger, frustration and resentment, and to the accumulated daily stresses of the Wood-type person.

Heart Fire and Stomach Fire can originate headaches. Heart Fire may arise from a life pattern of chronic overexcitement and overstimulation, or it may be associated with Stagnant Heart Qi and suppression of excitement or blocked affection. Stagnant Heart Qi may combine with Phlegm to give Heart Phlegm, and this may combine with Fire, to give Heart Phlegm Fire. All these Heart patterns can contribute to hypertension and headache, and eventually, to myocardial infarction or cerebrovascular accident.

Deficiency and Stagnation of Spleen and Stomach Qi, due to unwise eating, to worry or to mental overstrain, may result in Phlegm Damp which rises to the head, giving a headache with a heavy dull sensation. For this pattern, points which clear Phlegm, such as PC.6, ST.40 and ST.45 can be combined with local points such as ST.8, yìn táng and GV.20 to clear the mind.

INTERIOR DEFICIENCY

The patterns of Deficient Kidney Qi or Deficient Spleen Blood may give rise to a generalized dull ache in the head, perhaps with feelings of dizziness, faintness or emptiness in the head. These Deficiency syndromes are not as common in the clinic as the mixed syndromes of Deficiency and Excess.

INTERIOR EXCESS AND DEFICIENCY

The commonest headache patterns are those of Deficient Kidney with Hyperactive Liver Yang, the result of the commonest aetiology of all, the combination of tiredness and stress. The principle of treatment is to tonify Kidney and to calm Hyperactive Liver Yang. Combinations such as CV.4, KI.3 and ST.36, can be Reinforced for Deficient Kidney Qi, and KI.6 and SP.6 added for Deficient Kidney Yin, or KI.2 with Reducing method added for Deficiency Fire. Hyperactive Yang can be treated with combinations such as GV.20, GB.20 and GB.34 with Reducing method, or with GV.20, GB.20 and GB.40 with Even method if there is some Deficiency of Gallbladder Qi.

Another common pattern is Hyperactive Liver Yang with Deficient Spleen Qi, commonly seen as headache with hypoglycaemia, in those with this tendency who do not eat at sufficiently regular intervals. Hyperactive Yang can also arise when there is Deficient Spleen and Liver Blood, and in this case, points for Deficient Blood can be used such as ST.36, SP.6, SP.10, LR.8, BL.17, BL.18 and BL.20.

HEADACHES FOLLOWING TRAUMA

There must be thorough Western medical investigation of all headaches following trauma. Acupuncture can help headaches due to either neck or head injury. Where there may be delayed shock, KI.7 and ST.36 can be used with Reinforcing method and moxa, and HT.7 and LU.7 with Even method. The patient should be advised to rest after such a treatment.

Points such as LI.4, LR.3 and BL.17 can be used with Even or Reducing method to move Stagnant Blood, and local head points can be added near the site of the injury, providing there is not excessive scarring, sensitivity and pain in that area; if there is, then needles can be used to surround the area, with shallow insertion, but not used in the sensitive area.

SYNDROMES

Exterior
  Wind Cold
  Wind Cold and Interior Deficiency or Stagnation
Interior Excess
  Hyperactive Liver Yang and Stagnant Liver Qi
  Liver–Gallbladder Fire
  Retention of Phlegm Damp
  Stomach Fire
  Heart Fire
Interior Deficiency
  Deficient Kidney Qi
  Deficient Spleen Qi and Deficient Blood
Interior Excess and Deficiency
  Deficient Kidney Yin and Hyperactive Liver Yang
    and Fire
  Deficient Kidney Qi and Hyperactive Liver Yang
  Deficient Spleen Qi and Hyperactive Liver Yang
  Deficient Spleen Qi and Retention of Phlegm
  Stagnant Blood following trauma

TREATMENT

Treatment of the syndromes of headache and hypertension is summarized in Table 26.1. In mixed syndromes of Deficiency and Excess, during a severe acute attack, the emphasis is usually primarily on calming Hyperactive Yang with Reducing method. However, if there is no improvement during treatment of an acute attack, and if the Kidney pulse is empty, or wiry with an underlying emptiness, then reinforcing KI.3 or KI.6 may give immediate relief.

Obviously, between attacks the emphasis is on reinforcing Deficiency of Spleen or Kidney, but regulation

of the Liver with Even or Reducing method must also be done. Back Transporting point combinations can be alternated with other combinations. For example, for headache due to Excess Kidney Will and Deficient Kidney Qi and Hyperactive Yang, GV.20, BL.47 and BL.52 with Even method, can be used as an alternate treatment.

Chest pain syndromes due to heart disease

This section considers syndromes of chest pain due to heart disease, and not to digestive, lung or rib problems. The symptom under discussion is pain, and not feeling of heaviness, distension or oppression in the chest, although these symptoms may accompany the pain. Western syndromes include chronic heart disease, such as angina pectoris, and recovery from acute conditions, such as myocardial infarction. Pain may also be accompanied by dyspnoea or feelings of debility and exhaustion, depending on the syndrome.

AETIOLOGY

In Chinese medicine, the immediate cause of chest pain due to heart disease is Stagnant Heart Blood. Six main patterns may contribute to Stagnant Heart Blood:

Excess
Stagnant Heart Qi
  + Stagnant Lung Qi
  + Stagnant Liver Qi
Heart Phlegm
Heart Fire

Deficiency
Deficient Heart Qi and Yang
  + Deficient Kidney Qi
  + Deficient Spleen Qi
Deficient Heart and Spleen Blood
Deficient Heart Yin and Disturbed Heart Spirit

Heart disease may be predisposed in some cases by a physical heart defect that is inherited or follows an illness, such as rheumatic fever. Physical strain upon the heart can be an aggravating factor, whether from obesity, excessive physical work or excessive physical exercise, since it will tend to result in Deficient Qi of Heart and Kidneys. However, lack of physical exercise can cause obesity, Stagnant Heart Qi and Heart Phlegm.

Various nutritional factors, in excess, such as salt, sugar

and animal fats, can cause atheroma, the thickening of the walls of the coronary arteries, that may be associated with Heart Phlegm in Chinese medicine. Drugs such as tobacco, alcohol, amphetamines, and strong tea and coffee, may have a variety of effects. For example, coffee will tend to both disturb the Heart Spirit, and deplete Heart and Kidney Qi and Yin. Alcohol in excess can cause Stagnation of Liver Qi, Liver and Heart Fire, and Heart Phlegm.

Excessive activity, with long or irregular hours, no breaks, insufficient rest and lack of sleep, can result in Deficient Heart and Kidney Qi and Yin. Malnutrition and excessive strain of study or mental work, can result in Deficient Spleen Qi and Blood, and in Deficient Qi and Blood of the Heart, which must be nourished by Spleen.

PSYCHOLOGICAL FACTORS

Heart function is easily affected by emotional stress; it is not simply the number of hours of work, it is the degree of stress with which the work is done. Indeed it is the degree of stress with which the person lives their life. Those at risk are not only the hyperactive, energetic extroverts, but also the more Yin personalities who internalize high levels of worry, anxiety and anger, who 'take it all to heart'. Also, it is not only the more dynamic emotions of fear, anger and overexcitement that can predispose to heart disease, but also the more yin emotions of grief and depression. Particularly, it is difficulty in expressing feelings and affection, and in dealing with the problems and pressures of relationships, their disappointments and griefs.

THE ENERGY CENTRES AND HEART DISEASE

DAN TIAN CENTRE

If the Dan Tian centre, representing the stored energy of the body is weak, or its energy release is blocked by depression, heart disease due to Deficiency is more likely. CV.4 with Reinforcing method can be used with CV.17 to strengthen Deficiency, and CV.6 can be used with Even method, and maybe moxa, with CV.17 to move Stagnation in both Dan Tian and Heart centres.

SPLEEN CENTRE

If the Spleen centre is weak, then the Heart may not be supplied with sufficient Qi and Blood, or Damp may accumulate and turn to Phlegm, to obstruct the Heart system. In Deficiency of the Spleen centre, CV.12 may be combined with CV.17, and maybe also CV.4, with Reinforcing method. In Stagnation of the Spleen centre, CV.12 may be combined with CV.17, and maybe also CV.6, with Even method.

SOLAR PLEXUS CENTRE

The Solar Plexus energy centre is particularly important in the treatment of heart disease associated with the constant stress of the fear of loss of control. Increases in this constant daily fear can put extra pressure on the heart, for example, due either to expanded responsibilities, or to the fear of existing responsibilities being taken away. CV.14 with Even or Reducing method can be combined with CV.17. Also CV.4 can be added with Reinforcing method, to strengthen Kidney Deficiency and reduce fear.

LOVE AND FEAR

Much heart disease may be precipitated by the constant stress on the heart of the tension between love and fear. Ideally, the heart centre is open to give and receive love, but the spontaneity and power of these feelings may create fear. The ordered and familiar patterns of life may seem threatened by the overwhelming strength of feelings. If life is seen as a basically dangerous and threatening process, then a person may feel most vulnerable and afraid when they become open to the flows of love and affection.

In Kidney-type personalities particularly, there is a tendency to attempt to close the Heart centre, in order to feel less vulnerable, so that life is more easily controlled by the rational mind and the will. This tends to isolate such people from their fellows and from their own inner sources of love and affection. This creates great internal pressure, since the energies of love and spontaneous life are powerful forces which are not easily blocked. This internal pressure increases fear of loss of control. In Chinese medicine we can say that this is attempted overcontrol of Heart by Kidneys.

The combinations of CV.14, CV.17, HT.7, KI.3 E or BL.15, BL.23, BL.44, BL.52 are appropriate.

HEART CENTRE

Pain in the Heart area due to Stagnant Blood, may be linked to Deficiency or Stagnation of energy in the Heart centre. The obstruction or difficulty in the flow of love and affection may be due to Kidney fear; it may be due to Liver suppressed anger, resentment, frustration and depression; it may arise within the Heart itself from mixed

Table 26.1 Syndromes of headache and hypertension

Syndrome	Signs and symptoms	Pulse	Tongue	Point combination
Exterior				
Wind Cold	acute occipital headache, ache in muscles of neck and shoulders, e.g. with common cold or influenza	superficial, tight	thin white coat	LU.7, LI.4 Rd; GV.14, GV.15, BL.10, BL.11 Rd M
Wind Cold and Interior Deficiency or Stagnation	acute Wind Cold aggravation of chronic occipital headaches with pain and stiffness of neck and maybe shoulders, e.g. arthritis or sequelae of neck trauma	superficial, tight, empty	pale, flabby, thin white coat	SI.3, BL.62 E; GV.14, GV.15, jiā jǐ, BL.10, BL.11 Rd M + BL.23, KI.6 Rf for Deficient Kidney Qi + GV.3, GV.12 E for general spinal stiffness
Interior Excess				
Hyperactive Liver Yang and Stagnant Liver Qi	lateral or vertex headache, generalized muscular spasm, suppressed anger, frustration, depression, e.g. premenstrual headache	wiry, full	normal or purple	TE.5, GB.14, GB.20, GB.21, GB.41, SP.6 E or Rd or PC.6, GB.14, GB.20, GB.34, LR.3, LR.14 Rd
Liver–Gallbladder Fire	severe headache, or hypertension, violent anger, shouting, red face, feelings of heat, maybe epistaxis	wiry, full, rapid	dark red, yellow coat	GV.20, PC.8, LR.2, KI.1 Rd; tài yáng, PC.9, LR.1 B
Retention of Phlegm Damp	feelings of ache, dullness and heaviness in head and maybe limbs of body, or frontal headache with sinusitis	slippery, full	thick greasy coat	GV.20, yìn táng, LI.4, LI.10, ST.8, ST.40, ST.45 Rd or LI.4, LI.20, bí tóng, ST.2, ST.3, ST.40 Rd
Stomach Fire	generalized headache, aggravated by excess rich food or mental strain and worry, maybe burning pain in epigastrium and bad breath	wiry, slippery, full, rapid	red, thick greasy yellow coat	CV.12, LI.4, LI.11, ST.8, ST.21, ST.44 Rd + PC.6, ST.40 Rd for Phlegm + LR.3, LR.1 Rd for Liver invades Stomach + PC.3, HT.3 E for insomnia
Heart Fire	generalized headache, restlessness, red face, insomnia, with anxiety, overstimulation or suppressed excitement	full, rapid, maybe wiry, slippery or irregular	dark red, especially at tip, yellow dry coat	GV.20, CV.4, KI.1 Rd; HT.3, KI.10 Rf + PC.5, ST.40 Rd for Heart Phlegm + CV.17, PC.6 Rd for Stagnant Heart Qi
Interior Deficiency				
Deficient Kidney Qi	generalized headache worse with overwork and better with rest, tiredness, lower back pain, maybe tinnitus	empty, deep, maybe slow or choppy	pale, flabby, white coat	GV.20, CV.4, KI.3, ST.36, SP.6 Rf + BL.2, BL.64 Rf for mental exhaustion
Deficient Spleen Qi and Deficient Blood	generalized headache worse with study, lack of food, or loss of blood, e.g. after menstruation	thin, choppy	pale, flabby, maybe thin or swollen at edges	GV.20, CV.12, LI.4, ST.36, SP.3 Rf M + yìn táng, SP.1 E for poor memory + LR.8, SP.10 Rf for Deficient Blood
Interior Excess and Deficiency				
Deficient Kidney Yin and Hyperactive Liver Yang and Fire	lateral headache worse with tiredness or stress, tiredness, restlessness, irritability, insomnia, signs of Heat	wiry, thin, rapid	red or red edges, thin, dry	TE.5, GB.1, GB.14, GB.20, GB.38, LR.2 Rd; KI.6, SP.6 Rf + ān mián, yìn táng for insomnia + CV.4 Rf for Deficient Kidney Yin
Deficient Kidney Qi and Hyperactive Liver Yang	lateral headache worse with tiredness and overwork and better with rest, maybe dizziness, tinnitus	wiry, empty, maybe deep	pale, flabby	LI.4, GB.20, LI.3 Rd; CV.4, TE.4, KI.3, GV.40 Rf + GB.2, TE.17 E for tinnitus + CV.4 Rf for Deficient Kidney Yin
Deficient Spleen Qi and Hyperactive Liver Yang	lateral or generalized headache worse when hungry and better with eating, faintness and irritability	wiry, empty, maybe slippery	pale, flabby, white maybe greasy coat	GV.20, GB.20, LR.3 Rd; CV.12, ST.36 Rf M + PC.6, LR.13, SP.3 Rf M for Liver invades Spleen
Deficient Spleen Qi and Retention of Phlegm	frontal headache with mental dullness, sinusitis, tiredness, may be worse with fatty foods	empty, slippery	pale, flabby, thick white greasy coat	LI.4, LI.20, BL.2, ST.2, ST.40, ST.45 Rd; CV.12, SP.3 Rf M
Stagnant Blood following trauma	severe localized headache following trauma, maybe delayed shock or emotional withdrawal	wiry, choppy maybe thin	maybe purple spots or areas	Ah Shi points, GV.20, LI.4, LR.3, SP.8 Rd + LU.7, HT.7 E; KI.7, ST.36 Rf M for shock

Rd, Reducing method; Rf, Reinforcing method; E, Even method; M, moxa; B, bleeding.

feelings of love and hatred; it may be associated with the clinging attachment and overconcern of Spleen; or it may follow the shock and grief of bereavement, divorce or separation.

In each case, CV.17 and BL.15 form the basis of point combination, and points for the affected organ system are added, for example, BL.13, LU.1, LU.6 and LU.7 for Lung grief.

THROAT CENTRE

The Throat centre is responsible for the expression and communication of ideas, feelings and creativity. Where chronic heart pain is associated with difficulties in expressing feelings and needs in relationships, CV.23 with Even or Reducing method can be added to CV.17. If there is fear of expressing feeling, then CV.14 can also be added with Even or Reducing method.

HEAD CENTRES

GV.20 and yìn táng can be added to calm disturbance of the Heart Spirit, to allow the person to see the problems of their life more clearly, in a wider perspective, and, in combination with CV.17 to begin to balance mind and emotions.

SYNDROMES

Excess
  Stagnant Heart Qi
  Heart Phlegm
  Heart Fire
Deficiency
  Deficient Heart Qi and Yang
  Deficient Heart and Spleen Blood
  Deficient Heart Yin and Disturbed Heart Spirit

  very often Excess patterns are associated with underlying patterns of Deficiency, for example:

Excess	Deficiency
Stagnant Heart Blood	+ Deficient Heart Yang
Stagnant Heart Blood	+ Deficient Heart Blood
Heart Phlegm	+ Deficient Spleen Qi
Heart Fire	+ Deficient Heart and Kidney Yin

During aggravations, the emphasis of treatment is on dispersing Excess, with Even or Reducing method, and between aggravations, both reducing Excess and reinforcing Deficiency are emphasized.

TREATMENT

Point combinations for the main syndromes underlying heart pain are shown in Table 26.2.

MAIN POINTS

The main points for heart pain are those to move Stagnant Heart blood:

  CV.14, 15, 17
  BL.14, 15, 43, 44
  HT.3–8, especially HT.5, 6, 7
  PC.1–9, especially PC.4, 5, 6

These main points can be combined with points which treat the underlying syndrome, e.g. CV.12, ST.36, SP.6 Rf for Deficient Heart and Spleen Qi and Blood.

COMBINATIONS OF MAIN POINTS

Different combinations of the main points can be used according to the needs of the patient and the preference of the practitioner. For example:

  CV.17, BL.15, HT.6, PC.4 Rd
  PC.1, PC.6, SP.4, SP.21 Rd

In the first combination, HT.6 and PC.4 are used because they are Accumulation points for severe, acute, painful conditions, and CV.17 and BL.15 are used as a combination of points on front and back. This combination may be preferred for Excess acute conditions.

In the second combination, the Extra channel combination of SP.4 and PC.6 is chosen since the Thoroughfare and Yin Link vessels govern the Heart, and SP.21 and PC.1 are local points for chest pain on the same channels as SP.4 and PC.6. This combination may be preferred for heart pain with nervous anxiety and palpitations.

DURING AND BETWEEN AGGRAVATIONS

For severe episodes of chest pain, emergency Western medicine is required and acupuncture may not be appropriate, or only as secondary to Western medicine. For moderate aggravations of chest pain, where acupuncture is appropriate, the emphasis of treatment is on moving Stagnant Heart Blood to relieve heart pain, and on calming anxiety and fear. Between aggravations the principle of treatment is both to move Heart Blood and to treat underlying syndromes. For example:

  – during moderate aggravation: CV.14, CV.17, PC.1, PC.4, SP.4, SP.8, SP.21 Rd.

Table 26.2 Syndromes of chest pain due to heart disease

Syndrome	Signs and symptoms	Pulse	Tongue	Point combinations
Excess				
Stagnant Heart Qi and Blood	severe chest pain, maybe feeling oppression in chest, maybe cold extremities with blue lips and nails	wiry, maybe irregular	purple	CV.17, BL.15, HT.6, PC.6, SP.4 Rd + BL.13, LU.1, LU.6 Rd for Stagnant Lung Qi + LR.1, LR.3, LR.14 Rd for Stagnant Liver Qi + ST.36, KI.3 Rf for Deficient Qi and Blood
Heart Phlegm	chest pain with feeling of heaviness in chest and maybe head, lethargy and mental dullness or confusion	wiry, slippery, maybe irregular	purple, white or yellow greasy coat	CV.15, CV.17, HT.5, PC.5, ST.40 Rd + yìn táng, ST.45 E for mental confusion + CV.12, ST.36, ST.45 Rf M for Deficient Spleen + HT.8, PC.8 Rd for Phlegm Fire
Heart Fire	chest pain with severe agitation and anxiety, feelings of heat, restlessness and insomnia	wiry, rapid, full, maybe irregular	dark red, yellow dry coat	CV.14, CV.17, HT.8, PC.8 Rd; HT.9, PC.9 B + SP.6, KI.6 Rf for Deficient Yin + ST.40, ST.45 Rd for Phlegm
Deficiency				
Deficient Heart Qi and Yang	chest pain with dyspnoea and exhaustion, maybe cold extremities, blue lips and nails, palpitations	empty, maybe deep or slow, maybe wiry or irregular	pale purple, flabby, maybe moist white greasy coat	PC.4, HT.6 Rd; CV.4, CV.17, KI.3, ST.36 Rf M + KI.1 M; KI.27 Rf M for Deficient Kidney Qi + CV.12, SP.2 Rf M for Deficient Spleen Qi + GV.20, yìn táng, CV.14 E; KI.7 Rf for Excess Kidney Will and Deficient Kidney Qi
Deficient Heart and Spleen Blood	chest pain with palpitations, insomnia, tiredness, dizziness, poor memory	thin, choppy, maybe irregular	thin, pale, maybe purple	PC.6, SP.4 Rd; GV.20, CV.17, CV.12, ST.36, SP.6 Rf M + yìn táng, ān mián E for insomnia + CV.4 Rf M for Deficient Qi and Yang
Deficient Heart Yin and Disturbed Heart Spirit	chest pain with palpitations, tiredness, restlessness, insomnia, night sweats and anxiety	thin, rapid, maybe irregular	thin, red, maybe purple, dry, no coat	CV.14, CV.17, HT.6, PC.6, SP.4 E; KI.6, ST.36 Rf + GV.20, CV.24 for agitation + HT.8, KI.2 Rd for Deficiency Fire

Rd, Reducing method; Rf, Reinforcing method; E, Even method; M, moxa.

– between aggravations for Deficient Spleen and Heart Phlegm: CV.17, HT.5, PC.5, ST.40 Rd; CV.12, SP.3, ST.36 Rf M.

PREVENTION OF HEART DISEASE

Acupuncture can be used to assist in the prevention of heart disease in people who have been shown by medical examination to be at high risk. Chinese pulse diagnosis can assist in the medical screening process, by detecting anomalies of the Heart system. Acupuncture can also be used to reduce the likelihood of further myocardial infarctions in those who have already had a heart attack; it can be used to assist recovery from myocardial infarction; and it can assist recovery from heart surgery, such as heart bypass operations.

Point combinations for prevention are similar to those

for treatment between aggravations, in that they are treating the underlying syndrome in addition to moving Heart Qi and Blood. For example, for a man of 45 with a pattern of Stagnation of Liver and Heart Qi, hypertension and a family history of myocardial infarction, the following preventive combination could be used:

CV.15, CV.17, PC.6, TE.6, LR.1, LR.3, LR.14, GB.34 Rd alternating with BL.14, BL.17, BL.18, BL.43, BL.47 E

For recovery from heart attack or surgery, HT.7 and KI.7 Rf may be needed for shock, and LU.9 and ST.36 Rf may be helpful to strengthen Qi and Blood. If there is pain or discomfort from the scars from surgery, as after a bypass operation, needles can be inserted under the main painful areas of scarring, at about 1–2 unit intervals. Acupuncture can be part of a balanced programme of prevention or recovery, including nutrition, exercise, counselling and meditation.

Palpitation syndromes

Palpitations, the subjective sensation of heart beats of abnormal strength or pattern, is merely a symptom of underlying problems of the Heart system, which is treated by treating the underlying cause.

AETIOLOGY

The aetiology of palpitations and anxiety are very similar, since both symptoms reflect disturbance of the Heart Spirit. Palpitations, anxiety and insomnia may occur together as part of a pattern of Heart imbalance. The three main origins of disturbance of Heart Spirit are Excess, Stagnation and Deficiency.

EXCESS

The Excess is of Heart Fire, which may be aggravated by Stomach or Liver Fire, and be accompanied by Phlegm. Heart Fire is generated in the Yang Heart personality by constant restless overexcitement, overenthusiasm and general hyperactivity and social overstimulation. This is aggravated by coffee, strong tea and other stimulant drugs. Stomach Fire from chronic worry and overconcern, or from unwise eating, can aggravate Heart Fire, as can Liver Fire from suppressed anger, alcohol or drugs.

STAGNATION

The basic Stagnation is of Heart Qi, for example, from suppressed excitement or difficulty communicating or expressing affection in relationships. Stagnant Liver Qi from depression and frustration may add to this, and the Stagnation of Qi may interfere with the regular beating of the heart and in addition give a feeling of oppression or discomfort in the chest. Hyperactive Liver Yang, occurring with Stagnant Liver Qi, will further disturb the Heart Spirit.

Stagnation of Spleen and Stomach Qi, from mental and emotional congestion and worry, can result in Phlegm which can obstruct the channel system that circulates through and around the heart, so disturbing the heart beat.

DEFICIENCY

Deficiency of Heart Qi may be associated with Deficient

Qi of Spleen and Kidney. Deficient Heart Blood may be linked to Deficient Blood of Spleen, and Deficient Heart Yin is often together with Deficient Yin of Kidney. If Qi, Blood or Yin is Deficient the Heart Spirit is no longer properly controlled and may become disturbed. These Deficiencies may be due to lack of sleep and rest, overwork and emotional stress.

SYNDROMES

Excess
  Heart Fire
    + Liver Fire
    + Stomach Fire
    + Heart Phlegm
Stagnation
  Stagnant Heart Qi
    + Stagnant Liver Qi
    + Hyperactive Liver Yang
    + Heart Phlegm
Deficiency
  Deficient Heart Qi
    + Deficient Kidney Qi
    + Deficient Spleen Qi
  Deficient Heart Blood
    + Deficient Spleen Blood
  Deficient Heart Yin
    + Deficient Kidney Yin

TREATMENT

Table 34.9 shows basic point combinations, with modifications for the main syndromes of palpitation or anxiety. Palpitations do not always occur with anxiety, but the association is a common one.

Example

A woman of 60 had palpitations, anxiety and insomnia for many years, that were aggravated by stress. She had low energy and weak muscles, and was very sensitive to stress. Her pulse was thin and choppy and occasionally irregular. Her tongue was thin, pale and trembling.

The diagnosis was Deficient Blood of Heart, Spleen and Liver. The basic point combination and its alternation were:

CV.14, CV.17 Rd; CV.4, PC.6, SP.4, ST.36 Rf
alternate BL.44 Rd; BL.15, BL.18, BL.20

When the palpitations were the most distressing symptom, HT.6 was added with Reducing method; when insomnia was dominant, GV.20, ān mián and yìn táng were reduced.

Peripheral circulation syndromes

Syndromes of peripheral circulation, with cold extremities, here refers to problems of the peripheral arteries or their nervous control, but not to problems due to pressure of vertebrae or vertebral dics or spinal nerves. The most common pattern in the clinic is simple cold hands and feet, perhaps with chilblains. Raynaud's disease is less common and Buerger's disease is rare.

AETIOLOGY

There may be a strong inherited component which is exaggerated by factors causing Deficiency of Qi and Blood. Malnutrition, worry overwork, illness or exhaustion can cause Deficiency of Qi, Yang and Blood; and the lack of regular exercise, excessive consumption of greasy food, tobacco and suppressed emotion can cause Stagnation of Qi and Blood. In addition, nervous stress such as Kidney fear and Heart anxiety can affect nervous control of circulation causing sudden coldness of hands especially.

SYNDROMES

Stagnant Qi and Blood
Deficient Blood and Yang
Deficient Heart and Kidney Yang

In Raynaud's disease, fear and anxiety may be associated with Deficient Qi of Heart and Kidney.

TREATMENT

Point combination for the peripheral circulation syndromes are given in Table 26.3, but in addition to acupuncture, lifestyle changes are often essential, for example, giving up smoking and starting regular moderate exercise.

BASIC COMBINATION

The basic combination for all three syndromes is SP.4 + PC.6, since the Thoroughfare and Yin Link channels together control the balance between Heart, Spleen and Kidneys, and the quantity and movement of the Blood.

Example 1

A woman of 35 had cold hands and especially cold feet, which had become worse since the birth of her second child, after which she had been both exhausted and depressed. The cold extremities were aggravated by both tiredness and melancholy. Her pulse was thin, choppy, deep and hindered. Her tongue was very pale, thin and flabby.

The diagnosis was of Deficient Blood and Deficient Yang, with occasional Stagnation of Heart Qi. The point combination chosen was:

CV.4, PC.9, SP.1, SP.4, ST.36 Rf M; CV.17, CV.6 E M; PC.6 E

Table 26.3 Peripheral circulation syndromes

Syndrome	Signs and symptoms	Pulse	Tongue	Point combinations
Stagnant Qi and Blood	coldness mainly only at fingers and toes, maybe congested feeling in chest and abdomen, maybe inner feeling of heat in the body, with restlessness and irritability	wiry, maybe rapid and flooding	purple, maybe reddish, with yellow greasy coat	CV.6, CV.17, PC.6, PC.4 E + PC.4, HT.6 Rd for Stagnant Heart Qi + LU.1, LU.6 Rd for Stagnant Lung Qi + LR.3, LR.14 Rd for Stagnant Liver Qi + LI.11, ST.37 Rd for Interior Heat + KI.6 Rf; KI.2 Rd for Deficiency Fire + SP.1, SP.8 Rd for Stagnant Blood
Deficient Blood and Deficient Yang	coldness in hands, and feet, pallor, tiredness, maybe dizziness, blurred vision, insomnia, poor memory	choppy, maybe thin or empty, maybe deep	pale, thin, dry	CV.4, CV.12, CV.17, ST.36, SP.4 Rf; PC.6 E alternate with BL.17, BL.20, BL.43 Rf M
Deficient Heart and Kidney Yang	coldness extends into arms and legs, lower abdomen and back, or maybe even whole body, exhaustion, severe pallor, maybe depression and lack of drive, dyspnoea, back pain or urinary frequency	empty to minute	pale, flabby, moist, maybe white coat	CV.4, CV.6, CV.17, HT.8, KI.2, SP.4 Rf M; PC.6 E alternate GV.4, GV.11, GV.20, BL.15, BL.23 Rf M

Additional modifications	
+ PC.8, PC.9 Rf M	for cold hands
+ SP.1, SP.2 Rf M; KI.1 M	for cold feet
+ GV.20, CV.14, CV.24 Rd	for Raynaud's disease, with stress
+ SP.1, SP.8, ST.30, ST.31, ST.41 Rf M	for Buerger's disease

Rd, Reducing method; Rf, Reinforcing method; E, Even method; M, moxa.

Example 2

A man of 75, taking propanadol for hypertension, had cold extremities and depression, which were aggravated by the propanadol, and a sensation of oppression, restlessness and heat in the body. His pulse was wiry, rapid and flooding, with occasionally irregularity. His tongue was purple with some red spots, and a greasy yellow coat.

The diagnosis was of Stagnant Liver and Heart Qi, with Retention of Interior Heat. The Point combination was:

CV.6, CV.17, PC.6, SP.4 E; CV.10, PC.8, LI.10, ST.37 Rd

Varicose veins syndromes

The main complaints with varicose veins of the legs are the unsightly swollen veins themselves, aching pain or easy fatiguability of the calf muscles, itchy rash, or varicose ulcer.

AETIOLOGY

The main contributory patterns are Stagnation of Qi and Blood, Deficient Spleen with Sinking of Spleen Qi, and Damp Heat. There may be an inherited tendency to varicose veins which is aggravated by poor diet, obesity, pregnancy, long standing without moving, lack of exercise and general tiredness. Chronic worry and overconcern may weaken the Spleen, and suppressed irritation and anger may combine with Damp to produce Liver–Gallbladder Damp Heat.

In the case of varicose eczema, any factors, such as food additives, alcohol or food, that increase Damp and Heat, may aggravate. Sometimes, living and working in rooms that are too hot for the patient may exacerbate varicose eczema. Varicose veins may be combined with poor peripheral circulation, so that the toes and feet may be blue and cold, yet the patches of varicose eczema over the veins are hot. Treatment then aims at moving Qi and Blood and draining Damp Heat.

SYNDROMES

Stagnant Qi and Blood
Sinking of Spleen Qi
Damp Heat

These syndromes may occur together, sometimes also with Deficient Spleen Qi and Yang.

TREATMENT

BASIC COMBINATION

Points can be chosen from:

SP.1, 2, 4, 6, 8, 9, 10
ST.36, 37, 40, 41, 44
PC.6, 9
LR.1, 2, 3, 5
GB.34, 39, 41

For example: PC.6, SP.4, SP.6, SP.8, ST.36, ST.41 E.

Needles are not used in severely varicose areas, to avoid puncturing swollen veins, so if, for example, it is not possible to use SP.6 and LR.5 then SP.8 and LR.3 may be used instead. It may be possible also, to use SP.6 and LR.5 on the less-affected side.

MODIFICATIONS TO BASIC FORMULA

+ PC.9, SP.1, LR.1 Rd	for Heat in the Blood eczema
+ LI.4, ST.37, ST.44 Rd	for Heat in Stomach and Intestines type eczema
+ GB.34, GB.41, SP.9 Rd	for Damp Heat eczema
+ GV.20, CV.4, CV.12 Rf M	for Sinking of Spleen Qi

For varicose ulcers, needles can be inserted just outside the periphery of the ulcer, at shallow angles under it towards the centre, at intervals of about 1 unit. For varicose veins with poor peripheral circulation, and no systemic or local signs of heat, SP.1 and SP.2 can be used with moxa cones, to tonify Spleen Yang.

Locomotory syndromes 27

Back pain syndromes

Back pain may be acute or chronic, it may have aspects of Excess or Deficiency, Heat or Cold, Exterior or Interior factors, and it may involve different channels and organs.

AETIOLOGY

There is usually a mixed aetiology for back problems, and the relative importance of the contributing factors must be assessed, not only for effective treatment, but also for accurate advice on necessary changes in lifestyle. The channels involved in back problems are the Governor and Bladder channels, and to a lesser extent the Small Intestine and Gallbladder channels. The main organ systems involved are the Kidneys, and to a lesser extent the Liver.

CONTRIBUTING FACTORS

The main factors contributing to back pain are:

climatic factors
trauma, use and posture
chronic diseases
psychological factors
Deficient Kidneys.

CLIMATIC FACTORS

The main climatic factors are Exterior Wind, Cold and Damp. Once in the body, these factors may later give signs of Heat and inflammation. Local needling, moxa and cupping may be used to disperse the invading factor, as well as such distal points as SI.3, Bl.62, LI.4 and TE.5 with Reducing method. Patients should make every effort to avoid exposure to climatic factors; for example, avoiding getting chilled while swimming, standing around in cold, wet clothes or lying on cold, damp ground.

TRAUMA, USE AND POSTURE

Acute back sprain during work or sport, chronic strain on the back from constant bending and lifting, and poor posture while standing or sitting, can all contribute to back problems. Empirical or local points can be used for acute sprain, and local and distal points can be used for chronic problems relating to use and posture. Rest, gentle exercises and education on used and posture are necessary; for example, safe methods of lifting, avoidance of unsuitable beds and chairs, and minimal wear of high-heeled shoes.

CHRONIC DISEASES

Disorders such as spondylitis, arthritis, osteoporosis, multiple sclerosis and deformation or damage to the spine as a sequelae of trauma, can all contribute to chronic back problems. Acupuncture treatment of back problems must include points to treat the underlying chronic disorder, where this is possible.

PSYCHOLOGICAL FACTORS

These mainly relate to the Kidney and Liver organ systems. The Yin Kidney type has given up on life and spinal muscles will be flaccid and posture poor, hence the word 'spineless' to describe their character. The Yang Kidney type may be rigid and inflexible from fear of losing control, with stiff muscles and spine. Liver types may have general muscular tension associated with the suppression of anger and impatience, and although this can be especially marked in the areas of head, neck and shoulders, it can also include the back.

Acupuncture treatment can be combined with relaxation, meditation and Qi Gong exercises. For the Yin Kidney type, these exercises can focus on strengthening the Dan Tian centre, the back and the will, to improve the tone of spinal muscles. For the Yang Kidney type, it is necessary to strengthen the Dan Tian centre to control fear, so that the muscles can relax. For the Liver types, it is necessary to develop an inner peace, to relieve the pressures of impatience and anger, to relax the muscles.

DEFICIENT KIDNEYS

The Kidneys may be constitutionally weak, or may be depleted by illness, overwork, excessive exercise, excessive sex, childbirth, emotional stress, lack of sleep and old age. This Kidney Deficiency may manifest in general low resistance to disease, and specifically in a tendency to lower back problems. Self-help and Qi Gong exercises both aim to increase rest and conserve energy, to strengthen the back gradually.

SYNDROMES

The main syndromes of back pain are:

Acute
    Trauma with major disc protrusion
    Trauma without major disc protrusion
    Wind, Cold, Damp Invasion
Chronic
    Chronic diseases
    Deficient Kidneys
        Deficient Kidney Yang
        Deficient Kidney Yin
        Deficient Kidneys and Spleen
    Stagnant Liver Qi

TRAUMA WITH MAJOR DISC PROTRUSION

This pattern in rare in the acupuncture clinic. It is safest to avoid the needling method with patient movement, indeed the patient might find this too painful. The main points used are local GV and jiā jǐ points with Reducing method and perhaps moxa or electroacupuncture. Distal points may also be used with Reducing method or bleeding.

TRAUMA WITHOUT MAJOR DISC PROTRUSION

This syndrome is common in the acupuncture clinic. The difference between this and the previous pattern lies simply in the degree of disc protrusion and the degree of pain and incapacity. There is a choice between:

– Distal points with patient movement as the primary treatment

– Local points as the primary treatment with distal points as secondary.

The technique of using distal points with patient movement is outlined later. If the patient finds the method too painful, or if it is the first treatment and the patient has a history of fainting, local points can be used instead. Indeed, some practitioners often prefer the local treatment as primary. In this case, both local and distal points can be needled with Reducing method, with moxa also if required.

WIND, COLD, DAMP INVASION

Local and distal points are used with Reducing or Even methods, with moxa or cupping.

CHRONIC DISEASES

Local GV and jiā jǐ points can be used to treat vertebrae, vertebral joints and spinal nerves. Local points on the inner and outer Bladder lines can be used to treat muscular problems in a specific spinal segment. Distal points such as KI.3, KI.6, BL.23, BL.62, BL.64, GB.39 and SI.3 can be used to strengthen bones and marrow, and points such as BL.8, GB.34 and LR.3 used to nourish and relax the muscles.

DEFICIENT KIDNEYS

Local and distal points, such as GV.4, BL.23, BL.52, BL.60, BL.62, BL.64, KI.3, KI.6 and KI.7, can be used to tonify Deficient Kidneys. For Deficient Kidney Yang, moxa is used and points like BL.60 and KI.7 are emphasized. If there is general Deficient Yang, then GV.1, GV.2, GV.3, GV.14, GV.20, KI.1 or KI.2 may be added with Reinforcing method and moxa.

For Deficient Kidney Yin, no moxa is used and KI.6 and SP.6 are emphasized. It may be helpful to alternate treatments on the back with treatments including CV.4 on the front. For Deficient Kidneys and Spleen, SP.3, SP.6, ST.36 and BL.20 can be added with Reinforcing method and moxa. SP.3 can be helpful for chronic back weakness.

STAGNANT LIVER QI

Local, distal and Ah Shi points can be used to move systemic and local Stagnation of Qi and Blood due to Stagnant Liver Qi with frustration and suppressed anger and impatience. Points can be selected from GV.1, GV.8, GV.20, GV.26, BL.17, BL.18, BL.47, GB.21, GB.25, GB.34, LR.3, with Even or Reducing method, and moxa if appropriate.

MIXED SYNDROMES

Back pain is often due to combination of syndromes. For example, Deficient Kidney Yang may predispose to Exterior invasion of Cold and Damp. Initial treatment is to remove Cold and Damp, and when this is dispersed,

later treatments can tonify Kidney Yang to prevent further invasion.

Another example could be lower back pain associated with multiple sclerosis, from local Stagnation of Qi and Blood with underlying Deficient Kidney Yin. BL.22 could be used as a local point for the local pain in this area; GV.5 and the adjacent jiā jǐ points can be used to strengthen the spinal nerve in this segment; BL.23 and KI.6 could be reinforced to tonify Kidney Yin, and KI.2 reduced to drain Kidney Deficiency Fire.

POINTS FOR BACK PAIN

DISTAL POINTS USED WITH PATIENT MOVEMENT

Certain distal points can be manipulated whilst the patient moves the back. This method can be used for acute back sprain with no major disc protrusion. Great care must be taken on the first treatment with this method to avoid excessive pain or fainting. The method can be summarized:

- Ask patient to demonstrate the degree of limitation of movement.

- Insert needle into distal point on appropriate side and get gentle needle sensation.

- Ask patient to move body in the direction of limitation of movement as before, and to keep repeating this while you manipulate needle to produce needle sensation. Watch patient carefully for signs of fainting, and only manipulate for a few seconds, then stop and tell them to stop movement.

- Let patient rest for a few minutes, then repeat 1–2 times, depending on reaction of patient. With patients who appear more likely to faint, use gentler manipulation for shorter periods with fewer repeats.

- Remove needle from distal point and ask patient once again to demonstrate the degree of limitation and report on degree of pain. There should be improvement.

- Use needle, moxa, cupping etc. as required on local painful points if appropriate.

Different practitioners prefer different points; some examples follow.

yāo tòng diǎn

There are two of these points on the dorsum of each hand, located between the junction of either the second and third metacarpals or the fourth and fifth metacarpals. Needle vertically 0.5–1 unit and manipulate while patient moves their back. This point can also be used for stiff neck. It is for pain either side of midline, needling the affected side.

BL.40

This can be used for acute bilateral or unilateral pain, but not so much for pain on the midline. The patient is standing and moves the back around the area of pain. If the patient feels faint, remove needle and ask them to lie down.

GV.26

GV.26 is for pain on the midline only with difficulties of flexion and extension. Needle obliquely 0.3–0.5 unit toward the nose. The patient moves while the practitioner manipulates the needle.

BL.40 can also be bled, without patient movement, and ST.9 can be needled on the affected side 0.3–0.5 units, medial to the carotid artery, also without patient movement.

LOCAL POINTS

Local points can be used to disperse Exterior factors such as Wind, Cold and Damp; to move Stagnation due to trauma or Stagnant Liver Qi; or to tonify local Deficiency of Kidneys.

BL.22–19 and BL.52

All these points can be used with needle or moxa to treat local Excess, Stagnation or Deficiency. In addition, BL.23 and BL.52 tonify the Kidneys, and treat the weak knees, urinary frequency and tinnitus often associated with back pain due to Deficient Kidneys.

BL.31–34

These local points can treat back pain associated with menstruation or childbirth, and back pain associated with colon and bladder problems, as in multiple sclerosis.

yāo yǎo

This point, in the depression about 3–4 units lateral to the spinous process of the third lumbar vertebra, can be used for acute and chronic lower back pain, especially with dysmenorrhoea.

BL.54

This point can be used for pain in the lower back and sacrum, and for sciatic pain in the buttock and leg. It is specific for back pain associated with Damp Heat urinary problems.

GV.2–5

These points warm and tonify Kidney Yang and disperse Cold and Damp. They can be used for lower back and sacral problems associated with feelings of coldness, depression, exhaustion, impotence, urinary frequency and lack of will. GV.2 corresponds approximately to the sacral or reproductive energy centre, and GV.4 to the Dan Tian centre in its Yang aspect.

shí qī zhuī xià

Located below the spinous process of the fifth lumbar vertebra, this extra point on the Governor channel can be used with BL.26, at the same level, for lower back pain, or with BL.31 for sacral problems.

huá tuó jiā jǐ

Located at about 0.5–1 unit lateral to the inferior end of the spinous process of a vertebra, these points can be used for problems of individual vertebrae, vertebral joints, spinal nerves or spinal segments. They are often combined with GV or BL points at the same level.

DISTAL POINTS

The main general distal points for back pain are BL.40, 59, 60, 62 and KI.3, 6. 7. Also, SI.3 can combine with BL.62 for general problems of the spine, not so much the lower back. SP.3 can strengthen a weak lower back when there is Deficient Spleen Qi and Blood.

BL.40

This point can be used for chronic back problems as well as acute ones. For example, it can be combined with local Bladder points, such as BL.22, 23 or 24, for Stagnation and Deficiency in the Bladder channel, with chronic stiffness and pain in the back radiating down the Bladder channel on the leg.

BL.59

This is the Accumulation point of the Yang Heel vessel, useful for chronic unilateral weakness, stiffness and pain of leg and back, especially with headache or sensation of heaviness in the head.

BL.60

As the Fire point, this can be used for chronic patterns of Deficient Kidney Yang with invasion of Wind, Cold or Damp, and pain or stiffness in leg, back, shoulder, neck or occiput; especially with pre-existing injury or arthritis.

BL.62

As the Opening point for the Yang Heel channel, this point can be combined with SI.3, the Opening point of the Governor channel, to treat all problems of the spine, including ankylosing spondylitis, arthritis, multiple sclerosis and sequelae of accidents. BL.62 can also be used by itself, or in combination with SI.3, for Wind Cold invasion of the back, with stiff neck and occipital headache. BL.62 can be helpful for acute lower back pain, especially if unilateral, whether due to sprain or to Cold invasion.

Back pain syndromes are summarized in Table 27.1.

Hip pain and sciatica syndromes

Hip pain and sciatica can be due to local hip problems, vertebral problems or both. Hip pain often relates to inflammation; for example, osteoarthritis, rheumatoid arthritis, non-specific inflammation of a joint, or bursitis. Tumours of the hip must be excluded in the diagnosis. Vertebral problems, with pressure on spinal nerves, can result in pain in hips and legs, with or without concurrent back pain.

The aetiology of hip pain and sciatica is similar to that of back pain, e.g. trauma, Exterior invasion, chronic disease, Deficient Kidneys and Stagnant Liver Qi. The syndromes of hip pain and sciatica are similar to those for back pain shown in Table 27.1.

TREATMENT

VERTEBRAL ORIGIN

Where hip pain and sciatica are of vertebral origin, the point combinations are similar to those for lumbar pain but can include some of the additional points for hip pain and sciatica listed later.

Table 27.1 Back pain syndromes

Syndrome	Signs and symptoms	Pulse	Tongue	Point combination
Acute trauma (with major disc protrusion)	Severe, immobilizing pain following a trauma	wiry	various	local GV, jiā jǐ and BL points Rd or M E BL.40 Rd or B
Acute trauma (without major disc protrusion)	back pain and stiffness but more or less able to walk	wiry	various	first yāo tòng diǎn Rd with patient movement, then local points Rd or M, e.g. GV.5, BL.22 or: local, e.g. BL.24, BL.25 with distal e.g. BL.59
Invasion by Wind, Cold or Damp	acute back pain following exposure to Wind, Cold or Damp	maybe wiry, empty, deep or slow		local points, e.g. GV.3, BL.25 with Rd, with distal points e.g. BL.60 Rf M or C
Chronic diseases	chronic back pain associated with diseases such as arthritis, spondylitis, multiple sclerosis	maybe empty, thin or choppy, maybe wiry	thin or flabby	local GV, jiā jǔ, BL and SI points E (with moxa if no signs of heat) with BL.62, KI.6, SI.3 E + GB.14 Rd for signs of heat
Deficient Kidneys	chronic back pain with tinnitus, weak knees, impotence, urinary frequency, or other Kidney signs, aggravated by tiredness	empty or thin, maybe choppy deep or slow	thin or flabby	GV.4, BL.23, BL.52, BL.64, KI.3 Rf + GV.3, GV.20, BL.60, KI.2 Rf M for Deficient Kidney Yang + CV.4, KI.6, SP.6 Rf for Deficient Kidney Yin + KI.2 Rd for Deficiency Fire + SP.6, SP.9, BL.54 Rd for Damp Heat + SP.3, ST.36, BL.20 Rf M for Deficient Spleen
Stagnant Liver Qi	back stiffness and pain with stiff neck, frustration, suppressed anger and irritability	wiry, maybe full or empty, maybe rapid	maybe purple or red, especially at edges	local points Rd M; GV.8, GV.20, GB.21, GB.34; BL.18, SP.6, PC.6 E

Rf, Reinforcing method; Rd, Reducing method; E, Even method; M, moxa; B, bleeding; C, cupping.

HIP JOINT INFLAMMATION

Where hip pain and sciatica are due to inflammation of the hip joint, points on the lower back may not be necessary. However, if the hip joint inflammation is aggravated by tiredness and related to Deficient Kidneys, GV.4, BL.23 and BL.52 may be reinforced. If it is aggravated by stress and suppressed anger and related to Stagnation of Liver Qi, Liver–Gallbladder Damp Heat or Liver Fire, GV.8, BL.18 and BL.47 may be reduced.

RHEUMATOID ARTHRITIS

If the hip joint inflammation is associated with a systemic condition such as rheumatoid arthritis, distal points for Damp, Damp Heat and Deficiency Fire may be required in addition to points for hip and leg pain. For example, SP.6, SP.9, KI.2, KI.6, LR.2 and ST.44.

BURSITIS

Where the hip pain is due to bursitis, needles may be inserted obliquely around the bursa sac at intervals of about 2 cm. Moxa stick may be used on the affected area, but with caution if there are local signs of heat. In addition, local and distal points on the Gallbladder channel can be included in the treatment.

POINTS FOR HIP PAIN AND SCIATICA

These are primarily on the Bladder and Gallbladder channel and secondarily on the Stomach channel. Points are used on the channel or channels affected.

GB.30

This point may be needled to a depth of 1.5–2.5 units perpendicularly towards the genitals. Needle sensation may extend down the leg. If it does not, then the point can be needled 1 unit lower than the normal location.

GB.30 can be combined with local points such as GB.29 and zuǒ gǔ. It can be included in a chain of points for sciatica, on either the Gallbladder or Bladder channel, or both. For example:

GB.29, GB.30, GB.31, GB.33, GB.34
GB.30, GB.34, GB.39, GB.40
GB.30, BL.36, BL.37, BL.40, BL.60
GB.30, zuǒ gǔ, BL.36, BL.55, BL.57, BL.59

It can be combined with GB.34, GB.41, SP.6 and SP.9 for arthritis and hip pain from Damp Heat. It can be combined with GB.20, GB.21, GB.24, GB.27, SP.6 and TE.6 for Stagnant Liver Qi and Hyperactive Liver Yang

with pains down one side of the body from head to hip. For hip pain and sciatica from vertebral problems, GB.30 can be combined with Governor jiā jǐ and Bladder points at the level of the spinal lesion. For hip and sacral pain, GB.30 can be combined with BL.30, 31, 32, 33, 34 or 54.

GB.29, 31, 32, 33, 34, 39, 40, 41

Points can be selected from this group, for local pain in sciatica, to combine with GB.30. GB.34 has the general effect of relaxing the tendons, GB.39 nourishes the marrow, and GB.40, as the Source point tonifies the Gallbladder channel. GB.41, like GB.34, can be used to clear Damp Heat, and in combination with TE.5, can control the whole of the sides of the body.

Huán zhōng and zuǒ gǔ

Huán zhōng is midway between GB.30 and GV.2; zuǒ gǔ is one unit below the midpoint between the greater trochanter and the coccyx. Both can be needled perpendicularly to a depth of 1.5–2.5 units for sciatica, and combined with BL.37 and GB.34.

BL.36–60

One or more of these points can be combined with GB.30, jiā jǐ or sacral points, to treat sciatica. BL.58 is a distal point for pain on both Bladder and Gallbladder channels. BL.59 is the Accumulation point of the Yang Heel channel and can be used for pain in the lower back, hips and legs, with inability to stand. BL.60, the Fire point, can be used for pain on any part of the Bladder channel, from head to foot.

ST.31, ST.36, ST.41

ST.31 is especially for pain in groin and thigh, and can be combined with GB.30 if the pain is radiating from the hip. ST.36 is for problems of weakness, atrophy, stiffness or pain anywhere on the leg on the Stomach channel. ST.41 is more for problems of the lower leg and ankle. ST.31, 36 and 41 can be combined together with GB.30 for hip and leg pain.

Neck syndromes

Problems of the occipital and lateral neck area overlap with those of the back, shoulders and head, which are dealt with in separate sections. Arthritis also is discussed separately.

AETIOLOGY

The aetiology of neck problems is almost identical to the aetiology of the back syndromes. Where pain in the back, especially involving spinal nerves, frequently radiates through the hips and legs, neck pain may radiate through the shoulder area down into the arms and hands. While the Kidneys are the primary system involved in back problems, and the Liver is secondary, the Liver–Gallbladder system is of primary importance in the neck. Liver syndromes, such as Stagnant Liver Qi and Hyperactive Liver Yang, can be associated with stiff neck and shoulders with headache or migraine. In addition, the neck area is especially susceptible to invasion by Wind Cold, particularly when there are predisposing factors such as Deficient Kidney Qi or Stagnant Qi from previous injury or emotional stress.

The main channels involved are Governor, Bladder, Gallbladder, and secondarily Triple Energizer and Small Intestine.

SYNDROMES

Acute
Trauma
Wind Cold invasion
Chronic
Chronic diseases
Stagnant Liver Qi
Deficient Kidneys

TRAUMA

Trauma includes sprains, injury from falls, whiplash injuries and sequelae of neck surgery. It may involve muscles, tendons and bones, and when there is pressure on a cervical spinal nerve, there may be pain, numbness or tingling radiating down the arms into the hands. SI.3 or luò zhěn can be used as distal points with patient movement, as a preliminary to treatment of neck sprain, similar to the use of yāo tòng diǎn for back sprain.

WIND COLD INVASION

Wind and Cold may cause acute stiff neck, and they may also contribute chronic neck pain and stiffness from arthritis or sequelae of trauma, especially when Defensive Qi is low. In addition to local or adjacent points to disperse Wind (for example, GV.14, 15, 16, GB.20, BL.10, 11, 12), distal points (such as LI.4, SI.3, TE.5, GB.39, BL.62, BL.64, BL.65, BL.66, BL.67) can also be used to clear Exterior factors.

CHRONIC DISEASES

Diseases such as arthritis, spondylitis and osteoporosis may have associated chronic pain and stiffness of the neck. These patterns may be aggravated by Wind invasion emotional stress, and Kidney Deficiency. Local points are combined with distal points that are selected for:

pathogenic factors

Wind Cold	SI.3, BL.62 E M
Wind Heat	TE.5, GB.39 Rd
Heat	LI.4, LI.11 Rd
Damp	SP.3, SP.9 Rd M
Damp Heat	SP.6, GB.39 Rd

emotional stress

Kidney fear	KI.6 Rf; BL.62 Rd
Kidney–Heart nervous anxiety	KI.6 Rf; HT.6 Rd
Liver suppressed anger and impatience	SP.6, GB.21, GB.34 Rd

Kidney Deficiency

Deficient Kidney Jing	SI.3, KI.3, BL.62, GB.39 Rf
Deficient Kidney Yang with Cold	GV.4, KI.2, KI.7, BL.23, BL.60 Rf M
Deficient Kidney Yin with inflammation	BL.33, KI.6, SP.6 Rf; KI.2 Rd

STAGNANT LIVER QI

This may occur, together with Hyperactive Liver Yang, as a chronic condition with periodic aggravations that are related to peaks of emotional stress or to Wind invasion. Neck pain and stiffness often occur together with stiff shoulder muscles and headache. Local points such as TE.15, TE.16, GB.20 and GB.21, can be combined with such distal points as TE.5, PC.6, GB.34, GB.40, LR.3 and SP.6 to move Stagnant Liver Qi and calm Hyperactive Liver Yang.

DEFICIENT KIDNEYS

Deficient Kidney Jing contributes to neck problems in the elderly, and points such as GV.4, SI.3, BL.11, BL.23, BL.52, BL.6 and GB.37, can be used to tonify Jing, along with SP.6, and ST.36 to provide energy for the Kidneys to store. Deficient Kidney Yang is often associated with easy invasions of Wind into the neck and retention of Cold in the muscles. GV.4, GV.14, GV.16, GV.20, BL.10, BL.11, BL.12, BL.23, BL.60 and SI.3 can all be used with Reinforcing method and moxa to strengthen Kidney Yang and the Qi in the neck channels, to drive out Cold and Damp.

Deficient Kidney Yin may be associated with arthritis with inflammation and signs of Heat, which can be aggravated by lack of sleep, coffee and emotional stress. Points such as CV.4, BL.23, SP.6, ST.36, KI.3 and KI.6 to nourish Yin, may need to be combined with points such as ST.44, SP.1, KI.2, or HT.8 to disperse Deficiency Fire, where present.

POINTS FOR NECK SYNDROMES

Point combinations for neck syndromes are shown in Table 27.2.

DISTAL POINTS USED WITH PATIENT MOVEMENT

In cases of neck sprain or invasion of Wind Cold with stiff neck, SI.3 or luò zhĕn can be manipulated on the affected side while the patient repeatedly moves the neck into the position of greatest pain and restriction. The details of this method are the same as for yāo tòng diăn for back sprain on page 363. This method is done as the first stage of treatment, and is followed by the use of local points with Reducing method, moxa and massage.

AH SHI POINTS

Ah Shi points on or off the channels, in the neck area, can be used with needle and moxa for all neck syndromes, where appropriate. Ah Shi points both off the channels, in the muscles, and on the Governor, Bladder, Small Intestine and Gallbladder channels can be used, combined with distal points on the channels.

HUÁ TUÓ JIĀ JĬ POINTS

Huá tuó jiā jĭ points are especially useful to treat pressure on or inflammation of the cervical spinal nerves. These points are 0.5–1 unit lateral to the lower end of the spinous process of the vertebra. In the cervical region they can be inserted vertically, pointed slightly toward the spine, to a depth of 1.5 units. On patients with thicker neck muscles, 2 units may be necessary. There should be a definite needle sensation. The points are especially helpful when there is pressure on a spinal nerve due to trauma or degenerative disease.

Table 27.2 Neck syndromes

Syndrome	Signs and symptoms	Pulse	Tongue	Point combination
Trauma	acute neck pain and stiffness following trauma, maybe pain or numbness radiating into arms	wiry	various	first SI.3 or luò zhĕn Rd with patient movement, then local points Rd M, eg. Ah Shi, jiā jĭ, BL.10, GB.21
Wind Cold Invasion	acute neck pain and stiffness following exposure to wind and cold, especially when body resistance is low	wiry, maybe empty	maybe pale	local points, eg. GV.14, GV.15, GV.16, BL.10, BL.11, BL.12 or GB.20 Rd M, with distal points, e.g. LI.4, SI.3, BL.62 Rd
Chronic diseases	chronic neck problems from diseases such as arthritis, spondylitis, osteoporosis	wiry, maybe empty or thin, slow or rapid	maybe thin or flabby	local points, especially. jiā jĭ, distal points, e.g. BL.62 and SI.3 Rf to strengthen spine + GV.14, LI.4, SP.6, SP.9 Rd for arthritis with Damp Heat + GV.12, GV.14, GV.16, BL.10, BL.11, SI.15 for ankylosing spondylitis
Stagnant Liver Qi and Hyperactive Liver Yang	chronic neck stiffness and pain with acute aggravations from emotional stress, maybe stiff shoulder muscles and headaches	wiry or hindered, maybe full or empty, slow or rapid	maybe purple or red especially at edges	local points, eg. TE.15, TE.17, GB.21 Rd, with distal points eg. GV.20, TE.5, GB.34, GB.40, PC.6, LR.3, SP.6 Rd
Deficient Kidney	chronic neck problems, worse with tiredness, maybe with weak lower back, tinnitus or urinary frequency	empty or thin, choppy, maybe deep or slow	flabby	GV.14, GV.16, BL.10, BL.33, BL.64, KI.3, ST.36 Rf + BL.11, GB.39 for Deficient Kidney Jing + GV.4, GV.20, KI.7 Rf M for Deficient Kidney Yang + SP.6, KI.6 Rf for Deficient Kidney Yin + KI.2, HT.8 Rd for Deficiency Fire

Rd, Reducing method; Rf, Reinforcing method; M, moxa.

OTHER LOCAL POINTS

Apart from the jiā jǐ points, the main local points are GB.20, GB.21, TE.15 and TE.16 for lateral neck problems and GV.14, GV.15, GV.16, BL.10, BL.11, BL.12 and SI.15 for posterior neck problems.

DISTAL POINTS

Distal points are usually selected on the same channels as the local points used. Chains of points on the Small Intestine, Triple Energizer or Large Intestine channels may be used when there is pain or numbness down the arms as a result of pressure on a cervical nerve; the key points are SI.3, TE.5 and LI.4 respectively. BL.62, BL.64, BL.65, BL.66 and BL.67 can all be used for posterior neck problems, the most important being BL.62, since in combination with SI.3 it links the Governor, Bladder and Small Intestine channels. GB.34, GV.39 and GV.40 can all be used for lateral neck problems. GB.34 and GB.40 are mainly for tension in the neck muscles from Liver–Gallbladder Stagnation; GB.39 can both disperse Exterior Wind and strengthen the bones; and GB.40 is a point for general lateral neck stiffness. Where pain or numbness extends down into one or both arms, chains of points on the nearest channel to the path of the pain can be used, e.g. LI.4, LI.10, LI.16 or SI.3, SI.6, SI.8, SI.15.

Shoulder syndromes

Problems of the shoulder joint and the muscles of the shoulder area may relate to trauma, invasion by Wind Cold or Damp, chronic disease, Stagnant Liver Qi, and general Deficiency of Qi and Blood. Problems of the shoulder can be classified according to the channel affected, Lungs, Large Intestine, Triple Energizer or Small Intestine. Both local and distal points may be used on the affected channel, in addition to one or more points on the channel to which it is paired in the Six Divisions. For example, Large Intestine is paired to Stomach in the Bright Yang Stage of the Six Divisions, so that ST.38 can be added to LI.15. Also, two Extra channel relationships

may be used, TE.5 + GB.41 for shoulder arthritis with Damp Heat and lateral shoulder pain, or SI.3 + BL.62 for pain in posterior shoulder and upper back and neck from sprain, chronic disease or Wind Cold.

POINT COMBINATIONS

The first step is to ask the patient to move the arm in the direction of difficulty, to find the point of greatest pain, to determine the points and channels to be used. For example, if a location above jiān nèi líng is the most painful, it can be used as an Ah Shi point, jiān nèi líng as an adjacent point, LI.15 as the nearest local channel point, and LI.4 as a distal point.

DISTAL POINTS USED WITH PATIENT MOVEMENT

The most common point is ST.38, used according to the instructions for such points, on page 363. This is done as the first stage of the treatment, and can be followed, in the same treatment, by moxa and needle on local points. It can be effective not only for acute shoulder sprain, so-called 'frozen shoulder', but also, in some cases, for chronic shoulder restriction.

LOCAL AND DISTAL POINTS

In addition to Ah Shi points on and off the channels, local and distal channel points can be selected on the affected channel, as shown on Table 27.3.

EXTRA POINTS

Two important Extra points are jiān nèi líng and naò shàng.

jiān nèi líng

Midway between the top of the anterior axillary crease and LI.15, this point can be used for problems of the shoulder joint. The needle can be inserted perpendicu-

Table 27.3 Point combinations for shoulder syndromes

Channel	Shoulder	Shoulder and upper back	Neck	Distal	Paired channel
LU	LU.1, 2	–	–	LU.7	–
LI	LI.14, 15, 16	–	LI.17, 18	LI.4, 10, 11	ST.38
TE	TE.13, 14	TE.15	TE.16	TE.4, 5, 6	GB.34, 40, 41
SI	SI.9, 10	SI.11, 12, 13, 14, 15	–	SI.3, 6	BL.62
GB	–	GB.21	GB.20	GB.34, 40, 41	TE.4, 5, 15

larly 1–1.5 units to obtain needle sensation. If required the needle can then be lifted until just below the skin surface and reangled upwards at 45 degrees, to obtain needle sensation again. This point can be combined with LI.11 and TE.14 for shoulder problems.

naò shàng

This is an Extra point on the Large Intestine channel, in the middle of the deltoid muscle. It can be used for shoulder problems, and in combination with LI.4, LI.11, LI.15 and SI.9 for hemiplegia.

ADDITIONAL POINTS FOR RHEUMATOID ARTHRITIS

When shoulder problems occur in rheumatoid arthritis, in addition to local and distal arm points for shoulder problems, other points can be selected for arthritis. For example:

LI.4, ST.37, ST.44 Rd	for Heat in Stomach and Intestines
KI.2 Rd; KI.6, SP.6 Rf	for Deficiency Fire
TE.5, GB.34, GB.43 Rd	for Damp Heat in Liver–Gallbladder.

Arthritis syndromes

This section discusses those chronic problems of pain or loss of mobility in one or more joints, referred to as Bi syndromes in Chinese medicine. These problems can be roughly divided into two main groups. In osteoarthritis and related conditions, one or more joints may be involved, and the symptoms are confined to the affected joints. In systemic inflammatory conditions such as rheumatoid arthritis, a number of joints are affected, and in addition, there may be general signs such as weakness and low energy.

AETIOLOGY

OSTEOARTHRITIS

Osteoarthritis may be facilitated in joints that have been subjected to abnormal stresses, such as injury, excessive use, faulty posture, or excessive load-bearing as in obesity.

RHEUMATOID ARTHRITIS

Rheumatoid arthritis sufferers may inherit a physiological and psychological tendency to react to life stresses by the development of this particular syndrome. The condition may be aggravated by climatic factors, such as Wind, Cold, Damp, or Summer Heat, by emotional factors such as suppressed anger or grief, and by lifestyle factors such as diet or tiredness from overwork and lack of sleep. They may have feelings of guilt concerning the anger, and adopt a nice, pleasant caring manner. It is the internalization of the anger that results in the inflammation.

PERSONALITY TYPE

It may be that some rheumatoid arthritics have a personality type that includes the suppression of irritation and anger, and the inability to face their own aggression or to express it to the person with whom they have difficulty. The patient may feel trapped in close relationships with other people who are either more dominant and manipulative, or whose physical and emotional needs make them dependent upon the patient. In developing rheumatoid arthritis, the patient may become dependent on them in turn, and become immobilized both by their physical illness and their inability to express their anger and resentment.

This personality type relates to the balance between Liver and Spleen. The Spleen represents the worry and overconcern for others, and the unselfish, self-sacrificing pleasant personality. The Liver represents suppressed anger and resentment and the seemingly nasty, selfish unpleasant aspect of the personality, that the patient can't accept. However, the Liver also represents movement, independence and freedom, while the Spleen in this case represents stagnation, dependence and restriction. While this personality conflict remains unresolved, both Heat and Damp can be produced, with resulting inflammation.

DEFICIENT QI AND BLOOD

There is usually a background of Deficient Qi and Blood in rheumatoid arthritis, often aggravated by long-term steroid treatment, which increases Kidney Deficiency and further weakens the Defensive Qi. Also, continued use of anti-inflammatories may aggravate the existing condition of Deficient Blood, by causing gastric bleeding.

DEFICIENT YIN AND DEFICIENT YANG

Patients with both osteoarthritis and rheumatoid arthritis

tend to Deficient Kidney Qi, with symptoms of tiredness and low reserves of energy. This may manifest more as Deficient Yang, with cold extremities and depression, or more as Deficient Yin with restless anxiety and signs of Heat. There may be a mixture of Deficient Yin and Deficient Yang, with cold extremities but hot swollen joints. Deficient Heat signs are more common in rheumatoid arthritis, while signs of Damp are common in both types of arthritis.

TREATMENT OF OSTEOARTHRITIS

Treatment of osteoarthritis is primarily by the use of local points on and around the affected joint. Even method is often used with moxa to remove Cold and Damp. Bleeding can be used for heat and swelling. Treatment to strengthen Qi, Blood or Yang, and to reduce weight is done where necessary.

Example

An obese woman of 55 has osteoarthritis of the left knee, with pain and stiffness aggravated by tiredness, standing, Damp and Cold, and improved by warmth and rest.

ST.35 and ST.36 were chosen as local points, with ST.34 and ST.41 as distal points, and Ah Shi points in the painful area; all with Even method and moxa. In addition, CV.4 was combined with SP.4 bilaterally, with Reinforcing method and moxa, to raise metabolic rate to give energy and to help the patient lose weight. A nourishing but weight-reducing diet was recommended.

TREATMENT OF RHEUMATOID ARTHRITIS

Treatment has three aspects:

local points for affected joints
distal points for underlying causes
Back Transporting points for Deficiency and other factors.

LOCAL POINTS FOR AFFECTED JOINTS

Swollen joints can be tapped with plum blossom needles to produce slight bleeding, or points such as sì fèng or LU.5 and PC.3 can be bled to relieve local joint pain and immobility. The most tender points in tendons and muscles can be needled, either by deep insertion into the tendon, or by needling of the tender point in the muscle while the patient moves the limb, where this is possible.

DISTAL POINTS FOR UNDERLYING CAUSES

LIVER

Liver and Gallbladder points can be used to treat suppressed anger and resentment, and the Stagnation Heat and Damp Heat associated with these emotions:

Liver Fire   LR.2, GB.38 Rd
Stagnant Liver Qi   LR.2, GB.34, PC.6, TE.6 Rd
Liver–Gallbladder   LR.5, GB.34, GB.41 Rd.
Damp Heat

SPLEEN

Spleen, Stomach and Large Intestine points can be used to treat worry and overconcern, reactions to food and drink, general Deficiency, and the gastric side-effects of anti-inflammatory medicines:

worry   GV.20, SP.1, SP.2, yìn táng Rd
Stomach Fire   ST.21, ST.44, PC.3 Rd
Heat in Stomach   LI.4, LI.11, ST.37, ST.44 Rd
and Intestines
Deficient Stomach Yin   ST.44 Rd; SP.6, ST.36 Rf
Damp and Damp Heat   CV.6 E; SP.6, SP.9 Rd
Deficient Qi and Blood   SP.6, SP.10, ST.36 Rf.

HEART

Heart anxiety can be associated with Deficient Kidney Yin and Deficient Spleen Blood. One combination is GV.20, CV.14, PC.6 Rd; CV.4, SP.4, ST.36 Rf. Alternatively, HT.3, HT.7 and HT.8 can be used with Reducing method.

KIDNEY

CV.4 and KI.3 can be reinforced for Deficient Kidney Qi and KI.6 for Deficient Kidney Yin. KI.2 can be reduced for Deficiency Fire.

LUNGS

LU.7 and CV.17 can be reduced when the condition is aggravated by suppressed grief.

EXTERNAL FACTORS

GV.14, LI.11 and PC.9 can be reduced for aggravation by Summer Heat; GV.14, BL.11, TE.5 and LI.4 reduced for

Wind Cold or Wind Heat; and TE.6, SP.6, SP.9 reduced for Damp.

BACK POINTS FOR DEFICIENCY AND OTHER FACTORS

BL.23 can be reinforced for Deficient Kidneys, and BL.20 for Deficient Blood. BL.18 can be used with Even or Reducing method to regulate the Liver, and BL.27 can be reduced to clear Heat in the Intestines. GV.14 can be reduced to clear Heat, and GV.12, 11 and 8 reduced to regulate the emotions of Lungs, Heart and Liver respectively. SI.11 can be reduced by inserting the needle in different directions, for a wide radiation of needle sensation to treat problems of the arms. BL.40 can be bled or reduced to clear Heat and Damp Heat.

SUMMARY

First a selection of local points are used, with the patient sitting or lying on their back. Then the distal points on the limbs and front of the body are inserted and left for about 20 minutes, with occasional manipulation if required. Then these needles are removed, the patient lies on their front, and a selection of back points is inserted.

Example

A woman of 45 with rheumatoid arthritis, especially in the fingers and elbows, was first treated in a sitting position. The following local points were bled: PC.3, LU.5 and the sì fèng points on the second and third fingers of each hand. Since she had a recent aggravation due to excessive consumption of spicy food, LI.4, LI.11, ST.37, and ST.44 were reduced to clear Heat in the Stomach and Intestines. After 15 minutes, these needles were removed and the patient lay on her front. BL.20 and BL.23 were reinforced to counteract chronic Deficient Blood and Deficient Kidneys. GV.14, BL.27 and BL.40 were reduced to clear Heat in the Stomach and Intestines, and BL.18 and BL.47 were reduced to disperse suppressed anger. The needles were removed after 10 minutes.

Hemiplegia

Hemiplegia refers here to sequelae of cerebrovascular accident (CVA), the Windstroke of Chinese medicine. The author's experience is mainly of patients coming for treatment for hemiplegia 3 months or more after their cerebrovascular accident. Discussion will be limited to this category of patient, and for a fuller account of the different stages of CVA and sequelae, the reader is recommended to the article by Dr Sheng Canruo, *Journal of Chinese Medicine*, **22**, 1986.

AETIOLOGY AND SYNDROMES

CHINESE MEDICINE

In Chinese medicine, Windstoke is said to relate to four main factors:

Deficient Kidney Yin
Heart Fire
Liver Fire, Yang and Wind
Phlegm.

DEFICIENT KIDNEY YIN

If Kidney Yin becomes Deficient, through stress, overwork, etc., then Fire and Yang may not be properly controlled and rise up in the body.

HEART FIRE

If there is a pattern of long-term overexcitement and stressful overstimulation of the Heart Spirit, or if there is chronic Stagnation of Heart Qi, then Heart Fire may develop.

LIVER FIRE, YANG AND WIND

Liver Fire and Hyperactive Yang may arise from either chronic Deficient Kidney Yin or chronic Stagnation of Liver Qi. The disturbed movement of Liver Fire and Yang up the body is termed Liver Wind.

PHLEGM

If there is Deficiency or Stagnation of Spleen and Stomach Qi, the Damp and Phlegm may accumulate. If the obstructing effect of Phlegm combines with the disturbing effect of Liver Wind, and these two factors affect the brain, then Windstroke is possible.

Obviously, aspects of lifestyle such as stress, overwork, tobacco, alcohol and overconsumption of greasy, spicy food are likely to aggravate these four main factors and predispose to Windstroke.

PSYCHOLOGICAL FACTORS

The psychological stresses, predisposing to Windstroke arise primarily from the Liver, Kidney and Heart systems.

LIVER

Many Liver types continually generate stress by their tense, hasty and impatient style of work and life. Also, they easily feel obstructed and blocked, which in them generates frustration and anger. However, it is not only the Yang Liver types, with their externally expressed explosive anger, that are at risk, it can also be the Yin Liver types who internalize their anger, whilst presenting a pleasant or submissive face to the world.

KIDNEY

Much of this anger may arise from fear, especially the fear of losing control. For example, a domineering person may only feel safe if they have their own way in everything, or they may feel threatened and generate great anger. Another person, feeling themselves barely in control in a work situation, may feel threatened by change or by the pressures of increased responsibility. An older person might fear the loss of the ability to look after themselves, and fear being physically and emotionally dependent on others. Each of these individuals do not trust life or other people, and the pressure of their fear, frustration and resentment, may predispose them to Windstroke.

HEART

The chronically stressful, anxious, hyperactive, overexcited or even manic state of Yang Heart-type people may result in hypertension and predispose to CVA, especially if there is Phlegm in addition to Heart Fire.

It is important to have a clear understanding of the originating factors, in order to give the advice on lifestyle that can assist recovery and reduce chances of a further stroke.

TREATMENT

HEMIPLEGIA

Treatment here refers to patients who have not come for acupuncture until more than 3 months after their CVA. Points to treat muscle spasm or atrophy are used on the affected side, selected from such as the following:

GB.21, LI.15, TE.14, PC.2, LI.11, LI.10, TE.5, PC.7, LI.4, LI.3, SI.3, bā xié, GB.29, GB.30, GB.31, ST.32, BL.40, ST.36, GB.34, BL.57, GB.39, ST.41, LR.4, SP.5.

Especially important can be LI.10, PC.2, PC.3, ST.36 and GB.30. Points are mainly chosen from the Yang channels, but it is important to include one or more points from the Yin channels to maintain Yin–Yang balance.

MUSCULAR ATROPHY

If this is marked, LI.10 and ST.36 should be included in the combination, and used bilaterally, with additional points to tonify Spleen Qi as required, such as CV.12 and BL.20.

FACIAL PARALYSIS

LI.4 and ST.44 can be chosen as distal points and reduced bilaterally. Local points can be selected from GV.26, CV.24, ST.5, ST.6, SI.18, LI.20, GB.14 and BL.2, and used with Reinforcing method and moxa stick on the affected side.

SPEECH DIFFICULTIES

The main points are CV.23, TE.1 and HT.5 used with Even method. Scalp acupuncture may also be helpful.

TREATING THE UNDERLYING CAUSES

It is especially important to regulate the Liver, to relieve Stagnation of Liver Qi and to control Hyperactive Yang, if these are present. LR.3 and GB.20 can be used bilaterally with Reducing method if there is suppressed anger, impatience or dizziness, high blood pressure, wiry pulse, or other Liver signs. If there is Heart Fire, PC.3, the Water point, can be included in the treatment with Even or Reducing method. KI.6 with Reinforcing method can strengthen Kidney Yin and relieve fear. Both these points can be used bilaterally.

Example

A man of 50 came for treatment of hemiplegia 6 months after his CVA. He had been a very active and busy man, was very keen to exercise and help himself, but impatient and frustrated by the slow rate of recovery. Stagnant Liver Qi, Hyperactive Liver Yang and Heart Fire were diagnosed as the main underlying factors.

LR.3 and GB.20 with Reducing method were used bilaterally

to regulate the Liver, and PC.3 was used with Even method on the affected side to calm Heart Fire. In addition the following points were used with Even method on the affected side to treat the hemiplegia: PC.2, LI.10, LI.4, bā xié between third and fourth fingers, GB.30, ST.36, SP.5. Moxa stick was applied to LI.10 and ST.36. Progress was slow but definite, and at one stage was assisted by needling with Reducing method into the tense spinal muscles, to a depth of 0.5–0.8 units, in the area of BL.20–BL.22.

Qi Gong exercises, vizualizing inhaling to the Dan Tian centre and exhaling through the affected arm or leg were given to combine with physical exercises. Relaxation exercises were also given to help the basic pattern of overenthusiasm followed by impatience and frustration that was interfering with his progress.

Multiple sclerosis

Multiple sclerosis (MS), sometimes known as disseminated sclerosis, is the commonest of the demyelinating disorders. It mostly occurs between the ages of 20 and 40, beginning with weakness, most prominent in the legs, often with increasing disability. There may be visual disorders, vertigo, urinary and bowel problems, and the disease is often characterized by an alternation of remission and relapse.

AETIOLOGY

WESTERN MEDICINE

In Western medicine, the cause of MS is uncertain. There may be an inherited tendency, and the initial attack and major remissions may be preceded by infections such as influenza.

CHINESE MEDICINE

In Chinese medicine, MS is not well described, and could be included under the Wei syndrome group. In the initial stage of Wei syndrome, treatment may aim at clearing Wind Heat or Damp Heat, and in the later chronic stages, in tonifying Deficiency. In the opinion of the author, this problem is primarily linked to Kidney Deficiency, since the Kidneys govern the development and maintenance of the nervous system.

PERSONALITY TYPE

It is the author's opinion that some cases of multiple sclerosis relate to the Yin Kidney-type personality. The Kidneys are associated not only with the development of the nervous system and the strength of physical constitution, but also with the physiological and psychological development, especially at the main stages of the life cycle.

The Yin Kidney-type may lack the stamina and strength of character needed to make a developmental change. In this case, they may have deep feelings of inadequacy and lack the strength to enter fully into the world of adult responsibilities. They may feel overpowered or overwhelmed by either the prospect of adult responsibilities, increase in responsibilities, or the long-term continuation of responsibilities. They may feel fear of lack of capacity, or fear of failing in responsibilities. The tendency of the Yin Kidney-type is to give up, to let go of control, to surrender, and in this case retreat from the challenges of the adult world, into the dependent world of childhood. In MS, the incapacity of the body can make the patient greatly dependent on others.

The author would like to emphasize that although there may be a tendency to this personality type, there are many MS patients whose character is quite different.

TREATMENT

This is a disorder of the brain and spinal cord, in which both symptoms and points used will much depend on which of the spinal segments are affected. Governor, jiā jǐ, and inner Bladder channel points can be used in the affected spinal segment. BL.62 and SI.3 can be combined to strengthen the Governor channel and the brain and spinal cord. BL.23 and KI.6 can be added to this combination to strengthen the Kidneys. GB.20 and GV.16 can be added for visual disorders; BL.20 can be added for Spleen Deficiency with Deficient Blood and Damp; and BL.31, 32 or 33 can be used for urinary or bowel problems. GB.30, BL.40 and BL.57 can be added for weakness of the legs, while GV.14, LI.4 and LI.11 can be added for weakness of the arms. All points are used with Reinforcing method.

ALTERNATION

These points on the back can be alternated, in a separate treatment, with points on the front of the body. For example, CV.6 to strengthen the Kidneys and resolve Damp, CV.3 for urinary problems, CV.12 to strengthen the Spleen, ST.36 to tonify Qi and Blood, SP.6 and SP.9 to relieve Damp. All points are used with Reinforcing or Even method.

INITIAL ATTACK OR SEVERE RELAPSE

If initial attack or a severe relapse are associated with symptoms of Wind Heat, Heat, Damp Heat, or Damp, with rapid or slippery pulse, points can be used with Even or Reducing method until these symptoms are gone and the patient either recovers, or returns to the chronic Deficiency state. Points such as GV.14, TE.5 and LI.4 can be used for Wind Heat; GV.14, LI.4 and LI.11 for Heat; and LI.10, SP.6 and SP.9 for Damp and Damp Heat.

Digestive syndromes 28

Gastric syndromes

The gastric disorders discussed in this section include epigastric pain, discomfort or distension; sensations of heat, cold, emptiness, fullness or heaviness in the epigastrium, and nausea, vomiting, belching and hiccup.

Food allergies and disorders of eating and weight are discussed in separate sections, and although abdominal distension may accompany gastric disorders, it is not discussed here, but in the section on irritable bowel syndrome.

THE ORGAN SYSTEMS

SP
|
ST
|
Intestines

The digestive system is concerned with the transformation by the Spleen of the food and drink held in the Stomach into pure energy and wastes. The Small Intestine separates the pure from the impure and the Large Intestine eliminates the waste material. All this is dependent on a regular rhythmic flow of energy, and it is the function of the Liver to maintain this free flow.

AETIOLOGY

The two main factors affecting the Stomach and causing gastric disorders, are unwise eating habits and emotional disharmony. Unwise eating habits relate to:

type and amount of food consumed
regularity of eating
emotional state while eating.

The main emotions affecting the Stomach are:

worry	Spleen	Earth
anger	Liver	Wood
fear	Kidneys	Water

WORRY

The Earth element relates to the mother, to the nourishing, enfolding, caring and protection of the mother to the small child. If the child does not get this in solidity and strength, there may be patterns of deep insecurity and worry that last the rest of the life. Worry and fear of never having enough, insecurity about material possessions, the need for oral satisfaction, the need to eat, the need to be fat to feel safe, and the need to hold on to those in close relationship. Chronic worry may affect the gastric secretions, irritate the gastric lining and impair efficiency of digestion and absorption.

ANGER

Impatience, irritability and expressed anger, and suppressed anger and frustration all affect the Stomach. These emotions may result in oversecretion of stomach acid and in the inflammation of the gastric mucosa, or they may stagnate the stomach function, slowing the passage of food through the stomach into the intestines.

Yang effect
  oversecretion of stomach acid with gastric
  inflammation
  impatience, irritability, anger
Yin effect
  stagnation and slowing of the passage of food
  frustration, depression

Liver disharmony may involve both the Yang and Yin effects together, or an alternation between the two. The effects of the Liver on the Stomach can be divided into three main types:

- Liver Fire   Stomach Fire
- Stagnant Liver Qi   Stagnant Stomach Qi
    Excess e.g. Retention of Food
    Deficiency e.g. Stagnant Liver
      Qi and Deficient Spleen Qi

- Hyperactive Liver Yang   Rebellious Stomach Qi

These effects may occur together or convert into each other. For example, Stagnation and Rebellion of Stomach Qi, with distension and nausea.

FEAR

Fear has an immediate effect on the Solar Plexus centre and upon the Stomach. Fear may come in various combinations, requiring different point combinations:

fear and anxiety	Kidneys and Heart	CV.14, SP.4, PC.6 E
fear, worry and insecurity	Kidneys and Spleen	CV.14 E; KI.3, SP.3 Rf
fear and anger	Kidneys and Liver	CV.14, LR.2 E; KI.6 Rf

OTHER EMOTIONS

Depression may come not only from the Liver but also from Stagnation of the Qi of Heart or Lungs. However, it is the Liver that has the main effect upon the Stomach.

COMBINATIONS OF EMOTIONS

Where two or more emotions occur together, the emphasis of treatment is on the dominant emotion. For example, in a combination of anger and worry:

anger dominant   LR.1, LR.2, SP.6 Rd
worry dominant   CV.12, LR.13, SP.3 Rd.

SYNDROMES

Stagnant Stomach Qi
Retention of food
Rebellious Stomach Qi
Stagnant Stomach Blood
Stomach Fire
Deficient Stomach Yin
Fear and anxiety invade Stomach
Cold invades Stomach
Deficient Stomach and Spleen Qi
Deficient Stomach and Spleen Yang
Phlegm and Damp in Stomach

The syndromes are often found in combination with each other and are related as shown in Figure 28.1.

TREATMENT

Point combinations for the gastric syndromes are summarized in Table 28.1. Gastric syndromes are often found together in the clinic, as shown in the following example.

Example

A man of 30 had chronic gastric discomfort with epigastric and abdominal distension and belching. He occasionally had a burning sensation in the epigastrium, especially when tired or stressed. His pulse was wiry, thin and sometimes rapid. His tongue was slightly purple, with some red spots in the Stomach area.

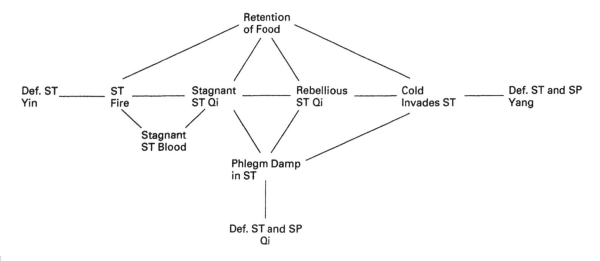

Fig. 28.1

The diagnosis was Stagnant Stomach Qi with some Rebellious Stomach Qi, and occasional Deficient Stomach Yin. The point combination was:

CV.12, PC.6, LR.3, ST.21 Rd; ST.36 Rf

to which SP.6 Rf; ST.44 Rd could be added for Deficient Stomach Yin.

Food allergy syndromes

INTRODUCTION

Allergy is an overreaction, or inappropriate reaction, of the body's defense mechanism to specific chemicals in:

air
food and drink
drugs and medicines
contact with the body surface
pathogenic organisms
the body's own tissues (autoimmune response).

Food allergy affects six main areas:

eyes, nose and throat
lungs
stomach
intestines
skin
joints.

The concept of food allergy is not a part of classical Chinese medicine, so that the organization of the syndromes in this section and the point combinations given for them, is based on the author's clinical experience, and not on Chinese texts.

ALLERGY AND INTOLERANCE

The immunological response involves the production of antibodies to inactivate antigens. The antigens of the allergic response, called allergens, are either proteins or chemicals which can bond to a protein, inducing the antibody response. Some of the body's adverse reaction to chemicals in food take place without the formation of antibodies, and these can be called food intolerances, to distinguish them from true allergic responses.

However, there is not always a clear division between allergy and intolerance, and indeed the two reactions may occur together to the same foodstuff. For example, the body may have an intolerance to the alcohol in red wine, and also an allergic reaction to some of the other chemicals contained in it. Therefore, in this section, the word allergy has been used very loosely to include both allergic and intolerance responses.

YIN AND YANG ALLERGIC RESPONSES

The allergy response may be roughly divided into Yin and Yang types.

YIN TYPE

The Yin type of allergic response may be associated with Deficient Qi, and is generally of slower onset, worse with tiredness, and with signs of Cold and Damp, rather than signs of Heat. It may be associated with Deficient Qi and Yang of Kidney, Lungs and Spleen. For example, the chronic diarrhoea of gluten allergy, or the chronic eczema associated with allergy to cow's milk products.

Table 28.1 Gastric disorders

Syndrome	Signs and symptoms	Pulse	Tongue	Point combination
Stagnant Stomach and Liver Qi	distending pain of epigastrium, hypogastrium or abdomen, worse with depression and frustration, sour belching, maybe headache	hindered or wiry, maybe slippery	maybe purplish	CV.12, PC.6, LR.3, LR.14 Rd + ST.36 Rf for Deficient Spleen Qi + GB.20, GB.34 Rd for headache + CV.17, LU.7 for Stagnant Lung Qi
Retention of food	no appetite, prolonged feeling of fullness in epigastrium related to excess or irregular eating, eating in a hurry or when upset	full or flooding, slippery, maybe wiry, maybe rapid or slow	thick greasy cost, maybe yellow or white	CV.10, CV.13, SP.4, PC.6, LI.10 Rd + ST.44, ST.45 for Heat + M on CV.10 and CV.13 for Cold invades Stomach ST.36 Rf M for Deficient Spleen Yang
Rebellious Stomach Qi	nausea, vomiting, belching, hiccup, epigastric discomfort	maybe wiry, rapid or slow	various	CV.10, CV.14, SP.4, PC.6 Rd + ST.36 Rf for Deficient Spleen Qi + GB.34 Rd for Hyperactive Liver Yang
Stagnant Stomach Blood	severe stabbing pain in epigastrium, maybe worse after eating, maybe blood in vomit or stools	wiry, maybe full or choppy	purple or purple spots	CV.12, ST.21, ST.36, SP.4, PC.6 Rd alternate with BL.17, BL.18, BL.21 Rd
Stomach Fire	burning sensation and pain in epigastrium, thirst, constant hunger, constipation, bad breath	rapid, full, maybe wiry or slippery	red, dry, yellow coat	CV.12, ST.21, ST.44, PC.8 Rd; ST.45 B; SP.6 Rf + LR.1, LR.2 Rd for Liver Fire + PC.3 Rd for Heart Fire + ST.37, LI.11 for constipation + LR.1, SP.1 B for gastric bleeding
Deficient Stomach Yin	epigastric discomfort and maybe buring sensation, patient is tired but restless	rapid, thin	red, maybe no coat, dry	CV.12, ST.36, SP.6, Rf; ST.44 Rd + CV.4, KI.6 Rf for Deficient Kidney Yin + yìn táng, ān mián for worry and insomnia
Fear and anxiety invades Stomach	epigastric pain and discomfort, nausea or loss of appetite aggravated by fear and anxiety, maybe insomnia and fear of places and people	maybe moving or irregular, empty or choppy	maybe trembling	CV.4, ST.36 Rf; CV.14, SP.4, PC.6 Rd or E alternate with BL.15, BL.21, BL.23 E
Cold invades Stomach	sudden epigastric pain and feeling of cold, usually following excess intake of cold food and drinks, preference for warmth and warm drinks	deep, slow, maybe flooding or tight	thick white coat	CV.10, CV.13, ST.21, ST.36, SP.4 Rd M
Deficient Stomach and Spleen Qi	epigastric discomfort worse with tiredness, weak limbs, mental tiredness, difficulty in studying, loose stools, change in appetite, loss of sense of taste	empty, maybe choppy or slippery	pale, flabby, white coat	CV.12, LR.13, ST.36, SP.3, LI.4 Rf M alternate with BL.20, BL.23, BL.49 Rf M + CV.4, KI.3, for Deficient Kidney Qi + SP.1, ST.45 Rf M for mental tiredness
Deficient Spleen and Stomach Qi and Hyperactive Liver Yang	gastritis with faintness, dizziness, mild headache, irritability when patient goes too long between meals	empty, wiry	pale	GV.20, CV.12, GB.34, LR.3 Rd; SP.3, ST.36 Rf
Deficient Stomach and Spleen Yang	epigastric discomfort and coldness, exhaustion and weak limbs, cold limbs, preference for warmth, maybe stomach prolapse or bleeding from Sinking of Spleen Qi	empty, slow deep	pale, swollen moist	CV.12, ST.21, ST.36, SP.2 Rf M; CV.6 M on ginger + CV.8 M on ginger on salt for exhaustion and cold alternate with GV.4, BL.20, BL.21, BL.23 Rf M + GV.20 M for stomach prolapse + SP.1 M for gastric bleeding
Phlegm Damp in Stomach	distension and fullness in epigastrium, heavy sensation in limbs or head, dizziness, mental dullness or confusion, maybe sinus headache	slippery	greasy white coat	CV.6, CV.12 E M; ST.40, SP.9, PC.6, LI.4 Rd + GV.20, GB.20, ST.8 for dizziness and headache + LI.20, ST.2 E for sinusitis

Rd, Reducing method; Rf, Reinforcing method; E, Even method; M, moxa; B, bleeding.

YANG TYPE

The Yang type allergic response may have aspects of Deficient Qi or Deficient Wei Qi, but is especially related to rapid onset attacks with signs of Heat. For example, Wind Heat urticaria, Wind Heat allergic rhinitis associated with pollen allergy, or Stomach Fire gastritis associated with red wine.

AETIOLOGY

Various factors can contribute to the development of allergies in childhood. These include inherited tendency, the health of the parents at conception, the state of the mother during pregnancy, childbirth and breast feeding, the change from breast to bottle, or bottle to solid food, and the emotional pressures that surround the child.

EXTERNAL WIND AND ALLERGIES

External Wind in Chinese medicine can mean exposure to wind or exposure to changing temperatures. It mainly involves the skin and the body surface or the respiratory system. However, it can also relate to food allergies which result in rhinits, asthma or urticaria, when these are associated with sudden onset, and in the case of urticaria, changing location. Therefore, LU.7 and LI.4 can be used in these cases to disperse Exterior Wind, or in the case of urticaria, GB.20, GB.31 and TE.5 can be used with Reducing method.

EMOTIONS AND ALLERGIES

Allergies of the Yin type may be associated with Deficient Qi and tiredness, which may be linked to overwork and stress. Allergies of the Yang type are often aggravated by suppressed excitement or anger, and can be a way of letting off accumulated emotional pressure.

The Heat associated with blocked emotions can be related to Deficient Yin, Stagnant Qi or Fire, which can be of Kidneys, Liver, Stomach and Heart especially.

- Kidneys: the force of the will does not find a suitable outlet, or the struggle of the will against fears.

- Liver: irritation, frustration and anger are unexpressed, and people and situations seem to block creativity and self-expression.

- Stomach: the pressure of worry, insecurity, overconcern and mental congestion.

- Heart: suppressed joy and excitement, or frustration

from inability to express feelings in relationships.

Basic combinations for the emotional component of food allergies can be:

Deficient Yin KI.6, SP.6 Rf
Fire PC.8, ST.44 Rd
Stagnant Qi CV.12, ST.21, PC.6 Rd

These basic combinations can be modified for each organ system:

	Deficient Yin	Fire	Stagnant Qi
KI	+ KI.10 Rf	+ KI.1 Rd	+ KI.8 Rd
LR	+ LR.8 Rf	+ LR.1 B, LR.2 Rd	+ LR.1, LR.3, LR.13 Rd
ST	+ ST.36 Rf	+ ST.45, PC.3 Rd	+ ST.40, ST.45 Rd
HT	+ HT.6 Rf	+ HT.3 Rf, HT.8 Rd	+ CV.17, BL.15 Rd

SYNDROMES

There are eight main food allergy syndromes, which can be divided into two groups:

Yang type (signs of Heat)	Yin type (no signs of Heat)
Wind Heat	Retention of Lung Phlegm
Stomach Fire	Deficient Spleen and Damp
Damp Heat in Intestines	Deficient Qi in Intestines
Liver Fire	
Heart Fire	

TREATMENT

Basic combinations and their modifications are given for each of these eight syndromes in Table 28.2. Syndromes may combine in the clinic as shown in the following example.

Example

A woman of 25 had urticaria and conjunctivitis of rapid onset as a reaction to a variety of foods. She sometimes got headache, restlessness and irritability as reactions to either foods or emotional stress. Her pulse was thin, wiry and rapid, with abnormal strength in the superficial level. Her tongue was thin and slightly red, with red spots along the edges. The diagnosis is of chronic Deficient Liver Yin and Liver Fire, which combines with Wind Heat during acute attacks.

The point combination for the chronic situation can be:

ST.21, ST.44, LR.2 Rd; CV.12, SP.6, KI.6 Rf

During acute attacks of urticaria and conjunctivitis, this can be changed to:

LI.4, TE.5, GB.1, GB.44, ST.44 Rd; SP.6 Rf

Table 28.2 Food allergy syndromes

Syndrome and signs	Pulse	Tongue	Basic combination	Modification	
				Points	Example
External Wind Heat rapid onset, maybe asthma, inflammation of eyes, nose or throat, or urticaria of variable location	superficial rapid or tight	maybe red	LU.7, LI.4, ST.36, ST.44 Rd	+ BL.2 E + LI.20, ST.2 E + SI.17 Rd + GB.20, GB.31 Rd + BL.13, BL.20, BL.23 Rf + LI.11, SP.6, SP.10 Rd	for conjunctivitis for rhinitis for sore throat for urticaria for Deficient Defensive Qi for Heat in the Blood
Stomach Fire Nausea, burning sensation, pain or discomfort in epigastrium, red, hot, itchy rash	rapid, maybe thin or full, wiry or slippery	red, dry yellow coat	CV.13, ST.21, ST.44, PC.3 Rd; SP.6 Rf	+ BL.2, ST.2 E; ST.45 Rd + LI.20, ST.40 Rd + LI.11, ST.25 Rd + LI.11, SP.10 Rd; BL.40 B	for conjunctivitis for sinusitis for constipation for Heat in the Blood eczema
Damp Heat in Intestine diarrhoea with bad smell, maybe with mucus and blood in stools, abdominal pain	slippery, rapid, full or flooding	red, greasy, yellow coat	CV.6, ST.25, ST.39, SP.6, SP.9, LI.11 Rd	+ CV.3 Rd + SP.1, SP.10 Rd	for lower abdominal pain for blood in stool
Liver Fire headache, irritability, impatience, anger, maybe gastritis or skin rash	wiry, rapid, full or flooding	red, especially at edges, dry yellow coat	CV.13, ST.21, ST.44, LR.2, GB.38 Rd; SP.6 Rf	+ BL.2, GB.1 E; GB.44 Rd + LR.1, PC.9 B; LI.4, LI.11 Rd + KI.1, GV.20, GB.20 Rd	for conjunctivitis for Heat in the Blood eczema for headache
Heart Fire suppressed excitement, anxiety, insomnia, palpitations, gastritis, maybe diarrhoea, skin rash	rapid, full or flooding, maybe irregular, maybe slippery	red, especially at tip, dry, maybe yellow coat	CV.13, ST.21, ST.44, HT.3, PC.3 Rd; SP.6 Rf	+ KI.1 Rd; HT.9 B + ān mián, ST.45 Rd + KI.6 Rf + ST.40, PC.6 Rd	for severe itching for insomnia for Deficient Heart Yin for Heart Phlegm
Retention of Phlegm in Lung catarrh in nose, throat or chest, maybe cough or asthma	slippery, maybe empty or full	greasy coat	BL.13, CV.12, ST.40 E M; LU.6 Rd	+ BL.2, ST.2, GB.20 E + CV.22 + CV.17, LU.1	for sinusitis for catarrh in throat for catarrh in chest
Deficient Spleen Qi and Damp chronic tiredness, weak limbs, respiratory catarrh, maybe fluid-filled or exuding skin eruptions	empty, slippery, maybe slow	pale, flabby, greasy white	CV.6, CV.12, ST.21, ST.36 Rf M; SP.6, SP.9 Rd	+ CV.17 Rf M; LU.1, LU.6 Rd + SP.1, SP.4 E M	for bronchial catarrh for loss of appetite or loss of weight
Deficient Qi of Intestine and Stagnant Qi of Intestine loose stools, diarrhoea, borborygmus, abdominal distension worse with tiredness or depression	empty, slippery, maybe slow, maybe wiry	pale flabby, greasy white, coat, maybe a little purple	CV.6, CV.12, ST.25, ST.39 Rf M; SP.6, SP.9 Rd alternate with BL.20, BL.22, BL.25, BL.27 E M; LI.10, ST.39 E	+ GV.20, SP.1 M	for loss of appetite, tiredness or blood in stool

Rd, Reducing method; Rf, Reinforcing method; E, Even method; M, moxa; B, bleeding.

Disorders of eating and weight

Weight reduction has become a multibillion dollar industry. Whilst unwise eating, obesity and lack of exercise increase the risk of diseases and a premature death, preoccupation with losing weight can be physically and psychologically destructive. The continual alternation between overeating and undereating can produce not only gastrointestinal disharmony and malnutrition, but can reinforce negative psychological patterns of poor self-image and low personal worth.

Acupuncture can help to balance the underlying causes of eating and weight disorders, but it is most effective when combined with counselling and mediation. Counselling is not only regarding sensible balanced nutrition and suitable moderate regular exercise, but also involving a deep and sympathetic understanding of personality and life pattern. In certain cases, specialist Western medical diagnosis may be necessary, since severe weight loss, for example, can relate to cancer or to serious malabsorption syndromes.

TYPES

There are two main overlapping problems, metabolic disorders and eating disorders.

METABOLIC DISORDERS

The two extremes are overweight, with food input normal or less, and underweight with food input normal or more.

OVERWEIGHT

This is usually associated with lowered metabolic rate. This can be related to Deficient Spleen Yang, with accumulation of fat and phlegm, or Deficient Kidney Yang with water retention. These two syndromes often occur in combination.

UNDERWEIGHT

This can be associated with either lowered or raised metabolic rate. Lowered metabolic rate can relate to Deficient Spleen Yang, with malabsorption of nutrients, underweight and muscular atrophy and weakness. (Deficient Spleen Yang can give rise either to overweight, if fat accumulates, or to underweight if there is malabsorp-

tion.) Raised metabolic rate, related to Deficient Yin and Fire, and often to chronic nervous tension, can cause underweight.

EATING DISORDERS

The two extremes are overweight related to overeating, and underweight related to undereating.

OVEREATING

The person is overweight from overeating, but may alternate periods of overeating with periods of fasting and perhaps vomiting after eating.

UNDEREATING

The anorexic eats very little, may vomit after eating, and is emaciated. The bulimic may be normal weight or less, and alternate reduced food intake with compulsive eating and vomiting.

THE BASIS OF WEIGHT

Assuming input is relatively normal, weight depends on output and constitutional metabolic and emotional type. If output is less than normal, the person will tend to be overweight, and if output is more than normal, the person will tend to be underweight. Raised metabolic rate may create underweight, and lowered metabolic rate may create either underweight or overweight as discussed earlier. The influence of emotional factors is discussed later.

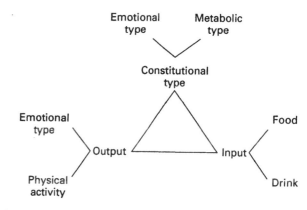

Fig. 28.2 The basis of weight.

INPUT

Weight depends on the types and amount of food eaten, and also on the food combination and the emotional state during eating and digestion. Input depends on metabolic rate, lifestyle and emotional imbalances. Also, intake and metabolic rate will vary with tobacco, alcohol or drug addictions, which are related to emotional state.

OUTPUT

Output is related to both physical activity and to the degree to emotional and mental stress. Physical activity is linked to metabolic rate. For example, if people do much athletic training when young they may eventually create Deficient Yang of Kidney or Heart, dropping their metabolic rate so that they gain weight.

PSYCHOLOGICAL ORIGINS OF EATING DISORDERS

THE BASIS

When the lower self, or ego, is in harmony with the higher self, eating and weight are in balance and eating is a pleasant and necessary part of life. When ego is not in harmony with the higher self, when the ego has lost contact with the love which is a natural part of the higher self, then there is pain or the unease of that separation.

FORMS OF COMPENSATION

To ease that pain, that sense of loss of love or alienation, a person may use the various forms of compensation listed on page 14. These compensations may become addictions. Addictions cannot be satisfied by more of the item, but only by re-establishing contact with the inner sense of peace, strength and love, the higher self. Addicts continually seek something outside themselves to satisfy the inner emptiness, which can only be filled from within.

THE YIN–YANG POLARITY

The two compensations that are important here are food and asceticism. This in fact is a Yin–Yang polarity:

hedonism	puritanism
indulgence	denial
sin	punishment
pleasure	pain
feasting	fasting
overweight	underweight

The two extremes are obesity due to overeating and anorexia due to undereating, but the two are merely part of the same phenomena and the obese may be obsessed with dieting and the anorexic with eating. Both extremes live in the tension of this polarity.

OBESITY

Obesity includes the related pressures to overeat and to be overweight.

PRESSURE TO BE OVERWEIGHT

The person may hide behind their fat and use their being overweight as a protection or a buffer between their self and the perceived threats of life. The more insecure the person feels, the more they fear life and need their protective fat. The more secure, the less they need it.

The person may feel more comfortable if they are overweight, the extra weight is reassuring and pleasant. They may not feel solid enough without it, even ungrounded and edgy. They may feel the extra weight enables them to be taken more seriously, giving their opinions greater weight and substance. The extra body weight, and perhaps the extra Damp and Phlegm in the brain, may give them the reassuring illusion that everything is slow, solid and stable, when in fact the world around them is in rapid change.

These feelings relate to the emotions of fear, insecurity and worry associated with weak or unstable Kidneys and Spleen, and can be treated by strengthening and stabilizing Kidney and Spleen Qi, and the Dan Tian and Spleen energy centres. It may be necessary to calm the Solar Plexus and Brow centres.

PRESSURE TO OVEREAT

Overeating is basically a compensation for loss of contact with the positive energies of the higher self. This has various facets.

LACK OF LOVE

Many of the obese have lost contact with the warmth and love within themselves, so that they do not feel love for themselves and are restricted in their exchange of love in relationships. Indeed, they may feel self-disgust and hatred for themselves, may despise themselves as weak, see themselves as basically unlovable. This gives them an excuse to avoid relationships or to avoid sex and sexuality. Treatment centres on strengthening Heart Fire and Heart and Spleen Qi.

DEPRESSION

In addition to Deficiency of Heart Fire, depression resulting in overeating can be associated with Stagnation of Liver, Heart or Lung Qi. Treatment involves moving Qi in the Stagnant organs.

INSECURITY

Emotional insecurity, perhaps linked to problems of inadequate feeding in infancy, can lead to a feeling of never having enough, or to the fear that there will not be enough. This can relate to food, love or material security. This can be aggravated under conditions of stress in the life, which will increase the food intake, especially of sweet things, and increase weight. This is especially linked to problems with the mother and the Earth element. There can be an exaggeration of the normal sensual pleasure of eating resulting in greed and excessive appetite. This can be helped by strengthening both Spleen and Kidney.

HUNGER FOR LIFE

The Heart Spirit manifests through the physical body in an excitement, interest and pleasure in the life experience, through which consciousness grows and expands. It is like a hunger for life. But if the person through fear and insecurity shuts themselves off from life experience, then this hunger may manifest as need for physical food. It is as if a spiritual need has been converted to a physical one, and the person simply expands in size instead of growing in character. Treatment involves calming the emotional pressure and loosening the blocks, so that the energy can be expressed outwards in participation in life and relationships.

NERVOUS TENSION

Sheer nervous tension may find an outlet in overeating, and treatment may involve tonifying Yin and dispersing Fire of Kidneys, Liver, Stomach or Heart.

ANOREXIA

Anorexia is not merely an emotional imbalance, it involves a rigid, fanatically held mental delusion by the patient about the size and shape of her own body. It is mainly a problem of young women of about 14–20 years.

Intake is restricted by the guilt that follows eating or the fear of becoming horribly fat. Also the patient may vomit, use laxatives or strenuous exercise to decrease bodyweight. In bulimics these activities may alternate with spasms of compulsive eating. The girl may withdraw from her social life, start solitary physical exercises, lose interest in her boyfriend and avoid sexual contact.

Weight loss can be followed by amenorrhoea, and in extreme cases death from suicide or the complications of malnutrition such as renal failure from potassium depletion.

ORIGINS OF ANOREXIA

There may be a disturbed relationship within the family, aggravating the emotional conflicts of puberty, but the basis is once again lack of love, yet in a framework of distorted beliefs. While overeating may include the need to root the person more firmly in the physical body, anorexia is the opposite. Anorexics are denying and attempting to reduce the demands of the physical body.

Treatment of anorexia aims at developing connection with the inner self, so that the person feels love and warmth with themselves. In addition to strengthening the Spleen, treatment involves strengthening Heart Fire.

TREATMENT

Point combinations for disorders of eating and weight are given in Table 28.3.

Constipation syndromes

Constipation can be described as hard stools or infrequent or difficult defecation.

AETIOLOGY AND SYNDROMES

The commonest form of constipation in the West is imaginary constipation. This is due to overconcern about bowel regularity, followed by laxative abuse, which leads to secondary constipation. Constipation may also be started by a diet of overly refined food with low fibre content, excessive fried food, irregular eating habits, travel, illness, enforced bed rest, lack of exercise, drugs and medications, such as the opiates, tricyclic antidepressants and anticholinergenics.

Constipation may start as a retentive reaction to overly forceful toilet training; it can be associated with depres-

Table 28.3 Disorders of eating and weight

Syndrome	Signs and symptoms	Pulse	Tongue	Point combinations
Metabolic overweight Deficient Spleen Qi and Yang	overweight, respiratory catarrh laziness, feelings of heaviness in limbs	empty, slippery	pale, white greasy coat	CV.6, CV.12, ST.25, ST.36, LR.13 Rf M + LI.10, TE.6 Rd for Stagnant Qi
Deficient Kidney Qi and Yang	overweight, fluid retention, coldness in back, legs and lower abdomen	empty, slow, slippery, deep	pale, moist white coat	CV.6, CV.9, CV.12 E M; SP.6, SP.9, TE.6 Rd alternate GV.4 GV.20, BL.20, BL.22, BL.23 Rf M
Metabolic underweight Deficient Spleen Qi and Yang	underweight, loose stools, muscular atrophy and weakness	empty, or minute, choppy	pale, flabby, hollow in SP–ST area	CV.4, CV.12, ST.21, ST.25, ST.36, LI.4 Rf M alternate BL.20, BL.23, BL.27, BL.43 Rf M
Deficient Yin and Fire	underweight, hyperactivity, signs of heat, restless nervous tension, restless sleep	rapid, thin or full, maybe wiry	red, especially at tip and edges, dry	CV.12, ST.36, SP.6, KI.6, Rf; KI.2, LR.2, ST.44 or HT.8 Rd, as appropriate
Overeating Deficient Heart Fire (lack of love)	overeating from lack of love of self, feel lonely, unlovable and disgusted with self	empty, maybe hindered or slow	pale	CV.12, CV.17, ST.36, HT.8, PC.8 Rf M
Stagnant Liver Qi (depression)	overeating from depression and frustration	wiry or hindered	maybe purplish	CV.12, CV.17, ST.36, SP.1, SP.2 Rf M; LR.1, LR.3, LR.13 Rd
Deficient Spleen Qi (insecurity)	overeating from fear, worry and insecurity, need fat as a buffer, to feel protected	empty or flooding, slippery	pale, greasy coat	CV.4, CV.12, ST.25, ST.36, SP.1, SP.2 Rf M alternate with GV.20, BL.44, BL.48, BL.52, LI.4, ST.36 Rf M
Suppression of Heart Spirit (hunger for life)	overeating from suppressed excitement, eating instead of participating in life	maybe rapid, hindered, irregular	maybe red, especially at tip, or trembling	ST.36, KI.4 Rf M; CV.23 E; CV.14, CV.17 E M; HT.5, PC.4 Rd
Deficient Yin and Fire (nervous tension)	overeating from restless nervous tension and hyperactivity	rapid, thin or full, maybe wiry	red, especially at tip and edges, dry	CV.12, ST.36, SP.6, KI.6 Rf; KI.1, CV.14, GV.20 Rd; KI.2, LR.2, ST.44 or HT.8 Rd as appropriate
Undereating – Anorexia Deficient Spleen Qi and Deficient Heart Fire	undereating, emaciation, deliberate vomiting after meals, amenorrhoea	empty, thin or choppy, maybe minute	pale, thin, flabby	GV.20, yìn táng E; CV.12, CV.17 M; SP.1, SP.2, ST.36, HT.8 Rf M

Rf, Reinforcing method; Rd, Reducing method; E, Even method; M, moxa.

sion; it can be aggravated by neurotic fears of contamination by public toilet seats; it may be concomitant of general stress and tension in those who feel rushed or unable to relax during defecation.

CHINESE AETIOLOGY

In Chinese medicine, constipation can be due either to Excess or Deficiency:

Excess	Deficiency
Heat	Deficient Qi, Blood and Fluids
Stagnant Qi	Deficient Yang and Cold

HEAT

Acute constipation, may be caused by fevers of the Bright Yang type. Chronic constipation due to Heat in the Stomach and Intestines may be associated with mental and emotional congestion and worry, or overconsumption of spicy foods and alcohol. Liver Fire from frustration and irritation can tend to aggravate constipation by increasing Stomach Fire.

STAGNANT QI

Stagnant Qi of Lungs or Liver may cause constipation. Both the Lungs and the Large Intestine, the Metal organs, are concerned with taking in and letting go. Liver is especially important in maintaining free-flow of Qi in the Lower Energizer. This type of constipation may be aggravated by depression, frustration or general repression of feelings. The uptight, tense and rigid person, afraid to let their feelings flow, trying to keep life under tight control.

DEFICIENT QI, BLOOD AND FLUIDS

Patients after illness, women after childbirth, or old people, may be very tired and deficient in the energy and fluids needed for defecation. If the dominant deficiency is Qi and Blood, the tongue will be pale, if the dominant deficiency is Yin, the tongue will be red and peeled as in old people of the Deficient Yin type.

DEFICIENT YANG AND COLD

This syndrome is found mainly in old, weak people, with exhaustion, cold limbs, and coldness and pain in the abdomen.

TREATMENT

Point combinations for constipation are summarized in Table 28.4. Back points such as BL.18, BL.20, BL.25, and BL.31–33 can also be used for constipation.

RECTAL PROLAPSE AND HAEMORRHOIDS

The main local point is GV.1, inserted perpendicularly. If required the needle can be directed towards the right and left to obtain a needle sensation radiating through the anus. Subsidiary local points can be chosen from BL.30, BL.32, BL.35 and BL.54. The main distal point is BL.57 used with Reducing method.

MODIFICATIONS

PC.8 Rd	for signs of Heat
SP.10 Rd	for bleeding from Heat
BL.25, ST.37 Rd	for constipation
GV.20 M	for haemorrhoids or rectal prolapse due to Sinking of Qi, moxa stick should be used for 15 minutes
CV.8 M	for Sinking Qi, moxa cones on ginger on salt

Diarrhoea and dysentery syndromes

GENERAL

Diarrhoea and dysentery are often given separate sections in Chinese texts. Diarrhoea is defined as increased frequency, looseness or liquidity of faeces. Dysentery is

Table 28.4 Constipation syndromes

Syndromes	Signs and symptoms	Pulse	Tongue	Point combination
Excess				
Heat	constipation with dry stools, maybe burning sensation in anus, maybe gastritis, dry mouth and bad breath	rapid and full or flooding	red, yellow or brown coat	ST.25, ST.37, ST.44, LI.11 Rd; CV.6 E; SP.6, KI.6 Rf
Stagnant Qi	constipation with abdominal distension, maybe discomfort in epigastrium and belching, emotional suppression	wiry, maybe full or flooding	various	CV.6, SP.15, ST.37, GB.34, LI.10, TE.6 E or Rd
Deficiency				
Deficient Qi, Blood and Fluids	constipation with dry stools, in tired, weak patients, e.g. after illness or childbirth or in old age	empty or thin, choppy	pale and thin, white coat, maybe dry	SP.15, LI.10, GB.34 E or Rd; CV.4, ST.36, SP.6, KI.6 Rf
Deficient Yang with Cold	constipation with sensation of coldness and pain in abdomen, cold limbs, in weak or old patients	empty, deep, slow	pale and flabby, white coat	CV.6, ST.25, ST.37 E M; GV.34, LI.10, TE.6 E; CV.4 Rf M

Rd, Reducing method; Rf, Reinforcing method; E, Even method; M, moxa.

defined as diarrhoea with abdominal pain, tenesmus and blood and mucus in the stools. Since the two diseases overlap and since the same point combinations are generally given for dysentery as for diarrhoea, these diseases are discussed together in this section. Abdominal distension with irregular defecation is dealt with in the later section on 'Irritable Bowel Syndrome and Abdominal Distension', and it is in that section that the psychological origins of irregular bowel movements are discussed.

IMPORTANCE

Changes in the pattern of bowel movements can be of relatively low importance, requiring simply an adjustment of lifestyle. However, these changes can also reflect serious disorders such as cancer of the bowel, so that thorough investigation by Western medicine may be necessary. Western medication may also be necessary in the treatment of diarrhoea or dysentery due to organisms such as *Entamoeba histolytica*, *Giardia*, *Shiegella* or *Salmonella*.

SYNDROMES

Acute diarrhoea or dysentery
Damp Heat
Cold Damp
Retention of food
Intermittent chronic dysentery
Chronic Diarrhoea
Deficient Spleen Qi
Deficient Kidney Qi
Stagnant Liver Qi
Fear and anxiety.

TREATMENT

Point combinations for diarrhoea and dysentery are shown in Table 28.5. Frequency of treatment varies with the severity. For severe acute cases treatment can be three times a day, reducing to one per day as the patient recovers, and then every other day. For intermittent chronic dysentery, treatments can be given once per day or every other day during an attack, and reduced to once per week between attacks. For chronic diarrhoea, treatment can be once or twice per week, depending on severity.

Table 28.5 Diarrhoea and dysentery syndromes

Syndromes	Signs and symptoms	Pulse	Tongue	Point combination
Acute diarrhoea or dysentery				**Basic Combination:** ST.25, ST.37 Rd
Damp Heat	diarrhoea with abdominal pain, burning sensation in anus, feverishness, thirst	rapid, slippery	red, yellow greasy coat	if Damp predominates, e.g. watery stools, add SP.6, SP.9 Rd if Heat predominates, e.g. fever, select from SI.1, LI.1, LI.11, ST.44, GV.14 Rd
Cold Damp	watery diarrhoea, with abdominal pain, sensation of cold and no thirst	deep, slow, slippery	pale, white greasy coat	Basic + CV.6, CV.12, SP.9 E M
Retention of food	diarrhoea with loss of appetite, distension in epigastrium and abdomen	slippery, wiry, maybe rapid	maybe red, yellow greasy coat	Basic + CV.12, PC.6 Rd
Intermittent chronic dysentery	intermittent dysentery over long periods, difficult to cure, less severe than acute type, tiredness, somnolence, weight loss	maybe empty, slippery	greasy coat	ST.25, ST.37 Rd if Deficient Yin, add KI.6, SP.10 Rf if Deficient Yang, add BL.20, BL.23 Rf M
Chronic diarrhoea Deficient Spleen Qi	loose stool with undigested food, tiredness, weight loss, loss of appetite	empty	pale, flabby	**Basic combination:** CV.12, ST.25, ST.36 Rf M Basic + BL.20 Rf M if worry, add BL.49 Rd if rectal prolapse, add GV.1 E; GV.20 M
Deficient Kidney Qi	diarrhoea with borborygmi and pain around the umbilicus, usually at dawn, aggravated by cold	empty, deep	pale, moist, white coat	Basic + GV.4, CV.4, BL.23, KI.3 Rf M
Stagnant Liver Qi	diarrhoea associated with mood changes, abdominal distension, belching and flatulence	wiry	various	Basic + LR.3, LR.13, BL.18 Rd
Fear and anxiety	diarrhoea associated with fear and anxiety, often before a specific event, e.g. public performance by the patient	maybe rapid, or irregular, moving	maybe trembling	Basic + CV.14, HT.7 Rd; KI.3 Rf

Rd, Reducing method; Rf, Reinforcing method; E, Even method; M, moxa.

Irritable bowel syndrome and abdominal distension

GENERAL

One of the commonest functional disorders is irritable bowel syndrome, IBS, which can be described as irregular bowel movements and abdominal discomfort without any organic disease. There may be constipation or diarrhoea, or an alternation between the two, abdominal pain and abdominal distension which are eased by defecation, sensation of incomplete defecation, or mucus in the stools. Irritable bowel syndrome usually occurs together with gastric symptoms, and is usually associated with emotional stress.

Abdominal distension has been included with IBS, since the same Chinese syndromes occur with each ailment.

IBS AND EMOTIONS

The four main emotions that aggravate IBS are fear, anger, anxiety and worry. Since these emotions may focus their effect around the Solar Plexus energy centre, IBS may occur together with urinary frequency, gastritis, palpitations or dyspnoea, as the stress also affects the Bladder, Stomach, Heart or Lung systems.

CV.14 is a key point to calm the Solar Plexus centre, and may be combined with acupressure on KI.1. It is most helpful for IBS patients to learn to relax deeply, and meditations linking breathing with concentration on the Dan Tian centre can be effective.

IBS is often a pattern associated with suppressed emotions, for example of anger and irritation, or excitement and anxiety, which the person is unable either to express or to eliminate from the system.

SYNDROMES

Stagnant Liver Qi
Deficient Spleen Qi and Yang
Stagnant Liver Qi and Deficient Spleen Qi
Kidney fear and Heart anxiety
Retention of food

TREATMENT

Point combinations for IBS and abdominal distension are given in Table 28.6. Points are selected mainly from the following:

CV.4, CV.6, CV.12, CV.14
ST.25, ST.36, ST.37
LR.3, LR.13
BL.18, BL.20, BL.25, BL.47, BL.49

In addition the Extra channel combinations of SP.4 + PC.6 can be effective.

Table 28.6 Irritable bowel syndrome and abdominal distension

Syndrome	Signs and symptoms	Pulse	Tongue	Point combination
Stagnant Liver Qi	abdominal distension, irregular bowel movements and gastritis aggravated by depression, frustration or anger	wiry or hindered	maybe slightly purplish	CV.6, CV.12, TE.6, ST.25, ST.37, LR.3, LR.13 Rd + PC.6 Rd for nausea + GB.27, GB.28 Rd for colon pain
Deficient Spleen Qi and Yang	abdominal distension, worse with tiredness or worry, loss of appetite, loose stools	empty, maybe slippery, maybe slow	pale, white greasy moist coat	CV.6, ST.25, LR.13 E M; CV.12, ST.36 Rf M alternate with BL.20, BL.25, BL.27 Rf M + CV.9, SP.6, SP.9 Rd for watery stools + GV.20, BL.49 E for worry
Stagnant Liver Qi and Deficient Spleen Qi	abdominal and epigastric distension, worse with tiredness or depression, worse with worry or anger	empty, wiry, maybe slippery	pale, maybe purplish, greasy white coat	CV.6, CV.12, ST.25, ST.37, LR.13 E M; LR.3 Rd alternate with BL.18, BL.20, BL.25 E M + LU.7, CV.17 or BL.13 Rd for Stagnant Lung and Large Intestine Qi
Kidney fear and Heart anxiety	abdominal distension and irregular bowel movements, aggravated by fear and anxiety, especially before important meetings, examinations, etc.	maybe rapid, irregular, moving	maybe trembling	CV.4 Rf; CV.12, ST.25, ST.37, SP.4, PC.6 E; CV.14 Rd alternate with BL.20, BL.25, BL.44, BL.52 E
Retention of food	abdominal distension and irregular bowel movements associated with excessive or irregular eating patterns	wiry, slippery, maybe flooding or rapid	greasy, maybe yellow coat	CV.6 E; CV.10, CV.13, ST.25, ST.37, LI.10, PC.6 Rd + ST.44. LI.4 for signs of Heat, e.g. constipation and bad breath

Rd, Reducing method; Rf, Reinforcing method; E, Even method; M, moxa.

Energy centres and digestive syndromes

The relationships between the energy centres and some common digestive syndromes are summarized in Table 28.7.

Table 28.7 Energy centres and digestive syndromes

Centre	Point	Method	Syndromes	Example
Crown	GV.20	M or Rf	Sinking of Qi	depression, lack of will, poor flesh tone, stomach prolapse, anal prolapse and haemorrhoids, diarrhoea
		E or Rd	Hyperactive Liver Yang Fire of Kidney Liver or Heart	overeating from stress, digestive headache
Brow	yìn táng	E	Stagnant Spleen–Stomach Qi	anorexia with rigid mental structures and lack of perspective, gastritis from mental congestion, IBS from worry and overconcern
Throat	CV.23	Rd	Stagnant Heart Qi	overeating from frustration at inability to express feeelings in relationships
Heart	CV.17	Rd Rf M	Stagnant Lung Qi Deficient Heart Fire	constipation, epigastric distension, overeating from loneliness and lack of love of self, anorexia from loss of interest in life
Solar Plexus	CV.14	Rd or E	Fear and anxiety invades Stomach, Rebellious Stomach Qi	overeating, gastritis, hiccup, irritable bowel syndrome or diarrhoea from fear, worry, insecurity, fear of loss of control
Spleen	CV.12	Rf M	Deficient Spleen and Stomach Qi Yang	underweight from malnourishment, lethargy and avoidance of exercise, Yin type food allergies, craving for food or for sweets due to insecurity
			Stagnant Spleen–Stomach	nausea, epigastric and abdominal distension with depression, or from mental congestion from overintensive study
Dan Tian	CV.4	Rf	Deficient Kidney Yin	underweight from raised metabolism, overweight from nervous eating, IBS and gastritis from fear and anxiety, constipation with dry stools
		Rf M	Deficient Kidney Yang	overweight from low metabolism and fluid retention, lack of energy or desire to exercise, depression and lack of interest in food, diarrhoea, food allergies from Deficient Defensive Qi
Reproduction	CV.3		Stagnant Spleen–Stomach Qi	anorexia or obesity from denial of sexuality or femininity, overeating from frustrations in expressing sexuality, reproduction, creativity

Rf, Reinforcing method; Rd, Reducing method; E, Even method; M, moxibustion.

Urinary and oedema 29 syndromes

Urinary syndromes

All the common urinary complaints are included in this section, such as cystitis, urethritis, enuresis and prostatitis, involving symptoms such as dysuria, haematuria, incomplete urination, frequency and incontinence.

AETIOLOGY

The basic aetiology is summarized in Figure 29.1.

DEFICIENT QI

Deficient Qi can be associated with reduced body resistance to infection, or with reduced ability to hold the urine in the body or the blood in the vessels. Deficient Qi may arise from physical and mental overwork, excess sex or childbirth, emotional stress, physical illness, surgical operation and shock.

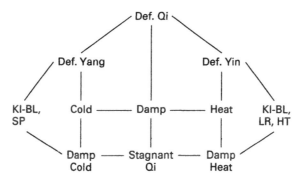

Fig. 29.1 Aetiological factors in urinary syndromes.

STAGNANT QI

Stagnant Qi may be associated with general stagnation of the emotions, especially of Kidneys, Liver and Heart, or with local stagnation due to lack of exercise, trauma, surgery or childbirth.

DAMP HEAT IN THE BLADDER

Damp may arise from Deficient Qi of Spleen and Kidneys, and from Stagnant Qi. Heat may arise as a progression of Stagnant Qi, especially in people whose constitution is of the Deficient Yin or Fire type. Damp and Heat may then combine to produce one of the commonest urinary syndromes, Damp Heat in the Bladder.

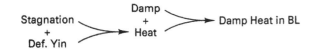

Fig. 29.2

EMOTIONS AND URINARY SYNDROMES

The main systems involved are Kidneys, Liver and Heart.

KIDNEYS

Fear, fright and shock can weaken the Kidneys and Bladder, with the resulting frequency, incontinence and enuresis associated with Deficient Kidney Qi and Yang. This weakness can also result in reduced resistance to infections, with dysuria and haematuria for example, and the Heat signs of Deficient Kidney Yin. Fear of change, fear of life, constant suspicions and paranoia, fearful holding in and holding on, can also result in Stagnation of Kidney-Bladder Qi, with feelings of distension and pain, or incomplete or difficult urination. Stagnation of Kidney Qi and Deficient Kidney Yin can combine to give the syndrome of Damp Heat in the Bladder.

LIVER

Depression, frustration, suppressed anger and the related feelings of bitterness, resentment and hatred, can be associated with Stagnant Liver Qi and Heat, and with Damp Heat in the Bladder. Liver Fire can result in dysuria with a burning sensation and haematuria.

HEART

Disturbance of Heart Spirit, associated with Deficient Heart and Kidney Qi, can result in enuresis or urinary urgency. Deficient Heart Yin and Heart Fire are often linked with cystitis and haematuria. Stagnant Heart Qi can relate to suppressed anxiety or excitement, or to difficulty in communicating in a relationship, especially where there are mixed feelings of love and hatred. These syndromes of Stagnation and Heat can then develop into Damp Heat in the Bladder.

SYNDROMES

Excess	Damp Heat in Bladder
Deficiency	Deficient Kidney Qi and Yang
Excess + Deficiency	Damp Heat in Bladder with Deficient Qi

ENURESIS

In Chinese medicine, enuresis is due either to Deficient Kidney Yang, or to Deficient Qi of Lung and Spleen. In the experience of the author, enuresis is mainly due to Kidney fear, which is often linked to Heart anxiety. The author therefore strengthens the Kidneys and calms fear and anxiety, choosing points from such as:

GV.20, CV.4, SP.6, KI.3, HT.7 Rf
alternating with GV.4, GV.20, BL.15, BL.23, KI.3, HT.7 Rf

For children up to about 8 years, minimum points are used, for example:

GV.20, KI.3, HT.7 Rf

For older children and teenagers, more points can be added. If there is a general Deficiency of Qi, then BL.13 and BL.20, with Reinforcing method or moxa, can be included in the treatment. It is often helpful to moxa or to massage KI.1 gently, to strengthen the Kidneys and to calm fear.

PROSTATITIS

Expert Western diagnosis must be made to exclude the possibility of prostate carcinoma. In Chinese medicine, prostatitis may be differentiated into Damp Heat and Deficiency as shown in Table 29.1. Many men with prostatitis have combined syndromes of Damp Heat and Deficient Qi, associated with stress, frustration, overwork, exhaustion and depression. It may be most effective to alternate treatments on the front of the body with treatments on the back, for example:

CV.1, CV.3, ST.29, SP.6, TE.6 Rd; CV.6, CV.12, ST.36 Rf
BL.28, BL.32, BL.39 Rd; GV.4, GV.20, BL.20, BL.23 Rf

Table 29.1 Urinary syndromes

Syndromes	Signs and Symptoms	Pulse	Tongue	Point combinations
Damp Heat in Bladder	cystitis or urethritis with dysuria, frequency, urgency or retention, maybe with distending sensation in lower abdomen, or burning sensation on urination, maybe, feverishness and restlessness, maybe emotional agitation or frustration	rapid, maybe slippery, wiry, full, flooding or thin	red, or red dots at tip or edges, yellow greasy coat	CV.3, ST.28, SP.6, SP.9 Rd alternate BL.23, BL.28, BL.32, BL.39, BL.64 Rd + LI.4, TE.5 for Wind Heat signs + SP.1, SP.10 (–SP.9) for haematuria + CV.6 E or Rd for Stagnant Qi in lower abdomen + CV.6, KI.8, SP.15, GB.25 Rd for Kidney stones + KI.2 Rd; KI.10 Rf for Kidney Deficiency Fire + LR.2, LR.11 Rd for Liver Fire and Damp Heat + HT.8 Rd; HT.3 for Heart Fire + KI.8 Rd for Stagnant Kidney Qi + LR.1, LR.3 Rd for Stagnant Liver Qi + CV.17, HT.5 for Stagnant Heart Qi
Deficient Kidney Qi	retention, frequency, incontinence, incomplete urination or enuresis, worse with tiredness, weak lower back, maybe tinnitus, depression, impotence and coldness of limbs, lower back and lower abdomen, maybe oedema	empty, maybe deep, slow choppy or changing	pale, flabby, moist white coat	CV.4, ST.28, ST.36, KI.3 Rf M; SP.6 Rd alternate GV.4, BL.20, BL.23, BL.28, BL.64 Rf M; BL.32 Rd + CV.12, SP.9 Rf M for Deficient Spleen + CV.14, CV.24 E or Rd for fear and anxiety + GV.20, HT.7 Rf for enuresis and reduce number of points for children — see notes
Damp Heat in Bladder with Deficient Qi	urinary disorders with both tiredness and restlessness or frustration, and with symptoms aggravated by both tiredness and stress	rapid, maybe slippery or wiry, thin or empty	maybe pale, flabby, with red dots at tip or edges, yellow coat	CV.3, ST.28, SP.6, SP.9 Rd; CV.4, ST.36, BL.64 Rf + KI.6 Rf for Deficient Kidney Yin + KI.3 Rf for Deficient Kidney Qi + CV.12 Rf for Deficient Spleen Qi

Rd, Reducing method; Rf, Reinforcing method; E, Even method; M, moxa.

Oedema syndromes

GENERAL

Oedema is swelling due to excess tissue fluid. It can have many different causes, and these causes must be treated. When oedema represents a serious organic condition, eg. failure of heart, liver or kidneys, acupuncture is secondary to Western medicine.

TYPES

In Chinese medicine, oedema is divided into acute Yang-type oedema with rapid onset, and chronic Yin-type oedema with gradual onset. Yang oedema is associated with Wind Heat invasion, as in acute nephritis, Yin oedema is associated with Deficiency of Spleen and Kidney Qi and Yang, as in chronic oedema of the lower body. Oedema may also be associated with systemic Stagnant Qi, as in premenstrual oedema, or with localized

Stagnant Qi and Blood due to injury, as in surgical closure of lymph vessels to prevent the spread of cancer.

SYNDROMES

Wind Heat
Stagnant Qi
Deficient Kidney and Spleen Qi
Stagnant Qi and Deficient Qi

Perhaps the most common is a combination of Stagnant Qi and Deficient Qi. Points are selected according to which of the two syndromes is dominant.

TREATMENT

Point combinations for the oedema syndrome are given in Table 29.2.

Table 29.2 Oedema synromes

Syndrome	Signs and symptoms	Pulse	Tongue	Point combination
Wind Heat	chills and fever, cough and sore throat, oedema of face and then generalized oedema, more severe in upper body, oliguria, maybe pain in lumbar area	superficial, rapid	thin white or yellow coat	ST.28, LI.4, LU.7, KI.7 Rd + GV.26, CV.24 Rd for facial oedema + ST.43, ST.45, LI.6 for facial and upper body oedema + BL.13, LU.1 E for Wind in Lungs + GV.14, TE.5 Rd for Wind Heat
Stagnant Qi	oedema of abdomen and legs especially, feeling of distension in epigastrium or abdomen, depression, frustration, maybe nausea or indigestion	hindered or wiry, slippery	purplish, maybe pale, greasy coat	CV.3, CV.6, ST.28, ST.40, SP.6, LI.10, TE.6 E or Rd + LR.3, LR.13 Rd for Stagnant Liver Qi + CV.17, LU.7 Rd M for Stagnation of Lung Qi with depression
Deficient Kidney and Spleen Qi and Yang	chronic oedema of abdomen and legs especially, tiredness, weak muscles and lower back, cold limbs, lower back and abdomen, depression, lack of drive, and worry	empty, slow, deep, slippery	pale, flabby, moist white coat	CV.4, CV.9, CV.12, ST.28, ST.36 Rf M; SP.6, SP.9, TE.6 Rd alternate GV.4, GV.6, BL.20, BL.22, BL.23, BL.29 Rf M; SP.6, LI.10 Rd + SP.1, SP.2 M for Deficient Spleen Yang syndrome + KI.1, KI.2 M for Deficient Kidney Yang
Stagnant Qi and Deficient Qi	chronic oedema of abdomen and legs especially, worse with either tiredness or depression	empty, hindered, slippery	pale, maybe purplish, flabby, moist white coat	CV.4, CV.12, ST.36 Rf M; CV.6, ST.28, SP.6, TE.6 E or Rd M

Rd, Reducing method; Rf, Reinforcing method; E, Even method; M, moxa

Male sexual syndromes 30

Impotence and male sexual syndromes

The problems considered in this section include lack of interest in sex, inability to obtain or to maintain an erection, premature ejaculation, failure to ejaculate, male infertility, and pain or irritation of the genitals. Problems due to structural or severe endocrine anomalies, to serious diseases such as carcinoma or to sexually transmitted diseases (STD), are not discussed here.

AETIOLOGY

In Chinese medicine, the main origins of male sexual problems are Deficiency, Stagnation, and Disturbance of Heart Spirit.

DEFICIENCY

Deficiency is primarily of Kidney Qi and Jing. Deficient Spleen Qi may be a secondary factor, since the replacement of Kidney energy derives from the food and drink processed by the Spleen. Exhaustion from illness, malnutrition, or excess of work, exercise, sex or emotional stress, can combine with inherited constitutional weakness and old age to give Deficient Kidneys. Medications, drugs and excess alcohol can also contribute to Kidney Deficiency.

DEFICIENT YANG AND DEFICIENT YIN

Whether a person shows signs of Deficient Kidney Yang or Deficient Kidney Yin, will depend on whether their constitution is Deficient Yin or Deficient Yang, and on the nature of the disease factor. Physical overwork, especially in cold, damp conditions with malnutrition is more likely to produce signs of Deficient Yang. Mental and emotional pressure in a hectic working environment, especially with a hot, dry atmosphere, is more likely to elicit Deficient Yin signs. However, eventually, a Deficient Yin person may become so totally exhausted that they burn out to become Deficient Yang. Deficient Yang constitutions will tend to have sexual disorders with Deficient Yang signs, such as lack of interest or impotence, whilst Deficient Yin types will tend more to Deficient Yin signs, such as stressed and restless sexual overactivity or premature ejaculation.

STAGNATION

Mental and emotional blocks and inhibitions cause a large proportion of male sexual dysfunction. Sex is simply one aspect of personal relationships, and emotions such as grief, depression, guilt, fear, suppressed anger and hatred, can affect sex just as much as they can affect any other form of sharing and communication.

If there are unresolved emotional difficulties between two people, and especially if the partners ignore and suppress these distortions of energy, instead of attempting to clear them, they may surface during sex. Table 30.1 shows suitable points for some emotional blockages that may affect sexual expression.

Table 30.1 Stagnation of the emotions and sexual expression

Organ	Emotions	Points
Heart	confusion between love and hate	CV.3, CV.14, CV.17, HT.5, SP.6 E
Spleen	clinging and dominating overconcern due to insecurity	yìn táng, CV.3, CV.12, LU.7, SP.1, SP.4, ST.29 E; ST.36 Rf
Lungs	grief, guilt	CV.3, CV.17, LU.1, LU.7, KI.6 E
Kidneys	fear of failure, fear of sex, fear of vulnerability, fear of surrender	GV.20, CV.3, CV.14, KI.8, KI.13 E
Liver	suppressed anger, bitterness, resentment	CV.3, CV.6, TE.5, GB.13, GB.41, SP.6 E

Rf, Reinforcing method; E, Even method

DAMP HEAT

Stagnation of Qi due to suppressed emotion can generate Heat, and this can combine with Damp to reduce Damp Heat, which can contribute to some types of impotence, to difficulties with orgasm, or to genital irritation and pain.

DISTURBANCE OF SPIRIT

Fear, worry, anxiety and restless, stressful overexcitement can all interfere with the harmonious unfoldment of the sexual process. Deficient Yin constitutions tend to Disturbance of Heart Spirit due to Deficiency Fire, and this may be exaggerated by concomitant Deficient Heart Qi and Blood.

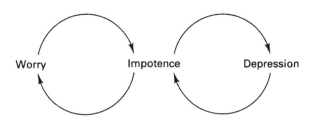

Fig. 30.1

Anxiety and depression can combine in impotence, for example, to produce a double vicious circle as shown in Figure 30.1.

SYNDROMES

Deficient Kidney Qi and Jing
   Deficient Kidney Yang
   Deficient Kidney Yin
Stagnation of Qi
Damp Heat
Disturbance of Heart Spirit

TREATMENT

If the Deficiency is extreme, then the patient needs to be advised that improvement may take a long time, and that they not only need to be patient, but also carefully to build up their reserves of energy. Qi Gong exercises focusing on the Dan Tian centre and emphasizing energy storage and conservation are appropriate. Patients with the syndrome of Excess Kidney Will with Deficient Kidney Qi are particularly likely to set themselves unrealistic goals, and to burn out energy as soon as it is accumulated — see Chapter 34. The combination of GV.20 + KI.1 Rf M may be necessary at some stage in treatment to relax the will, to allow them to recover. Deficient Kidney Yin patients can also pose a problem since they tend to suffer from tense restless insomnia, and either use sex to relax and assist sleep, or else become sexually overactive, further exhausting themselves and depleting their Yin. It is therefore important to reduce Kidney Fire and to calm the Spirit, using such points as:

HT.8, KI.2 Rd; HT.3, KI.10 Rf; yìn táng, ān mián E

Counselling can be an important part of treatment for those patients with Stagnant Qi, simply to talk about their problems to help to get the emotions moving, and also to give them a feeling of support and confidence to gradually let go of blocks.

Table 30.2 Impotence syndromes

Syndrome	Signs and symptoms	Pulse	Tongue	Point combination
Deficient Kidney Yang	lack of interest in sex, impotence or low sperm count, with exhaustion, depression, cold body and extremities	empty or minute, deep, slow, choppy	pale, swollen, moist white coat	GV.20, CV.2, CV.4, KI.2, KI.7, ST.30, ST.36 Rf M; SP.6 Rf alternate GV.4, GV.11, GV.20, BL.23, BL.31 Rf M
Deficient Kidney Yin	impotence or premature ejaculation, with tiredness and depletion, restlessness and signs of heat, worse with stress	thin, choppy, rapid, maybe deep	thin, red, maybe flabby	CV.4, HT.6, KI.6, ST.29, ST.36, SP.6 Rf alternate GV.4, BL.23, BL.44, BL.52 Rf + KI.2, HT.8 Rd for Deficiency Fire
Stagnation of Qi	problems of impotence, orgasm or genital pain, with depression or suppressed emotions	wiry or hindered	maybe purple	CV.3, CV.6, CV.17, SP.6, ST.29 E or Rd M + HT.5, SI.3 Rd for Stagnant Heart Qi + CV.12, LR.13 Rd for Stagnant Spleen Qi + LU.1, LU.7 Rd for Stagnant Lung Qi + KI.8, KI.13 Rd for Stagnant Kidney Qi + LR.1, LR.11 Rd for Stagnant Liver Qi + LR.1, KI.8 Rd for genital pain
Damp Heat	genital pain or itching rash, problems with erection or orgasm, heavy feeling in legs or body, maybe suppressed anger or depression	wiry, slippery, rapid	red, greasy yellow coat	CV.3, LR.1, LR.5, LR.11 Rd + SP.9 Rd for discharge
Disturbance of Spirit	impotence or premature ejaculation worse with fear, worry or anxiety, maybe restlessness, insomnia	thin, rapid, maybe irregular	red, thin, dry, no coat, maybe centre crack or trembling	CV3, CV.14, CV.17, HT.7, ST.29 E; KI.6, SP.6 Rf + GV.20, yìn táng E for worry + GV.24, GB.13 Rd for mental disturbance + HT.8, KI.2 Rd; HT.3, KI.10 Rf for Deficiency Fire

Rf, Reinforcing method; Rd, Reducing method; E, Even method; M, moxa.

Gynaecological and 31
obstetric syndromes

Premenstrual syndromes

AETIOLOGY

The main syndromes involved are summarized in Figure 31.1. Stagnant Liver Qi and Liver Fire are basically Excess syndromes. Hyperactive Liver Yang can have aspects of Excess, especially when it is associated with Stagnant Liver Qi or Liver Fire, or aspects of Deficiency, especially when it is associated with one or more of the four Deficiency syndromes shown in Figure 31.1.

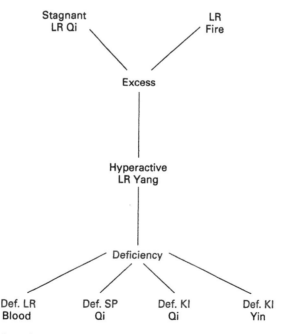

Fig. 31.1 Premenstrual syndromes

HYPERACTIVE YANG AND DEFICIENCY

Liver Yang needs a sufficiency of Yin, Blood and Spleen and Kidney Qi to hold it down and to hold it stable, so that it can perform its proper function of maintaining free-flow of Liver Qi, so necessary in menstruation. If any one of the four controlling factors become Deficient, then Liver Yang becomes Hyperactive and can rise up the body with headache, dizziness, irritability and mood swings.

HYPERACTIVE LIVER YANG AND STAGNANT LIVER QI

In the time after ovulation, Yang is increasing in order to initiate and maintain the flow of Blood in menstruation. If there is not enough movement, e.g. Stagnation of Liver Qi, there may be depression, distending sensation in breasts and abdomen, and painful menstruation. If there is too much disturbed movement, e.g. Hyperactive Liver Yang, then there may be headaches with a moving feeling in the head and dizziness.

LIVER FIRE

Since the premenstrual phase can magnify existing tendencies, women with Liver Fire can find this characteristic exaggerated in the days before menstruation, with anger, shouting and sometimes physical violence. If the Liver Fire is combined with Deficient Liver Yin, there may be insomnia, restlessness and difficulty in concentration. If the Liver Fire is associated with Stagnant Liver Qi, there may be depression alternating with explosions of anger.

SYNDROMES

Stagnant Liver Qi and Hyperactive Liver Yang
Liver Fire and Deficient Liver Yin
Hyperactive Liver Yang and Deficient Liver Blood
Hyperactive Liver Yang and Deficient Spleen Qi
Hyperactive Liver Yang and Deficient Kidney Qi

The five paired syndromes above are not the only possibilities, and other combinations are seen in the clinic, such as Stagnant Liver Qi and Deficient Spleen Qi, with nausea and indigestion. See Table 31.1.

TREATMENT TIMING

Point combinations to regulate Hyperactive Yang, Stagnant Qi and Fire of the Liver, can be used especially at two times: postovulation and premenstruation.

POSTOVULATION

Points can be used with Even method a few days before premenstrual signs begin, or just as they are starting, in order to prevent full development of premenstrual syndrome.

PREMENSTRUATION

Points can also be used with Reducing method in the premenstrual phase, when symptoms are at their worst. If symptoms are particularly severe, or if the premenstrual phase is prolonged, it may be necessary to treat twice or more in this phase.

POSTMENSTRUATION

Point combinations to treat Deficiency of Qi, Blood or Jing are most effective in the postmenstruation phase, when Yin and Blood are increasing, but can be incorporated into treatments at any time in the cycle.

Example

A patient has premenstrual signs due to Stagnant Liver Qi and Hyperactive Liver Yang combined with Deficient Kidney Qi and Deficient Liver Blood. There can be two basic point combinations:

Stagnant Liver Qi + Hyperactive Liver Yang	GV.20, CV.6, CV.17, LR.3, LR.14, PC.6 Rd; SP.6, ST.36 Rf
Deficient Kidney Qi + Deficient Liver Blood	BL.18, BL.20, BL.23, ST.36 Rf; LR.3, LI.4 Rd

The two combinations each treat both Excess and Deficiency, but the emphasis is different. The first combination can be used postovulation and premenstruation, and the second combination can be used postmenstruation.

Table 31.1 Premenstrual syndromes

Syndrome	Signs and symptoms	Pulse	Tongue	Point combination
Stagnant Liver Qi and Hyperactive Liver Yang	depression, irritability, sore breasts, abdominal pain and distension, maybe nausea or headache	wiry	maybe purplish	GV.20, CV.6, CV.17, LR.3, LR.14, SP.6, PC.6 E or Rd + ST.18, SI.1 Rd for sore breasts + CV.12, ST.36 E for nausea + CV.12, SP.1, SP.2 E M for increased or decreased appetite + LU.1, LU.7, BL.13 E or Rd for grief + HT.6, BL.15 E for frustration in relationships + GB.20, GB.21, tài yáng for headache + GB.27, GB.34, TE.6 E for irritable bowel syndrome or constipation
Liver Fire and Deficient Liver Yin	violent anger, irritability, restlessness, signs of heat, maybe insomnia or headache	wiry, rapid, thin or full	red, dry	GV.20, LR.2, LR.3, PC.6, PC.8 Rd; CV.6; KI.6 Rf + KI.1 Rd; LR.1, PC.9 B for severe anger + HT.6, ān mián E for insomnia
Hyperactive Liver Yang and Deficient Kidney Qi	hypersensitivity, touchiness, irritability, headache, dizziness or tinnitus, worse with tiredness or stress, maybe lumbar pain	wiry, thin or empty, maybe deep, maybe changing	pale, maybe flabby, maybe red edges	GV.20, GB.20, GB.34, PC.6 E or Rd; CV.4, SP.6, KI.3 Rf + CV.9, TE.6 E or Rd for oedema
Hyperactive Liver Yang and Deficient Spleen Qi	moodiness, irritability, headache or dizziness, worse with lack of food and improved by eating, maybe oedema or craving for sweets	wiry, empty, maybe slippery	pale, flabby, greasy white coat	LR.3, LR.13, SP.6 Rd; GV.20, CV.12, ST.36 Rf + GB.14, GB.20, tài yáng E or Rd for headache + PC.6, ST.21 E or Rd for nausea or gastritis + CV.6, ST.40 E for oedema
Hyperactive Liver Yang and Deficient Liver Blood	physical and mental tiredness, depression, irritability, feelings of weakness and vulnerability, maybe dizziness, headache, loss of concentration	hindered, wiry, choppy, or thin	pale, maybe thin	GV.20, GB.34, LR.3 E; CV.4, SP.6, LR.8 Rf alternate with GV.20, BL.18, BL.20, ST.36, SP.6, LI.4 Rf + SP.1, yìn táng E for loss of concentration

Rd, Reducing method; Rf, Reinforcing method; E, Even method; M, moxa.

Amenorrhoea and infertility syndromes

Both these disorders require specialist Western medical diagnosis. Acupuncture can be effective when dysfunction relates to physiological or psychological causes, unless there is severe endocrine imbalance, e.g. pituitary tumour, when acupuncture may be appropriate only as a secondary support to Western medicine.

AETIOLOGY AND SYNDROMES

The main syndrome of amenorrhoea and infertility are:

Excess
Stagnant Qi and Blood
Phlegm Damp

Deficiency
Deficient Kidney
Deficient Blood and Qi
Deficient Blood and Jing

Stagnant Qi and Blood can relate to emotional stagnation,

lack of exercise, poor posture, trauma or surgery. Phlegm Damp can relate to the tendency of some women of the Spleen constitutional type to form fat and phlegm, so that phlegm blocks the Fallopian tubes or the general reproductive process.

Some women have constitutionally weak Kidney Qi and so find conception difficult, especially if the Kidney Deficiency is aggravated by overwork, lack of sleep or excessive exercise. Others become deficient in Blood and Jing due to childbirth, illness or strain, and yet others become deficient in Qi and Blood due to malnutrition, as in anorexia. See Table 31.2.

PSYCHOLOGICAL FACTORS

Emotional stresses may inhibit both menstruation and conception, and mainly relate to Liver, Kidneys, Lungs, Heart and Spleen.

LIVER

Stagnation of Liver Qi may relate to general depression,

Table 31.2 Amenorrhoea and infertility syndromes

Syndrome	Signs and symptoms	Pulse	Tongue	Point combination
Excess Stagnant Qi and Blood	amenorrhoea or infertility with depression, frustration, fear or sadness, maybe distension and discomfort in chest, epigastrium or abdomen, maybe nausea	wiry or hindered	maybe purplish	CV.3, CV.6, ST.29, SP.8, LR.3, LI.4 E or Rd + LR.1, LR.14 Rd for Stagnant Liver Qi + KI.8, KI.13 Rd for Stagnant Kidney Qi + CV.17, LU.1, LU.7 Rd for Stagnant Lung Qi + CV.17, PC.6, HT.5 Rd for Stagnant Heart Qi + CV.12, SP.4 E M for Stagnant Spleen Qi
Phlegm Damp	amenorrhoea or infertility with obesity or respiratory catarrh, lethargy, maybe lack of exercise	slippery	greasy, white or yellow coat	CV.3, CV.6, CV.12, ST.30, ST.40, SP.6, SP.9 TE.6 E or Rd; moxa if no signs of Heat alternate with BL.20, BL.22, BL.32 Rd
Deficiency Deficient Kidney Qi	amenorrhoea or infertility with chronic tiredness, lower back ache, urinary frequency, maybe cold extremities, lower abdomen and lower back	empty, deep, slow	pale, flabby, moist, white coat	CV.4, ST.29, ST.36, KI.3, KI.13, SP.6, LI.4 Rf M alternate with GV.4, BL.20, BL.23, BL.32 Rf M + GV.20, KI.2 M for Deficient Kidney Yang
Deficient Blood and Deficient Jing	amenorrhoea or infertility especially after one or more childbirth, particularly if birth is difficult, prolonged and with much loss of blood, exhaustion, dizziness, tinnitus, depression	thin, choppy	pale, thin	CV.4, KI.6, KI.13, BL.62, ST.36, SP.6, LI.4 Rf alternate with BL.17, BL.20, BL.23, BL.43 Rf; BL.32 E
Deficient Qi and Deficient Blood	amenorrhoea or infertility with emaciation, tiredness and weakness from dieting, e.g. anorexia, or from prolonged or severe illness, depression	thin, choppy or minute	pale, thin, flabby	CV.4, CV.12, ST.29, ST.36, SP.1, SP.6, LI.4 Rf M alternate with BL.17, BL.20, BL.23, BL.43 Rf; BL.32 E + GV.20, yìn táng for anorexia

Rd, Reducing method; Rf, Reinforcing method; E, Even method; M, moxa.

frustration and suppressed anger, or more specifically to resentment of femininity and resistance to the physiological and psychological changes of adult sexuality.

KIDNEYS

For many women the major developmental stages of puberty, pregnancy, childbirth and motherhood are surrounded by fear, the fear of the unknown, fear of pain, fear of death, fear of responsibility, fear of failure. This can cause Stagnation of Qi just as much as anger and frustration.

LUNGS

Closely related to the fear of the unknown, are grief and the fear of loss. Holding on to the past, trying to stop time, and unwillingness to let go of old relationships and fully participate in new ones, are associated with Stagnant Lung Qi.

HEART

There may be an unwillingness to participate in any

relationships at all, with an attempt to block the flow of love, life and sexuality, as in anorexia nervosa, with amenorrhoea. Or in some cases of infertility there may be stresses and fluctuating affections within the relationship, with mixed feelings about conception. One part of the woman wants to conceive, while other stronger parts do not want a child at all, or a child with this man, or at this time. It seems that these mixed emotions and mixed motivations can prevent conception, which then only occurs when the desire to conceive becomes dominant.

SPLEEN

If there was not a solid, warm, caring relationship between the woman and her own mother, the woman may feel a great lack and emptiness within, a feeling of rejection and lack of support, and may withdraw into anorexia, or subconsciously or consciously avoid motherhood herself. She may feel that she has nothing to give a child, especially if it is a daughter.

TREATMENT

Amenorrhoea can initially be treated once per week. In infertility, when the syndrome is one of Stagnation of Qi and Blood requiring Reducing method on points with strong moving action, treatment can be once per week only if no attempt at conception is made or if contraception is used. If conception is being attempted during the period of treatment, then treatments can be given only after menstruation and before ovulation. If treatments with a strong moving action are given between ovulation and menstruation time, then if conception has occurred, there may be a chance of miscarriage. However, gentle tonifying treatments can be given throughout the cycle, if points on the sacrum and lower abdomen are avoided, and moving points like SP.6 and LI.4 are omitted.

Irregular menstruation syndromes

There are three main types of irregular menstruation:

short cycle (increased frequency of menses)
long cycle (decreased frequency of menses)
irregular cycle.

AETIOLOGY

STAGNANT QI

Stagnation of any of the five emotions, especially those of the Liver, may result in long cycles or irregular cycles, or if Stagnation turns into Heat, in short cycles.

HEAT IN THE BLOOD

Stagnation of Qi of Heart or Liver, associated with suppressed emotions, may generate Heat in the Blood, shortening the cycle.

COLD

If there is Cold, due to Deficient Yang, excess raw food, excess cold food and drink, or exposure to cold and damp

during menstruation, the movement of Blood is slowed by the Cold, and the cycle is longer.

DEFICIENT BLOOD

If there is insufficient Blood, due to childbirth, menorrhagia, malnutrition, illness or worry, then the cycle can become longer.

DEFICIENT QI

Malnutrition or overwork may lead to Deficiency of Spleen Qi, and then of Heart Qi, so that the Qi fails to control the Blood, resulting in a short cycle.

SYNDROMES

The main syndromes are shown in Figure 31.2.

TREATMENT

The point combinations for these syndromes are summarized in Table 31.3.

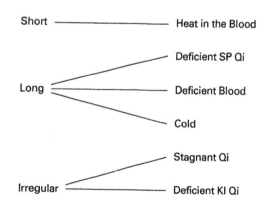

Fig. 31.2 Irregular menstruation aetiology.

Table 31.3 Irregular menstruation syndromes

Type	Syndrome	Signs and symptoms	Pulse	Tongue	Point combination
Short	Heat in the Blood	much dark red thick blood irritability, restlessness, insomnia, dark urine	rapid, full,	red, dry yellow coat	CV.3, LI.11, SP.6, SP.10 Rd + LR.1, LR.2 Rd for Liver Heat + KI.2 Rd; KI.10 Rf for Deficient Kidney Yin
Long	Deficient Spleen Qi	much thin light red blood, tiredness, weakness, low appetite, loose stools	thin, choppy, changing	pale, thin, maybe flabby	CV.4, CV.12, SP.6, ST.36 Rf M + SP.1 M for severe bleeding + GV.20 M; yìn táng E for worry
	Deficient Blood	scanty light red menses, sallow skin, dizziness, blurred vision, palpitations	thin, choppy	pale, thin, dry	CV.4, LI.4, SP.6, SP.10, ST.36 Rf M alternate with BL.17, BL.20, BL.43 Rf M + GV.20, HT.7 E for insomnia
	Cold	scanty dark menses, pain and sensation of cold in lower abdomen	empty, deep, slow	pale, flabby, moist white coat	CV.4, CV.6, ST.29. ST.36, SP.4 E M
Irregular	Stagnant Qi	delayed or irregular menses, maybe think purple blood, maybe distension and pain in breasts or abdomen, depression	wiry	maybe purplish	CV.6, TE.6, ST.29. SP.8, LR.3 Rd + CV.17, PC.6 Rd for Stagnant Heart Qi + CV.3, LI.4 Rd for dysmenorrhoea + GB.20, LR.13 Rd for Stagnant Liver Qi
	Deficient Kidney Qi	scanty light red menses, tiredness, dizziness, tinnitus, lumbar ache	empty, deep	pale, thin white coat	GV.20, CV.4, KI.8, KI.10, ST.36 Rf M alternate with GV.4, GV.20, BL.23, BL.32 Rf M

Rd, Reducing method; Rf, Reinforcing method; E, Even method; M, moxa.

Dysmenorrhoea syndromes

AETIOLOGY

The main cause of pain during menstruation is Stagnation of the flow of Qi and Blood in the uterus. Two origins of this Stagnation may be Liver and Kidneys.

STAGNANT LIVER QI

This may be associated with suppressed anger, frustration and depression, arising from the stresses of daily living, especially if the person is of the Wood constitutional type. More specifically, there may be resentment at the surrender of self, limitation of ego and restriction of freedom and independence that is involved in femininity and is symbolized by menstruation.

STAGNANT KIDNEY QI

Kidney fear may also cause Stagnation of Qi and Blood in the uterus. There is the ongoing fear of failure and fear of loss of control involved in daily living, which is felt more acutely by personalities of the Water type. Specifically, there is fear of femininity with fear of letting go and fear of the unknown, which may involve fear of sexuality, fear of pregnancy, fear of pain and fear of motherhood.

DEFICIENCY OF QI AND BLOOD

Whilst the main syndrome associated with dysmenorrhoea is Stagnation of Qi and Blood, Deficiency of Qi and Blood may be a secondary syndrome, where Qi and Blood have become Deficient due to illness, overwork, stress, blood loss, and so on. In some cases Cold and Damp, and in other cases Damp Heat, can also interfere with the movement of Qi and Blood, causing pain.

SYNDROMES

The main syndrome is Stagnation of Qi and Blood, but there are three minor syndromes, and as usual two or more syndromes may be mixed together.

Stagnation of Qi and Blood
Accumulation of Cold and Damp
Downward flow of Damp Heat
Deficient Qi and Blood

TREATMENT

DURING AND BETWEEN

There are two types of treatment for dysmenorrhoea, firstly during or just before the time of pain, and, secondly between menses. Treatment during or just before the pain concentrates on moving Stagnation to relieve pain. Treatment between menses includes moving Stagnation, but also involves tonifying any Deficiency and balancing psychological factors.

TIMING OF TREATMENT

The 'during' treatment can be given either during the pain itself or, usually more effective, a few days before its onset in the premenstrual stage. This applies to pain associated with Stagnant Qi and Blood especially. If the pain is severe, treatment can be given both a few days before and also during menstruation. The 'between' treatments can be given, one per week, in the time between menses.

BASIC TREATMENT

An effective basic combination for all four syndromes is:

CV.3, ST.29, LI.4, SP.6 Rd

This basic combination can be modified according to the syndrome and the changing needs of the patient.

OTHER POINTS

Some other points which can be useful in dysmenorrhoea and endometriosis are:

CV.4	RF M to strengthen Qi and Blood, to warm and move Stagnation from Cold
CV.6	E M to strengthen and warm Qi and to move Stagnant Qi in depression
KI.8	E or Rd to move Stagnation from Stagnant Kidney Qi and fear
KI.12, KI.13	E or Rd to move Stagnation in uterus
ST.28, ST.29	Rd to move Stagnant Blood in uterus
SP.4, SP.8	Rd to move Statnant Blood in uterus
SP.10	Rd to disperse Heat in the Blood, and to move the Blood, Rf to tonify Blood
LR.2	Rd to disperse Heat in the Blood
LR.3	Rd to move Stagnant Qi and Blood from Stagnant Liver Qi
LR.5	Rd to disperse Damp Heat
LR.8	Rf to strengthen Liver Blood

BL.17	Rd to move Stagnant Blood, and calm Stagnation due to fear
BL.18	E to regulate Liver Qi; Rf to strengthen Liver Blood
BL.20	Rf to strengthen Qi and Blood
BL.23, BL.52	Rf to strengthen Qi; E to calm Kidney fear
BL.32	Rd to move Stagnant Blood or Damp Heat in uterus
zǐ gōng	Rd to move Stagnant Blood or Damp Heat in uterus

(Rf, Reinforcing method; Rd, Reducing method; E, Even method)

Example

A woman of 35 had severe pain the day before menstruation, and also the first day of menstruation until she had passed some large clots of blood. She then had no pain, but for 3–4 days after menstruation felt very tired with some dizziness and a generalized dull headache. Her pulse was wiry, thin and choppy, and her tongue was pale and thin.

The diagnosis was Stagnant Blood and Deficient Blood. The following combination was used premenstrually, or on the first day of menstruation, if the pain was severe and she was able to come to the clinic:

CV.3, ST.29, LI.4, SP.6 Rd M; ST.36 Rf M

After menstruation, the following combination was used, primarily to strengthen Blood, and secondarily to regulate the Liver:

CV.4, SP.10, ST.36 Rf M; CV.6, E M; PC.6, LR. 3 Rd alternating with BL.17, BL.20, BL.43 Rf M; BL.18, BL.32 Rd

ENDOMETRIOSIS

Endometriosis is endometrium growing outside the uterus, usually attached to the pelvic organs. There is pain during or between periods, and maybe pain during intercourse, pain with bowel movements, infertility, tiredness or exhaustion. There may also be heavy uterine bleeding.

TREATMENT

As for dysmenorrhoea, treating regularly for 3–9 months. It is helpful to treat in the last 2 weeks of the cycle, when Stagnation of Blood is increasing, unless the syndrome is Deficient Qi and Blood, which needs tonification in the first 2 weeks of the cycle.

Table 31.4 Dysmenorrhoea and endometriosis syndromes: basic combination CV.3, ST.29, LI.4, SP.6 Rd

Syndrome	Signs and symptoms	Pulse	Tongue	Point combination
Stagnation of Qi and Blood	distending pain before or severe pain during menses, often relieved by the passage of clots, maybe suppressed anger, suppressed fear, frustration or depression, maybe nausea	wiry	normal or purplish	**During** Basic + CV.6, CV.17, PC.6, LR.3 Rd for Stagnant Liver Qi Basic + KI.8, KI.13 Rd; KI.1 M (no SP.6) for Stagnant Kidney Qi **Between** BL.18, BL.24, BL.32, LI.4, SP.6 E for Stagnant Liver Qi BL.17, BL.23, BL.32, BL.52, LU.7, KI.8 for Stagnant Kidney Qi
Accumulation of Cold and Damp	severe pain during menses, with cold lower abdomen, alleviated by warmth	wiry, maybe slow and deep	purplish, white coat	**During** Basic + CV.4, SP.4 Rf M **Between** GV.4, BL.20, BL.23, BL.32 E M; LI.4, SP.6 E
Downward flow of Damp Heat	abdominal pain worse with pressure, maybe feverish during menses, with restlessness and thirst	wiry, rapid, maybe slippery	red, yellow coat	**During** Basic + GB.34, LR.5, LR.2 Rd **Between** BL.18, BL.32, TE.5, GB.41, LR.2, SP.6 Rd
Deficient Qi and Blood	dull pain after menstruation, tiredness, pallor, maybe dizziness, blurred vision, poor memory	thin, choppy, maybe minute	pale	**During** Basic Rd + CV.4, ST.36, SP.10 Rf **Between** BL.18, BL.20, BL.23, BL.43, LI.4, ST.36, SP.6 Rf

Rd, Reducing method; Rf, Reinforcing method; E, Even method; M, moxa.

Abnormal uterine bleeding syndromes

Abnormal uterine bleeding (AUB) refers in this section only to excessive bleeding at menstruation. Irregularities of length or timing of menstruation are dealt with separately on pages 403–404. AUB here refers to dysfunctional uterine bleeding, when gynaecological examination has excluded other causes of bleeding, such as tumour, infection, systemic disease or foreign body.

AETIOLOGY

Stagnation of emotions can be associated with Stagnant Qi and the accumulation of Heat, as depression and frustration can retain the pent-up energy and Heat of anger. This is especially so where the person has Deficient Yin and Fire of Kidneys, Liver or Heart. The Excess Heat can then cause the Blood to leave the vessels. Deficiency of Spleen Qi can affect the ability of the Spleen to hold the Blood in the vessels, and in this case, there may be haemorrhage with signs of Deficiency and Cold. Deficiency of Kidney Qi and Yang can contribute to this. Excessive physical work, worry and too much study can contribute to Deficient Spleen Qi and to anaemia from loss of blood.

SYNDROMES

Excess
  Stagnant Qi and Heat
Excess + Deficiency
  Stagnant Qi + Deficient Qi
Deficiency
  Deficient Qi

TREATMENT

The immediate aim is to stop bleeding. Treatment may need to be once or even twice daily in severe acute situations. Once the bleeding has stopped, treatment can be once per week, to correct the cause of bleeding, e.g. Heat or Deficient Qi, and, if there is Deficiency of Blood as a result of the bleeding, this may also be corrected.

Points for Deficient Blood can be:

BL.17, BL.20, BL.43, ST.36, SP.6, LI.4 Rf

At the next menstruation, once again the aim is to stop bleeding.

Example

A woman of 22 had severe uterine bleeding after sleeping on cold wet ground while camping. Previously, she usually had heavy bleeding at menstruation but not so severe. She was usually tired, depressed and sometimes irritable. Her pulse was thin, choppy, and slightly wiry. Her tongue was pale and thin.

The diagnosis was chronic Deficient Qi and Blood with some Stagnant Liver Qi, and acute Cold invasion. To stop the bleeding, the following combination was used:

GV.20, CV.4, TE.4, SP.6, SP.10, ST.36 Rf M;
SP.1 M (15–20 cones)

Later, once the bleeding had stopped, the following combination was used to tonify Blood and Qi, and to regulate the Liver:

CV4, SP.6, SP.10, ST.36 Rf M
alternate with GV.4, GV.20, BL.20, BL.23 Rf M; BL.18 Rd

Table 31.5 Abnormal uterine bleeding

Syndrome	Signs and symptoms	Pulse	Tongue	Point combination
Stagnant Qi and Heat	deep red blood, depression or irritability, restlessness, insomnia, maybe dizziness	wiry, rapid, thin or full	red, especially at tip and edges	CV.3, SP.1, SP.6 Rd + LR.3 Rd for Stagnant Liver Qi + LR.1, LR.2 Rd for Liver Fire + HT.5 or HT.8 Rd for Heart Fire + SP.9 Rd for Damp Heat + SP.10, KI.5 Rd for Heat in the Blood + KI.2 Rd; KI.10 Rf for Deficient Kidney Yin
Stagnant Qi and Deficient Qi	menstrual or mid-cycle bleeding with both depression and tiredness, maybe abdominal pain and distension, loss of appetite or lumbar pain	wiry or hindered, empty	flabby, maybe pale, with red edges	LR.1, LR.3, SP.1, SP.6 Rd; CV.4, KI.3, ST.36 Rf M
Deficient Qi and Blood	light red and thin blood, tiredness, weakness, shortness of breath, pallor and maybe cold extremities	empty or thin, choppy, maybe slow and deep	pale, flabby or thin, maybe moist white coat	GV.20, CV.4, ST.36, SP.6, TE.4 Rf M; SP.1 M (15–20 moxa cones) alternate with BL.17, BL.20, BL.23, BL.43 Rf M + KI.7 Rf M for Deficient Kidney Yang + yìn táng for worry

Rd, Reducing method; Rf, Reinforcing method; M, moxa.

Vaginitis syndromes

Vaginitis is here defined as vaginal inflammation which may be associated with excessive discharge (leucorrhoea), itching, or dryness and pain. Western gynaecological examination is necessary to check for carcinoma and sexually transmitted diseases (STD).

LEUCORRHOEA

Providing the patient really has excessive discharge and is not merely oversensitive about normal secretions, acupuncture can be effective, but especially when combined with basic self-help and hygiene precautions.

SELF-HELP

HYGIENE

The patient should avoid potentially irritant chemicals, e.g. bath salts, bubble baths, deodorants and strong or scented soaps, and use only mild soaps. The patient should keep the area as dry as possible, use clean dry towels, wipe from front to back, wear clothes which allow air to circulate to the area, avoid tights and tight jeans, and use cotton rather than nylon underwear. In the case of STD, it is preferable to abstain from intercourse until the infection has gone.

NUTRITION

The patient should eat plenty of green vegetables, both raw and cooked, but if the syndrome is Deficient Spleen Yang, avoid raw foods or cold food and drink. Excess coffee, strong tea or alcohol are to be avoided. Moderate intake of sugars, dairy products and highly spiced or greasy foods is recommended.

MEDICATION

It may be necessary to use alternative birth control methods to the contraceptive pill if there are chronic vaginal problems. Also, if the patient is taking antibiotics then live yoghurt can be taken vaginally and also as food, to restore the balance of microorganisms.

AETIOLOGY

DEFICIENT KIDNEY QI

Chronic Deficient Kidney Qi, from the usual causes, can weaken the Conception and Belt vessels and lead to discharge.

DEFICIENT SPLEEN QI AND DAMP

Chronic Spleen Deficiency, from the usual causes, can lead to the accumulation of Damp, and also weaken the circulation of Qi, leading to Stagnation of Qi.

Damp Heat

In a person of the Deficient Yang type, Deficient Qi of Kidney or Spleen tends to lead to Cold Damp leucorrhoea. In a person of the Deficient Yin type, Damp Heat is more likely; for example, when suppressed emotions transform into Stagnant Qi and Heat.

SYNDROMES

Excess
Damp Heat

Deficiency
Deficient Spleen Qi and Damp
Deficient Kidney Qi

VAGINAL AND GENITAL ITCHING

In Chinese medicine, this is related mainly to Damp Heat, or to Heat in the Blood. Damp Heat is generally linked to Stagnant Liver Qi, and Heat in the Blood may be linked to Liver and Heart Fire, and to emotional irritation, frustration, suppressed anger and excitement. It is helpful to determine the underlying emotional cause and to treat this whenever possible.

VAGINAL DRYNESS AND PAIN

Vaginal dryness may be due to Deficient Yin, and also to Deficient Jing and Blood in the postmenopausal woman. Pain during intercourse is often linked to vaginal dryness, which in many cases is not due to pathology, but to incomplete sexual arousal. Treatment then relates more to counselling and less to acupuncture.

POINTS FOR VAGINITIS

The main points have been given in Table 31.6. The following points can be used in addition or as alternatives:

CV.1, CV.2	for Damp Heat or Heat in the Blood
LU.7 (with KI.6)	for itching with menopausal syndrome
LR.5	as alternative to SP.6 for Damp Heat
GB.27, GB.28	as additions to GB.26 for Damp Heat
HT.7, HT.8	for severe itching, with distress and insomnia, from Heat in the Blood
TE.6	for itching with menopausal syndrome.

Table 31.6 Vaginitis Syndromes

Syndromes	Signs and symptoms	Pulse	Tongue	Point combination
Damp Heat	sticky yellow discharge with foul smell, itching vulva, maybe restless, feverish, irritability	wiry, rapid, slippery	red, yellow greasy coat	CV.3, GB.26, ST.29, SP.6, LR.3 Rd alternate: BL.18, BL.32 Rd
Heat in the Blood	severe genital irritation with red inflamed areas, restless irritability, insomnia, maybe skin rashes in other areas	rapid, thin or full	red, especially tip or edges, dry	CV.3, LI.4, LI.11, SP.6, SP.10 Rd; KI.6 Rf + SP.1, LR.1, B; LR.2 Rd: LR.8 Rf for Liver Fire + PC.9, HT.9 B; HT.3, PC.3 Rf for Heart Fire
Deficient Kidney Yin	vaginal dryness with soreness and irritation or pain on intercourse, restless but tired	thin, rapid	red, thin, dry no coat	CV.2, KI.2 Rd; CV.4, KI.6, SP.6, ST.36 Rf alternate: BL.20, BL.23 Rf; BL.32 Rd
Deficient Kidney Jing and Deficient Liver Blood	vaginal dryness during or after menopause, dry skin, tiredness, dizziness tinnitus, blurred vision, poor memory	thin, choppy, maybe deep	pale, thin, dry	CV.4, LI.4, LR.8, SP.6, KI.6, ST.36 Rf alternate: BL.18, BL.20, BL.23 Rf
Deficient Spleen Qi	much thick white or pale yellow discharge, tiredness, poor appetite	empty, slippery	pale, flabby, greasy white	CV.3, SP.6, SP.9, GB.26 E; CV.6, ST.36 E M alternate: BL.20, BL.32 E M
Deficient Kidney Qi	much thin white discharge, exhaustion, low back pain, cold limbs and abdomen, urinary frequency	empty, deep, slow	pale, flabby, moist white coat	GV.20, CV.4, ST.28, ST.36, KI.7 Rf M alternate: GV.4, GV.20, BL.20, BL.23, BL.32 Rf M

Rd, Reducing method; Rf, Reinforcing method; E, Even method; M, moxa.

Breast syndromes

Breast problems are primarily due to Stagnant Qi in the chest and breasts, whether the Stagnation is of Liver Qi, Lung Qi, Heart Qi or a combination. Deficiency of Qi and Blood may also contribute to some breast problems, for example insufficient lactation.

TYPES OF BREAST PROBLEMS

Four main types will be considered here:

    premenstrual syndromes
    lactation problems
    breast lumps
    breast abscess.

Point combinations are shown in Table 31.7.

PREMENSTRUAL SYNDROMES

This has been discussed earlier, and distension and soreness of the breasts at this time is usually due to a combination of Stagnant Liver Qi and Hyperactive Liver Yang.

LACTATION PROBLEMS

The main problem is insufficient lactation, which is associated with Stagnant Liver Qi, Deficient Qi and Blood, or a combination of both syndromes. Excessive lactation can be treated by reducing:

    CV.17, ST.18, GB.37. GB.41

BREAST LUMPS

Breast lumps require specialist diagnosis with Western medicine, before treatment with acupuncture, to check the possibility of carcinoma. Whether benign or malignant, breast lumps may be said to have four main contributing factors in Chinese medicine: Stagnant Liver Qi, Stagnant Lung Qi, Stagnant Heart Qi, and Phlegm.

STAGNANT LIVER QI

Stagnant Liver Qi may be associated with resentment of femininity, resentment at the limitations of freedom and independence imposed upon the ego by menstruation,

pregnancy and motherhood. There may also be resistance to change, an unwillingness to flow with the changes of life and to adapt to the new roles and identities associated with such major developmental stages as puberty, motherhood and menopause. Resistance to change and stagnation of the flow of Qi can be associated with depression, frustration and suppressed anger.

STAGNATION OF LUNG AND SPLEEN QI

The Lungs and the Metal element are associated with the formation of bonds between individuals, for example between partners, between mother and child. When partners separate, or when children leave home there is grief, the pain of letting go, of allowing the bonds to dissolve, so that each individual, alone, can reach a new identity and a new level of understanding and perspective. Stagnant Lung Qi occurs when there is a suppression of grief, a holding on from fear of letting go because of fear of the pain of loss, fear of being alone, fear of the unknown, fear of facing the truth.

The Spleen and Earth element are associated with nourishment, caring and protection, whether physical, emotional or mental. The breasts are the physical organ through which the physical substance milk flows from the mother to nourish the physical body of the child, just as her enfolding, caring, concern and sympathy nourish the child's emotional needs for comfort and security.

For the mother, it gives a sense of satisfaction and fulfilment to be needed, and to enfold another person and have them near. Stagnant Spleen Qi can occur when the children leave home, or the partner leaves, since the mother can feel that she is no longer needed and no longer able to find fulfilment outside herself by physically and emotionally caring for others. Unless she is able to find contentment within herself, or to find a new role in caring for others, she may become insecure, clinging, possessive and intrusive into the lives of her children, driving them further away from her. Earth is now moving into Metal, sympathy into grief, as the pleasure in enfolding becomes the need to hold on and the fear of letting go.

Stagnation of Lung and Spleen Qi can act closely together.

STAGNANT HEART QI

The Heart and the Fire element rule the expression of warmth and affection, the joy in giving and receiving love, the pleasure in communication with others and in a feeling of oneness and communion with all life. If this expression is blocked, if the person suppresses affection,

Table 31.7 Breast syndromes

Syndrome	Signs and symptoms	Pulse	Tongue	Point combination
Stagnant Liver Qi and Hyperactive Liver Yang	premenstrual syndrome with depression, irritability, sore breasts, abdominal pain and distension, maybe nausea or headache	wiry	maybe purplish	GV.20, CV.6, CV.17, PC.6, SI.1, LR.3, LR.14, ST.18, SP.6 E or Rd
Stagnation in Liver and Stomach channels	breast abscess with redness, swelling, pain and maybe purulent discharge, maybe feverish, restlessness, thirst	wiry, rapid, slippery, flooding	red, greasy yellow coat	CV.17, ST.1, ST.18, ST.36, GB.21, LR.3, LR.14, Rd + LI.4, LI.10 Rd for Heat in Stomach and Liver + LI.4, TE.5 Rd. for fever + LR.5, GB.41 Rd for Damp Heat
Stagnant Liver Qi	insufficient lactation or breast lumps with depression, frustration, suppressed anger, resistance to change, soreness and distension in the breasts	wiry	maybe purplish	CV.17, PC.6, ST.18, GB.21, LR.3, LR.14 Rd + SI.1 for insufficient lactation + TE.6 for breast lumps
Stagnant Lung and Spleen Qi	breast lumps, suppressed grief, needing to care for others with difficulty in caring for and nourishing self, holding on to the past	wiry or hindered, maybe flooding and deep	maybe purplish, white greasy coat	CV.17, PC.6, LU.1, LU.7, ST.18, ST.40, SP.4 Rd alternate BL.13, BL.16, BL.20, BL.42, BL.49 Rd
Stagnant Heart Qi	breast lumps, suppressed affection, difficulty in communicating or giving and receiving love in relationships	hindered, maybe deep	maybe swelling in Heart area	CV.17, PC.1, HT.6, SI.1, ST.18 Rd alternate BL.15, BL.16, BL.44, SI.11 Rf
Deficient Qi and Blood	deficient lactation with tiredness, depression, weak muscles, loose stools, dry skin, especially after much loss of blood in childbirth	empty or thin, choppy	pale, flabby, maybe dry	CV.17, ST.18, SI.1 E; CV.4, LI.4, SP.6, ST.36 Rf alternate BL.18, BL.20, BL.23, BL.43 Rf, moxa if no Heat signs

Rd, Reducing method; Rf, Reinforcing method; E, Even method; M, moxa

or finds difficulty in communicating or giving and receiving love in a relationship, then there may be Stagnant Heart Qi and Stagnation of Qi in the chest and breasts. There may be sadness, loneliness and a great need to express feelings and affection but difficulty in finding or developing relationships in which this can happen.

BREAST ABSCESS

In Chinese medicine, breast abscess is mainly associated with Stagnation in the Liver and Stomach channels that govern the breast, and in the Liver and Stomach organs, perhaps with Stomach Fire or Liver–Gallbladder Damp Heat.

POINTS FOR BREAST PROBLEMS

Combinations for breast syndromes are summarized in Table 31.7. In addition the main points for breast problems are:

CV.17
LU.1, LU.6, LU.7
LI.10

ST.18, ST.36
BL.16
LR.3, LR.14
GB.21, GB.41
PC.1, PC.6
TE.6
SI.1, SI.11

Menopause and midlife syndromes

INTRODUCTION

There are three related factors in the treatment of menopause:

menopause
midlife changes
personality type.

MENOPAUSE

The physiological changes of menopause may have less importance than is generally supposed. Firstly, the main midlife factor for women may not be menopause, but the psychological stresses resulting from the life changes at that time. Secondly, the signs and symptoms commonly associated with menopause may have less to do with hormonal changes, and more to do with lowered self-image arising from how women see their changing status in society.

MIDLIFE CHANGES

Between the ages of 40 and 55 come main life changes requiring considerable psychological adaptations to changing roles and self-image. Children may leave home, there may be disillusionment with job, fears of loss of femininity or attractiveness, estrangement or separation from partner, midlife crisis of partner, retirement of self or retirement of partner, arrival of grandchildren or death of parents.

There is a need to change and to let go of the past, but there can be great fear of change, fear of the unknown, and fear of being alone, with feelings of not being loved or needed. The tension between the need to change and the fear of change can create great depression and anxiety. The Yin personality tending to hold on to the past and let go of the present, and the Yang personality tending to hyperactivity, busying themselves with external things to avoid facing the need to change.

The menopause can be an extremely positive time, when a woman can integrate her past experience, and as the dross is burned away, discover a new inner strength and beauty within herself. Menopause can be a time of increasing wisdom and a deeper sense of purpose and fulfilment.

PERSONALITY TYPE

How a woman reacts to the hormonal changes of menopause and, perhaps more important, to the psychological changes of the midlife period, will depend on her constitutional and personality type.

HEART TYPE

At menopause the Heart type will either tend to rush about in restless hypomania, with ceaseless overstressed activity, or become lonely, melancholy and depressed. The gift of the Fire element is a new level of consciousness, feeling a new enthusiasm and awareness of life, but centred in peace within herself.

SPLEEN TYPE

During midlife, the Spleen type may either feel great insecurity, worry and self-pity within herself, or feel empty and rejected as those she cares for move away from her. Learning to care for and nourish herself, and then to find plesure in caring for others without mutual dependence, is the gift of the Earth element.

LUNG TYPE

At midlife, the Lung type will tend to hold on to her previous identity, try to avoid facing the truth, and resist letting go of her previous life patterns. But if she can let go, the gifts of the Metal element are a clear wisdom and deep perception, free of the confusion and griefs of the past.

KIDNEY TYPE

The water type may fear the changes of menopause and may try to resist or ignore them. She may fear getting old or losing her physical attraction, she may fear the unknown. If in the menopause she can learn to overcome her fears, she will gain the gift of the Water element and find a new source of strength and identity deep within herself.

LIVER TYPE

Liver type personalities will tend to react to menopause either with increased irritation and anger, which may be expressed or suppressed, or with depression. If Liver type woman can accept menopause and come to terms with the changes within herself, and around her in her life, then she may gain the great positive gifts of the Wood element. These are the development of intuition and the ability to flow harmoniously through life.

AETIOLOGY

As shown in Figure 31.3, three basic syndromes of menopause can be Deficient Yin with Deficiency Fire, Deficient Yang or Deficient Blood. Whether a woman manifests the Deficient Yin or the Deficient Yang syndrome in menopause will depend on whether her constitution is Deficient Yin or Deficient Yang. The syndrome of Deficient Heart and Spleen Blood may arise from blood in childbirth or menstruation, illness, worry, and so on.

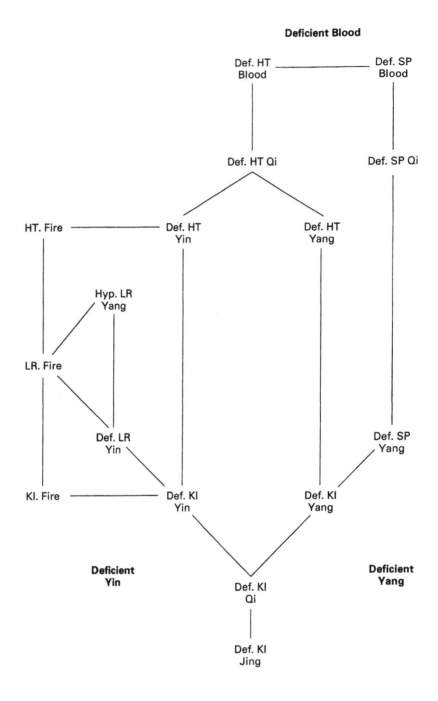

Deficient Blood

Def. HT ——————————— Def. SP
Blood   Blood

Def. HT Qi   Def. SP Qi

HT. Fire ——————— Def. HT   Def. HT
                              Yin   Yang

Hyp. LR
Yang

LR. Fire

Def. LR
Yin

Def. SP
Yang

KI. Fire ——————— Def. KI   Def. KI
                              Yin   Yang

**Deficient
Yin**

**Deficient
Yang**

Def. KI
Qi

Def. KI
Jing

Fig. 31.3

A syndrome that is characteristic of menopause is the oscillation between Deficient Yin with anxiety and over-excitement and signs of Heat, and Deficient Yang with depression and signs of Cold. This often has an under-lying pattern of Deficient Kidney Qi, where the Qi is no longer strong enough to hold stable the body temperature and emotions. Deficient Kidney Jing and Liver Blood is a natural concomitant of the ageing process, but occuring at menopause it may represent a constitutional tendency which is aggravated by childbirth, and by dietary defi-ciency of, or malabsorption of, nutrients such as calcium, iron and the essential fatty acids.

MENOPAUSE AND THE EXTRA CHANNELS

There are three additional menopausal syndromes which relate to the symptomatology of the three Extra channel pairs:

Conception + Yin Heel	Deficient Heart Qi, Blood and Yin
Thoroughfare + Yin Link	Deficient Kidney Qi and Stagnant Lung Qi
Belt + Yang Link	Deficient Kidney Yin and Hyper-active Liver Yang

The symptom patterns of these Extra channel pairs are summarized in Table 31.8. The combination of SI.3 + BL.62 for Governor + Yang Heel, is less used in menopausal situations. It might be used for osteoporosis or arthritis linked with menopause, but would then be combined with KI.6 and HT.6, to tonify Yin to balance an otherwise Yang treatment, and to reduce hot flushes.

SYNDROMES

Deficient Yin with Fire
Deficient Yang
Deficient Yin and Deficient Yang
Deficient Heart and Spleen Blood
Deficient Kidney Jing and Liver Blood
Deficient Heart Qi, Blood and Yin
Deficient Kidney Qi and Stagnant Lung Qi
Deficient Kidney Yin and Hyperactive Liver Yang

Table 31.8 Extra channels, menopause and midlife changes

Extra channel pair	Opening points	Signs and symptoms	Combination
Conception + Yin Heel	LU.7 + KI.6	fear of change, fear of letting go, depression and suppressed grief, maybe lumps in breasts or uterus	CV.6, CV.17, LU.1 E M; LU.7, KI.6 E
Thoroughfare + Yin Link	SP.4 + PC.6	anxiety depression, emotional lability, hot flushes, cold hands and feet, palpitation	CV.4, ST.36 Rf; GV.20, CV.14, SP.4, PC.6, HT.6 E
Belt + Yang Link	GB.41 + TE.5	uncertainty of self or of direction in life, touchiness, irritability, depression, headaches, hot flushes	CV.6, KI.6, HT.6 Rf; GV.20, GB.20, GB.41, TE.5 E

Rf, Reinforcing method; E, Even method; M, moxa.

Table 31.9 Menopause syndromes

Syndrome	Signs and symptoms	Pulse	Tongue	Point combination
Deficient Yin with Fire (Kidney, Liver, Heart)	hot flushes, hyperactivity, restlessness, insomnia, overexcitement, irritability, maybe weight loss, dry skin	thin, rapid, maybe wiry thin, dry	red, especially at tip or edges	CV.4, SP.6, KI.6 Rf; GV.20, KI.2 Rd + HT.3 Rf: HT.8 Rd for Heart Fire + LR.8 Rf; LR.2 Rd for Liver Fire + CV.3, ST.29 E for vaginal dryness
Deficient Yang (Kidney, Spleen, Heart)	exhaustion, depression, loneliness, cold limbs, maybe oedema, weight gain, arthritis with feeling of coldness	empty, deep, slow, maybe slippery	pale, flabby or swollen, moist white coat	GV.20, CV.4, KI.7, ST.36 Rf M; SP.6 E + CV.12, SP.2 Rf M for Deficient Spleen Yang + CV.17, HT.8 Rf M for Deficient Heart Yang + CV.9, SP.9, TE.6 Rd M for oedema
Deficient Yin and Deficient Yang (Kidney, Heart)	sometimes hot flushes, sometimes cold limbs, sometimes depression and withdrawal, sometimes hyperactivity and manic restlessness	variable speed and force, maybe irregular	various, maybe pale with red tip, maybe trembling	CV.4, ST.36, SP.6, KI.3 Rf; GV.20, HT.6 E + CV.14, KI.2 Rd for Deficient Yin phase + KI.2, HT.8 Rf for Deficient Yang phase
Deficient Heart and Spleen Blood	emotional vulnerability, insomnia, depression, tiredness, dry skin, blurred vision, dizziness	thin, choppy, maybe rapid or slow	pale, thin, dry	CV.4, CV.12, CV.17, ST.36, LI.4, SP.6, SP.10 Rf alternate with BL.17, BL.20, BL.43 Rf + yìn táng, ān mián, BL.44 for insomnia
Deficient Kidney Jing and Deficient Liver Blood	osteoporosis, arthritis, dizziness, tinnitus, dry skin, withdrawal, maybe palpitations	thin, choppy, maybe deep	pale, thin, dry	CV.4, CV.12, ST.36, KI.6, LR.8, HT.6 Rf alternate with BL.11, BL.18, BL.20, BL.23, GB.39, KI.6, HT.6 Rf
Deficient Heart Qi, Blood and Yin	anxiety, depression, emotional lability, weak and nervous people, some hot flushes, maybe cold hands and feet	thin, choppy, maybe irregular, moving or changing	pale, thin or flabby with red tip	CV.4, ST.36 Rf; GV.20, CV.14, SP.4, PC.6, HT.6 E
Deficient Kidney Qi and Stagnant Lung Qi	fear of change, fear of letting go, depression and suppressed grief, maybe dyspnoea or oedema, maybe lumps in breasts or uterus	empty or flooding at deep level, hindered, slippery	pale, maybe hollow or swelling in Lung area	CV.6, CV.17, LU.1 E M; LU.7, KI.6 E + ST.40, LU.6 Rd for breast lumps + CV.3, KI.13, ST.29 for uterine fibroids
Deficient Kidney Yin and Hyperactive Liver Yang	hot flushes, mood swings, irritability, touchiness, uncertainty of self, headaches, stiff muscles	thin, rapid, wiry, maybe slippery	red, especially at edges, thin, dry, yellow coat	CV.6, KI.6, HT.6 Rf; GV.20, GB.20, GB.41, TE.5 E

Rd, Reducing method; Rf, Reinforcing method; E, Even method; M, moxa.

Example 1

A woman of 45 had a cold lower body and oedema, and was exhausted, depressed and emotionally labile. She had a pulse speed of 68 and the pulse was short, deep, empty and changing. Her tongue was pale and flabby.

The diagnosis was Deficient Kidney Qi and Yang, with Stagnant Lung Qi. The Deficiency of Qi was responsible for the labile emotions and the changing pulse. The basic point combination was:

CV.4, KI.6 Rf; CV.9, CV.17, LU.1, LU.7 E or Rd

Example 2

A woman of 48 had a weak constitution with insomnia and occasional hot flushes. She was restless, anxious, fearful and easily startled. Her pulse speed was 85 and the pulse was thin, choppy and moving. Her tongue was pale, with only a few red spots and trembling.

The diagnosis was Deficient Spleen and Heart Blood, and Deficient Heart and Kidney Yin. The point combination was:

CV.4, SP.4, ST.36 Rf; CV.14, CV.17, PC.6, HT.6 E or Rd

Obstetric syndromes

MORNING SICKNESS

Acupuncture can be effective and safe for morning sickness, provided that certain precautions are observed:

• Minimum number of points should be used.

• Strong needle stimulation should be avoided. Reinforcing or Even method should be used rather than Reducing method.

• For women with a history of miscarriage, needling in pregnancy should be done with great caution, if at all.

• Points with strong moving effect, e.g. LI.4, SP.6 and SP.8, should be avoided. In the first 3 months, points on the lower abdomen and sacrum are contraindicated, and after 3 months, no points on the abdomen or lower back should be used.

POINT COMBINATION

A good basic combination is CV.12, ST.36, PC.6 Rf or E. SP.4 can be added with Reinforcing method and moxa, when tiredness, sleepiness and an empty pulse indicate Deficient Spleen Qi. CV.17 can be added with Even method for depression. CV.13 can be used as an alternative or an addition to CV.12 for nausea and vomiting.

PC.6 can be used with Reducing method if necessary, since this point affects the stomach and upper body, rather than the lower abdomen, and the patient can be taught to use finger pressure on this point when needed.

MALPOSITION OF FETUS

Malposition of the fetus may be treated by the use of moxa stick on BL.67 bilaterally for 15–20 minutes daily until the fetal position is corrected. The underlying cause of the malposition must be known, to exclude such problems as deformities of pelvis or uterus.

ACUPUNCTURE IN CHILDBIRTH

This section is contributed by Lilleba Olsen, who organizes hospital training on acupuncture in childbirth for midwives in Sweden.

COOPERATION WITH MIDWIVES

If the acupuncture practitioner is not a midwife, it is essential to have good communication and cooperation between acupuncturist and midwife. If there is not cooperation, the parents-to-be will feel it, and this may complicate the labour. If there is good communication, then the midwife may be able to inform the acupuncturist of details of labour with which they are not familiar, so that they can use acupuncture more effectively,

METHOD OF NEEDLING

In this system, electroacupuncture is not used in normal childbirth. It is sometimes used to initiate contractions and sometimes to control pain during stitching. Usually, needles are inserted at an oblique angle, and needle sensation is obtained. The needles can then be taped to the skin, for example in the first stage, so that the woman can walk about, or they can be left untaped so that the practitioner can manipulate them, during delivery for example. Needles can be retained for as long as they are effective, from 10 minutes to 3 hours or more, as required.

SELECTION OF POINTS

The minimum number of points is used. The points higher on the body are used initially, to be replaced by points lower on the body as the pain changes during the progress of labour. For example, BL.24, BL.25 or BL.26 may be used for back pain in the first stage, changing to BL.27, BL.30 or BL.35 in the second stage.

FIRST STAGE

Pain

GB.25	pain in lower back and in abdomen
BL.24, BL.25 or BL.26	pain in lower back
GB.27, GB.28	pain in groin
CV.3, CV.4	pain in central lower abdomen
jiaǒ líng, SP.11	pain down front of thighs

(jiaǒ líng (chiao ling) is 1 unit below LR.10)

Two or three points can be used bilaterally as required. One needle can be inserted after a contraction, waiting one or two contractions to see if it is effective. The woman should immediately feel some relief. The practitioner can start with GB.25, then proceed with BL.24 or GB.27 or CV.3, depending on the locations of the pain.

Other Problems

LU.7	worry, anxiety, hypertension
GV.20	worry, anxiety, hypertension, but try LU.7 first; if GV.20 is used at the beginning of labour, remove after 20 minutes, so it can be used again later if needed
PC.6	lingering constant nausea
GV.20, BL.22 or LI.4	ineffective, painful contractions

SECOND STAGE

If any point is still effective it can be retained and used, otherwise the points from the first stage should be removed and the following points used, which are lower on the body, as the second stage proceeds.

BL.27, BL.28, BL.29, BL.30, BL.35	select one or two of these points for back pain at the end of the second stage
CV2, CV.3, KI.11, jiaǒ líng	frontal pain
LR.5 + wei mo	ineffective contractions (electro-acupuncture can be used with this combination if necessary (wei mo is on the lateral calf, opposite LR.5)
LR.3 + LI.4	generalized pain and ineffective contractions

CV.2, KI.11, BL.35 or jiaǒ líng	perineal pain during delivery; only one or two needles should be used, e.g. BL.35 and CV.2, or jiaǒ líng and KI.11, with continual manual stimulation

THIRD STAGE

KI.11	KI.11 can give good analgesia during stitching if the needles are stimulated for 1 or 2 minutes before the midwife starts to examine and stitch
LR.5 + wei mo	retained placenta, using all these points together and stimulating LR.5 and wei mo manually or with electroacupuncture

POSTNATAL PAIN AND BLEEDING

PRINCIPLE OF TREATMENT

It is necessary to treat the effect, for example, to relieve pain or to stop bleeding; any underlying Deficiency can then be treated, as with postnatal exhaustion and depression.

POINT COMBINATIONS

The following combinations can be effective, but must be modified to fit the needs of the individual patient. Pain and bleeding after termination can also be treated with these combinations.

Retained placenta

CV.3, ST.29, KI.6, GB.21, TE.5 Rd

Postnatal abdominal pain

CV.3, ST.30, SP.6 Rd; ST.36 Rf M

Postnatal bleeding

CV.3, SP.1, SP.6, LR.3 Rd for Stagnant Qi and Heat
CV.4, ST.36, SP.6, TE.4 Rf M; SP.1 M for Deficient Qi

Postnatal exhaustion

CV.4, CV.12, CV.17, ST.36, SP.6, LI.4 Rf (+ M if no signs of Heat) alternate with BL.15, BL.18, BL.20, BL.23 Rf (+ M if no signs of Heat)

POSTNATAL EXHAUSTION AND DEPRESSION

There may be great physical exhaustion if the birth was difficult and tiring, if there was much loss of blood, or if this birth followed closely a previous birth or illness from which the mother has not fully recovered. In addition to this Deficiency of Qi and Blood, there may be an exhaustion of Yang and Fire.

DEFICIENCY AND DEPRESSION

These Deficiencies may be associated with depression:

Deficient Kidney	exhaustion, depression, fear, withdrawal
Deficient Heart	lack of warmth, interest in and excitement about the baby
Deficient Spleen	feeling of lack of capactiy to nourish baby, either physically or emotionally, insecurity and worry.

All these Deficiencies can lead to feelings of guilt which increase the depth of depression.

STAGNATION AND DEPRESSION

Depression may also be associated with Stagnation of Qi, for example of Liver, Heart or Lungs:

Stagnant Liver Qi	resentment of the baby, of the suffering of birth, of the loss of freedom
Stagnant Heart Qi	mixed feelings about the baby or the relationship with partner, blocking the flow of affection
Stagnant Lung Qi	grief, feelings of guilt and self-blame.

POINT COMBINATIONS

Combinations are summarized in Table 31.10. However, often, rather than occurring as individual syndromes, these different Deficiencies and Stagnation may combine to contribute to the depression. The emphasis of treatment then depends on the relative importance of the contributing syndromes.

UTERINE PROLAPSE

Uterine prolapse is seen in Chinese medicine as Deficiency of Qi; specifically, failure of the normal function of Qi to hold up the organs. Uterine prolapse may occur after childbirth, in which case it should be treated about 2 weeks afterwards, since delay may decrease the effectiveness of treatment. Acupuncture may be helpful in some cases of uterine prolapse, and in addition gentle exercises may be helpful. Vigorous exercise or lifting of heavy weights should be avoided during treatment, and the patient should rest as much as possible to allow the Qi to recover.

POINT COMBINATION

GV.20 M; CV.6, ST.36 Rf M; SP.6, KI.6 Rf; GB.28 Rd

METHOD

Approximately five moxa cones can be used on GV.20 to raise the Qi. CV.6, ST.36, SP.6 and KI.6 aid this function. GB.28, and ST.30 which may be added to assist this point, are located over the ligaments which support the Fallopian tubes and the uterus.

CV.6 is inserted 1.5–2 inches in the direction of the external genitals. GB.28 is inserted at an oblique angle, along the groin towards the genitals, and is rotated to cause a pulling sensation. ST.30 can be inserted at an oblique angle, directly upwards away from the groin. Both GB.28 and ST.30 can be inserted 1.5–3 inches, when used at an oblique angle.

If there are signs of Damp Heat, SP.9 and LR.8 can be added with Reducing method.

Table 31.10 Postnatal exhaustion and depression syndromes

Syndrome	Signs and symptoms	Pulse	Tongue	Point combination
Deficient Qi and Blood	depression and lack of interest with exhaustion, weakness and pallor, maybe feelings of cold or faintness	empty, thin or minute, choppy, maybe slow and deep	pale, flabby	GV.20, CV.4, CV.12, CV.17, ST.36, KI.3, HT.7 Rf alternate with BL.15, BL.18, BL.20, BL.23 Rf + KI.7 or GV.4 and BL.52 Rf for Deficient Kidney + HT.8 or GV.11 and BL.44 Rf for Deficient Heart + SP.6 and SP.10 or BL.49 Rf for Deficient Spleen Moxa in all cases if no Heat signs
Stagnant Qi	depression with suppressed emotions and feelings of fullness in chest, epigastrium or abdomen, maybe nausea and indigestion	wiry or hindered, maybe empty choppy or slippery	maybe purplish	CV.6, CV.12, CV.17, SP.6, LR.3, PC.6 E or Rd alternate with BL.15, BL.18, BL.20, BL.31 E + LR.14 or BL.47 E for Stagnant Liver Qi + TE.6 or BL.44 E for Stagnant Heart Qi + LU.7 or BL.42 E for Stagnant Lung Qi

Rd, Reducing method; Rf, Reinforcing method; E, Even method.

Eye, ear and facial 32
syndromes

Eye syndromes

INTRODUCTION

This section discusses the treatment of two main types of eye disorder: inflammatory conditions, such as conjunctivitis, and conditions of progressive loss of vision, such as glaucoma and cataracts. Acupuncture can be effective for some of the inflammatory disorders, and can assist treatment of glaucoma and cataract in the early stages. Acupuncture treatment of myopia, squint, colour blindness and retinal disorders, although performed in China, is outside the experience of the author and therefore not included in this section.

AETIOLOGY

Factors contributing to eye disorders include inherited predisposition to optic problems, prolonged exposure to wind, chemical or mechanical irritants, allergens in air or in food, toxins (e.g. medicines, drugs, alcohol and tobacco), overuse of the eyes (e.g. excess reading or use of a computer screen), working in conditions of lighting that is too dim or too bright, psychological stress, old age, and any factor that contributes to Deficiency (e.g. excess work, excess sex, lack of sleep, malnutrition or illness).

THE DEFICIENCIES

The main Deficiencies affecting vision are related mainly to Kidney, Liver and Spleen:

Deficient Kidney Jing, Deficient Kidney Yin
Deficient Liver Blood, Deficient Liver Yin
Deficient Spleen Blood, Deficient Spleen Qi.

As Kidney Jing and Liver Blood decrease, e.g. with old age, so does visual acuity. This process is aggravated by a Deficient Spleen which does not supply sufficient Qi and Blood to be stored by Kidneys and Liver respectively. If Kidney and Liver Yin are Deficient, then Liver Yang and Fire may not be properly controlled by Yin and may rise up the body to affect the eyes.

OVERUSE

Overuse of the eyes, from excessive reading or use of a computer screen, is often associated with mental strain from too much study or mental work. Eye disorders may be part of a pattern of poor posture, tense eye muscles, tense muscles of the shoulders and neck, headache or migraine, and mental strain and exhaustion. In this pattern, Hyperactive Liver Yang is often combined with Deficient Spleen and Kidney Qi.

PSYCHOLOGICAL FACTORS IN EYE DISORDERS

THE INWARD FLOW

Energy and information flow into the eye from the external environment, but individuals may not like what they see, and may attempt to limit their perceptions. For example, some people wish to restrict the field of their perception, so that they only see what they want to see, and perceive the world as if through blinkers. It is possible that by habitually reducing the field of their perception they gradually reduce their field of vision, as in glaucoma.

Others may wish to blur their perception of the outside world so that they do not have to look at the unpleasant details of life, which they may find threatening or exhausting to deal with. They prefer to live in a pleasant haze, avoiding looking at or dealing with the truth, and withdrawn from full participation in life. This habitual dulling of perception may result in an increasing dulling of vision, as in cataracts.

As another example, if people are only interested in themselves and restrict the area of their perceptions to the area immediately surrounding themselves, this may lead to a restriction in the depth of vision and aggravate myopia.

THE OUTWARD FLOW

The eyes are often called 'the windows of the soul', in which we can perceive the feelings of others – love, hate, anger, withdrawal, grief, worry, insanity. It is as if there is an outward stream of energy and information from the eyes, from one person to another. Some people seem consciously to make use of the exchange of energy in eye contact to manipulate others. Some try to use eye contact to dominate others, some try to dump their fear, aggression and bitterness, and some seem to use eye contact to drain the energy of other people.

If this outflow exists, it may be that those who use it to express bitterness or hatred, or to dominate, create a pressure in the eye which may translate into either inflammation, as in conjunctivitis, or into raised intra-ocular pressure, as in glaucoma. However, if the outflow through the eyes is blocked, as in suppressed grief, the pressure of suppressed tears may affect the tear ducts, resulting in either dry eyes or excessive lachrymation.

THE MAIN ORGAN SYSTEMS

The Kidneys supply the Jing to the eyes, and contact them via the Conception, Yin Heel and Yang Heel channels, which run to the eyes. The Liver supplies Blood to the eye system, and contacts the eyes via its internal pathway.

In addition to this, some people of the Water–Wood type whose dominant emotions are fear and anger may, by attempting to express their aggressions and to dominate others with their eyes, precipitate eye problems for themselves.

The Spleen is another potential component of eye problems, partly due to eye strain from excessive study and work, and partly due to Deficient Qi and Blood from excessive worry, study and malnutrition. The Lungs may be a component of eye disorders in the special case of blocked grief, and the Heart may be associated with inflammatory eye conditions from Heart Fire related to manic behaviour or suppressed excitement.

In summary, the main Excess eye disorders are related to Liver, and the main Deficiency disorders to Kidneys, Liver and Spleen.

SYNDROMES

Whatever their name in Western medicine, eye disorders can be subdivided into the following Chinese syndromes:

Excess
  Wind Heat
  Liver Fire and Liver Yang
    + Stagnant Liver Qi
    + Deficient Kidney and Liver Yin
    + Heart Fire
    + Phlegm
  Stagnant Blood

Deficiency
  Deficient Kidney and Liver Yin
  Deficient Jing, Qi and Blood

Therefore, whether the disease is labelled conjunctivitis, blepharitis, optic neuritis, cataract or glaucoma, acupuncture treatment is based on:

selection of local points
point combination according to Chinese syndrome.

Table 32.1 Eye syndromes

Syndromes	Signs and symptoms	Pulse	Tongue	Point combination
Excess Wind Heat	sudden acute eye inflammation with redness, itching and dryness of the eyes, aversion to wind maybe lachrymation, e.g. allergies	superficial, rapid, maybe tight	maybe red	BL.1, GB.1 E; LI.4, TE.5, GB.20 Rd + SP.6, KI.6 Rf for Deficient Kidney and Liver Yin + GB.43, LR.2 Rd for Liver Fire and Yang + LU.7, LI.20 Rd for allergic conjunctivitis and rhinitis + LI.11, ST.44 Rd for conjunctivitis with food allergy
Liver Fire and Hyperactive Liver Yang	red, dry, hot, painful eyes, irritability, anger, frustration, maybe feeling of pressure in the eyes, photophobia or lachrymation, maybe headache or tense muscles	rapid, wiry, full	red, especially at edges, maybe dry yellow coat	BL.1, GB.1, TE.23 E; TE.5, LR.2, GB.43 Rd + LR.1 B; KI.1 Rd for severe Liver Fire + GB.14, GB.20, GB.21 Rd for Hyperactive Liver Yang + LR.3, LR.14 Rd for Stagnant Liver Qi + LR.8, KI.3, SP.6 Rf for Deficient Kidney and Liver Yin + HT.5 Rd for Heart Fire + ST.40 for Phlegm
Local Stagnant	local eye injury with pain, redness or burning	maybe wiry	various	local points E; LI.4, GB.20, LR.3, SP.8, BL.62 Rd
Deficiency Deficient Kidney and Liver Yin	chronic dryness, soreness and redness of eyes, maybe irritability, tiredness, restlessness, weak lower back, tinnitus and night sweats	thin, rapid	red, dry, maybe peeled	CV.4, TE.3, KI.6, BL.2, BL.62, SP.6 Rf alternate BL.10, BL.18, BL.23, BL.62 Rf
Deficient Jing Qi and Blood	chronic or increasing blurring or diminishing of vision, maybe worse with tiredness, maybe floaters, dizziness or tinnitus	empty or thin, choppy, maybe deep	maybe pale and thin or flabby	CV.4, LI.4, KI.3, BL.2, BL.62, SP.6, ST.36 alternate BL.17, BL.18, BL.20, BL.23 Rf + SI.3, BL.10, GB.37 Rf for Deficient Jing + CV.12, SP.3, for Deficient Spleen Qi + LR.8, SP.10 for Deficient Liver Blood

Rd, Reducing method; Rf, Reinforcing method; E, Even method.

COMBINATIONS OF SYNDROMES

Some common combinations are:

Wind Heat + Liver Fire and Yang, e.g. some conjunctivitis
Liver Fire and Yang + Deficient Kidney and Liver Yin, e.g. some glaucoma
Deficient Kidney and Liver Yin + Deficient Jing, Qi and Blood, e.g. some cataracts.

The basic principle is to disperse Excess and tonify Deficiency.

POINTS FOR EYE DISORDERS

LOCAL POINTS

Local points for eye disorders include:

BL.1, BL.2, GB.1, ST.1, ST.2, TE.23, yìn táng, tài yáng, qiú hòu, yú yáo

In the opinion of the author, it is personal preference as to which local points are selected. Obviously, for eye disorders related to Kidney and Bladder, BL.1 and BL.2 are appropriate, for Liver–Gallbladder, GB.1 and TE.23, and for Stomach, ST.1 and ST.2.

For eye disorders related to worry, excessive study and mental strain, yìn táng is suitable, and for eye problems related to hypertension, tài yáng. Qiú hòu and yú yáo are of general application, although yú yáo can be joined to GB.14 for eye strain with migraine.

DISTAL POINTS

Some of the main distal points for eye disorders are:

LI.4	all, especially Wind Heat, Hyperactive Liver Yang, Deficient Blood, Stagnant Blood
TE.3	all, especially Wind Heat
TE.5	Wind Heat
HT.5	Heart Fire with sensation of congestion and heat in the eyes
SI.3	Wind Heat, Deficient Jing (in combination with BL.62)
SP.6	Deficient Yin, Deficient Blood, Stagnant Liver Qi
ST.8	Wind Heat, also eyelid spasms
ST.36	Deficient Qi and Blood

ST.40	Phlegm (discharges)
ST.44	Stomach Fire, as in conjunctivitis associated
ST.45	with food allergies
LR.1	Liver Fire
LR.2	Liver Fire, Hyperative Liver Yang
LR.3	Stagnant Liver Qi, Hyperactive Liver Yang, Liver Wind
LR.8	Deficient Liver Yin, Deficient Liver Blood
GB.14	Hyperactive Liver Yang
GB.20	all, especially Wind Heat and Hyperactive Liver Yang
GB.37	all
GB.41	Wind Heat, Liver Fire, Liver–Gallbladder Damp Heat
GB.43	Wind Heat with Liver Fire and Hyperactive
GB.44	Yang
KI.1	Fire of Kidney, Liver, Heart
KI.3	Deficient Kidney Jing Qi and Yin
KI.6	Deficient Kidney Jing and Yin
BL.10	Wind Heat
BL.17	Deficient Blood
BL.18	all, especially Deficient Liver Blood, Deficient Liver Yin
BL.20	Deficient Spleen Qi and Blood
BL.23	Deficient Kidney Jing and Yin, excessive Kidney will producing eye strain and inflammation
BL.62	all, especially Wind Heat and Deficient Jing
BL.63	general points for eye problems, including
BL.67	inflammation and congestion, obstruction of the tear ducts and corneal opacity
CV.4	Deficient Qi Jing, Blood and Yin
yì míng	myopia, optic nerve atrophy, night blindness

Ear syndromes

The ear disorders discussed in this section are otitis media, Menières disorder, tinnitus and deafness.

OTITIS MEDIA

Otitis media is inflammation of the middle ear, usually as a result of infection of the mucous membranes of the nose spreading to the middle ear via the Eustachian tube. Common symptoms are earache, discharge of pus into the external ear, fever and other symptoms of systemic infection. Otitis media may occur in severe acute form, or in chronic form with periodic aggravations. While acupuncture can be effective for the severe acute form, the use of antibiotics may be preferred, due to the potential serious complications of acute otitis media. Alternatively, acupuncture and antibiotics can be used together.

AETIOLOGY

Four important predisposing factors are Deficient Defensive Qi, Deficient Kidney Qi, Deficient Spleen Qi with accumulation of Phlegm, and Liver Fire.

DEFICIENT DEFENSIVE QI

This is especially important in children, where lowered resistance facilitates repeated common colds, leading to catarrhal infections of the nose, which progress to otitis media. The principle of treatment is to treat incidents of otitis media when they occur, but between attacks build up the Defensive Qi as a preventive measure. This can be done with combinations such as BL.13, BL.20, BL.23, LU.7, ST.36, KI.7 Rf, which by tonifying Lungs, Spleen and Kidneys, strengthen the Defensive Qi system.

DEFICIENT KIDNEY QI

This is more important in adults, where Deficient Kidney Qi and Jing predisposes to ear infections and to tinnitus and deafness. Here, local points must be combined with points that tonify the Kidneys, such as CV.4, KI.3, ST.36, BL.23.

DEFICIENT SPLEEN QI AND PHLEGM

Deficient Spleen Qi may lead to Deficient Qi and Blood, and Deficient Defensive Qi, allowing repeated infections. The other importance of Deficient Spleen Qi, is the accumulation of phlegm that can block the nasal passages and Eustachian tube, forming a background for infection.

It is essential, especially in children, for patients to greatly reduce their intake of mucus-forming foods and to increase their intake of fresh fruit and vegetables. Some children have a strong reaction to cow's milk products, and these should be avoided, as should excessive intake of sugars and chocolate.

LIVER FIRE

An existing condition of Liver Fire, or Liver–Gallbladder Damp Heat, predisposes to invasion of Wind Heat. Liver Fire may arise from chronic tension, frustration, ambition and suppressed anger.

In children, emotional tensions between the parents may result in emotional tensions within the child, with generation of Heat. Also, at the age when children are being given much verbal instruction and commands, there may be a resistance to learning and obedience, and a desire not to hear, to shut out the voices. It is possible that this resistance creates Heat and inflammation both within the ear and systemically, predisposing to otitis media.

It is also important to reduce intake of anything likely to increase Liver Fire and Liver–Gallbladder Damp Heat. For example, tobacco, alcohol, and greasy spicy foods.

The principle of treatment is primarily to disperse Wind Heat and to disperse Liver–Gallbladder Fire or Damp Heat, both systemically and locally in the ear. In addition it is helpful to move Stagnant Liver Qi or to tonify the Deficient Yin, which predispose to Liver Fire.

SYNDROMES

Excess
Liver Fire and Wind Heat
Deficiency
Deficient Defensive Qi
Deficient Spleen and Phlegm
Deficient Kidney Qi

In chronic otitis media, there may be a background of chronic Deficiency, with periodic Wind invasion or aggravations of Liver Fire.

TREATMENT

Initially, in severe acute cases, treatment can be once or twice per day, reducing to once per day, where logistically possible. In acute moderate aggravations of chronic cases, treatment can be once or twice per week, depending on severity. In chronic conditions, between attacks, treatment can be once per week until there is definite improvement, such as reduced number of colds, reduced phlegm, increased energy and so on. Preventive treatment to tonify Qi, move Stagnant Liver Qi, or to disperse Liver Fire, can then continue on a monthly basis, if required.

In babies and young children, 2–4 distal points may be enough, for example TE.5 and GB.41 on the affected side and LI.4 and ST.36 on the other. In older children, TE.5, TE.17 and GB.41 Rd on the affected side, can be combined with ST.36 and KI.3 Rf on the opposite side, or whatever other points are appropriate. In adults, the full number of points shown in Table 32.3 can be used, using TE.17 and GB.2 on the affected side, and the other points bilaterally or unilaterally as preferred.

MENIÈRE'S SYNDROME

Menière's syndrome is an affection of the inner ear with disturbance of both hearing and balance. It is commonly periodic attacks of vertigo, tinnitus and deafness, in which the vertigo may be accompanied by nausea, vomiting and an inability to stand. Vertigo indicates that the subject feels that he or his surroundings are rotating. It can be distinguished from dizziness, which indicates a feeling of light headedness, faintness or vague movement in the head, by the criterion of definite rotation. Menière's syndrome is not the only cause of vertigo, but vertigo is the characteristic feature of the disorder.

AETIOLOGY

The aetiology of Menière's syndrome in Western medicine is not clear, but in Chinese medicine, the three main factors are said to be Hyperactive Liver Yang, Phlegm, and Deficient Kidney Yin.

HYPERACTIVE LIVER YANG

The irregular movement of Hyperactive Liver Yang and Liver Wind can give rise to both dizziness and vertigo, and may be associated with a sudden increase of emotional pressure in an ongoing situation of suppressed anger and frustration. Liver Yang and Wind may be associated with Excess, Liver Fire arising from Stagnation of Liver Qi, or they may be associated with Deficiency of Kidney Qi and Yin.

The principle of treatment is primarily to calm Hyperactive Liver Yang and Wind, and secondarily to treat underlying conditions of Liver Fire and Stagnation, or Deficient Kidney Yin.

PHLEGM

Phlegm may cause dizziness or vertigo by obstructing the channels of the head. There may also be sensations of dullness and heaviness in the head, and nausea and vomiting. Phlegm may combine with Hyperactive Liver Yang and Wind, and may arise from a Deficient Spleen. For an Excess condition with Phlegm, PC.6 and ST.40 Rd are appropriate, for a Deficient Spleen with Phlegm, CV.12 and ST.36 Rf may be necessary.

DEFICIENT KIDNEY YIN

Deficient Kidney Yin, or a combination of Deficient

Kidney Yin with Deficient Qi and Blood, may mean that Liver Yang is not under proper control, and rises up the body to the head.

SYNDROMES

Hyperactive Liver Yang and Wind
Phlegm
Deficient Kidney Yin

The syndromes of Hyperactive Liver Yang, Phlegm and Deficient Kidney Yin are often combined in cases of Ménière's syndrome. Treatment during an attack emphasizes calming Liver Yang and Wind, treatments between attacks emphasize resolving Phlegm, tonifying Deficiency and regulating the Liver.

TINNITUS AND DEAFNESS

Tinnitus and deafness may result from damage to the auditory nerve or its deterioration with age. Reduced hearing may also result from wax in the external ear, or from catarrh in the Eustachian tubes and inflammation of the middle ear. A useful guide to prognosis lies in whether or not the deafness or tinnitus varies with time. If there is no variation in the degree of deafness or in the volume and quality of the tinnitus, it may be that the auditory nerve is severely damaged and that acupuncture will give only limited assistance. If the deafness or tinnitus varies with the presence of catarrh, or with tiredness or stress, for example, this may indicate that the auditory nerve is intact or that it has at least partial function, and that acupuncture may give considerable help.

AETIOLOGY

In Chinese medicine, tinnitus and deafness is divided into two main types: Excess and Deficiency. The Excess type is mainly associated with Liver–Gallbladder Fire, and the Deficiency type with Deficient Kidney Jing. In addition there is catarrhal deafness, sometimes associated with otitis media where the pressure of catarrh in the sinuses and Eustachian tubes, associated with acute or chronic sinusitis, reduces the level of hearing. In Chinese medicine, this relates to a mixed syndrome of Deficiency and Excess: Deficient Spleen Qi with Phlegm which accumulates in the sinuses and Eustachian tubes.

Deafness may arise from a variety of physical causes; for example, working in very noisy situations, medicines, head injuries, illness, and so on. However, there may be a psychological component of impaired hearing, and it

may be possible to differentiate two groups, as shown in Table 32.2. It may be that the Yin personality type can't be bothered to listen to or to respond to much of what is said to them, they only want to hear the pleasant things, and prefer to withdraw inside themselves. With increasing age and decreasing Jing, many people lose their adaptability, and no longer have the interest or the energy to respond to the constant changes and challenges of life. Many become conveniently deaf. The Yang personality type, with strong Kidney will and strong Liver assertion and dogmatism, may strongly disagree with what they hear, with the opinions, instructions or criticism of others, and may try to block it out, while increasing in anger, frustration and resentment. This may originate and aggravate deafness, tinnitus and ear infections, by raising Liver–Gallbladder Fire.

Table 32.2 Deafness and personality type

	Yin	Yang
Personality type	passive	active
Syndrome type	Deficiency, e.g. Deficient Kidney and Liver Qi	Excess, e.g. Liver – Gallbladder Fire, Hyperactive Liver Yang
Type of deafness	gradual deafness or tinnitus	sudden deafness or tinnitus, maybe inflammation

SYNDROMES

Liver–Gallbladder Fire
Deficient Kidney Jing
Deficient Spleen Qi with Phlegm

TREATMENT

Treatment is based on a combination of local and distal points. The Excess pattern of Liver–Gallbladder Fire may require more local points with Reducing method, and the pattern of Deficient Jing requires less local points, with more emphasis on reinforcing distal points.

LOCAL POINTS

The most effective local point is usually TE.17. GB.2, TE.21, SI.9 and yì míng are also effective. There are also various special points around the ear which can be used according to personal preference. zhì lóng gǔ, for sudden tinnitus and deafness, is located by pressing the tragus until its tip touches the inside surface of the ear. It is needled perpendicularly to a depth of 0.8 – 1 unit. For tinnitus especially, points from the Gallbladder and Triple Energizer channels above the ear can be added to the basic treatment, e.g. TE.18–22 and GB.6–12.

DISTAL POINTS

Pairs or chains of distal points can be used in conjunction with one or more local points on the same channel, for example:

SI.3, SI.4, SI.5, SI.19
TE.3, TE.5, TE.17, TE.21
GB.2, GB.20, GB.34, GB.43

The basic principle is to start with the minimum number of points and add points if necessary.

Table 32.3 Ear syndromes

Syndromes	Signs and symptoms	Pulse	Tongue	Point combination
Otitis media Wind Heat, Liver Fire or Liver–Gallbladder Damp Heat	Acute, severe earache, yellow discharge, maybe fever, headache	rapid, maybe wiry, maybe slippery	red, maybe greasy yellow coat	LI.4, TE.5, TE.17, GB.2, GB.20, GB.41 Rd + GV.14, LI.11 Rd for high fever + LR.3, LR.14 Rd for Stagnant Liver Qi + SP.6, KI.6 Rf for Deficient Kidney and Liver Yin + SP.9, GB.34 Rd for Damp Heat
Deficient Defensive Qi	recurrent colds, nasal infections and otitis media	usually empty, maybe slippery during infections	pale, flabby maybe white greasy coat	TE.17, GB.2, GB.40, ST.36, KI.3 Rf between attacks BL.13, BL.20, BL.23, LU.7, ST.36, KI.3 Rf
Deficient Spleen Qi with Phlegm	chronic otitis media with much sinus catarrh and feeling of blockage in ear and maybe catarrhal deafness	slippery, maybe full or wiry	pale, white or yellow thick greasy coat	LI.4, TE.17, GB.2, GB.20, ST.40 Rd; CV.12, ST.36 Rf
Deficient Kidney Qi	chronic otitis media with dizziness, tinnitus and impaired hearing aggravated by tiredness	empty, deep maybe slow	pale	CV.4, TE.17, GB.2, GB.40, ST.36, KI.3 Rf
Menière's syndrome Hyperactive Liver Yang and Wind	vertigo and maybe distending headache, headache induced or aggravated by anger and frustration	wiry, maybe rapid, maybe full	maybe red, maybe thin yellow coat	TE.17, PC.6, LR.3, GB.20, GB.43 Rd + LR.2, KI.1 Rd for Liver Fire + SP.6, KI.6 Rf for Deficient Kidney Yin + SI.3, SI.19 Rd for severe vertigo
Phlegm	vertigo with sensation of dullness and heaviness in the head, nausea and vomiting, maybe mental confusion	wiry, slippery, full or empty	pale or red, thick greasy coat	TE.17, PC.6, GB.20, GB.34, ST.8, ST.40 Rd; + ST.36, CV.12 Rf for Deficient Spleen Qi
Deficient Kidney Yin	vertigo with tinnitus or impaired hearing, worse with tiredness, maybe weak lower back or insomnia	thin, rapid, maybe deep, maybe choppy	red, thin, dry, no coat	GV.20, CV.4, TE.17, GB.34, ST.36, KI.3 Rf + ST.36, SP.10 Rf for Deficient Blood
Tinnitus and deafness Liver–Gallbladder Fire	tinnitus and deafness, often of sudden occurrence and related to suppressed anger and frustration, maybe headache, red face, restlessness	rapid, full, wiry	red, especially at edges	TE.3, TE.5, TE.17, GB.2, GB.20, GB.41 Rd + LR.3, LR.14 Rd for Stagnant Liver Qi + yìn táng, tài yáng for dizziness and headache + zhì lóng gǔ for sudden deafness and tinnitus + PC.5, ST.40 for Phlegm Fire
Deficient Kidney Jing	gradual tinnitus or deafness, maybe of variable degree and aggravated by tiredness, maybe dizziness and low back pain	empty, thin or choppy, maybe deep	pale	CV.4, TE.17, GB.2, KI.3, ST.36 Rf alternate GV.4, SI.2, BL.18, BL.23, BL.62 Rf
Deficient Spleen Qi with Phlegm	see Otitis media, above			

Rd, Reducing method; Rf, Reinforcing method.

Facial syndromes

FACIAL PARALYSIS

Facial paralysis, sometimes known as Bell's palsy, is a disorder of the facial nerve, which may be associated in Western medicine with cerebrovascular accident, head injury, or infection, or it may have no obvious origin. In Chinese medicine, facial paralysis, with deviation of the mouth and eye, is associated with invasion of the channels of the face by Wind Cold, leading to a Stagnation of Qi and Blood, resulting in malnourishment of the muscles. The initial invasion by Wind Cold may be facilitated by Deficient Qi and Blood.

TREATMENT

Treatment is mainly of local points on the affected side, with Even method and maybe moxa, with one or more distal points used bilaterally.

LOCAL POINTS

A number of local points can be selected from the following list, according to the main area of difficulty:

tài yáng, GB.14, TE.23, BL.2, yú yáo, SI.18, ST.2, ST.3, ST.4, ST.6, ST.7

LONG NEEDLE TECHNIQUE

One local point can be needled horizontally, just underneath the skin, towards a second point, for example, GB.14 to yú yáo, ST.4 to ST.6, or tài yáng to ST.6.

DISTAL POINTS

LI.4 is usually used bilaterally with Reducing method. In addition, ST.36 can be used with Reinforcing method and moxa, if there is Deficient Qi and Blood. GB.20 can be used bilaterally with Reducing method to disperse Wind Cold, especially if there is also headache. For earache or tenderness of the mastoid, TE.5 with Reducing method and TE.17 with Even method can be added on the affected side.

GV–CV METHOD

SI.3 + BL.62 to open the Governor channel may be combined with LU.7 + KI.6 to open the Conception channel, and GV.26 + CV.24 added to these, to open all the channels of the face. Suitable local points may be added to the basic combination of GV.26, CV.24, LU.7, SI.3, KI.6, BL.62.

TRIGEMINAL NEURALGIA

Trigeminal neuralgia is treated partly according to which branch or branches of the trigeminal nerve are affected, and partly according to underlying causes.

SYNDROMES

External
　Wind Cold
　Wind Heat
Internal
　Liver Fire
　Stomach Fire
　Deficient Kidney Yin

Trigeminal neuralgia, in Chinese medicine, may originate from Wind Cold invasion of the face, which may be facilitated by a pre-existing condition of Deficient Qi and Blood. Wind Cold may convert to Wind Heat in the face. It may also originate with dental problems, or from Liver Fire and Stomach Fire, associated with suppressed anger and worry, or with unwise eating habits. Deficient Kidney Yin from stress or overwork, may predispose to a Fire condition.

TREATMENT ACCORDING TO NERVE BRANCH

Table 32.4 Treatment of the trigeminal nerve branches

Branch	Local points	Distal point
1st branch (ophthalmic)	tài yáng towards ST.7, BL.2 towards BL.1, GB.14, TE.23, ST.8	TE.5
2nd branch (maxillary)	LI.20 towards ST.3, ST.3 towards ST.7, ST.2, SI.8	LI.4
3rd branch (mandibular)	ST.6 towards ST.5, CV.24 towards jiá chéng jiāng, ST.7	LI.4

Points are selected from Table 32.4 according to the area of greatest pain. Local points are used on the affected side with Even method, and TE.5 and LI.4 can be used bilaterally with Reducing method. Jiá chéng jiāng, also known as Keliao, located 1 unit lateral to CV.24, directly below ST.4, is needled to a depth of 0.5 unit into the mental foramen of the mandible.

LONG NEEDLE TECHNIQUE

When one point is needled towards another, for example, tài yáng towards ST.7 in Table 32.4, the needle can either be inserted just subcutaneously horizontally under the skin for 0.5 – 1.0 unit, or can be run horizontally under the skin at a deeper level, close to the bone surface, for a longer distance, to connect the two points. It is personal preference, but the author would usually try the shallower shorter insertion technique first, and only if this proved inadequate use the deeper insertion.

BLEEDING

Where trigeminal neuralgia is associated with Heat, whether Interior or External, bleeding may be used. For example, for pain in the ophthalmic branch, tài yáng, TE.1 and LI.1 can be bled. For trigeminal neuralgia with Liver–Gallbladder Fire, TE.23, TE.1, GB.44 and LR.1 could be bled; for Stomach Fire, LI.1 and ST.45 would be appropriate. Bleeding is usually combined with acupuncture needling of other points, for example, LI.4 and GB.20 with Reducing method, to clear Wind invasion.

ELECTROACUPUNCTURE

A local point on the affected branch can be connected with a distal point on the arm, usually LI.4 or TE.5. The frequency can depend on the patient's preference, but can initially be about 20 cps. It is the experience of the author that electroacupuncture is best reserved for acute Excess conditions of severe pain, and only after ordinary acupuncture has not given sufficient relief. If the intensity or duration is excessive, the condition may be aggravated in some cases, especially in Deficient and nervous patients. Electroacupuncture is strongly reducing, and can be balanced with bilateral needle and moxa on ST.36, if the patient is Deficient.

TREATMENT ACCORDING TO UNDERLYING CAUSES

In addition to local points chosen according to the nerve branch affected, distal points can be selected from the following list to treat underlying cause:

Wind Cold or Wind Heat	LI.4, LU.7, TE.5, GB.20 Rd
Deficient Qi and Blood	ST.36 Rf
Liver Fire	LR.2, GB.38 Rd
Stomach Fire	LI.4, ST.44 Rd
Deficient Kidney Yin	KI.6 Rf.

Skin syndromes 33

Skin disorders may be seen in the clinic as primary ailments, such as psoriasis or eczema, or as secondary signs of systemic disease such as diabetes, thyroid disease, systemic lupus erythematosus, carcinoma and sexually transmitted diseases. This section deals only with primary skin disorders, and not with the systemic diseases.

AETIOLOGY

Four main factors predisposing to skin disorders are: inherited tendency, illness, lifestyle and psychological stress. In Chinese medicine, the main types of skin disorders are:

Heat
Stagnation
Deficient Blood.

Any factor that increases Heat, Stagnation or Deficient Blood will therefore tend to precipitate or aggravate skin disorders.

HEAT

Any factor that increases Heat in the body can aggravate skin lesions of the red, hot itchy type. For example, sugar, alcohol, greasy or spicy food, certain drugs and medicines, illness, psychological stress and allergens whether contact, airborne or in food and drink.

STAGNATION

Factors that increase Stagnation of Qi and Blood can aggravate skin lesions associated with Stagnant Blood, or with the accumulation of Damp or Heat. For example, suppression of emotions, lack of exercise and greasy food.

DEFICIENT BLOOD

Factors that increase Deficient Blood can aggravate the associated pattern of pale, dry rough skin that is thin or scaly, and easily invaded by Exterior Wind. For example, excessive worry, study or mental work, illness, and loss of blood, as in surgery, childbirth, menstruation or chronic gastric bleeding.

LIFESTYLE

Many skin disorders can be improved simply by changes in lifestyle. For example, in some adults, the skin disorder improves when they reduce coffee, tea, alcohol, drugs and spicy or greasy food and adopt a balanced nutrition, eating and sleeping at regular times, and taking moderate regular exercise. In some children, the skin greatly improves when they reduce cow's milk products, and avoid all foods with the potentially allergenic chemical additives.

PSYCHOLOGICAL STRESSES

In skin disorders, as in other illnesses, there is a question for the patient: 'What am I doing that is causing this problem, and what measures can I take to solve it?' This question relates to lifestyle and leads to the further question: 'What imbalances in my personality are associated with this illness, what are the life lessons underlying it, and how can I use this illness for personal growth?' Many patients do not wish to deal with either of these questions and simply request acupuncture treatment for the immediate problem of their skin symptoms. Other patients are willing to make changes in lifestyle, for example in nutrition and exercise, but are not willing to go deeper into the origins of their skin disorder within their personality.

EMOTIONAL PRESSURES

It is the opinion of the author that many skin disorders in both children and adults are directly linked to emotional pressures, for which they act both as an indicator and a safety release. In children, skin disorders are often an indication of the emotional pressures within the home between the parents. In this situation, treating one or both parents, where this is possible, can improve the skin disorder of the child.

Skin disorders may start after a physical illness, a shock, a stressful incident, or after a long period of emotional disturbance. In adults, it may be difficult to relate aggravation of skin disorders to a specific incident, since adults tend to suppress emotions more than children, and their reactions to stress may be delayed and cumulative.

SOURCES OF HEAT

Four main sources of Heat in skin disorders relate to the emotional pressures within the systems of Kidneys, Liver,

Heart and Spleen, as shown in Table 33.1. Both the skin disorder itself and the underlying emotional pressures can be treated.

Table 33.1 Emotions and Heat in skin disorders

System	Emotion
KI	pressure of will when linked to unrealistic goals, pressure of trying to keep control, fear of failure
LR	irritability, intolerance, frustration, suppressed anger
HT	suppressed excitement, restless overexcitement, frustration and disappointment over difficulties in communication in relationships
SP	worry, mental strain, intrusive overconcern in the lives of others

SKIN DISORDERS IN CHINESE MEDICINE

TEN MAIN FACTORS

We can say that there are 10 main factors involved in skin diseases:

Wind Heat	Stagnation of Qi and Blood
Deficient Blood	Damp
Dryness	Damp Heat
Deficient Yin	Excess Heat
Heat in the Blood	Fire poison

These factors are related as shown in Figure 33.1.

FACTOR COMBINATIONS

Often, a patient may have two or more of these factors working together, for example:

Wind Heat, Deficient Blood, Dryness
Wind Heat, Damp, Damp Heat
Heat in the Blood, Deficient Yin, Damp Heat,
Fire poison.

The point combination is determined by the relative importance of the different factors, and by which are better treated first and which can be left for later. For example, severe itching and distress due to Wind and Heat are generally treated before attempting to remedy Dryness, due to Deficient Blood and Deficient Yin, which can take much long to improve.

WIND HEAT

This refers not only to exposure to wind, or to changes in

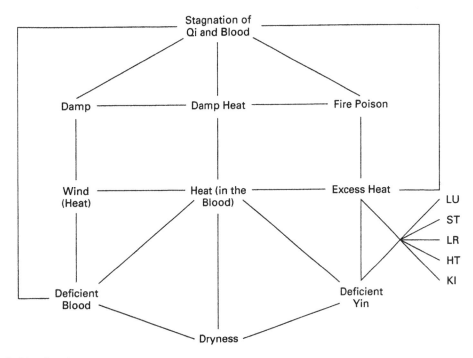

Fig. 33.1 Aetiology of skin disorders.

environmental temperature, but to skin disorders of variable location which suddenly come and go, for example acute urticaria or eczema. Wind Heat skin problems are characterized by itching. The skin lesions may be of a short duration, and may not have redness and heat.

Wind Heat skin disorders are often associated with allergic reactions; for example, to substances in contact with the skin, airborne allergens, food, alcohol and drugs, or to medications. These allergic skin reactions may be associated with respiratory disorders, such as asthma and hayfever, digestive disorders, such as gastritis and enteritis, and with some forms of rheumatoid arthritis.

DEFICIENT BLOOD

Deficient Blood can lead to Wind invasion of the skin, so that the factors of Deficient Blood and Wind Heat often occur together. The principle of treatment would be to disperse Wind Heat, and to tonify Blood to prevent further Wind invasion. Deficient Blood can also result in dryness of the skin, which may become pale, rough, and thin or scaly. If Deficient Blood is combined with Deficient Yin, then both Blood and Yin must be tonified to moisten and nourish the skin.

DRYNESS

Dryness can of course come from excessive use of strong detergent or other chemicals which remove the natural oils from the skin. However, Dryness is often a secondary factor resulting from Deficient Blood, Wind Heat, Deficient Yin or Fire. The primary factor must always be treated.

DEFICIENT YIN

The two main skin factors associated with Deficient Yin are Dryness and Heat. The principle of treatment is to tonify Yin and Disperse Heat in the affected organ systems.

HEAT IN THE BLOOD

In the context of skin disorders, Heat in the Blood involves acute or chronic skin lesions which are red, hot, itchy and maybe sore or painful. The itching may be intense, with severe emotional distress and insomnia, the skin may be dry and rough. Heat in the Blood may be a progression of Wind Heat in the skin, or it may arise from Deficient Yin or Excess Heat of one or more organ systems. While such points as SP.6, SP.10, LI.4, LI.11 and BL.40 are specific for Heat in the Blood skin problems, other points may need to be added to tonify Yin, or to disperse Heat in the affected organ systems.

EXCESS HEAT

This pattern is a precursor to Heat in the Blood, and treatment will depend on which organ systems have Excess Heat.

DAMP AND DAMP HEAT

Damp can arise from a combination of Deficient Spleen Qi and Stagnation of Qi in the channels. It is characterized by fluid-filled or exuding skin lesions, and is most commonly seen as Damp Heat, where the lesions have yellow fluid and may also be red, hot and itchy. The principle of treatment is to tonify Spleen to transform Damp, move Stagnation of Qi and to drain Damp Heat.

STAGNATION OF QI AND BLOOD

Stagnation may lead to accumulation of Damp, Heat and Fire poison, but in addition some Chinese practitioners consider that Stagnation can be a major factor in such stubborn skin diseases as psoriasis, especially where the lesions are purple and resistant to treatment. Points which move the Blood are selected, such as SP.8 and BL.17

FIRE POISON

This is a concept which includes boils, abscesses and mumps, and is characterized by skin problems with swellings that are painful and hot, where the patient may also have general sensations of heat, sickness or lethargy. Examples are boils and some forms of acne.

WESTERN SKIN DISORDERS

Each of the Western skin diseases can be classified according to the 10 factors just discussed. Table 33.2 shows some common Western categories.

POINTS FOR SKIN DISORDERS

Points for skin disorders are selected according to the combination of factors involved, and according to the underlying psychological stresses.

SELECTION OF POINTS

Various types of points can be selected as shown in Tables

Table 33.2 Western skin disorders and the 10 factors

Western disease	Chinese factors
sunburn	Summer Heat, Heat in the Blood
urticaria	Wind Heat
eczema	Wind Heat, Deficient Blood, Dryness, Heat in the Blood, Deficient Yin, Excess Heat, Damp, Damp Heat
varicose eczema	Heat in the Blood, Damp Heat, Deficient Blood, Stagnant Blood
herpes zoster	Wind Heat, Damp Heat, Liver–Gallbladder Fire
psoriasis	Heat in the Blood, Deficient Yin, Excess Heat, Stagnant Blood, Damp Heat
acne, boils	Fire poison, Damp Heat, Heat in the Blood, Stagnant Blood

33.6 and 33.7. Well and Spring points are commonly used with Reducing method for acute Excess patterns of Heat and Stagnation. Back Transporting points can be used for all types of skin disorders, but are especially useful for chronic Deficiency patterns, e.g. Deficient Defensive Qi, Deficient Blood and Deficient Yin with Dryness.

WELL AND SPRING POINTS

Well points and Spring points, either singly or in combination, are effective in many acute skin disorders due to Heat in the Blood. Some examples are given in Tables 33.3 and 33.4. In addition, Well points can be incorporated into combinations to move Stagnant Qi and Blood; for example, LI.1, LI.4, ST.37, ST.45 for acne due to Heat in Large Intestine and Stomach.

Table 33.3 Well point and skin problems

Well point	Combination	Syndromes	Example
LU.11	+ LI.1	Heat in Lung and Liver	urticaria
LI.1	+ ST.45	Heat in Liver and Stomach	food allergy
PC.9	+ BL.40	Heat in Blood	sunburn
TE.1	+ GB.44	Wind Heat	facial eczema
HT.9	+ HT.3	Heat in Blood	acute eczema
SP.1	+ SP.10	Heat in Blood	acute psoriasis
ST.45	+ SP.1	Stomach Fire	eczema and gastritis
LR.1	+ LR.5	Liver Fire	genital eczema
GB.44	+ GB.38	Liver–Gallbladder Fire and Damp Heat	acute eczema
KI.1	+ HT.9	Heat in Blood from Heart and Kidney Fire	acute eczema
BL.67	+ BL.2	Wind Heat	generalized itching

Table 33.4 Well and Spring point combinations for the skin

Well point	Spring point	Additional combination	Syndromes	Example
PC.9	PC.8	HT.8	Heat in the Blood	eczema of palms
HT.9	HT.8	KI.1	Heart Fire, Heat in the Blood	acute eczema and insomnia
SP.1	SP.2	LR.2	Heat in the Blood	varicose eczema
ST.45	ST.44	LI.11	Stomach Fire	food allergy
LR.1	LR.2	CV.3	Liver Fire and Damp Heat	genital itching
KI.1	KI.2	SP.6	Kidney Fire and Damp Heat	genital eczema

CHAINS OF POINTS

Chains of points on a channel are only used when single points or pairs of points on that channel are not sufficiently effective. Chains of points on paired channels is especially useful for the Lesser Yang and Bright Yang pairs of the Six Divisions, for example:

TE.1, 5, 10 + GB.20, 34, 41 for eczema on sides of body with Damp Heat
LI.1, 4, 11 + ST. 25, 37, 44 for psoriasis with Heat in Liver and Stomach.

LOCAL POINTS

Local points are often used to treat skin disorders in specific areas; for example, PC.8 for palmar eczema, CV.24 for chin acne, LI.18 for neck boils, or BL.40 for eczema in the popliteal crease.

Table 33.5 Chains of points for skin disorders

Channel	Points	Syndrome	Example
LI	1,4,11	Heat in Blood	eczema
	1,4,15	Wind Heat	eczema
	4,11,18	Fire poison	acne
	4,11,20	Wind Heat	facial eczema
PC	3,8,9	Heat in Blood	acute eczema
	7,8,9	Damp Heat	palmar eczema
HT	3,8,9	Heat in Blood	eczema and insomnia
SP	1,2,4	Damp Heat	varicose eczema
	1,6,10	Heat in Blood	eczema
	1,8,10	Stagnant Blood	psoriasis
ST	3,4,44	Stomach Fire	acne
	25,37,45	Heat in Stomach and Liver	acute psoriasis
LR	1,5,11	Damp Heat	eczema of legs and genitals
GB	20, 31, 44	Wind Heat	allergic eczema
	24, 34, 41	Damp Heat	eczema of sides of body
BL	17, 40, 67	Fire poison, Heat in Blood	boils
CV	6,12,17	Stagnant Qi and Blood	psoriasis on chest and abdomen
GV	10,12,14	Fire poison, Stagnant Blood	boils

SUPERFICIAL NEEDLING

For skin problems with large lesions, such as psoriasis, herpes zoster or varicose ulcer, needles can be inserted just outside of the periphery of the lesion, at a shallow angle under the lesion, towards its centre, at intervals of about 0.5–1 inch around the lesion. This is in addition to conventional point combination. For chronic skin disorders with dry, scaly lesions with unbroken skin, for example psoriasis, plum blossom needle may be used to break up the scaly surface and prick the underlying skin to produce slight bleeding. This is to move Stagnant Blood in the local area and is combined with local and distal points to move the Blood.

Table 33.6 Skin Syndromes

Syndrome	Signs and symptoms	Pulse	Tongue	Point combination
Wind Heat	acute itchy skin lesions of variable location that quickly come and go, e.g. allergic urticaria or eczema	superficial, tight, rapid	red, thin yellow coat	choose from GV.14, GB.20, GB.31, BL.2, BL.10, BL.13, LU.7, LI.4, TE.5 Rd + BL.13, BL.20, BL.23, ST.36, KI.7, LU.7 Rf for lowered resistance + PC.7, HT.7 for severe itch
Deficient Blood	chronically pale, dry, rough skin that may be thin or scaly, maybe tiredness, dizziness or dry grey, thinning hair	thin, choppy	pale, thin dry	choose from ST.36, SP.6, SP.10, LR.8, BL.17, BL.20, BL.43 Rf + HT.7, BL.15 Rd for severe itch + LU.7, LI.4 Rd for Wind Heat
Dryness	dry, rough, maybe red, hot, itchy skin, maybe thirst, dry mouth	thin, maybe rapid	dry, maybe red	choose from BL.22, BL.23, SP.6, SP.10, KI.3, KI.6, LU.5, LI.4, TE.6 Rf + KI.2, LU.10 Rd for Heat
Heat in the Blood, Deficient Yin, Excess Heat	dry, red, hot skin lesions, maybe sore or painful, maybe severe itching with severe distress and insomnia, e.g. sunburn or acute eczema	full, rapid, maybe wiry	red or dark	BL.40, SP.6, SP.10, LI.4, LI.11 Rd + bleed Spring and Well points for Excess Heat + Rf Water points for Deficient Yin
Damp, Damp Heat	fluid-filled or exuding skin lesions, maybe red or sore if Damp Heat	slippery, empty or full, maybe rapid	pale or red, greasy coat	choose from CV.3, CV.6, SP.6, SP.9, ST.40, LI.4, TE.6 Rd + SP.3, ST.36, BL.20 Rf for Damp + BL.39, BL.40, GB.34, GB.41, LR.5 Rd for Damp Heat
Stagnant Qi and Blood	purple skin lesions resistant to treatment, e.g. chronic psoriasis	wiry or hindered	purple, maybe greasy yellow coat	choose from CV.6, CV.17, BL.13, BL.15, BL.17, BL.18, SP.1, SP.4, SP.6, SP.8, ST.40, LR.1, LR.3, GB.34, LI.4, LI.10, PC.6, TE.6 Rd
Fire poison	raised, hot, red, often painful swellings, e.g. boils or acne	maybe full or flooding, maybe wiry or rapid	maybe red or purple, maybe yellow greasy coat	choose from GV.10, GV.12, BL.17, BL.40, GB.20, GB.21, ST.37, LI.4, LI.11, LU.11 Rd + CV.24, ST.4, LI.18 for acne

Rd, Reducing method; Rf, Reinforcing method.

Table 33.7 Points for skin disorders

Point	Point type	Type of skin problem	Point combination
LU.5	Water	Wind Heat	+ LU.7, LI.4 Rd
		Dryness	+ KI.6, SP.10 Rf
		Heat in Lung and Large Intestine	+ LU.11, LI.4 Rd
LU.7	Connecting	Wind Heat	+ LI.4, BL.13, GB.20 Rd
	Opening point of CV	Damp Heat in CV. e.g. abdominal itching	+ KI.6, CV.3 E
LU.11	Wood, Well	Wind Heat	+ GV.14, LI.4 Rd
		Heat in Blood	+ PC.9, PC.3 B
		Summer Heat	+ LI.11, BL.40, GV.14 Rd
LI.4	Source	Wind Heat	+ TE.5, GB.20, GB.21 Rd
		Dryness	+ LU.5, SP.6 Rf
		Heat in Large Intestine and Stomach	+ LI.11, ST.44 Rd
		Damp Heat	+ LR.5, CV.3 Rd
		Summer Heat	+ PC.9, CV.14 Rd
		Stagnant Qi and Blood	+ SP.4, SP.8, BL.17 Rd
LI.5	Fire	Wind Heat	+ LI.11, LU.5, LU.7 Rd
LI.10		Stagnant Qi in Stomach and Intestines	+ ST.40 Rd
LI.11	Earth	as for LI.4 also Fire poison, e.g. boils	+ LI.4, ST.37 Rd
LI.15		Wind Heat	+ LI.4, LI.11 Rd
LI.20	Crossing point (ST)	Heat in the Blood/Fire poison	+ CV.24, LI.18, ST.44 Rd
		Wind Heat facial skin problems	+ LU.7, LI.4, ST.3 Rd
PC.3	Water	Summer Heat, Heat	+ PC.9, BL.40, LI.4 Rd
PC.7	Source, Earth	Summer Heat, Heat as for PC.3	
		Stomach Fire, e.g. acne	+ LI.4, LI.20, CV.24 Rd
PC.8		Heat, Damp Heat, e.g. fungal infections of hands and feet	+ HT.8, PC.3, PC.7, LI.4 Rd hands + SP.2, LR.2, SP.6 Rd feet

Table 33.7 *(cont'd)*

Point	Point type	Type of skin problem	Point combination
PC.9		Summer Heat, Heat as for PC3	
TE.5	Connecting	Wind Heat	+ LI.4, GB.20, GB.31 Rd
	Opening point Yang Link	Damp Heat	+ GB.41, CV.3, LR.5 Rd
TE.6	Fire	Wind Heat, as for TE.5	
		Damp Heat	+ GB.34, LI.4, LI.11 Rd
		Dryness	+ SP.6, SP.10, BL.22 Rd
TE.7	Accumulation	Wind Heat, Heat, e.g. painful skin problems	+ LI.4, SP.6, LR.3 Rd
TE.10	Earth ⎱	Wind Heat, Damp Heat	+ TE.5, LI.4, SP.6 Rd
TE.14	⎰		
HT.3	Water	Heat	+ HT.7, SP.6, SP.10 Rd
HT.7	Source, Earth	Heat (calms the mind — for eczema with severe itching)	+ PC.3, PC.9, BL.40 B
HT.8	Fire	Heat, e.g. pruritus	+ HT.7, CV.3, LR.2 Rd
		e.g. boils	+ LI.4, PC.4, BL.17, BL.40 Rd
SP.6	Crossing point (LR, KI)	Dryness	+ SP.10, KI.6, LU.5 Rf
		Heat	+ LI.4, LI.11, SP.10 Rd
		Damp Heat	+ SP.9, GB.34, GB.38 Rd
		Damp	+ SP.9, CV.6, CV.9 Rd
		Deficient Blood	+ SP.10, ST.36, LR.8 Rf
SP.8	Accumulation	Stagnant Blood	+ LI.4, SP.6, BL.17 Rd
SP.9	Water	Damp and Damp Heat, as for SP.6	
SP.10		Dryness, Heat, Deficient Blood as for SP.6	
ST.2 ⎱		Wind Heat, e.g. allergic facial swellings	+ ST.44, ST.45, LI.20 Rd
ST.3 ⎰			
ST.36	Earth	Deficient Defensive Qi, e.g. to prevent allergies	+ KI.7, LU.7 Rf
		Deficient Blood	+ SP.6, SP.10, LR.8 Rf
ST.37	Lower Sea	Damp Heat/Fire poison, e.g. with constipation	+ LI.4, LI.11, TE.6 Rd
ST.40	Connecting	Damp	+ CV.6, CV.9, SP.9 E
ST.44	Spring, Water	Stomach Fire, e.g. food allergy	+ LI.4, ST.36, ST.45 Rd
ST.45	Well, Metal	as for ST.44	
LR.1	Wood, Well	Damp Heat, e.g. genital rashes	+ CV.2, CV.3, LR.5 Rd
		Heat, e.g. varicose inflammation	+ SP.1, SP.2, LR.2, SP.6, SP.9 Rd
LR.2	Fire	Liver Fire	+ KI.1, LR.8, SP.6, LI.4, LI.11
LR.3	Source, Earth	Stagnation of Liver Qi, Liver Fire	+ GB.34, SP.6, SP.9, CV.6, TE.6 Rd
		Liver–Gallbladder Damp Heat	
		Stagnant Blood	+ SP.4, SP.8, CV.6, LI.4, LI.11 Rd
LR.5	Connecting	Damp Heat	+ CV.3, CV.6, SP.9, GB.34 Rd
LR.8	Water	Deficient Liver Blood, Deficient Liver Yin	+ KI.6, SP.6 Rf
GB.20	Crossing (TE, Yang Link)	Wind Heat, e.g. urticaria of upper body	+ TE.5, LI.4, KI.7 Rd
GB.21	Crossing (TE, Yang Link)	Fire poison, e.g. boils	+ GB.20, BL.10, BL.11, SI.3 Rd
GB.31		Wind Heat, e.g. unilateral itching	+ GB.30, TE.5 Rd
		Damp Heat, e.g. herpes zoster	+ GB.41, TE.5 Rd
GB.34	Earth	Damp Heat, e.g. weeping eczema	+ SP.6, SP.9, LR.1, LI.4 Rd
	Gathering Point (sinews)		
GB.41	Opening point of Yang Link	Damp Heat, Wind Heat	+ TE.5, GB.24 Rd
GB.44	Well, Metal	Wind Heat Liver–Gallbladder Fire	+ TE.5, GB.38 Rd
KI.1	Well, Wood	Excess Fire of Kidney, Liver, Heart	+ SP.6, KI.2, LR.2, HT.8 Rd
KI.2	Spring, Fire	Kidney Deficiency Fire, e.g. genital itching	+ CV.3 Rd; SP.6, KI.10 Rf
KI.6	Opening point of Yin Heel	Deficient Yin and Dryness	+ CV.4, SP.6, SP.10 Rf
		Dryness	+ KI.6 Rf
KI.10	Water	Kidney Deficiency Fire, as for KI.2	
BL.2		Wind Heat, e.g. itching around eyes	+ TE.23, GB.1, TE.5 E
BL.10		Wind Heat, e.g. eczema on neck	+ SI.3 Rd
BL.13	Back Transporting (LU)	Wind Heat	+ LU.7 Rd
		Stagnation of Lung Qi	+ LU.7 Rd
		Dryness	+ LU.5, KI.6 Rf
BL.15	Back Transporting (HT)	Heat (calms mind)	+ HT.7, SP.6, SP.10 Rd
BL.16		Heat, e.g. psoriasis	+ SP.6, SP.10, LI.4, LI.10 Rd

Table 33.7 *(cont'd)*

Point	Point type	Type of skin problem	Point combination
BL.17	Gathering (Blood)	Heat, as for BL.16	
		Deficient Blood	+ BL.20, SP.6, SP.10 Rf
		Dryness	+ BL.23, BL.22, KI.6 Rf
		Stagnant Blood	+ SP.4, SP.8, LR.3 Rd
		Fire poison	+ GV.10, GV.12, BL.16, BL.40
BL.18	Back Transporting (LR)	Liver Heat	+ KI.1, LR.3, SP.6 Rd
BL.19	Back Transporting (GB)	Liver–Gallbladder Heat	+ GB.41, TE.5 Rd
BL.20	Back Transporting (SP)	Damp	+ BL.23, TE.6, ST.40 Rd
		Deficient Blood, as for BL.17	
BL.23	Back Transporting (KI)	Deficient Yin and Dryness	+ KI.6, SP.6, LU.5 Rf
		Deficient Yin and Deficiency Fire	+ KI.2 Rd; SP.6, HT.3 Rf
BL.25	Back Transporting (LI)	Damp Heat and Fire poison	+ LI.4, LI.11, ST.37 Rd
BL.39	Lower Sea (TE)	Damp Heat, e.g. eczema in popliteal crease	+ BL.40, BL.67 Rd
BL.40	Earth	Damp Heat, as for BL.39	
		Wind Heat, e.g. allergic urticaria	+ LI.4, LU.7, SP.6 Rd
		Summer Heat, e.g. sunburn	+ PC.9, PC.3, GV.14, LI.4 Rd
		Heat	+ LI.4, LI.11, SP.6, SP.10 Rd
BL.43	Outer BL (PC)	Fire poison	+ BL.16, BL.17, GV.10, GV.12 Rd
		Deficient Blood, e.g. dry skin	+ BL.20, LI.4, ST.36 Rf
CV.2	Crossing point (LR) ⎫ Crossing point (LR, SP, KI) ⎬ Alarm (BL) ⎭	Damp Heat, e.g. genital itching	+ LR.1, SP.6, SP.9 or + LR. 5, LR.11
CV.6		Stagnant Qi Blood	+ LR.3, TE.6 Rd
CV.24	Crossing point (ST, LI)	Heat and Fire poison, e.g. acne	+ LI.4, LI.20, ST.3, ST.44
GV.10		Fire poison	+ GV.12, BL.40, LI.4 Rd
GV.12		Wind Heat, Fire poison, e.g. boils	+ BL.17, LI.4, GB.21 Rd
GV.14		Wind Heat, e.g. urticaria and eczema	+ LI.4, LI.11, LU.7 Rd

Rd, Reducing method; Rf, Reinforcing method; E, Even method; B, bleeding.

Psychological and related 34 syndromes

Depression syndromes

Depression can be said to be the subjective experience of feeling down, negative, miserable, melancholy, low in spirits, and unable to cope with life.

DEPRESSION AND QI

Depression is usually associated with either Deficiency, where there is simply not enough energy for positive feelings, or Stagnation, when there is energy, but the flow of energy and emotions is blocked. Deficiency can also be associated with Excess, as in manic depression, or with Irregularity, as in anxiety depression.

DEPRESSION AND THE FIVE ORGAN SYSTEMS

Table 4.2 summarizes the Yin and Yang emotional aspect of each of the five organ systems. Depression corresponds more to the Yin aspect and may be linked to each of the five systems. Since depression can be due to either Deficiency or Stagnation, there are 10 main possibilities:

Deficiency
    Deficient Heart Qi and Yang
    Deficient Spleen Qi and Yang
    Deficient Lung Qi and Yang
    Deficient Kidney Qi and Yang
    Deficient Liver Qi and Yang

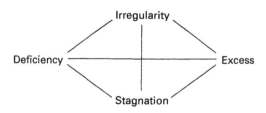

Fig. 34.1

437

Stagnation
Stagnant Heart Qi
Stagnant Spleen Qi
Stagnant Lung Qi
Stagnant Kidney Qi
Stagnant Liver Qi

While depression itself is Yin, depression due to Stagnation is Yang relative to depression due to Deficiency, since in Stagnation there is energy, it is just blocked. These 10 main types of depression are detailed in Table 34.1

Table 34.1 Depression Deficiency and stagnation

System	Deficiency	Stagnation
Fire Heart	loneliness, lack of joy, lack of interest, lack of warmth and affection, lack of love for self and others	difficulty in expressing needs or affection in close relationships, blockage of the flow of affection
Earth Spleen	depression from worry and insecurity, lost in an internal world of obsessive thoughts, without pleasure in the physical body or the outer world	obstruction in feelings of caring and sympathy, or the apparent rejection of these feelings by others, mental congestion with difficulty in converting thought into action
Metal Lungs	withdrawal, lack of participation in life from lack of ability to form or maintain bonds, or from fear of loss	suppression of grief, unwillingness to let go or to face the truth, stagnation in relationships from fear of change and fear of loss
Water Kidney	feeling helpless or powerless, feeling of failure and low self-worth, lack of drive, giving up on life, easily discouraged	strong will but depression from inability to achieve goals from lack of energy, inappropriate goals, or unrealistic time scale
Wood Liver	self-doubt, uncertainty, lack of confidence, lack of self-assertion, weak boundaries, allowing others to intrude or dominate	depression, frustration, feeling of being blocked in life in general, and in self-expression and creativity in particular, internal pressure and desire to act, but uncertain of path in life

DEPRESSION AND DEFICIENCY

SINGLE SYNDROMES

Depression may be associated with a single syndrome, for example, depression due to Deficient Kidney Qi and Yang. In these patterns, depression may be linked with such signs as exhaustion, cold, weak lower back, urinary frequency and impotence. The principle of treatment is to tonify the Deficiency.

COMBINATION OF TWO SYNDROMES

It is very common in the clinic to find that depression is

due to Deficiency of two or more organ systems. Some common duos are:

- Deficient Kidney and Liver: lack of drive, lack of assertion, no clear goals, uncertain as to identity or path in life.

- Deficient Kidney and Heart: apathy, lack of drive, lack of energy, lack of interest in work and achievement, life in general and sex and relationships in particular.

- Deficient Heart and Spleen: need for warmth and caring, but difficulty in maintaining relationships due to feeling of lack of love and solidity.

COMBINATION OF THREE SYNDROMES

Some common combinations of three systems are:

- Deficient Kidney, Heart and Spleen: depression associated with fear, worry and anxiety from lack of strength of self, lack of self-love and lack of solidity; need for, but inability to give warmth and caring, due to fear and insecurity.

- Deficient Heart, Spleen and Lungs: depression associated with difficulties in relationships due to lack of warmth, lack of ability to give consistent support and sympathy, and difficulty to form and maintain bonds.

DEPRESSION AND STAGNATION

Depression may be linked with Stagnation in one or more of the organ systems. The patient may claim physical tiredness but this is a sensation rather than an actual Deficiency, and the feeling of tiredness and the depres-

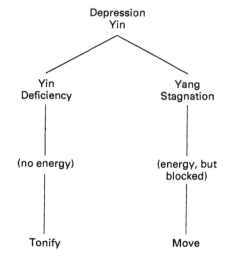

Fig 34.2

sion itself may be temporarily relieved by the movement of physical exertion. The principle of the treatment is not to tonify, but to move the Qi.

DEFICIENCY AND STAGNATION

The two commonest causes of depression may combine, for example:

- Deficient Kidney Qi + Stagnant Kidney Qi: weak energy, constitutionally or due to burnout, but strong will, so depression at not achieving goals.
- Deficient Liver Qi + Stagnant Liver Qi: poor planning and poor decisions create problems, and lead to depression with feelings of obstruction and inability to see way out of the mess.
- Deficient Heart Qi + Stagnant Heart Qi: need for warmth and affection, but shy and embarrassed, with difficulty in easy communication and in starting relationships, thus much pent up feelings.

EMPHASIS OF TREATMENT

The emphasis of treatment will depend on whether the Stagnation or the Deficiency is dominant. For example, a patient has depression associated with Deficient Kidney and Heart Qi and Stagnation of Heart Qi. The patient is primarily fearful, anxious and shy due to Deficiency, and secondarily inhibited due to Stagnation of Qi. A combination could be:

CV.4, KI.3, HT.7 Rf; KI.1 M; CV.14 E; CV.17, PC.6 Rd

The emphasis is therefore primarily on reducing shyness by strengthening Heart and Kidney, and by calming fear with CV.14, and secondarily on moving Stagnation of Heart Qi.

DEPRESSION AND EXCESS

MANIC DEPRESSION

Manic depression can be seen as an example of alternation between Excess + Irregularity and Deficiency + Stagnation.

Excess	+ Irregularity	Deficiency	+ Stagnation
Heart Fire	+ Disturbance of Spirit	Deficient Heart Fire	+ Stagnant Heart Qi
hyperactivity, overexcitement mania, foolish behaviour		exhaustion, loneliness, self-disgust, despair, depression	

DEPRESSION AND AGGRESSION

Another example of the alternation of depression with Excess is found in the alternation between the depression of Stagnant Liver Qi and the anger and violence of Liver Fire. Often this is an alternation between emotional suppression and expression.

This can be a general characteristic of Wood, the type which may be exaggerated by such factors as alcohol or menstruation.

DEPRESSION AND ANXIETY

ANXIETY

Anxiety, as discussed on pages 453–457, is the feeling of apprehension, often with jumpiness, restlessness and insomnia, that is associated with Disturbance of Heart Spirit. Anxiety is often based on Deficiency of the Qi, Blood or Yin needed to keep the Heart Spirit stable. Three common syndromes of anxiety are:

Deficient Heart and Kidney Qi
Deficient Heart and Kidney Yin
Deficient Heart and Spleen Blood.

TWO MANIFESTATIONS OF DEFICIENCY

Deficiency can be associated with depression, reduced emotional movement due to lack of energy; or with anxiety, disturbed emotional movement due to lack of sufficient Qi, Blood or Yin to stabilize Heart Spirit. The difference in principle of treatment is: for Deficiency with depression, primarily tonify and secondarily move; for Deficiency with anxiety, tonify and calm. The relative emphasis on tonifying or calming in the case of Deficiency with anxiety will depend on the severity of the agitation. In acute agitation it may be necessary initially to emphasize calming.

DEFICIENT YANG AND DEFICIENT YIN

While Deficient Qi or Blood can be associated with either depression or anxiety, Deficient Yang is more likely to be associated with depression due to lack of emotional movement, and Deficient Yin with anxiety due to Heat and the restless movement of Spirit.

Depression: Deficient Yang
Anxiety: Deficient Yin
Either: Deficient Qi or Blood.

MIXED SYNDROMES OF DEPRESSION AND ANXIETY

Three common syndromes can give mixtures of depression and anxiety, or alternation between the two:

Deficient Qi and Blood
Deficient Heart Qi, Blood and Yin
Deficient Heart Yang/Deficient Heart Yin.

DEFICIENT QI AND BLOOD

General Deficiency of Qi (Kidney, Spleen, Heart) and of Blood (Spleen, Liver, Heart) may give rise to depression with anxiety, especially after childbirth, during menopause, or in old age.

DEFICIENT HEART QI, BLOOD AND YIN

When Kidney, Spleen and Heart are Deficient, Heart may suffer from Deficiency of Qi, Blood and Yin, with both depression and anxiety. This pattern can be treated with SP.4 + PC.6, the Opening points for the Thoroughfare–Yin Link combination. CV.4, CV.12 and CV.17 may be added, to strengthen Kidneys, Spleen and Heart.

DEFICIENT HEART YIN/DEFICIENT HEART YANG

The basis of this oscillation is Deficiency, usually Deficient Qi of Kidneys and Heart. It is a very common syndrome at menopause, but can occur at other times. In this syndrome, depression due to Deficient Yang alternates with anxiety due to Deficient Yin. This syndrome is based on Deficiency, and so is less extreme than manic depression, although the two syndromes may overlap. Generally, anxiety is more related to Deficiency and mania is more related to Excess.

SYNDROMES

Fifteen main depression syndromes are summarized in Table 34.3:

Deficient Heart Qi and Yang
Deficient Spleen Qi and Yang
Deficient Lung Qi and Yang
Deficient Kidney Qi and Yang
Deficient Liver Qi and Yang

Stagnant Heart Qi
Stagnant Spleen Qi
Stagnant Lung Qi
Stagnant Kidney Qi
Stagnant Liver Qi

Stagnant Liver Qi/Liver Fire
Deficient Heart Fire/Heart Fire
Deficient Heart and Kidney Yang/Deficient Heart and Kidney Yin
Deficient Heart Qi, Blood and Yin
Deficient Qi and Blood

DEPRESSION AND RELATED DISORDERS

Table 34.2 lists some common disorders related to depression.

Table 34.2 Some common depressive disorders

Disorder	Syndromes
manic depression	Deficient Heart Fire/Heart Fire
depression and aggression	Stagnant Liver Qi/Liver Fire
anxiety depression	Deficient Heart Qi, Blood and Yin
menopausal depression	Deficient Heart and Kidney Yang/ Deficient Heart and Kidney Yin
premenstrual depression and emotional lability	Stagnant Liver Qi/Hyperactive Liver Yang
postnatal depression	Deficient Qi and Blood
impotence and depression	Deficient Kidney Yang and Deficient and Disturbed Heart Spirit
burnout and depression	Excess Kidney will and Deficient Kidney Qi

Table 34.3 Depression syndromes

Syndrome	Signs and symptoms	Pulse	Tongue	Point combination
Deficient Heart Yang	lack of joy, sadness, loneliness, lack of interest in life, feeling unloved and unlovable	empty or thin, deep, slow	pale, flabby maybe a hollow at tip	CV.4, CV.17, ST.36, SP.6, HT.7, HT.8 Rf Moxa with caution
Stagnant Heart Qi	frustration in relationships from difficulty in expressing warmth and feelings, with sadness and misery	hindered or wiry, maybe choppy	various, maybe pale purple at tip	CV.17, BL.14, BL.44, SP.4, PC.6, HT.5 Rd
Deficient Spleen Qi	preoccupied with endless thoughts, worry and mental arguments, too much thinking and not enough action	empty or thin, maybe choppy and deep	pale, maybe thin and dry	GV.20, yìn táng, CV.4, ST.36, ST.45, SP.1, SP.2 Rf
Stagnant Spleen Qi	isolated, lonely people, avoided by others due to their clinging, dominating possessiveness which interferes and intrudes into the lives of others, always complaining	slippery, maybe full or flooding with underlying emptiness	pale, flabby or swollen, maybe deep groove in Spleen area	CV.12, ST.40. ST.45, LR.1, LR..3, LR.13 E
Deficient Lung Qi	withdrawal and lack of participation in the present, difficulty in or fear of forming lasting bonds with others, living in memories of the past	empty, deep	pale, flabby maybe a hollow in Lung area	CV.4, CV.17, ST.36, KI.3, LU.1, LU.9, LU.10 Rf M
Stagnant Lung Qi	suppressed grief, unwillingness to let go of past relationships, difficulty in dealing with the pain of loss	hindered, maybe flooding at the deep level	pale or purplish	CV.17, ST.40, BL.13, BL.42 Rd M; LU.1, LU.7, PC.6 Rd
Deficient Kidney Yang, Kidney Qi	collapsed personality, given up on life, oversurrendered, let go of control, weak-willed, apathetic	empty or thin, slow, deep, choppy maybe scattered	pale, flabby, moist	GV.20, CV.4, KI.2, KI.7, ST.36, HT.8 Rf M; KI.1 M
Excess Kidney will and Deficient Kidney Qi	continual disappointment due to will being stronger than energy reserves, or to unrealistic ambitions, maybe burnout	wiry, thin, choppy, changing maybe flooding	pale, flabby maybe red spots	GV.20, ST.36, KI.3, BL.64 Rf M; BL.2 Rf
Deficient Liver–Gallbladder Qi	self-doubt, uncertainty, insecurity, touchiness and hypersensitivity with depression and a weak sense of self	empty or thin, choppy, maybe changing or hindered	pale, maybe thin, maybe red spots at edges	GV.20, CV.4, GB.13, GB.40, TE.4, KI.3 Rf
Stagnant Liver Qi	depression and frustration, feeling obstructed by circumstances, liking for movement and hatred of blockage, maybe angry or irritable	wiry, maybe slow or rapid, full or empty	purplish maybe red or red spots at edges	CV.6, CV.17, LR.1, LR.3, LR.14, PC.1, PC.6 Rd
Stagnant Liver Qi/Liver Fire	alternation of depression with aggression and anger, alternation of suppressed anger with expressed anger	wiry, full or flooding, maybe rapid	purple, red, maybe deviated or trembling	LR.2, LR.14, PC.8 Rd; GV.20, CV.6, SP.6 E + KI.1 Rd, LR.1 B for anger
Deficient Heart Fire/Heart Fire	manic depression; alternation of exhilaration, enthusiasm and sociability, with depression which may be desperate and suicidal	rapid, full or empty, maybe irregular or slippery	red, especially at tip, maybe trembling, maybe greasy coat	CV.17, PC.6 E; SP.6, KI.3 Rf ı HT.3, HT.8 E for manic phase + GV.20, KI.1 Rd for severe manic phase + ST.36, HT.7 Rf for depressive phase + CV.4 Rf; KI.1 M for severe depressive phase
Deficient Heart and Kidney Yang/Deficient Heart and Kidney Yin	tiredness with feelings of cold, alternating with restless anxiety, insomnia and feelings of heat	variable speed, thin or empty, maybe irregular	pale with red tip, maybe toothmarks and trembling	CV.4, CV.17, ST.36, SP.6 Rf + CV.14, HT.6 E; KI.6 Rf for anxiety + GV.20, KI.4, HT.8 Rf for depression
Deficient Heart Qi, Blood and Yin	anxiety, depression, emotional lability, weak and nervous, easily tired and easily emotionally upset	thin, choppy maybe irregular, moving or changing	pale, thin or flabby with red tip and irregular shape at tip	CV.4, ST.36 Rf; CV.14, CV.24, SP.4, PC.6 E
Deficient Qi and Blood	anxiety and depression with exhaustion, weakness and maybe dizziness, e.g. after childbirth	empty, thin or minute, choppy, deep	pale, flabby, toothmarks	GV.20, CV.4, CV.12, CV.17, ST.36, SP.6, LR.8, LI.4 Rf alternate GV.4, GV.20, BL.15, BL.20, BL.23, SP.6, LI.4 Rf Moxa if no Heat signs

Rf, Reinforcing method; Rd, reducing method; E, Even method; M, moxa.

Tiredness and exhaustion syndromes

There is a strong tendency in modern society to overemphasize Yang, activity, and to disregard the need for Yin, rest. One result of this is that vast numbers of people live their lives in a state of tiredness bordering on exhaustion. Also, for many people, their dissatisfaction with themselves and their lives can create a feeling of tiredness, even if they have sufficient energy. Tiredness can therefore be differentiated into Deficiency, with a genuine lack of energy, and Stagnation, where the energy is there but blocked. This differentiation has been discussed in the previous section on Depression.

Chinese medicine can be effective in cases of tiredness, but many patients are highly likely to relapse unless they effect changes in their personality which reflect in their lifestyles.

AETIOLOGY

It is especially helpful, where appropriate, for the practitioner to give patients a detailed understanding of the origins of their tiredness, and a clear insight into the nature of their personality and the overall patterns of their lives. Those patients who are sufficiently motivated can then apply self-help measures more effectively.

Some of the main origins of tiredness are:

constitutional type
climatic factors
life pressures
hormonal and life changes
childbirth
psychological disorders
physical illness
medicines
drugs
nutrition
exercise
work
lack of sleep
sex.

CONSTITUTIONAL TYPE

A person's physical and psychological constitutional type depend on the interaction between their genetic makeup and their environment from conception onward. In Chinese medicine, poor parental health during conception or pregnancy can result in weak constitution in the child. Emotional pressures in the parents during pregnancy,

childbirth, childhood and puberty, can affect both the physical strength and psychological structure of the child.

One classic combination for such generalized constitutional weakness is:

CV.4, PC.6, SP.4, ST.36 Rf

CV.12 can be added for Deficient Spleen and CV.17 added for Deficient Heart or Lungs. This combination can be alternated with:

BL.13, BL.20, BL.23, BL.43 Rf

Moxa can be added to both combinations if there are no signs of Heat.

CLIMATIC FACTORS

Climatic factors, such as living in cold damp rooms or working in hot damp climates, can sap the strength, as can working in air-conditioned concrete buildings with artificial lighting. Obviously the patient needs to avoid or take precautions against the Exterior factor. In addition, if the factor has invaded the body, or is lingering in the body, it needs to be removed, and then the body needs to be tonified to treat the tiredness, and to prevent further invasion.

For example, a student living in a damp cold basement flat and suffering repeated colds which progress to chronic bronchitis with exhaustion, needs to find another flat. Points like LU.7, LI.4 and BL.12 can be used with Reducing method and moxa, to disperse Wind Cold and Damp, then points like CV.17, LU.9, LU.1, BL.13 and ST.36 can be used with Reinforcing method and moxa to strengthen the Lungs, and to treat the tiredness.

LIFE PRESSURES

Life pressures such as start of school, change of house, loss of job, difficulties in a relationship, car accident, bereavement, and so on can both deplete and stagnate the energy, resulting in tiredness. The way that a person reacts to psychological stresses will depend on their personality type.

For example, an Earth-type person may experience extreme insecurity and worry about losing their job, being unable to pay for the mortgage on their house, being homeless and destitute, and not knowing where the money for their next meal is coming from — one of the deepest fears of an Earth-type person. The endless worrying thoughts prevent sleep and rest, and so create tiredness.

It can be helpful for such patients to make affirmations in great detail, for each area of their lives, and so utilize their analytical ability and active mind in a positive way. Points like GV.20, ān mián, yìn táng, HT.7, SP.1, SP.2 and ST.45 can be used with Reducing method to calm the mind and reduce insomnia. Points such as CV.4, CV.12 and ST.36 can be used with Reinforcing method to increase energy.

HORMONAL AND LIFE CHANGES

Tiredness often follows the major life stages, such as puberty, pregnancy, childbirth and menopause, not only because of the hormonal changes at these key times, but also because of the difficulties in adapting to the new role. For example, at menopause, women with Deficient Qi and Blood may suffer both tiredness and depression. They may feel that they are becoming old and grey and physically unattractive, and may find it difficult to adapt to the changes within themselves and their lives.

Meditation exercises which develop a sense of inner beauty and strength can be most helpful, in conjunction with acupuncture treatments to tonify Spleen and Heart Qi and Blood. For example, GV.20, CV.4, CV.17, HT.7, LI.4, SP.6, SP.10, ST.36 and KI.6 with Reinforcing method.

CHILDBIRTH

Childbirth is often followed by severe tiredness and depression, especially when the mother has not completely recovered from a previous childbirth and has lost much sleep with the previous child. It is important that the mother has a nourishing diet, and has as much sleep, rest, and help with the baby as possible. In addition, acupuncture combinations such as GV.20, CV.4, CV.17, PC.6, SP.4, ST.28 and ST.36, can be alternated with BL.15, BL.17, BL.20 and BL.23, both combinations with Reinforcing method and moxa.

PSYCHOLOGICAL DISORDERS

Everyone has potential or minor imbalances in their psychological makeup. Under sufficient pressure these imbalances can manifest in minor or major psychological disorders, of type depending on the type of personality – anxiety, depression, manic depression, schizophrenia and so on. These disorders often involve tiredness as a major component.

For example, of a Wood-type person separates from their partner, in addition to unprocessed grief, there may also be anger, resentment and bitterness. Such a person, may then feel depressed, tearful and irritable, and may

greatly benefit from a combination such as CV.6, CV.17, LU.7, LR.3, LR.14 with Reducing method, which helps the blocked emotions flow, releasing the grief and anger, and clearing the feeling of tiredness and depression.

PHYSICAL ILLNESS

Chronic pain, hypothyroidism, diabetes, cancer and many other physical conditions can result in severe tiredness. An excellent example is severe skin rashes of the Heat in the Blood type, with sore red hot skin lesions with extreme itching, emotional distress, insomnia and resulting physical and nervous exhaustion. It is essential that such a person avoids all heat-producing foods and drinks, and avoids further emotional stress whenever possible. Initial treatments would aim to reduce acute Heat, by bleeding points such as PC.3, PC.9, BL.40 and LR.1, and after this, in the same treatment, reducing yìn táng, ān mián, HT.3, HT.7, LI.4, LI.11, SP.6, SP.10 and maybe KI.1, to cool the skin and assist sleep. Later treatments would aim at nourishing the skin and the nervous system by tonifying Yin and Blood, for example, GV.20, CV.4, CV.14, HT.3, HT.6, SP.6, SP.10, KI.6 and ST.36 with Reinforcing method.

MEDICINES

Various medical drugs have tiredness or drowsiness as a side-effect; for example, various benzodiazepines, many analgesics, antihistamines and antibiotics. Also, many hypnotics, if taken over long periods, will cause chronic tiredness by interfering with the natural sleep rhythms. For example, many people have been prescribed benzodiazepine tranquillizers for bereavement. Apart from blocking the natural process of grieving, such medicines may have side-effects of drowsiness, tiredness and mental dullness.

Unless there are special severe problems, acupuncture combined with gentle supportive counselling is preferable to tranquillizers. If the patient is taking tranquillizers and wishes to come off them, this process can be gradual and assisted by ear acupuncture to reduce the stress during withdrawal. Points such as LI.1, ST.8, ST.45, LR.1, GB.13 and GB.43 can then be used to clear the drug side-effects of drowsiness and mental disorientation and congestion.

DRUGS

Stimulants such as strong tea, coffee, amphetamines and cocaine will drain the energy and may also interfere with the sleep patterns. Some other drugs, such as alcohol and marihuana can create tiredness by causing both Stagnation of Qi and confusion of the mind. For example, in the opinion of the author, marihuana taken to excess over a long period of time can lead to Stagnant Liver Qi, with depression and tiredness; Damp Heat, with itching skin; Stagnant Heart Qi, with poor circulation; and scattering of the Spirit, with poor concentration and a less-focused grasp on reality.

To assist the person to come off marihuana, especially if it has been smoked with tobacco, ear acupuncture points may be helpful. Then, to treat tiredness and other effects of long-term use, combinations such as yìn táng, CV.6, TE.5, GB.13, GB.41, SP.6, SP.9 can be used with Even method.

NUTRITION

Malnutrition, from poverty, ignorance or unwise dieting can cause tiredness, since the Spleen cannot produce enough Qi and Blood for the body to use or the Kidneys to store. For example, many people become so obsessed with losing weight that their intake of proteins, vitamins and iron especially, becomes so low as to cause severe tiredness and loss of concentration. Obviously, adopting a nutritional pattern that gives them all their requirements, while minimizing weight gain is essential, if they will adopt it. Also, regular moderate exercise once their energy has returned will help to reduce weight.

A combination for this problem can be CV.6, CV.12, LI.1, LI.10, ST.8, ST.25, ST.36, SP.6 and SP.9 with Even method, to strengthen Qi, reduce Damp and Phlegm, and help concentration.

EXERCISE

Lack of exercise can produce a feeling of tiredness and depression. For example, lack of exercise in a person tending to Stagnant Liver Qi with Deficient Spleen Qi and Damp, can lead to a feeling of tiredness, lethargy and lack of interest, especially if the diet contains too much Damp- and Phlegm-forming foods, for example excessive carbohydrates and dairy products. Moderate exercise will move the Stagnation, raise the metabolism and help to clear accumulating Damp and Phlegm. Combinations such as CV.6, CV.12, CV.17, TE.6, LI.10, ST.40, SP.9 and LR.3 with Even method and moxa will complement the effect of the exercise.

Excessive exercise can result in exhaustion due to Deficiency of Kidney and Heart Qi and Yang. What constitutes excessive exercise will depend on a person's capacity at a particular time. One problem is that to preserve macho self-image, or to reduce weight, many people are reluctant to reduce the amount of exercise, even when exhausted. This problem can sometimes be solved if it is suggested to them that less of the vigorous exercise, and more of such nourishing exercise as Qi Gong or Yoga, will make them stronger, and younger-looking and more attractive. These more Yin exercises can be combined with relaxation and meditation exercises that make them feel good as they are, so they are less inclined to pursue a false self-image.

Combinations such as GV.20, CV.4, CV.17, HT.7, PC.6, SP.4, SP.21 and ST.36 with Reinforcing method can be used for exhaustion, provided the patient has reduced the strenuous exercise and started energy-strengthening Qi Gong techniques. If they have not, CV.4 should not be used, since they will merely burn out their last reserves of energy.

WORK

It is not simply the quantity of work that is exhausting, it is the degree of stress with which it is performed, and the degree of dissatisfaction with the work situation. Unemployment, redundancy, retirement, job insecurity in time of recession, a boring repetitive or unchallenging job, can all lead to depression and a feeling of tiredness. However, a person in a 'good' job may feel just as dissatisfied, depressed and tired, if the job does not match their abilities and personality, if they detest their colleagues, if they are not shown sufficient appreciation of their effort, or if they feel they cannot express their creativity through their work.

For example, for some people, retirement constitutes an enormous change. They may find themselves with less physical exercise, less mental challenge, less social stimulation, less meaning or direction in life, and spending far more of their time in the company of their partner, who may be less than pleased to have them hanging around the house. Apart from the obvious suggestions of part-time work, voluntary work and new social outlets, counselling can be helpful in assisting a new understanding of self, and a reappraisal of life pattern and goals.

Acupuncture can be helpful in giving energy, lifting depression and in assisting the person to let go of old patterns and see new possibilities. One possible combination is yìn táng, CV.6, CV.17, LU.1, LU.7 and KI.6 with Even method and moxa. Another combination is GV.23, CV.6, SI.3, BL.2, BL.62, KI.6 with Even method.

LACK OF SLEEP

One of the most obvious causes of tiredness is lack of sleep. Either the patients do not permit themselves sufficient hours of sleep, or their rhythms are broken by the irregular hours of shift work, or they have insomnia — difficulty getting to sleep or staying asleep. The use of hypnotics is no long-term solution, as discussed in the later section on insomnia.

For example, people with Deficient Qi and Yin of Heart and Kidney often feel tired, and attracted to stimulants such as coffee, which mobilize Kidney energy and stimulate Heart Spirit. This tends to create more severe tiredness as Kidney energy is burned out, and also restlessness and insomnia due to disturbance of Heart Spirit. The insomnia further aggravates the tiredness, increasing desire for coffee to 'get started' in the morning and to 'keep going' during the day.

For Heart–Kidney types with insomnia and exhaustion, it is essential to stop the coffee, if necessary substituting with a non-caffeine drink of a bitter taste. So called caffeine-free tea and coffee are not advisable, since the residual amounts of caffeine in them are enough to affect many of those sensitive to this chemical. Point combinations need to calm Heart Spirit and also to nourish Kidney and Heart Qi and Yin. For example, GV.20, CV.14, ān mián, HT.7, SI.3, with Reducing method, plus CV.4, KI.6, SP.6 and BL.62 with Reinforcing method.

In extreme cases of restlessness and insomnia, GV.20, HT.8, SP.1, KI.1 and KI.2 with Reducing method can be combined with HT.3 and KI.10 with Reinforcing method.

SEX

It is not only the amount of sex that is depleting, it is the degree of stress with which it is performed. Also, lack of satisfaction and completion in sex can lead to great frustration and depression, and to a feeling of tiredness and despondency. Excessive sex may aggravate tiredness due to Deficiency, but sexual problems may give rise to a feeling of tiredness, associated with depression and Stagnation. One combination for impotence, tiredness and depression can be CV.3, CV.6, CV.17, LU.7, LR.5, LR.12, LR.14, ST.30 with Even method and moxa on CV.3, CV.6 and CV.17 unless there are signs of Heat.

TIREDNESS SYNDROMES

As with depression, there are 10 basic syndromes of Deficiency and Stagnation:

Deficiency
Deficient Heart Qi and Yang
Deficient Spleen Qi and Yang
Deficient Lung Qi and Yang
Deficient Kidney Qi and Yang

Deficient Liver Qi and Yang

Stagnation
Stagnant Heart Qi
Stagnant Spleen Qi
Stagnant Lung Qi
Stagnant Kidney Qi
Stagnant Liver Qi

The principle of treatment is to tonify Deficiency and to move Stagnation. The point combinations for these syndromes are given in Table 34.3.

EXCESS BECOMES DEFICIENCY

The reason that some Deficient patients become depleted, is an Excess of activity in their lives. This hyperactivity, whether of work, socializing, exercise or sex, can burn out the energy and eventually result in Deficiency.

BURNOUT

Burnout refers to exhaustion resulting from overactivity. Burnout can occur even to a strong constitution if the pattern of excess activity and insufficient rest goes on for too long. It will simply occur more quickly in those who are constitutionally generally Deficient. It is more likely to occur in Deficient Yin constitutions, than in those with Deficient Yang. This is because the Deficient Yang type does not have enough Yang energy to enter a burnout situation. In Deficient Yin types, the Yang energy is not properly controlled. So despite the tiredness of Deficiency there is a restless hyperactivity that can lead to burnout.

BURNOUT AND PERSONALITY TYPE

Of the 10 personality types discussed in Chapter 4, three are particularly attracted to burnout situations, Yang Kidney, Yang Liver and Yang Heart.

YANG KIDNEY

The Yang Kidney type has a strong focused will, and a ceaseless drive to achieve, and in some cases, is driven by inner fear and insecurity to dominate and gain power over others, in order to control their surroundings. This type may have little consideration for their own health or that of others. By setting themselves unrealistic goals, they burn themselves out in an attempt to achieve them and then feel great self-disgust at their own supposed weakness and inadequacy.

The most extreme result of burnout here is Deficient Kidney Yang, with total exhaustion, lowered metabolism, cold limbs and body, and deep depression at the loss of self-image and feeling of uselessness. If burnout is this severe, convalescence may take years. In less severe cases, there is a pattern of Excess Kidney will and Deficient Kidney Qi. Here the person feels very tired, with scant reserves of energy, but their will is still strong, and on those occasions, for example, after an acupuncture treatment, when they do feel more energetic, they will immediately overwork again.

YANG LIVER

The Yang Liver type has a forceful fiery energy. Such people are quick and decisive, tending to be impatient, intolerant and critical of those who are slower or less perceptive than themselves. They easily feel frustrated by apparent obstructions in their lives and may make hasty decisions which lead them into greater difficulties, aggravated by the effect of their abrupt abrasive personalities on others. The pressure of their inner restless fiery drive against these apparent obstacles, may lead to severe stress and eventual burnout. This may take the form of a retreat into depression, or into the so-called nervous breakdown pattern of anger, tears, feelings of shakiness, weakness and being unable to cope, followed by withdrawal.

YANG HEART

Yang Heart people can be inspiring, popular leaders, initiators and social entertainers, but in extreme the Yang Heart type tends to classic hypomania, with feelings of excitement, enthusiasm, elation and ceaseless hurried overactivity. Yang Heart people tend to overwork by becoming involved in too many different projects. They start many things in their initial bursts of enthusiastic energy, but can be easily depressed if other people's enthusiasm wanes and they themselves lack the energy to continue the project. Burnout in this case can result in both exhaustion and depression, and in extreme cases, manic depression with suicidal tendencies.

In the case of the three personality types of Yang Kidney, Liver and Heart, burnout comes as a result of overactivity directed to basically selfish ends. In the case of Yang Spleen, exhaustion from overwork can come from the apparently selfless activity of caring for others.

YANG SPLEEN

This personality type can expend much energy in worry, concern and caring for others and in giving them nourishment and support. In Chinese theory, this is the Earth element, it is a more feminine aspect, and is more the role of the mother, although it can be performed by either parent, since both men and women have their feminine aspect.

This caring can be given to those within the family, or to people outside the family through the fields of medicine, teaching or social work, for example. It can be given through a feeling of love and compassion for others, with a feeling of pleasure in caring for them; it can be given through a sense of duty and obligation; it can be given through a feeling of insecurity in order to keep people close to the giver, or to control them, and as such may be felt as an intrusion and an interference by the receiver, although the receiver may have come to be dependent on the help given.

In many who exhaust themselves in caring of others, there is not only a mixture of love and duty but also, to varying degrees, the adoption of the role of the martyr and victim.

YANG LUNG

The Yang Spleen personality can be linked to the Yang Metal Type in people who feel their own inner griefs so acutely that the sorrows of the world move them to take action in helping others in tragic and desperate circumstances of homelessness, hunger, disease and persecution. Some of those working in this way are so driven by their feelings of compassion, grief, pity and guilt, that they burn themselves out physically and mentally by their efforts.

TREATMENT OF BURNOUT

A major problem in the treatment of burnout is that the modern world so strongly supports the ethos of ceaseless activity – 'work hard, play hard'. Burnout patients face two great challenges: firstly, in resting sufficiently to allow recovery, and secondly, in changing their whole life patterns to a better balance of activity and rest. The principle of acupuncture treatment is not merely to tonify Deficiency, but simultaneously to treat the causes of the overactivity that produced the Deficiency. This cannot be done without the cooperation of the patient. The practitioner needs to give the patient a clear perspective of the origins of burnout within their personality and the understanding that the only way out is personal change. Each personality type has a different life lesson to learn from the burnout situation.

YANG KIDNEY

The Kidney type needs to find and develop a deep inner feeling of strength within themselves. This relieves the inner fear that drives them to attempt to dominate, control and gain power over others. This feeling of strength, faith in self, and self-worth allows them to form more realistic goals, so that they are not driven so hard by a need to achieve to prove self-worth. This allows them to find a new balance between doing and being.

In meditation and Qi Gong, they need to focus on the Dan Tian centre, to build up reserves of energy, to overcome fear, and to bring the will into harmony with their need to create a balance between rest and activity. Two points must be used with caution for the Kidney Yang type, KI.1 and CV.4.

KI.1 is likely, even with Reinforcing method, to relax the will so strongly that they feel the underlying exhaustion that they have been trying to overcome or hide from themselves. It is preferable to use combinations that both gently relax the will and gradually increase the energy, for example:

GV.20, CV.14, PC.6, SP.4, ST.36, KI.3 Rf

CV.4 should be avoided in early treatment until the patient has reduced work load and increased rest. It is unwise to use CV.4 to mobilize the patient's last reserves of energy, if they are simply going to use this energy in further burnout.

Once the patient has more energy and has adopted a suitable pattern of energy storage, then CV.4 and KI.1 can be used:

GV.20, CV.4, PC.6, SP.4, ST.36, KI.1, KI.7 Rf

KI.7 will strengthen Kidney Qi to balance the relaxing effect of KI.1. This can be alternated with:

GV.4, GV.20, BL.20, BL.52 Rf

YANG LIVER

The Yang Liver type needs to find within themselves an inner peace which they then allow to project out into every aspect of their lives, giving them the patience to listen both to their own intuition and to the needs of others, so that they begin to flow through life in harmony with it, rather than trying to force their way through it.

A great problem for the Yang Liver type is impatience with the speed of improvement in their treatment. They have to learn to do things slowly. They have to learn to slow down sufficiently to experience peace within themselves, and to act out of a feeling of peace rather than out of impatience. They have to slow down enough to allow things to unfold naturally so that they can put themselves in harmony with this unfolding. This will reduce their feelings of obstruction and frustration.

In meditation and Qi Gong, they need initially to focus on the Dan Tian centre to develop relaxation and to develop a self-discipline of inner peace. They can then use exercises to balance the Dan Tian, Heart and Head centres, to harmonize will, compassion and intuition.

Acupuncture combinations aim at relaxing tension, moving Stagnation, and strengthening Blood and Yin to control Hyperactive Liver Yang. An initial combination can be:

GV.20, CV.17, PC.6, LR.3, LR.14, SP.6, KI.1 E

which can be alternated with:

GV.8, GV.20, BL.47 E; BL.20, BL.23 Rf

If there is severe Liver Fire, then LR.1 and PC.9 can be bled, and LR.2 and PC.8 used with Reducing method.

YANG HEART

The Yang Heart type also needs to learn the lesson of inner peace, that joy can come in peace and strength, simply from the pleasure of being, rather than from restless excitement and a hectic search for stimulation. They need to learn to act from a point of stillness, after contemplating in calmness the possible consequences of their actions, otherwise they are prone to impulsive, foolish, irresponsible and reckless behaviour.

Meditation and Qi Gong exercises focusing on the Dan Tian centre and the centres around KI.1 on the soles of the feet, can help to ground their joys and affections in strength, sobriety and practicality.

Acupuncture points are selected to clear Heart Fire and calm the Spirit, and to tonify Heart and Kidney Qi and Yin to give stability. For example:

GV.20, CV.14, HT.8, KI.2 Rd; CV.4, SP.6, KI.10 Rf

which can be alternated with:

GV.20, KI.1 Rd; BL.23, BL.44 Rf

YANG SPLEEN

If the person is overworking in caring for others from genuine love and the pleasure of helping, then they need to learn that they cannot nourish others without also nourishing themselves. They need to spend time in caring for themselves, not only to recover from exhaustion, but to prevent it happening again. It is often helpful for them to organize a detailed daily routine which they then adopt as the basis of their life.

If they are overworking from a sense of duty, rather than love or pleasure in helping, they can become tired and depressed from the feeling of unavoidable burden and both helper and helped can develop a deep mutual resentment.

If they are compensating for their own insecurities, and avoiding facing their own problems, by busying themselves with the problems of others, they need to develop their own inner strength to overcome their insecurities. Otherwise they will overwork because they create a situation where they become dependent on helping others and the helped are dependent on them.

Each of these three Yang Spleen tendencies, can benefit from meditation and Qi Gong exercises that focus on the Dan Tian centre for strength and storage of energy, and on the Spleen centre for nourishment. In addition, those driven by duty can be helped by Heart centre exercises which may help to transform an onerous burden into a labour of love.

Point combinations will vary according to the situation. For example:

GV.20, yìn táng E; CV.4, CV.12, LI.4, SP.6, ST.36

which can be alternated with:

GV.20, BL.20, BL.21, BL.23, BL.47 Rf

Additional points can be selected from SP.3, SP.21, ST.25, ST.30 to strengthen the Spleen, and from CV.17, GV.11, BL.44 to move Stagnant Heart Qi.

YANG LUNG

People of this type may say that if they stop and rest even for a short time, people in that time may die or be in misery. The answer to this is that if they do not take a break they will become so exhausted that they will not be able to work at all. Treatment focuses on two areas, on recovery of strength and the development of reserves of energy, and on the reduction of feelings of pain, grief and guilt at the suffering of others. These feelings do not help other people, they simply make the helper stressed and unhappy, and lead to eventual burnout.

Qi Gong exercises focus on the Dan Tian centre to build energy reserves, and on the Heart centre to relieve feelings of grief and distress.

Acupuncture treatment can be:

GV.24, CV.4, LU.7, KI.6, GB.13 E

which can be alternated with:

GV.4, GV.11, BL.23, BL.44, BL.42 E

MYALGIC ENCEPHALITIS

Otherwise known as ME, postviral syndrome or chronic Epstein–Barr virus disease, the distinguishing features of this illness are exhaustion, poor memory and concentration, severe muscular ache, fatigue and an intermittent feeling like influenza. Is it the muscle ache and feverish symptoms that distinguish ME from other patterns of tiredness and exhaustion.

This pattern may occur gradually without a previous obvious infection, or it may appear after an infection, hence the name postviral syndrome. Its occurrence without obvious previous infection can be explained in Chinese medicine by the concept of Latent Heat. Exterior Wind can invade the body without immediate symptoms, convert to Latent Heat, and emerge later with feelings of fatigue, muscular aches and fever.

The reoccurrence of the symptoms of ME is explained in terms of residual pathogenic factors, which have been incompletely eliminated by the body, and activate whenever the defensive energy becomes Deficient or there is further Wind invasion. Underlying the invasion of the body by the pathogenic factors, their retention in the body, or their activation, is a chronic Deficiency of Defensive Qi, often linked to Deficient Kidneys.

TREATMENT OF ME

This has two aspects: that of dispersing Latent Heat or residual pathogenic factors, and that of tonifying the Kidneys and Defensive Qi.

If the pulse is of Excess type, i.e. full, flooding, wiry or slippery, then the main principle is to use Reducing method to clear Wind Heat, Heat or Damp Heat, using points such as:

Wind Heat: TE.5, LI.4
Heat: GV.14, LI.11
Damp Heat: SP.6, SP.9.

If the pulse is of the Deficiency type, i.e. thin, empty, minute or choppy, then the main principle of the treatment is to use Reinforcing method to tonify Deficient Defensive Qi and Defensive Kidney, using points such as:

Deficient Defensive Qi: LU.7, ST.36, KI.7 or BL.13, BL.20, BL.23
Deficient Kidney Yin: CV.4, CV.12, SP.6, KI.6 or BL.20, BL.23, BL.52
Deficient Kidney Yang: CV.4, CV.12, CV.17, ST.36, KI.7 or GV.4, GV.20, BL.20, BL.23.

If the patient has an infection such as influenza during the course of treatment, this infection must be treated immediately, or the patient may suffer a relapse which can be very discouraging, since the progress is often slow in any case. If the acupuncturist is available then points such as LI.4, TE.5, LU.7, and BL.12 can be reduced. It is often safer to give the patient a supply of Yin Qiao San, as pills or powder, which they can take immediately they have signs of infection. It is also most important that they rest during any infections.

ME AND PSYCHOLOGICAL FACTORS

ME is distressing in itself since it can lead to a loss of a job or difficulties in a relationship, but it can also be precipitated or aggravated by emotional factors. One common pattern is Deficiency of Heart and Kidney Qi and Yin, with restless anxiety, insomnia, emotional lability and over-reaction to small stresses. In this case, points such as HT.6, and KI.2 with Even method can be added to the treatment for Deficient Yin.

With this illness it is best to use the minimum number of needles, to use only mild needle sensation, and to adopt caution with the Back Transporting points, since some patients with this pattern are very sensitive to acupuncture and may have adverse reactions if these precautions are not taken.

Gentle meditation technique using guided imagery, and gentle and gradual strengthening of the Dan Tian centre, can help to reduce stress and the emotional lability which is often associated with feelings of feverishness or cold. In patients with this lability, which is due to Deficient Qi and Yin, Qi Gong and meditation techniques which tend to generate Heat or to loosen emotional blocks should be avoided. Warming meditation techniques can be used for Deficient Yang patients with depression, providing this pattern does not alternate with one of Deficiency Heat.

Table 34.4 Summary of combinations for burnout

Syndrome	Point combination
Yang Kidney	GV.20, CV.14, PC.6, SP.4, ST.36, KI.3 Rf M progress to
	GV.20, CV.4, PC.6, SP.4, ST.36, KI.1, KI.7 Rf M
Yang Liver	GV.20, CV.17, PC.6, LR.3, LR.14, SP.6, KI.1 E alternate
	GV.8, GV.20, BL.47 E; BL.20, BL.23 Rf
Yang Heart	GV.20, CV.14, HT.8, KI.2 Rd; CV.4, SP.6, KI.10 Rf alternate
	GV.20, KI.1 Rd; BL.23, BL.44 Rf
Yang Spleen	GV.20, yìn táng, LI.4, SP.6 Rd; CV.4, CV.12, ST.36 Rf alternate
	GV.6, GV.20, BL.20, BL.21, BL.23 E
Yang Lung	GV.24, LU.7, GB.13 Rd; CV.4, KI.6 Rf alternate
	GV.12, BL.42, BL.43 E M; GV.4, BL.23 Rf

Rf, Reinforcing method; E, Even method; Rd, Reducing method; M, moxa.

Insomnia syndromes

Insomnia is the most common sleep disorder and is here defined as difficulty in getting to sleep or in staying asleep, or sleep that is disturbed, restless or otherwise of poor quality.

THE IMPORTANCE OF SLEEP

Sleep is vital to replenish Yin. It is not merely rest in terms of cessation of activity, it is a different form of being. It is an entry into the world of Yin, the world of feeling and intuition, sometimes said to be governed by the right brain. The daytime world is the domain of physical activity and the analytical mind, said to be governed by the left brain.

YIN–YANG IMBALANCE

In the modern world there is enormous emphasis on the development of the rational intellectual mind, and a pressure to maintain ceaseless stressful activity in the outside world. There is a tendency to prolong the day into the night. It is rare to find darkness away from artificial lighting, and it is difficult for most people not to carry their daytime mental activity into the world of sleep. This creates a great imbalance between Yin and Yang, with Yang generally increased and Yin greatly reduced, with the daytime world effectively extended far into that of night.

FUTURE OF INSOMNIA

In the opinion of the author, the world-wide prevalence of insomnia will increase until in homes, schools and in society, individuals learn to develop the intuitive mind to the same degree as the analytical mind. Until people learn to find an inner peace and stillness within themselves, which pervades both daytime activities and sleep.

SWITCHING OFF

It is not simply a matter of turning off the rational mind at the end of the day, it is also necessary to nourish and develop the intuitive mind and the realm of imagination and feelings. This can only be done when the mind and body are still, by an act of surrender, a letting go of control of the analytical mind. This is the first stage of meditation.

AETIOLOGY

In Chinese medicine, insomnia relates to disturbance of Heart Spirit and the aetiology and syndromes of insomnia are therefore similar to those of anxiety and palpitation. The aetiology of insomnia and anxiety has been summarized in Figure 34.3. Insomnia depends on the related factors of constitution, personality type and lifestyle. Any factor that leads to the irregular movement of Heart Spirit can aggravate insomnia.

THE MAIN ORIGINS OF INSOMNIA

One of the main causes of insomnia is nervous tension, anxiety, worry, and the projection of these daytime stresses into the world of sleep. Also important is depression and, especially in children, fear; that is, insecurity, fear of dark, and night terrors.

ILLNESS

The pain, discomfort or emotional distress associated with illness may result in difficulties with sleep. For example, nocturnal cough, pulmonary insufficiency or itching skin disorder. Both the illness and the insomnia must be treated, in the context of the patient's needs.

MEDICATION CAN PERPETUATE INSOMNIA

In 1991, the world sales of hypnotics reached 400 million dollars. A general opinion is that the hypnotics, used to treat sleeping problems, are grossly overprescribed, do nothing to cure the basic problem, can have adverse side-effects, and can have great problems of dependence and addiction. Some studies have shown that the quality of sleep is worse on hypnotics than off them, and there is the major difficulty of insomnia of increased severity when patients try to stop these drugs. It may be necessary to treat such drug withdrawal problems with ear and electroacupuncture, as for heroin addiction.

In summary, hypnotics should only be used for severe acute insomnia, for the briefest possible time, and the patient made aware of all possible measures of self-help.

LIFESTYLE

Stimulants such as tea, coffee, cocaine and amphetamines can aggravate or cause insomnia, especially in persons with Deficient Kidney and Heart Yin. Alcohol, that common unofficial prescription for insomnia, can help relaxation and sleep in some people, but if taken to excess, the person may wake in the night as the alcohol starts to manifest as Heat. This is especially likely if the person tends to Heart, Liver or Stomach Fire. Irregular eating, eating late at night and excessive consumption of rich, spicy foods can all aggravate Stomach Fire and prevent sleep. However, for some people it may be impossible to get to sleep on an empty stomach, so moderation is advisable.

For those with Stagnation of Heart, Lungs or Liver Qi, moderate exercise in the evening may disperse Stagnation and Heat and assist sleep. Moderate exercise can also disperse Heat from patients with Deficient Yin and Deficiency Fire, but should not be done too close to bedtime, to allow the Heat released a chance to disperse before sleep.

Excessive study or mental work, without adequate regular breaks can cause Stagnation of Spleen and Stomach Qi, and also Deficient Heart and Spleen Blood. Mental work too late in the evening may result in the mind being active into the night, preventing or disturbing sleep.

Relaxation and meditation exercises at the beginning and end of the day are perhaps the most important way to prevent insomnia.

SYNDROMES

Fire
Heart Fire and Deficient Heart and Kidney Yin
Liver Fire and Hyperactive Liver Yang
Stomach Fire

Stagnation
Stagnant Heart Qi and Heart Phlegm
Stagnant Liver Qi
Stagnant Lung Qi

Deficiency
Deficient Heart and Spleen Blood
Deficient Kidney and Gallbladder Qi

TREATMENT

A list of points for insomnia are given in Table 34.5, and Table 34.6 associates the energy centres with the main insomnia syndromes. Point combinations for insomnia syndromes are summarized in Table 34.7.

Table 34.5 Points for insomnia (n.b. all these points calm Heart Spirit)

Point	Syndromes
ST.36	Stagnant Stomach Qi, Stomach Fire, Deficient Blood
ST.40	Stagnant Stomach Qi, Heart Phlegm
ST.45	Stomach Fire
SP.1	Stagnant Stomach Qi
SP.2	Stomach Fire
SP.4	Stagnant Heart Qi, Deficient Blood
SP.6	Heat in the Blood, Deficient Blood, Deficient Yin
HT.3	Heart Fire, Deficient Heart Yin
HT.5	Heart Fire, Heart Phlegm
HT.6	Deficient Heart Yin
HT.7	Heart Fire, Heart Phlegm, Deficient Heart Qi and Blood
HT.8	Heart Fire
SI.3	Heart Fire, Heart Phlegm
BL.1	Yin–Yang imbalance
BL.13, 42	Stagnant Lung Qi, Lung Fire
BL.15, 43, 44	Heart Fire, Heart Phlegm, Stagnant Heart Qi, Deficient Heart Blood or Yin
BL.18,47	Liver Fire, Stagnant Liver Qi, Hyperactive Liver Yang, Deficient Liver Qi
BL.19, 48	Gallbladder Fire, Deficient Gallbladder Qi
BL.20, 49	Deficient Blood
BL.23, 52	Deficient Kidney Qi and Yin
BL.62	Deficient Kidney and Heart Yin, Heart Fire
KI.1	Kidney, Liver or Heart Fire
KI.2	Deficiency Fire of Kidney
KI.3	Deficient Kidney Qi or Yin
KI.6	Deficient Kidney Yin
PC.3–8	Heart Fire, Stagnant Heart Qi, Heart Phlegm
GB.12	Liver–Gallbladder or Heart Fire
GB.20	Liver–Gallbladder Fire or Hyperactive Liver Yang
GB.40	Deficient Liver–Gallbladder Qi
GB.44	Gallbladder Fire, Hyperactive Liver Yang
LR.2	Liver Fire
LR.3	Stagnant Liver Qi, Hyperactive Liver Yang
LR.14	Stagnant Liver Qi
CV.4	Deficient Qi, Blood or Yin
CV.6	Stagnant Qi
CV.12	Stomach Fire, Stagnant Stomach Qi
CV.14, 15	Heart Fire, Heart Phlegm, Heart Deficiency Fire (insomnia with fear and anxiety)
CV.17	Heart Phlegm, Stagnant Heart Qi, Stagnant Lung Qi
CV.24	Deficient Heart Yin (insomnia with anxiety)
GV.11	as for BL.15
GV.16	Deficient Kidney Qi (insomnia with fear and depression)
GV.20	Heart and Liver Fire, Hyperactive Liver Yang, Deficient Qi and Blood
yìn táng	all forms of insomnia

Table 34.6 Main energy centres for insomnia

Centre	Point	Use
Crown	GV.20	Heart and Liver Fire, Hyperactive Liver Yang, Deficient Heart and Spleen Blood (balance Excess and Deficiency of energy in head)
Brow	yìn táng	all insomnia syndromes (calms tense and overactive mind)
Heart	CV.17	Stagnant Heart or Lung Qi, Heart Phlegm (moves Stagnation and depression)
Solar Plexus	CV.14 CV.15	Heart Fire, Heart Phlegm, Deficient Heart and Kidney Yin (calms fear and anxiety)
Spleen	CV.12	Stomach Fire, Stagnant Stomach Qi (harmonizes digestion)
Dan Tian	CV.6 CV.4	Stagnant Qi (moves Stagnation and depression) Deficient Qi of Kidney, Gallbladder or Heart Deficient Yin of Kidney and Heart Deficient Blood (tonifies Deficiency, balances Yin–Yang, stabilizes the Spirit to prevent fear and anxiety)

Table 34.7 Insomnia syndromes

Syndrome	Signs and symptoms	Pulse	Tongue	Point combinations
Fire Heart Fire and Deficient Heart and Kidney Yin	insomnia with anxiety, restlessness, sensations of heat especially in chest and face, night sweats, maybe palpitations	rapid, full or thin, maybe irregular	red, dry, maybe cracked	GV.20, CV.17, HT.8, KI.1 Rd; HT.3, KI.6, SP.6 Rf
Liver–Gallbladder Fire and Hyperactive Liver Yang	insomnia with irritability, restlessness, sensations of heat especially in the head, maybe headache	rapid, wiry, full or thin	red, especially at edges	GV.20, HT.7, GB.12, GB.44, LR.2, KI.1 Rd KI.6, SP.6 Rf
Stomach Fire and Stagnant Stomach Qi	insomnia with intense worry and mental congestion, maybe gastritis with burning sensation	rapid, full	red, dry thick yellow coat	CV.12, PC.3, PC.6, SP.1, ST.40, ST.44 Rd HT.6, SP.6 Rf
Stagnation Stagnation Heart Qi and Heart Phlegm	insomnia with melancholy and depression, maybe sensation of fullness in chest, maybe mental confusion	full, wiry or hindered, maybe slippery	maybe swollen in Heart area, or greasy coat	GV.20, CV.12, CV.17, PC.6, HT.5, SP.4, ST.40 Rd
Stagnant Lung Qi	insomnia following grief or bereavement, maybe sensation of fullness in chest, maybe crying	full or flooding, wiry or hindered, slippery	greasy coat	CV.17, CV.22, LU.1, LU.6, LU.7, ST.40 Rd
Stagnant Liver Qi	insomnia with depression, frustration, suppressed anger, maybe indigestion, maybe muscular tension	wiry, full	maybe purple	CV.6, CV.17, PC.6, HT.6, LR.1, LR.3, LR.14 Rd
Deficiency Deficient Heart and Spleen Blood	insomnia with worry, tiredness, maybe dizziness, palpitations, poor memory, worse with excessive study	thin, choppy	pale, thin, dry	yìn táng ān mián, HT.7, SP.36, SP.6, SP.10 Rf or, if also Deficient Heart and Kidney Yin: GV.20, CV.14, PC.6, SP.4 Rd; CV.4, ST.36 Rf
Deficient Kidney Qi and Deficient Liver-Gallbladder Qi	insomnia with jumpiness, timidity, night terrors, maybe grinding of teeth in sleep, maybe muscular tension	empty or thin, wiry	maybe pale	GV.20, HT.7, GB.12, GB.13, GB.40, KI.3, KI.7 Rf alternate GV.4, GB.12, BL.18, BL.23
Deficient Kidney and Bladder Qi	insomnia with depression, fear, fright, anxiety or disorientation, maybe headache and stiff neck and shoulders	empty, maybe wiry or moving	maybe pale	GV.16, GV.20, SI.3, HT.6, BL.10, BL.62, KI.6 E

Rd, Reducing method; Rf, Reinforcing method; E, Even method.

Anxiety syndromes

Anxiety can be defined as a subjective state of unpleasant restless, tension and apprehension, in which it is difficult to relax, or to find calmness and peace. Anxiety may have no apparent cause or it may be related to a specific ongoing situation or past event.

UNKNOWN CAUSE

When there is no apparent cause, the fears may be vague and formless, or they may be clear and vivid, although imaginary. Sometimes anxiety with apparently unknown cause relates to a past event which the person does not wish to face or remember, for example, sexual abuse.

KNOWN CAUSE

Anxiety can occur with postconcussion syndrome, it can follow withdrawal from drugs or medicines, it may occur with hallucinogenic drugs such as LSD, it may involve apprehension about a specific event such as an examination or an operation, and it is certainly aggravated by tiredness and general stress.

Anxiety may arise in daily life when a person has to perform difficult tasks at high speed in an atmosphere of conflict and uncertainty. A person may become anxious when there is great pressure to make a decision, their future rests on that decision, but it is far from clear what decision to make.

Some people are more prone to anxiety than others, and the different Five Element types will manifest anxiety in different ways

ANXIETY AND THE FIVE EMOTIONS

BIOLOGICAL SIGNIFICANCE OF FEAR AND ANXIETY

Fear and anxiety have survival value to an animal under threat. The response to these emotions, increase in alertness, respiration rate, heart beat rate and muscle tone, prepare the animal for flight or fight. In humans, anxiety can be a healthy response which enables people to avoid danger or unsuitable situations, or to achieve high levels of performance. However, if the state of anxiety becomes chronic or out of proportion to the stimulus, this healthy response can become pathological. Overalertness may progress to mental strain, insomnia and exhaustion, raised breathing rate to dyspnoea or panic attack, raised heart rate to palpitations, and increased muscle tone to muscular tension, pain or tremors.

ANXIETY AND THE HEART SYSTEM

In Chinese medicine, anxiety is linked with the Heart and Kidney systems. It may be associated with other Heart emotions, such as agitation, panic and hysteria, but anxiety differs from mania, in that anxiety is unpleasant, while mania may be associated with feelings of well-being and euphoria. Anxiety may occur with other Heart signs such as insomnia, palpitations, hypertension, cardiac pain, pallor and cold extremities.

ANXIETY AND THE KIDNEY SYSTEM

Heart anxiety is rooted in Kidney fear, with marked feelings of apprehension, the fear that something terrible is going to happen. Anxiety may then be combined with jumpiness and fearfulness, and with physical signs such as trembling, urinary frequency or loose bowels.

FEAR, ANGER AND ANXIETY

Fear may give rise to both anxiety and anger, involving the Kidney, Heart and Liver systems. These three emotions may each cause mental, emotional and physical tension, so that the person feels and looks strained and tense. If there is Liver–Gallbladder involvement, there may be additional feelings of uncertainty, indecision, irritability, touchiness and hypersensitivity, and there may be headaches and pain, stiffness or tremors in the muscles of face, neck, shoulders, back and limbs.

FEAR, ANXIETY AND WORRY

In addition to the fearful apprehension associated with the Kidney system, anxiety may also be linked to worry for the present and future, and anticipation of problems which may never occur. In severe cases, the sense of insecurity may become very great, and the person may become lost in an inner world of fears, worries and obsessional thoughts, which may bear little relation to actual events in the outer world.

FEAR, ANXIETY AND GRIEF

The Lung system may be involved with Kidney and Heart in situations where there is great insecurity and fear of loss; for example, a parent's fear that a sick child may die, or a wife's fear that her husband may leave her for another woman.

Table 34.8 Anxiety and the five systems

System	Emotion	Typical signs
Heart	anxiety	palpitations, insomnia
Spleen	worry	gastritis, nausea
Lungs	fear of loss	dyspnoea, asthma
Kidneys	fear and apprehension	urinary frequency, loose bowels
Liver	uncertainty and irritability	muscular tension, headache

TYPES OF ANXIETY

In terms of Chinese medicine, anxiety is one manifestation of Disturbance of Heart Spirit. This disturbance, this irregularity of movement, may derive from Excess, Deficiency or Stagnation.

EXCESS

The main form of Excess that gives rise to Irregularity is Fire. Heart Fire makes the Spirit more intensely and irregularly active, resulting in anxiety or manic behaviour. Heart Fire, and the Liver Fire and Stomach Fire that are often associated with it, can come from suppression of emotions or from an overly rushed, stressed and hectic lifestyle.

Heart Phlegm Fire is a form of Excess that may lead to anxiety and confused thinking, speech and behaviour. It is essentially Phlegm, from Spleen Deficiency and Stagnation, combining with Heart Fire. It can arise from emotional stress or excessive tobacco, alcohol and greasy foods with lack of exercise.

STAGNATION

Stagnation may give rise to disturbance of movement; for example, Stagnation of Heart and Liver Qi, from emotional stagnation, may lead to Disturbance of Heart Spirit and to Hyperactive Liver Yang, leading to anxiety. Stagnation of Qi may result in accumulation of Phlegm, which may disturb the free circulation of Spirit, causing anxiety.

DEFICIENCY

Anxiety increases when the energy is low, when there is Deficiency from lack of sleep and rest, overwork, stress, illness, malnutrition, and so on. Deficiency of Heart and Kidney Qi, of Heart and Kidney Yin, and of Heart and Spleen Blood, may each give rise to anxiety, since Qi, Yin and Blood are needed to keep the Spirit stable.

ANXIETY AND DEPRESSION

While Deficiency can be associated with depression and slower movement of Spirit, it can also be associated with anxiety and increased irregular movement of Spirit, due to reduced control of Spirit by Qi, Blood and Yin. The principle of treatment is to calm and tonify.

Similarly, while Stagnation can be associated with depression and retardation of the movement of the Spirit, it can also be associated with anxiety when Stagnation and blockage disturb the regular movement of Qi. Also, Stagnant Qi may give rise to Excess Fire, which further

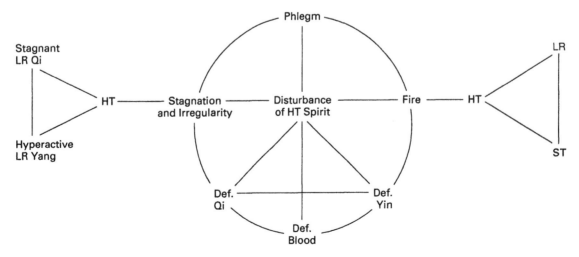

Fig. 34.3 Aetiology of anxiety and insomnia.

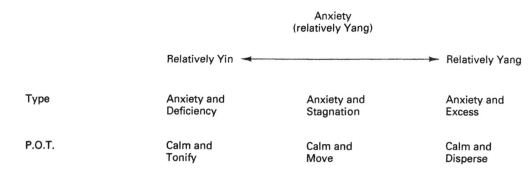

Fig. 34.4. Types of anxiety and principles of treatment.

disturbs the Spirit. The principle of treatment is to calm, to move Stagnation and to disperse Phlegm where present.

Anxiety and depression differ in that depression is not usually associated with Excess Fire. Manic depression and depression with aggression are alternations between depression and a more active state. In anxiety due to Excess Fire, the Heat causes increased, faster, more irregular movement of the Spirit. The principle of treatment is to calm and to disperse Excess Fire.

SYNDROMES

Excess
Heart Fire + Liver Fire
        + Stomach Fire
        + Heart Phlegm

Stagnation
Stagnant Heart Qi + Stagnant Liver Qi
                   + Hyperactive Liver Yang
                   + Heart Phlegm

Deficiency
Deficient Heart Qi   + Deficient Kidney Qi
                      + Deficient Spleen Qi
                      + Deficient Liver Qi
Deficient Heart Blood + Deficient Spleen Blood
Deficient Heart Yin   + Deficient Kidney Yin

TREATMENT

Point combinations for anxiety are given in Table 34.9.

Example

A woman of 21, a final-year student, taking her final examinations in one week's time, required an acupuncture treatment to calm her anxiety and increase her concentration. Her pulse was empty and choppy.

The diagnosis was Deficient Qi of Kidney, Heart and Spleen and Disturbance of Heart Spirit. The point combination was:

GV.20, yìn táng, PC.6, SP.4 E

Example 2

A woman of 65 was in a constant state of worry and anxiety, over-reacting to even the smallest problem so that she had no joy or pleasure in her life. Her pulse was thin, rapid, choppy and slightly moving. Her tongue was pale and thin with some red spots.

The diagnosis was extreme disturbance of Heart Spirit from Deficient Blood of Heart and Deficient Yin of Heart and Kidney. The point combination was:

GV.20, CV.14, CV.24, PC.6, HT.6, KI.1 Rd; CV.4, SP.4 Rf

Panic attacks

So-called panic attacks are a specific form of severe anxiety occurring suddenly in response to a specific stimulus; for example, an important meeting, or a phobic situation such as an enclosed space or a crowded supermarket. The attack may come on suddenly with little warning, especially if the precipitating situation has not been anticipated, or in an anticipated situation there may be a steady build up of anxiety preceding the attack.

Symptoms include feelings of increasing anxiety, reaching panic proportions, hyperventilation, palpitations, profuse perspiration, dizziness and maybe fainting. There is usually an intense desire to leave the precipitating situation, and if the person can do this they usually feel better, although the feelings of anxiety and panic can linger for days.

PHOBIC ANXIETY SYNDROME

This can occur in obsessional people, following a severe fright or emotional disturbance. There may be an overwhelming feeling of dread, vague fears and a most unpleasant feeling of unreality. They may be afraid to leave their homes, and indeed may not do so unless accompanied by someone close to them, or they may be afraid of falling asleep because of a feeling they are going to die.

Table 34.9 Anxiety and palpitation syndromes (palpitations may occur with any of the syndromes in this table)

Syndrome	Signs and symptoms	Pulse	Tongue	Point combination
Heart Fire	agitation, feelings of desperation, rapid restless movements, nervous talking, red face, whole body hot	full, rapid	red or dark red, maybe dry yellow coat	GV.20, CV.17, HT.8, PC.8, KI.1 Rd, HT.3, PC.3 Rf + LR.2 Rd; LR.1 B for Liver Fire + ST.44, ST.45 B for Stomach Fire + PC.6, HT.5 Rd; - PC.3, HT.3 Rf for Heart Phlegm
Stagnant Heart Qi	feelings of anxiety, depression and irritability, sensation of fullness and discomfort in chest and epigastrium	hindered, wiry, maybe full	maybe normal or slightly purple	CV.6, CV.12, CV.17, PC.6, SP.4, SP.21 E or Rd + LR.3, LR.14 Rd for Stagnant Liver Qi + LR.3, GB.34 Rd for Hyperactive Liver Yang + HT.5, PC.4 Rd for Heart Phlegm
Deficient Heart Qi	anxiety and emotional lability, worse with tiredness, maybe palpitations and cold hands and feet	empty	pale	CV.4, CV.17, HT.7, ST.36, KI.3 Rf M alternate BL.15, BL.20, BL.23, BL.64, SI.3 Rf M + KI.27 Rf M for Deficient Kidney Qi + SP.3 Rf M for Deficient Spleen Qi + GB.40 Rf M for Deficient Liver–Gallbladder Qi
Deficient Heart Blood	anxiety, insomnia and palpitations, maybe tiredness, dizziness, poor memory, feelings of vulnerability and weakness	thin, choppy	pale, thin, dry	CV.4, CV.12, CV.17, HT.7, ST.36, SP.6 Rf alternate BL.15, BL.20, BL.43 Rf + SP.10 Rf for Deficient Spleen Blood
Deficient Heart Yin	tired but restless, anxiety and insomnia with sensations of heat, maybe night sweats	thin, rapid maybe irregular	red, no coat, maybe cracks	CV.4, SP.6, KI.6 Rf; CV.14, CV.17, HT.7 Rd + GV.20, CV.24 Rd for severe anxiety HT.8, KI.2 Rd for Heart and Kidney Deficiency Fire

Rd, Reducing method; Rf, Reinforcing method; E, Even method; M, moxa; B, bleeding.

AETIOLOGY

Fear is the basis of these syndromes, and may manifest as anxiety or worry and obsessional patterns. The organ systems involved are mainly Kidney, Heart and Spleen. There may be an inherited predisposition and certain emotionally powerful events in childhood may form the nuclei for future phobic patterns. Attacks can be made more likely by a background of tiredness and stress, and a general feeling of insecurity.

TREATMENT

Treatment aims firstly at calming the fear, anxiety, panic or worry, and secondly at tonifying the underlying Deficiency.

CALMING POINTS

Sometimes the best results are gained by using KI.1 on the feet with needle, moxa or massage, and at other times the best results come from using mainly head points such as GV.18, GV.20, GV.24, GV.26, CV.24, BL.2, BL.7, BL.9, GB.13, GB.20 or yìn táng. Generally, it is advisable to use combinations of points at both head and feet, such as

GV.20 and KI.1, or BL.2 and BL.67, or GB.13 and GB.40. CV.14 is a useful point for calming fear, but should be used gently at first, and with moxa if the patient feels cold. This point combines well with either KI.1, or with SP.4 and PC.6.

Sometimes calming is produced by points with tonifying effect, such as CV.4, or KI.3 with Reinforcing method, which calm fear by tonifying the Kidneys. Generally, the Back Transporting points have less immediate calming effect, and are best used for tonifying the underlying Deficiency, when the acute anxiety has reduced.

EXTRA CHANNEL COMBINATIONS

SP.4 + PC.6 can be used, especially if palpitation is a main symptom, and LU.7 + KI.6 can be used, especially if hyperventilation or asthma is a main symptom. For example:

CV.14, PC.6, SP.4   or   CV.17, LU.7, KI.6

Example 1

A man of 50 had panic attacks during important business meetings, especially when he had to present his own work. His face became extremely red and hot, and he had extreme difficulty stopping his hands and voice from shaking. His pulse was full, rapid, wiry and slightly irregular.

The diagnosis was Deficient Heart Yin with Heart Fire. The point combination was:

sì shén cōng, CV.24, CV.14, PC.6, HT.8, KI.1 Rd; ear apex, PC.9 B

Example 2

A woman of 35 developed a phobic anxiety syndrome after an emotional crisis with her partner. She felt extremely anxious and depressed, with severe feelings of unreality and constant thoughts that she was going to die. Her pulse was thin, choppy, hindered and slightly irregular.

The diagnosis was Deficiency of Heart and Kidney Qi and scattering of Heart Spirit. The point combination was:

GV.20, LU.7, KI.1, KI.6, BL.6, BL.8, GB.13 E

Emotional lability

In emotional lability, the person's emotional responses are exaggerated and out of proportion to the stimuli, also the person is more than usually disturbed by them, and takes longer to recover from their after-effects.

AETIOLOGY

One of the functions of Qi is to control the emotions and to keep their movement stable and within suitable limits. If Qi becomes Deficient, the emotions become disturbed and exaggerated. Qi can give both stability and adaptability in times of change and crisis. If Qi is Deficient, then emotional lability will occur, especially at times of increased movement within the body (for example, before menstruation), or increased change in the person's life (for example, menopause).

DEFICIENCY

If Qi, Blood or Yin is Deficient, then there is reduced control of the Heart Spirit, resulting in emotional distur-

bance. Emotional lability includes anxiety of the Deficiency type, but in a broader sense, also covers patterns of irritation, touchiness, tearfulness and vulnerability. Emotional lability is a pattern of Deficiency where the emotional responses are exaggerated, but the person feels weak, shaky, tired, and often unable to cope with life. The principle of treatment is to calm the disturbed emotions and tonify the underlying Deficiency.

TREATMENT

Some examples of point combinations are given in Table 34.10.

Table 34.10 Point combinations for emotional lability

Syndrome	Emotion	Combination
Deficient Kidney Qi	fearful jumpiness	CV.4, KI.7, ST.36 Rf; CV.14 Rd
Deficient Gallbladder Qi	touchiness, uncertainty	CV.4, KI.3, GB.13, GB.40 Rf; GV.20 Rd
Deficient Liver Blood	vulnerability	CV.4, LR.8, SP.6, ST.36 Rf; LI.4, LR.3 Rd
Deficient Liver Yin	irritability	CV.4, SP.6, KI.6 Rf; GV.20, LR.2 Rd
Deficient Heart Qi Deficient Heart Blood	anxiety, overexcitement	CV.4, SP.4, ST.36 Rf; PC.6, HT.7 Rd
Deficient Heart Yin		
Deficient Lung Qi	tearfulness	CV.4, KI.6, ST.36; CV.17, LU.7 Rd

Rd, Reducing method; Rf, Reinforcing method.

Example 1

A woman of 30 was emotionally labile, becoming easily irritable or tearful under stress. She had been working very hard on many projects and was thoroughly exhausted. Her pulse was empty in the Kidney position, empty and wiry in the Gallbladder position and flooding and empty in the Lung position.

The diagnosis was Deficient Qi of Kidney, Gallbladder and Lung. The point combination was:

CV.4, KI.7, GB.40, ST.36 Rf; LU.7, GB.13 E

Appendix: pulse qualities

CHANGING

The pulse is constantly changing in volume or quality, for example from stronger to weaker or from harder to softer, so that the quality or volume is difficult to assess. This usually means Deficient Qi, with not enough Qi to hold the pulse stable. This is not the same as sudden changes in speed or quality, due to the patient becoming emotionally upset or excited while their pulse is being taken, e.g. if they are talking about emotionally charged topics. A Changing pulse seems to drift from one volume or quality to its opposite and then drift back again.

HINDERED

This pulse should be clearly distinguished from the Wiry and the Choppy pulses. It is harder than normal but not as consistent and hard as the Wiry pulse. The Hindered pulse does not flow smoothly and freely, but seems to have some restraint or hesitation in its movement. It is due to suppression of the emotions of anger, excitement or grief, so the person thinks, hesitates or holds back, instead of responding spontaneously to an emotional impulse. The person is to some degree repressed.

Hindered
   relatively Yin
   tends to keep emotions inside
   less forceful personality
   relatively Deficient

Wiry
   relatively Yang
   can explode into anger, etc.
   more forceful personality
   relatively Excess

The Choppy pulse has all beats softer than normal and all beats weaker than normal, whereas the Hindered pulse has all beats harder than normal, and may be normal or more than normal strength.

PREIRREGULAR

A pulse which actually misses or adds a beat is relatively uncommon in an acupuncture practice, and is usually associated with a physical heart problem, a Heart-type personality disharmony, or both. It can be non-pathological, as a result of a heart birth defect or damage to heart in early life, with no current symptoms. However, many pulses *almost* miss a beat, they hesitate but do not actually miss, usually associated with Heart-type emotional stress. They may develop into Irregular if not treated, or if the patient does not change lifestyle. They often represent Deficient Qi, Blood or Yin of the Heart, perhaps with Deficiency Heart Fire and Disturbance of Spirit.

Index

Page numbers in bold refer to illustrations.

461

Points index

Alphabetical list of points

An mian (extra)

Ba xie (extra)
Bai huan shu (BL 30)
Bai hui (GV 20)
Ben shen (GB 13)
Bi guan (ST 31)
Bi nao (LI 14)
Bi tong (extra)
Bing feng (SI 12)

Chang qiang (GV 1)
Cheng fu (BL 36)
Cheng jiang (CV 24)
Cheng qi (ST 1)
Cheng shan (BL 57)
Chi ze (LU 5)
Chong yang (ST 42)
Ci liao (BL 32)

Da bao (SP 21)
Da chang shu (BL 25)
Da du (SP 2)
Da dun (LR 1)
Da he (KI 12)
Da heng (SP 15)
Da ling (PC 7)
Da zhong (KI 4)
Da zhu (BL 11)
Da zhui (GV 14)
Dai mai (GB 26)
Dan shu (BL 19)
Di cang (ST 4)
Di ji (SP 8)
Du bi (ST 35)

Er jian (LI 2)
Er men (TE 21)

Fei shu (BL 13)
Fei yang (BL 58)
Feng chi (GB 20)
Feng fu (GV 16)
Feng long (ST 40)
Feng men (BL 12)
Feng shi (GB 31)
Fu bai (GB 10)

Fu liu (KI 7)
Fu tu (LI 18)
Fu yang (BL 59)

Gan shu (BL 18)
Gao huang shu (BL 43)
Ge shu (BL 17)
Gong sun (SP 4)
Gu gu (CV 2)
Guan chong (TE 1)
Guan yuan (CV 4)
Guan yuan shu (BL 26)
Guang ming (GB 37)
Gui lai (ST 29)

He gu (LI 4)
Heng gu (KI 11)
Hou xi (SI 3)
Hua tuo jia hi (extra)
Huan tiao (GB 30)
Huan zhong (extra)
Hui yang (BL 35)
Hui yin (CV 1)
Hui zong (TE 7)
Hun men (BL 47)

Ji mai (LI 12)
Ji men (BL 63)
Ji zhong (GV 6)
Jia che (ST 6)
Jia cheng jiang (ke liao) (extra)
Jian jing (GB 21)
Jian liao (TE 14)
Jian ne ling (extra)
Jian shi (PC 5)
Jian wai shu (SI 14)
Jian yu (LI 15)
Jian zhen (SI 9)
Jian zhong shu (SI 15)
Jie xi (ST 41)
Jiao ling (extra)
Jiao xin (KI 8)
Jin suo (GV 8)
Jing gu (BL 64)
Jing men (GB 25)
Jing ming (BL 1)
Jiu wei (CV 15)
Ju gu (LI 16)
Ju liao (ST 3)

Ju que (CV 14)
Jue jin shu (BL 14)

Kong zui (LU 6)
Kun lun (BL 60)

Lao gong (PC 8)
Li dui (ST 45)
Li gou (LR 5)
Lian quan (CV 23)
Liang men (ST 21)
Liang qiu (ST 34)
Lie que (LU 7)
Ling xu (KI 24)
Luo zhen (extra)

Ming men (GV 4)

Nao shang (extra)
Nao shu (SI 10)
Nei ting (ST 44)

Pang guang shu (BL 28)
Pi shu (BL 20)
Pian li (LI 6)
Po hu (BL 42)

Qi chong (ST 30)
Qi hai (CV 6)
Qi hai shu (BL 24)
Qi men (LR 14)
Qi xue (KI 13)
Qian gu (SI 2)
Qiu hou (extra)
Qiu xu (GB 40)
Qu bin (GB 7)
Qu chi (LI 11)
Qu quan (LR 8)
Qu yuan (SI 13)
Qu ze (PC 3)
Quan liao (SI 18)
Que pen (ST 12)

Ran gu (KI 2)

Ren ying (ST 9)
Ren zhong (GV 26)
Ri yue (GB 24)
Ru gen (ST 18)
Ru zhong (ST 17)

San jian (LI 3)
San jiao shu (BL 22)
San yang luo (TE 8)
San yin jiao (SP 6)
Shang ju xu (ST 37)
Shang liao (BL 31)
Shang wan (CV 13)
Shang xing (GV 23)
Shang yang (LI 1)
Shao chong (HT 9)
Shao fu (HT 8)
Shao hai (HT 3)
Shao shang (LU 11)
Shao ze (SI 1)
Shen cang (KI 25)
Shen dao (GV 11)
Shen mai (BL 62)
Shen men (HT 7)
Shen shu (BL 23)
Shen tang (BL 44)
Shen ting (GV 24)
Shen zhu (GV 12)
Shi qi zhui xia (extra)
Shi xuan (extra)
Shou san li (LI 10)
Shu fu (KI 27)
Shuai gu (GB 8)
Shui dao (ST 28)
Shui fen (CV 9)
Shui quan (KI 5)
Si bai (ST 2)
Si shen cong (extra)
Si zhu kong (TE 23)

Tai bai (SP 3)
Tai chong (LR 3)
Tai xi (KI 3)
Tai yang (extra)
Tai yuan (LU 9)
Tan zhong (CV 17)
Tao dao (GV 13)
Tian chi (PC 1)
Tian chong (GB 9)

Tian chuang (SI 16)
Tian fu (LU 3)
Tian jing (TE 10)
Tian liao (TE 15)
Tian rong (SI 17)
Tian shu (ST 25)
Tian tu (CV 22)
Tian you (TE 16)
Tian zhu (BL 10)
Tian zong (SI 11)
Tiao kou (ST 38)
Ting gong (SI 19)
Ting hui (GB 2)
Tong li (HT 5)
Tong tian (BL 7)
Tong zi liao (GB 1)
Tou qiao yin (GB 11)
Tou wei (ST 8)

Wai guan (TE 5)
Wan gu (GB 12)
Wan gu (SI 4)
Wei dao (GB 28)
Wei mo (extra)
Wei shu (BL 21)
Wei yang (BL 39)
Wei zhong (BL 40)
Wen liu (LI 7)
Wu shu (GB 27)

Xi men (PC 4)
Xi yang guan (GB 33)
Xia guan (ST 7)
Xia ju xu (ST 39)
Xia liao (BL 34)
Xia xi (GB 43)
Xiao chang shu (BL 27)
Xiao hai (SI 8)
Xin shu (BL 15)
Xing jian (LR 2)
Xuan li (GB 6)
Xuan lu (GB 5)
Xuan zhong (GB 39)
Xue hai (SP 10)

Ya men (GV 15)
Yang bai (GB 14)
Yang chi (TE 4)

Yang fu (GB 38)
Yang gu (SI 5)
Yang lao (SI 6)
Yang ling quan (GB 34)
Yang xi (LI 5)
Yao shu (GV 2)
Yao tong dian (extra)
Yao yang guan (GV 3)
Yao yao (extra)
Ye men (TE 2)
Yi feng (TE 17)
Yi ming (extra)
Yi she (BL 49)
Yin bai (SP 1)
Yin gu (KI 10)
Yin lian (LR 11)
Yin ling quan (SP 9)
Yin men (BL 37)
Yin tang (extra)
Yin xi (HT 6)
Ying xiang (LI 20)
Yong quan (KI 1)
Yu ji (LU 10)
Yu yao (extra)
Yu zhong (KI 26)

Zan zhu (BL 2)
Zhang men (LR 13)
Zhao hai (KI 6)
Zhi bian (BL 54)
Zhi gou (TE 6)
Zhi long gou (extra)
Zhi shi (BL 52)
Zhi yang (GV 9)
Zhi yin (BL 67)
Zhi zheng (SI 7)
Zhong chong (PC 9)
Zhong fu (LU 1)
Zhong ji (CV 3)
Zhong liao (BL 33)
Zhong wan (CV 12)
Zhong zhu (TE 3)
Zhu bin (KI 9)
Zi gong (extra)
Zu lin qi (GB 41)
Zu qiao yin (GB 44)
Zu san li (ST 36)
Zu tong gu (BL 66)
Zu wu li (LR 10)
Zuo gu (extra)

Printed and bound by CPI Group (UK) Ltd, Croydon, CR0 4YY

03/10/2024

01040360-0020